ANTIHYPERTENSIVE THERAPY

PRINCIPLES AND PRACTICE

AN INTERNATIONAL SYMPOSIUM

PROCEEDINGS

EDITED BY

F. GROSS

WITH THE ASSISTANCE OF

S. R. NAEGELI AND A. H. KIRKWOOD

BASLE

WITH 225 FIGURES

SPRINGER-VERLAG

BERLIN · HEIDELBERG · NEW YORK

1966

The Symposium took place at Siena, Italy
28th June - 3rd July, 1965
under the chairmanship of
C. Bartorelli, Siena
and was sponsored by
CIBA

 Library of Congress Catalog Card Number 66-17 551
Softcover reprint of the hardcover 1st edition 1966

ISBN 978-3-642-49456-7 ISBN 978-3-642-49737-7 (eBook)
DOI 10.1007/978-3-642-49737-7

Title No. 1329

Preface

Hypertension has certainly been one of the topics most frequently discussed at symposia, meetings, and congresses during recent years. There may be several reasons for this; three of them are obvious: firstly, the fact that a large proportion of the world's population is suffering from various forms of hypertensive disease; secondly, increasing knowledge of the pathogenesis of hypertension and of the disturbances underlying it; and, thirdly, the marked progress which has been made in antihypertensive therapy over the past fifteen years. When plans for the present symposium were being drawn up, it was felt that it should not simply bring forth just another meeting on hypertension, but should place particular emphasis on those aspects which had not been adequately discussed at previous symposia of this kind. Curiously enough, the topic which appeared to have received least attention in the past was therapy, although from the practical point of view this is by far the most important. The choice of therapy as the main theme of the whole symposium also seemed to be warranted in view of the relatively long period that had elapsed since effective antihypertensive treatment became available; the time had in fact come now to pass judgement on the benefits as well as the shortcomings of drug treatment as available today.

An assessment of the value of antihypertensive therapy must of necessity be based to a substantial degree on work undertaken some time ago – work which has therefore to some extent already been published. Nevertheless, although some of the data contained in this volume may previously have appeared in print elsewhere, there is much to be said for looking at them again in the context of a symposium at which all the different aspects of the subject have been treated. For once, it is also useful to have the numerous data assembled in a single volume, instead of scattered throughout the abundant literature.

Long-term therapy of hypertension, to which much of this volume is devoted, has undergone various modifications during the one and a half decades since the first antihypertensive drugs appeared. It is not so much the individual compound, but rather the beneficial effect of lowering elevated blood pressure by drug treatment, which is responsible for the better chance of survival that the patient suffering from hypertension has today. For this reason no special treatment schedules for the various drugs are given. It is evident from some of the papers read at this symposium that the hypertensive patient whose blood pressure is brought down to within normal limits has the best life expectancy and that this aim can now be achieved by the most active of the drugs at present available.

There remains the question whether it is worth while to publish the proceedings of such a meeting. During the symposium, one evening, one of the participants expressed the opinion in the course of an informal chat that their publication would be unnecessary and that those attending the gathering would be only too glad not to have to face the burden of preparing a manuscript for printing or of revising what they had said during the discussions. Recently, however, the Editor was gratified to receive a letter indicating that the speaker in question had meanwhile become "converted" to the idea of printing the proceedings: "When I was in Siena I made a comment that perhaps publication of papers was not necessary. After thinking it over I realise that these publications are very important not only as a reference for the participants but even more so to those who were unable to attend."

The success of a meeting of this type depends to a decisive degree upon the organiser, upon the man who, together with his advisers, determines who should speak about what and is responsible for all the necessary preparations. Prof. BARTORELLI and Prof. ZANCHETTI, working in close collaboration, drew up an excellent programme and, together with their young and enthusiastic collaborators, proved most charming and attentive hosts.

In a place like Siena, where the working sessions and the many discussions following them were held in most beautiful surroundings and in a congenial and stimulating atmosphere, fascinating impressions and exciting episodes to which participants at the symposium were treated may bewitch the critical intellect. The book which contains the proceedings provides a more sober record than may the memories of those who had the pleasure of participating at the meeting – and it is up to the reader to decide what it has achieved and whether or not it has made a valuable contribution to the chosen subject. Between the picture and its frame there has to be a well balanced relationship. The small group who had the privilege of being in Siena on this occasion saw both the picture and the frame, whereas the great majority to whom this book is addressed can only imagine the blue sky of Tuscany, the slender tower of *La Mangia* rising majestically above the warm brick façades of Siena brown, and the magnificent, colourful spectacle of the *Palio*. It remains to be seen, however, whether the proceedings of the symposium and the scientific progress achieved by it stand the test of deframing as well as the unforgettable *La Maestà* by Duccio in the *Museo dell'Opera del Duomo*.

The Editor of such a volume tends, alas, to prove a rather unpopular person – at least during the period when he has to remind the authors to submit their manuscripts, corrected galley proofs, summaries, etc. Moreover, in trying to "edit" he may do too much of a good thing and inflict additional strain on authors whose patience and goodwill have already been sorely taxed. He apologises for any annoyance he may inadvertently have caused them and expresses his warmest thanks to all contributors to the volume who so patiently dealt with his many queries and requests. Without their understanding help it would not have been possible to publish the volume so soon after the meeting.

We should also like to extend our sincerest thanks to Dr. R. Deguillaume, who translated the summaries into French, to Dr. Wiltrud Hatzinger, who prepared the subject index, and – last but by no means least – to Springer-Verlag, who, as in former years, did their utmost to ensure rapid publication of the volume and whose staff made every effort to meet all our wishes.

Basle, November 1965 *F. G.*

Contents

Long-term treatment

Diagnosis and treatment of renovascular and other forms of renal hypertension

Participants in the Symposium

Bartorelli, C.	Istituto di Patologia Speciale Medica e Metodologia Clinica, Università di Siena, Siena (Italy)
Bein, J. H.	Forschungslaboratorien der CIBA Aktiengesellschaft, Basel (Switzerland)
Bloch, H.	Forschungslaboratorien der CIBA Aktiengesellschaft, Basel (Switzerland)
Bock, K. D.	Medizinische Klinik und Poliklinik, Klinikum Essen der Wilhelms-Universität Münster, Essen (Germany)
Brest, A. N..	Department of Medicine, Hahnemann Medical College and Hospital, Philadelphia, Pa. (U.S.A.)
Brod, J..	Ústav pro Choroby Oběhu Krevního, Praha-Krč (Czechoslovakia)
Brunner, H..	Forschungslaboratorien der CIBA Aktiengesellschaft, Basel (Switzerland)
Byrom, F. B..	Medical Unit, The London Hospital, London (Great Britain)
Califano, L..	Istituto di Patologia Generale, S. Andrea delle Dame, Napoli (Italy)
Carlsson, A..	Farmakologiska institutionen, Göteborgs universitet, Göteborg (Sweden)
Cottier, P. T.	Medizinische Abteilung, Bezirksspital, Interlaken (Switzerland)
Cranston, W. I.	Department of Medicine, St. Thomas's Hospital Medical School, London (Great Britain)
Deming, Q. B.	Department of Medicine, Albert Einstein College of Medicine, Bronx, N. Y. (U.S.A.)
Dengler, H. J..	Medizinische Universitäts-Klinik, Heidelberg (Germany)
Dollery, C. T..	Department of Medicine, Postgraduate Medical School, London (Great Britain)
Dontas, A. S.	Department of Clinical Therapeutics, University of Athens, Athens (Greece)
Dustan, Harriet P. . .	Research Division, Cleveland Clinic Foundation, Cleveland, Ohio (U.S.A.)

FREIS, E. D.	Veterans Administration Hospital, Washington, D. C. (U.S.A.)
GENEST, J..	Département de recherches cliniques, Hôtel-Dieu de Montréal, Montréal (Canada)
GROSS, F.	Forschungslaboratorien der CIBA Aktiengesellschaft, Basel (Switzerland)
HAMILTON, M.	Chelmsford and Essex Hospital, Chelmsford, Essex (Great Britain)
HARTMANN, F.	Medizinische Klinik der Medizinischen Hochschule Hannover, Hannover (Germany)
HOOBLER, S. W.	Department of Internal Medicine, The University of Michigan Medical Center, Ann Arbor, Mich. (U.S.A.)
HOOD, B.	Medicinska kliniken I, Göteborgs universitet, Sahlgrenska sjukhuset, Göteborg (Sweden)
HUMERFELT, S. B. . . .	Medisinsk avdeling A, Universitetet i Bergen, Haukeland sykehus, Bergen (Norway)
IMHOF, P.	Forschungslaboratorien der CIBA Aktiengesellschaft, Basel (Switzerland)
KINCAID-SMITH, PRISCILLA	Department of Medicine, The University of Melbourne, Royal Melbourne Hospital, Melbourne, Victoria (Australia)
KIRKENDALL, W. M.. . .	Department of Medicine, University of Iowa Hospitals, Iowa City, Iowa (U.S.A.)
LAGERLÖF, H.	Medicinska kliniken, Karolinska sjukhuset, Stockholm (Sweden)
LEE, R. E..	Department of Medicine, Cornell University Medical Center, The New York Hospital, New York, N. Y. (U.S.A.)
LEISHMAN, A. W. D.. . .	United Sheffield Hospitals, Sheffield (Great Britain)
LEONETTI, G..	Istituto di Patologia Speciale Medica e Metodologia Clinica, Università di Siena, Siena (Italy)
LIBRETTI, A..	Istituto di Patologia Speciale Medica e Metodologia Clinica, Università di Siena, Siena (Italy)
MACH, R. S.	Clinique universitaire de thérapeutique, Hôpital cantonal, Genève (Switzerland)
MILLIEZ, P..	Hôpital Broussais, Paris (France)
MORRIS, N. F.	Department of Obstetrics and Gynaecology, Charing Cross Hospital Medical School, London (Great Britain)
MORUZZI, G.	Istituto di Fisiologia, Università di Pisa, Pisa (Italy)

MULL, R. P. . . . . . . Chemical Research Department, CIBA Pharmaceutical Company, Summit, N. J. (U.S.A.)

PAGE, I. H. . . . . . . Research Division, Cleveland Clinic Foundation, Cleveland, Ohio (U.S.A.)

PEART, W. S.. . . . . . Medical Unit, St. Mary's Hospital, London (Great Britain)

PETERS, G.. . . . . . . Institut de Pharmacologie de l'Université, Lausanne (Switzerland)

PICKERING, SIR GEORGE . The Radcliffe Infirmary, University of Oxford, Oxford (Great Britain)

PLUMMER, A. J.. . . . . Macrobiology Department, CIBA Pharmaceutical Company, Summit, N. J. (U.S.A.)

PUDDU, V. . . . . Divisione Cardiologica A. Cesalpino, Ospedale San Camillo, Roma (Italy)

REUBI, F. C. . . . . . . Medizinische Universitätspoliklinik, Bern (Switzerland)

SJOERDSMA, A. . . . . . National Heart Institute, National Institutes of Health, Bethesda, Md. (U.S.A.)

SMIRK, SIR HORACE . . . Wellcome Medical Research Institute, University of Otago Medical School, Dunedin (New Zealand)

STAMEY, T. A. . . . . . Division of Urology, Stanford University School of Medicine, Palo Alto, Calif. (U.S.A.)

TAQUINI, A. C. . . . . . Centro de Investigaciones Cardiológicas, Facultad de Ciencias Médicas, Universidad de Buenos Aires, Buenos Aires (Argentina)

TCHERDAKOFF, P. . . . . Hôpital Broussais, Paris (France)

TRAEGER, J. . . . . . . Service des maladies métaboliques et rénales, Hôpital de l'Antiquaille, Lyon (France)

WERKÖ, L. . . . . Medicinska kliniken I, Göteborgs universitet, Sahlgrenska sjukhuset, Goteborg (Sweden)

WILSON, C.. . . . . . . Medical Unit, The London Hospital, London (Great Britain)

WOLFF, H. P.. . . . . . II. Medizinische Universitatsklinik und Poliklinik, Homburg/Saar (Germany)

ZAIMIS, ELEANOR . . . . Department of Pharmacology, The Royal Free Hospital School of Medicine, London (Great Britain)

ZANCHETTI, A. . . . . . Istituto di Patologia Speciale Medica e Metodologia Clinica, Università di Siena, Siena (Italy)

Opening remarks

By

C. Bartorelli

It is a great honour for me to open this symposium and to welcome all of you who are participating in what I am sure will prove a most interesting and stimulating week of lectures and discussions.

It is also a pleasure for me to acknowledge with gratitude the support we have received from CIBA Basle, which has enabled us to assemble such a large gathering of distinguished specialists and scientists. I should also like to express sincere thanks to our friend Franz Gross for his valuable advice and help in connection with this meeting.

I think that first of all I owe you – as well as future readers of the proceedings of this symposium – a few explanations:

Why was arterial hypertension chosen as the subject of our deliberations and, more particularly, why did we decide to place the main emphasis on the treatment of hypertension? And what have been our chief aims in planning the programme?

I feel that you are the last people in the world to whom I need explain why we have selected hypertension as the topic of our symposium, since the very reason why we are gathered here today is because we all share a mutual interest in the study and treatment of this disease. If anybody is to be blamed for the fact that we have all been "bitten by the hypertension bug", then I suggest it is some of the senior members of our group, whose intriguing work it was which first induced so many of us to embark on research in the field of hypertension.

But why a symposium on the *treatment* of hypertension?

I have to admit that I had long cherished the idea of a meeting devoted to the *pathogenesis* of arterial hypertension, because – as I feel sure you will agree – the prospect of searching deeply into the mechanisms underlying the disease is indeed a most fascinating one. However, not long ago, while preparing a chapter on hypertension for an Italian textbook of medicine, I was forcibly struck by the fact that, compared with recent advances in the management of hypertension, precious little progress has been made in our understanding of hypertensive mechanisms.

As in authoritative studies published two or three decades ago, we are still confronted with several hypotheses concerning the pathogenesis of hypertensive disease — some implicating the kidneys, some the brain, and others the endocrine system, as well as our ancestors. But, unlike the authors of such older works, we are nowadays becoming less and less convinced that each of these factors alone can account for the causation of hypertension. Our present confidence does not go beyond saying that all these factors are merely pathogenetic elements on which to construct what — with characteristic academic caution — is referred to as a working hypothesis. This caution, of course, does not extend to our belief in the responsibility of our ancestors, who — whether because of a single gene or several genes — are always considered guilty by the younger generation.

I am not suggesting, of course, that for many years there has been no real progress in our understanding of the pathogenesis of hypertension. In this connection, I need only remind you, for example, of the identification of renovascular hypertension as a clinical entity — a discovery which stemmed from well-known experimental studies — and of our increasing knowledge concerning the role played by such substances as renin, angiotensin, and aldosterone; on the other hand, however, we still do not know whether these humoral substances are involved only in renovascular disease or also in other types of hypertension. I think that what was said five years ago at the Symposium in Prague (*1*) still conveys quite an accurate picture of the state of our knowledge . . . and of our ignorance . . . in this field — except, of course, for the progress that has meanwhile been made in studies on the renin-angiotensin system and aldosterone, a very interesting review of which was presented only eighteen months ago at the excellent symposium organised by JACQUES GENEST in Ste Adèle-en-Haut (*2*). Be that as it may, there are many of us who feel that, as regards the mechanisms responsible for hypertensive disease, we are now probably on the brink of some new and important developments along these or possibly other lines and that we are therefore justified in hoping that in one or two years' time there may well be ample scope for a fruitful symposium on the pathogenesis of hypertension.

When, on the other hand, we turn to the treatment of hypertension, there is no doubt that here substantial changes have been, and are still being, made. Those of us who already had the frustrating privilege of dealing with hypertensive patients some twenty years ago or more, have no need to consult such classics as the 1945 edition of PAGE and CORCORAN's "Arterial Hypertension" (*3*) in order to remind ourselves that thiocyanate, nitrites, kidney extracts, and vitamins were then the only medical means available for controlling hypertension; and I need hardly add that the therapeutic effectiveness of such substances was not much greater than could have been expected from the procedures suggested in VAQUEZ's famous "Diseases of the Heart" at the beginning of the century (*4*).

Although it is true that no basically new antihypertensive preparation has appeared during the last year or two, I am convinced that our knowledge of the mechanisms by which antihypertensive drugs exert their actions is steadily growing and that more and more reliable testing procedures are being developed. In this context, I am thinking particularly of the increasing possibilities which we now have of assessing the long-term effects – both desirable and undesirable – of antihypertensive medication, which, owing unfortunately to the chronic nature of the disease, has to be continued uninterruptedly for an indefinite number of years.

It was considerations of this kind which guided us in drawing up the scientific programme of the symposium. As regards the experimental basis upon which modern antihypertensive therapy is founded, we decided to concentrate on two categories of drug that have proved most effective in lowering elevated blood pressure, i.e. firstly, the various substances acting at different levels on the autonomic nervous system and, secondly, the diuretics. The functional, biochemical, and morphological changes produced by the prolonged administration of antihypertensive drugs to animals will also be discussed.

Reports describing spontaneous blood-pressure fluctuations under physiological conditions both in hypertensive animals and in patients suffering from hypertensive disease have also been included in the programme, because they provide a fitting introduction to discussion of the new techniques for assessing the results of antihypertensive therapy by means of frequently repeated measurements of arterial pressure, carried out either by the doctor in the surgery or by the patient himself at home – a procedure which seems likely to make for better controlled and more successful treatment.

Several problems relating to clinical biochemistry and pharmacology will also be dealt with in the programme, as well as the results of treatment in conditions such as hypertensive crises and hypertension during pregnancy, which call for short-term drug therapy. A full session will likewise be devoted to the assessment of long-term treatment, which is one of the cardinal questions concerning us in this symposium.

After discussing certain technical aspects connected with the organisation of these studies, we shall try to determine to what extent effective antihypertensive therapy, which has now been available for almost fifteen years, has succeeded in improving the prognosis not only in cases of severe and malignant hypertension, but also in patients with mild to moderate hypertension.

Special attention will, in addition, be paid to several of the metabolic changes which the diuretic agents now in wide-spread use have been found to induce. Needless to say, in a broad evaluation of long-term antihypertensive treatment such as we propose to undertake here, we shall also have to consider the possible indications for sympathectomy and adrenalectomy, in order to decide whether there are sound reasons for the fact that in most circles these surgical solutions to the problem of hypertension have now fallen into disrepute.

Since we felt that it would be impossible to assess the long-term results of antihypertensive therapy without first considering the relationship between hypertension and vascular disease as such, we have included in the second session of the symposium several papers dealing with this stimulating topic.

Finally, in view of the increasing importance attached in recent medical literature to renovascular hypertension, an additional session will be devoted to a discussion of various specialised methods used in the diagnosis of this disease and to a comparison of the results which medical and surgical treatment have yielded in renovascular hypertension.

Now, having tried to give you a broad outline of the programme upon which we are about to embark, it only remains for me to express once again the earnest hope that our meeting will prove a fruitful and stimulating one . . . not only for all of us who are attending it, but also for those who will later have an opportunity of reading the published proceedings. May you enjoy these few days in Siena as much as we enjoyed preparing this symposium!

References

1. The Pathogenesis of Essential Hypertension. Proc. of the Prague Symposium, 1960. Ed. by J. H. Cort, V. Fencl, Z. Hejl, and J. Jirka. State Medical Publishing House, Prague, 1961. — 2. International Symposium on Angiotensin, Sodium, and Hypertension, Ste Adèle-en-Haut, P.Q., 1963. Canad. Med. Ass. J. **90**, No. 4, 1964. — 3. Page, I. H., and A. C. Corcoran: Arterial Hypertension. Its diagnosis and treatment. The Year Book Publishers, Chicago, 1945. — 4. Vaquez, L. H.: Diseases of the Heart. Transl. and ed. by G. F. Laidlaw. W. B. Saunders Company, Philadelphia and London, 1924.

Experimental basis of antihypertensive treatment

Pharmacology of the sympathetic nervous system

By

A. CARLSSON

Drugs may interfere with the efferent sympathetic system, mainly at four different levels: 1) the sympathetic centres (and these in turn are located at different levels), 2) the sympathetic ganglia, 3) the postganglionic sympathetic nerve-endings, and 4) the effector cells (smooth muscle, heart, glands, etc.). In general their actions are brought about by interference with neurohumoral transmission mechanisms – at least peripherally, but probably also centrally. In the periphery, essentially two transmitters are involved, namely noradrenaline (N.A.) in the postganglionic fibres, and acetylcholine in the preganglionic fibres. However, some postganglionic sympathetic fibres are cholinergic. Some of them have a vasodilator function, but there are certain reasons to doubt that they are of any great importance in primates (UVNÄS, 1964). To complicate the matter further, N.A.-containing fibres have been found, with the aid of the new histochemical fluorescence method of visualising N.A. and related compounds developed by the late N.-Å. HILLARP and his co-workers, to terminate in sympathetic ganglia (HAMBERGER et al., 1963, 1965), and in parasympathetic ganglia, too, for that matter (NORBERG, 1964; HAMBERGER and NORBERG, 1965). The origin and function of these nerve-terminals in the sympathetic ganglia are unknown, but they are probably derived from cell bodies located in the same ganglia, and there is some evidence that they have an inhibitory function. In other words, they may cause some degree of physiological ganglionic blockade. To what extent these neurones are involved in the action of drugs remains to be elucidated. It has been suggested that reserpine facilitates, and monamine-oxidase inhibitors suppress, ganglionic transmission – which is what one might expect. However, in the case of reserpine the findings of different laboratories are contradictory (COSTA et al., 1961; REINERT, 1963), and it is uncertain whether monamine-oxidase inhibitors cause any significant degree of ganglionic blockade when administered in therapeutic doses (Pletscher et al., 1960). These ganglionic N.A.-containing fibres undoubtedly merit further investigation.

It is, of course, the sympathetic postganglionic fibres innervating vessels that are of greatest interest for our present topic. By means of the histochemical fluorescence method it has been found that all parts of the arterial tree, including the arterioles, have a rich supply of N.A. fibres (with certain exceptions, e.g. the intracerebral vessels), whereas innervation on the venous side is variable and sometimes scarce, particularly at the level of the venules (Fuxe and Sedvall, 1965). This may help to explain why drugs causing sympathetic inhibition tend to give rise to marked orthostatic reactions, the scarce innervation of the venules being most vulnerable. One might ask what can be done to avoid this side effect. Such reactions are pronounced after treatment with agents acting at different levels of the *peripheral* sympathetic system, i.e. the ganglia, the nerve-terminals, and the α-receptors, and, even theoretically, it is doubtful whether they can be avoided, as far as drugs acting at these levels are concerned. Perhaps a more promising line of approach would be to make use of the fact that the sympathetic centres are able to act selectively on different parts of the sympathetic system. It thus seems theoretically possible to influence the sympathetic centres by drugs in such a way as to obtain selective inhibition of the resistance vessels, with only a slight concomitant action on the capacitance vessels. Unfortunately, our knowledge of the central control of the sympathetic system is fragmentary. In fact, very little is known about the importance of possible central components in the actions of some of the antihypertensive drugs now in use. From the low incidence of orthostatic reactions to some of these drugs it might be inferred that they act partly centrally. I am thinking particularly of reserpine and α-methyldopa. In both cases there is some evidence to support this assumption. It should be borne in mind, however, that the incidence of orthostatic reactions to hydralazine, which appears to act chiefly peripherally (Åblad, 1963), is also low. However, this drug seems not to interfere directly with the peripheral sympathetic system, but to act on the vascular smooth muscle, and thus falls beyond the scope of this paper.

Before concluding this general part of my talk, I should perhaps say a few words about the different levels of central control of the sympathetic system. The lowest sympathetic centre from which preganglionic fibres emanate is located in the intermediolateral column of the spinal cord. Other important centres are located in the medulla, in the hypothalamus, in various parts of the limbic system, and even in the neocortex, at least if we use the term "sympathetic centres" in a broad sense, which I think we should in this context. Sometimes the statement is found in the literature that the sympathetic centres are adrenergic, just as the post-ganglionic sympathetic fibres are. This is, no doubt, a considerable over-simplification. In all probability, several transmitters are involved, and N.A. may even be inhibitory at certain levels. Other transmitters to take into consideration are dopamine, 5-hydroxy-tryptamine, and acetylcholine, to say nothing of further, as yet unknown, transmitters; again, they may be excitatory and inhibitory at different levels. For example, there is evidence that the descending 5-hydroxytryptamine-containing axons terminating in the intermediolateral column of the spinal cord are inhibitory (CARLSSON et al., 1964; ANDÉN et al., 1964). An accumulation of 5-hydroxytryptamine in this structure might play a role in the hypotensive action of monamine-oxidase inhibitors. However, there are indications that N.A. may exercise an excitatory function at certain higher integrative levels, e.g. in the hypothalamus (VOGT, 1954). Here, as well as in the limbic system, changes in sympathetic tone may form part of complex reaction patterns (LÖFVING, 1961). Interference with such reactions may possibly account to some extent for the action of drugs such as reserpine and α-methyldopa.

Since many of the antihypertensive drugs have an influence on the brain catecholamines and 5-hydroxytryptamine, it is interesting to note the wide-spread distribution of the neurones containing these substances and probably using them as transmitters (Fig. 1). Interference with these amines may result in functional changes in the sympathetic centres at different levels.

I should now like to discuss very briefly the mode of action of drugs interfering with the sympathetic system. I shall confine myself essentially to three drugs, namely reserpine, guanethidine, and α-methyldopa.

Reserpine. It has been shown that reserpine specifically inhibits the adenosine triphosphate-Mg^{++} (A.T.P.-Mg^{++})-dependent incorporation of N.A. and related compounds into a storage complex held in specific intracellular particles ("granules"or "vesicles") in adrenal medullary cells as well as in adrenergic nerves (for detailed discussion and references cf. CARLSSON, 1965a). This blockade leads to depletion of transmitter and consequently to inhibition of transmission. However, the storage particles do not seem to be homogeneous but contain different fractions of stored amines. In experiments on adrenal medullary granules *in vivo* and *in vitro* and on adrenergic nerve-terminals *in vivo*, it has been shown that one small labile fraction recovers from reserpine more quickly than the

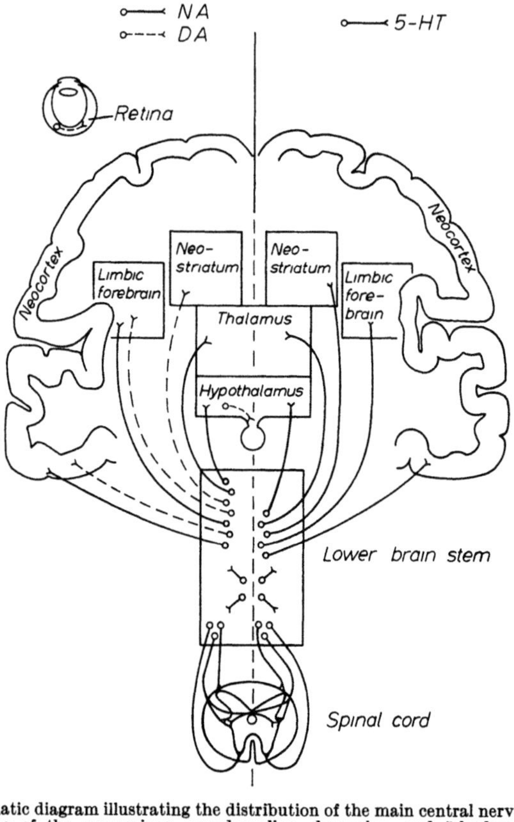

Fig. 1. Schematic diagram illustrating the distribution of the main central nervous pathways containing one of the monamines, noradrenaline, dopamine, and 5-hydroxytryptamine. Noradrenaline- (N.A.) and dopamine- (D.A.) pathways are shown on the left, 5-hydroxytryptamine- (5-H.T.) pathways on the right. *Note:* The cell bodies are generally located in the lower brain stem. From here the axons radiate to various parts of the central nervous system and terminate, *inter alia*, in several regions of importance for blood-pressure control.

bulk of stored transmitter, and this seems to be temporally correlated with functional recovery (Fig. 2). In the central neurones, storing N.A., dopamine, and 5-hydroxytryptamine, the biochemical, and thus probably also the functional, changes are similar to those found in the peripheral adrenergic neurones. By means of long-term treatment the large inert portion can be removed, thus unmasking the small labile, functionally essential fraction (HÄGGENDAL and LINDQVIST, 1963).

Guanethidine also causes depletion of the transmitter store. The mechanism of this depletion has not been studied very extensively,

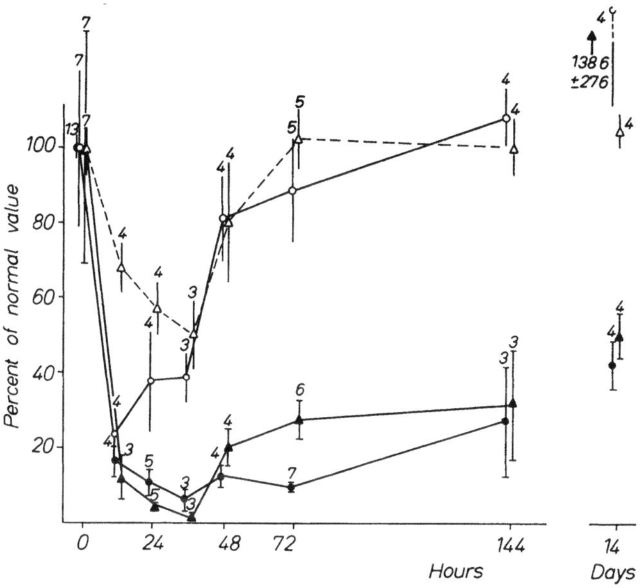

Fig. 2. Effect of a single dose of reserpine (0.1 mg./kg. s.c.) on the adrenergic nerves of the cat's nictitating membrane. *Note:* The response to sympathetic nerve stimulation (two upper curves, representing two different frequencies of stimulation) is lowered 12—36 hours after the injection. Simultaneously, both the N.A. level of the nictitating membrane and the uptake of injected ^{3}H-N.A. are lowered. The response to nerve stimulation recovers 36—72 hours after the injection. During this interval, N.A. remains unchanged at a low level, whereas the uptake of injected ^{3}H-N.A. shows partial recovery, indicating the existence of a very small, but functionally essential, N.A. fraction in the adrenergic nerves, probably located in the storage particles. Figures indicate numbers of experiments (from ANDÉN and HENNING, 1965).

0.2 imp./sec.
20 imp./sec.
N.A. nictitating membr.
^{3}H-N.A. nictitating membr.
} mean ± S.E.M.

but it has many features in common with reserpine. It is thus possible that it acts in the same way, i.e. by blocking the amine uptake by the storage granules. Guanethidine also causes blockade of adrenergic transmission, but the block may set in long before depletion is complete (for detailed discussion and references cf. MUSCHOLL, 1965). This does not mean that the two actions are not causally related. It seems quite possible that guanethidine primarily depletes the small, labile, functionally essential fraction of the transmitter store. — Guanethidine differs from reserpine in certain other respects. It is not lipid-soluble and therefore does not readily pass through biological membranes in general. It does not penetrate through the blood-brain barrier, and the basis for its penetration of, and accumulation in, sympathetic nerve-endings is the existence of a special amine-concentrating mechanism probably located at the level of the cell membrane (for detailed discussion and references; cf. Malmfors, 1965; Carlsson and Waldeck, 1965; Carlsson, 1965b). This amine "pump" normally recaptures some of the N.A. released from the nerve-terminals. It is blocked by desipramine, for example, and consequently this drug appears to block all the known actions of guanethidine on adrenergic nerve-endings. When utilising the "pump", guanethidine acts as a competitive inhibitor and thus blocks the recapture of N.A. This dual action of guanethidine, on the storage particles and on the amine "pump", probably explains the initial, often very pronounced, sympathomimetic action of the drug. Reserpine has no such effect, because it acts on the particles only. However, if the membrane pump is first blocked by desipramine, then reserpine causes an initial, sympathomimetic response. Reserpine is highly soluble in lipids and is thus able to penetrate into the nerve-endings independently of the membrane pump. It thus seems possible to explain the paradox that pretreatment with one and the same drug, desipramine, induces a sympathomimetic activity of reserpine but blocks the sympathomimetic activity of guanethidine.

The model depicted in Fig. 3 serves to illustrate, *inter alia*, the two amine-concentrating mechanisms operating in peripheral (and also central) N.A.-storing neurones: one located in the storage particles and blocked by reserpine, the other occurring at the level of the cell membrane and blocked by desipramine, cocaine, and amphetamine. It should be noted that blockade of the two mechanisms results in opposite functional effects: reserpine inhibits, whereas desipramine potentiates, the response to sympathetic nerve stimulation.

α-Methyldopa was introduced as a dopa-decarboxylase inhibitor. Certainly, it does act in this way, but it is doubtful whether this activity alone explains any of the effects of the drug. Other, at least equally potent, dopa-decarboxylase inhibitors are known, but they do not seem to possess any of the pharmacological properties of α-methyldopa. Like guanethidine and reserpine, α-methyldopa causes a pronounced decrease in tissue N.A., but unlike these drugs it does not appear to cause any inhibition of the peripheral adrenergic transmission mechanism, as judged by the response to nerve stimulation. This should be related to the fact that the mechanisms by which α-methyldopa and reserpine cause N.A. depletion are entirely different. α-Methyldopa does not block the amine uptake by the storage granules, but is converted to α-methyl-N.A. (via α-methyldopamine), which displaces the N.A. from the stores

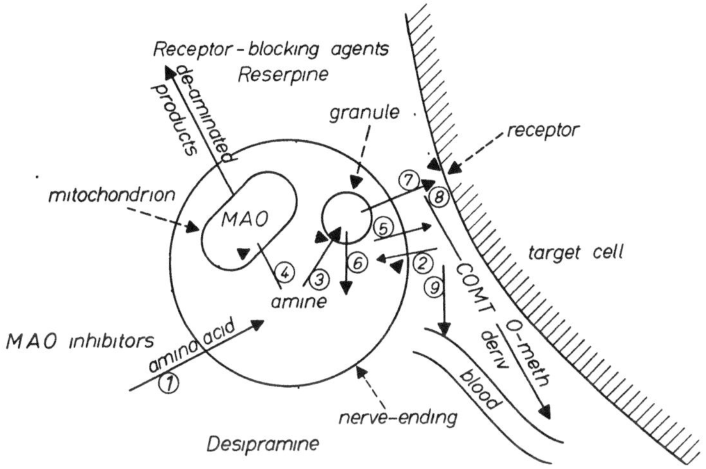

Fig. 3. Schematic diagram illustrating the various processes involved in monamine transmission and the sites of attack of four different types of drugs. An amino acid, in the case of catecholamines, tyrosine, enters the nerve-terminal (*1*). Tyrosine is hydroxylated on the ring to dopa, which is decarboxylated to dopamine. In adrenergic nerves, dopamine is hydroxylated on the side chain to N.A., probably within the storage granules. By means of an A.T.P.-Mg^{++}-dependent process (*3*), which is specifically blocked by reserpine, even in very low concentrations (10^{-7}M), the amines formed are incorporated into a complex held in the storage granules. The monamine oxidase (M.A.O.), occurring in the mitochondria of the nerve terminals, competes with this incorporation process for cytoplasmic amines (*4*). It appears that the amines must be incorporated into the storage complex in order to become available for release by the nerve impulse (*7*). Part of the amine released into the synaptic cleft (*5*) is recaptured by means of a very potent amine-concentrating mechanism (*2*), probably located at the level of the cell membrane, and can thus be utilised again. This mechanism is blocked by imipramine, desipramine, cocaine and amphetamine.

(Carlsson and Lindqvist, 1962). α-Methyl-N.A. is released by nerve stimulation, just as N.A. is, and may thus serve as a "false transmitter" (Muscholl, 1965). Now, the physiological activity of α-methyl-N.A. on peripheral tissues appears to be broadly the same as that of N.A., so there is no reason why the adrenergic nerves should not continue to function normally. In fact, even if N.A. is largely replaced by a "false transmitter" of lower activity, such as *d*-adrenaline or metaraminol, the adrenergic nerves appear to function normally (Andén and Magnusson, 1965). From this it may be inferred that if the synthesis of N.A. is unimpaired and if the amine uptake by the storage particles is not inhibited, then transmission can function normally, even if the bulk of the store is occupied by an amine of low activity. This is in agreement with the concept of a small, functionally essential transmitter pool, by-passing the bulk of the store.

Thus, if α-methyldopa were devoid of any pharmacological activity, it would be easy to explain. But how can we explain the actions that it has? For example, is the antihypertensive action due to the drug itself or to its decarboxylation products? According to one report, the antihypertensive activity in rats with renal hypertension is abolished if decarboxylation is prevented by treatment with a decarboxylase inhibitor of different structure – which supports the second alternative (DAVIS et al., 1963). If this is so, and if the sympathetic nerves still function normally, we should perhaps start to look for central neurones more susceptible to this kind of treatment than the peripheral adrenergic nerves. The amine turnover is, in general, much more rapid centrally than peripherally. It may be that the combination of replacement by a false transmitter and inhibition of synthesis leads more easily to interference with central than with peripheral amine-transmission mechanisms. In connection with the inhibition of synthesis we have to consider not only dopa decarboxylase – and 5-hydroxytryptophan decarboxylase, with which it may be identical (ROSENGREN, 1960) – but also aromatic hydroxylases, such as tyrosine hydroxylase, and tryptophan hydroxylase, which seem to be inhibited by α-methyldopa (ROOS and WERDINIUS, 1963).

However, there is one recent report that does not readily fit in with this interpretation, namely that orally ingested metaraminol, which in many respects behaves like α-methyl-N.A., biochemically as well as pharmacologically, has an antihypertensive effect in man (CROUT and SHORE, 1965). Metaraminol does not readily penetrate through the blood-brain barrier. If metaraminol possesses such activity and if it acts by the same mechanism as α-methyldopa, then we have to look for a site of attack outside this barrier.

Summary

Several antihypertensive drugs have been shown to interfere with adrenergic transmission in the peripheral sympathetic nervous system, and the mechanisms by which the effects are brought about have been partly elucidated. Thus, reserpine has been shown to block the incorporation of the adrenergic transmitter into a complex held in specific, intracellular storage particles, leading to depletion of transmitter and block of transmission;

guanethidine may act by a similar mechanism. No satisfactory explanation of the antihypertensive action of α-methyldopa has been given so far, although it has been shown to interfere with both the formation and storage of noradrenaline and related amines. Several antihypertensive agents are able to penetrate into the central nervous system and interfere with amine-transmission mechanisms in sympathetic centres at different levels. Central effects may play an important role in the antihypertensive actions of drugs such as reserpine and α-methyldopa.

Zusammenfassung

Verschiedene blutdrucksenkende Substanzen beeintrachtigen die adrenergische Erregungsübertragung in peripheren sympathischen Nerven. Die diesen Effekten zugrundeliegenden Mechanismen sind heute zum Teil geklärt. So ließ sich zeigen, daß Reserpin den Einbau des adrenergischen Überträgerstoffes in einen Komplex hemmt, der in einer spezifischen intrazellulären Speicherform vorliegt, und auf diese Weise zu einer Entleerung des Überträgers und zu einer Hemmung der Übertragung führt. Guanethidin dürfte uber einen ähnlichen Mechanismus wirken. Bisher ist keine befriedigende Erklärung für die blutdrucksenkende Wirkung von α-Methyldopa zu geben, obwohl nachgewiesen werden konnte, daß es nicht nur mit der Bildung, sondern auch mit der Speicherung von Noradrenalin und verwandten Aminen interferiert. Verschiedene blutdrucksenkende Stoffe dringen in das Zentralnervensystem ein und beeinträchtigen dort die Amin-Überträgermechanismen in sympathischen Zentren auf verschiedenen Ebenen. Bei der blutdrucksenkenden Wirkung bestimmter Stoffe wie Reserpin und α-Methyldopa konnen zentrale Effekte eine wichtige Rolle spielen.

Résumé

On a montré, pour plusieurs substances antihypertensives, que leur mode d'action est une intervention sur la transmission adrénergique au niveau du sympathique périphérique, et certains des mécanismes de production de leurs effets ont été élucidés. Ainsi, on a montré que la réserpine bloque l'incorporation du médiateur adrénergique dans un complexe contenu dans des particules spécifiques intracellulaires de mise en réserve, avec pour conséquence l'épuisement de ce médiateur et le blocage de la transmission; il est possible que la guanéthidine agisse de cette façon. Il n'existe encore aucune explication satisfaisante de l'action antihypertensive de l'α-méthyldopa, bien que l'on ait montré qu'elle intervienne à la fois sur l'élaboration et la mise en réserve de la noradrénaline et des amines apparentées. Plusieurs agents antihypertenseurs sont capables de pénétrer dans le système nerveux central et d'influencer les phénomènes de transmission assurés par les amines aux différents étages des centres sympathiques. Les effets centraux peuvent jouer un rôle important dans l'action antihypertensive d'une substance, comme c'est le cas pour la réserpine et l'α-méthyldopa.

Acknowledgements

The research reported in this document has been sponsored by the Air Force Office of Aerospace Research under Grant AF EOAR 65-56 through the European Office of Aerospace Research (OAR), United

States Air Force, from a Public Health Service Research Grant (NB 04359-02) from the National Institute of Neurological Diseases and Blindness, and the Swedish State Medical Research Council (14x-155-01).

References

ÅBLAD, B.: Acta pharmac. tox. **20**, Suppl. **1** (1963). — ANDÉN, N.-E., A. CARLSSON, and N.-Å. HILLARP: Acta pharmac. tox. **21**, 183 (1964). — ANDÉN, N.-E., and M. HENNING: to be published (1965). — ANDÉN, N.-E., and T. MAGNUSSON: In: Pharmacology of Cholinergic and Adrenergic Transmission. Proc. 2nd Internat. Pharmacol. Meeting, Prague, 1963. Ed. by G. B. KOELLE, W. W. DOUGLAS, and A. CARLSSON. Pergamon Press, Oxford, 1965, **3**, p. 319. — CARLSSON, A.: In: Handbuch der experimentellen Pharmakologie. Ergänzungswerk. Ed. by V. ERSPAMER. Springer, Berlin, 1965a, in press. — CARLSSON, A.: Physiological and pharmacological release of monoamines in the central nervous system. Paper read at Internat. Symposium on Release of Biogenic Amines. Stockholm, Sweden, February 1965b. — CARLSSON, A., B. FALCK, K. FUXE, and N.-Å. HILLARP: Acta physiol. Scand. **60**, 112 (1964). — CARLSSON, A., and M. LINDQVIST: Acta physiol. Scand. **54**, 87 (1962). — CARLSSON, A., and B. WALDECK: Acta pharmac. tox. **22**, 293 (1965). — COSTA, E., A. M. REVZIN, R. KUNTZMAN, S. SPECTOR, and B. BRODIE: Science **133**, 1822 (1961). — CROUT, J. R., and P. A. SHORE: Personal communication (1965). — DAVIS, R. A., D. J. DRAIN, M. HORLINGTON, R. LAZARE, and A. URBANSKA: Life Sc. **3**, 193 (1963). — FUXE, K., and G. SEDVALL: Acta physiol. Scand. **64**, 75 (1965). — HAMBERGER, B., and K. A. NORBERG: Internat. J. Neuropharmacol. **4**, 41 (1965). — HAMBERGER, B., K. A. NORBERG, and F. SJÖQVIST: Internat. J. Neuropharmacol. **2**, 279 (1963). — HAMBERGER, B., K. A. NORBERG, and U. UNGERSTEDT: Acta physiol. Scand. **64**, 285 (1965). — HÄGGENDAL, J., and M. LINDQVIST: Acta physiol. Scand. **60**, 351 (1963). — LÖFVING, B.: Acta physiol. Scand. **53**, Suppl. **184** (1961). — MALMFORS, T.: Acta physiol. Scand. **64**, Suppl. **248** (1965). — MUSCHOLL, E.: In: Pharmacology of Cholinergic and Adrenergic Transmission. Proc. 2nd Internat. Pharmacol. Meeting, Prague, 1963. Ed by G. B. KOELLE, W. W. DOUGLAS, and A. CARLSSON. Pergamon Press, Oxford, 1965, **3**, p. 291. — NORBERG, K. A.: Internat. J. Neuropharmacol. **3**, 379 (1964). — PLETSCHER, A., K. F. GEY, and P. ZELLER: Fortschr. Arzneimittelforsch. **2**, 417 (1960). — REINERT, H.: J. Physiol. **167**, 18 (1963). — ROOS, B.-E., and B. WERDINIUS: Life Sc. **2**, 92 (1963). — ROSENGREN, E.: Acta physiol. Scand. **49**, 364 (1960). — UVNÄS, B.: Personal communication (1964). — VOGT, M.: J. Physiol. **123**, 451 (1954).

Mode of action of antihypertensive drugs

By

H. J. Bein and H. Brunner

In view of the many reviews on the pharmacology of antihypertensive drugs that have already been published, we do not feel justified in presenting yet another compilation; instead, we propose to discuss just a few aspects relating to the pharmacological analysis of antihypertensive agents.

First of all, it should be said that the term "antihypertensive agents" comprises substances which are clinically active in lowering chronically elevated blood pressure and are of therapeutic usefulness. In this respect, it is irrelevant whether the compound in question lowers the blood pressure of animals in which hypertension has been induced by some means or other. The selection of those clinically effective agents that are currently employed in the treatment of hypertensive patients has not been based on pharmacological tests in chronically hypertensive animals, but on observation of their action in normotensive ones; alternatively, it has been based on biochemical speculation – which may or, as in the case of α-methyldopa for instance, may not subsequently have proved correct; or, last but not least, the drug's antihypertensive action has been discovered quite empirically from clinical observation.

Since the discovery of the first antihypertensive agents, experience has shown that the blood-pressure-lowering activity of some antihypertensive agents could not have been predicted solely from observations in normotensive animals (Table 1). α-Methyldopa, for example, which is practically inactive in normotensive animals, displays a marked antihypertensive effect in the renal hypertensive rat, whereas ganglionic blocking agents show only moderate activity under the same conditions. The example of isocaramidine (Abrams et al., 1964) illustrates that a chemical analogy – in this case with guanethidine – does not guarantee identical responses in different hypertensive models.

One question arising at this point is that of drawing a distinction between hypertensive and non-hypertensive blood pressure. Within certain limits at least, the choice of a "critical" blood-pressure

Table 1. *Blood-pressure-lowering activity of some antihypertensive drugs in normotensive and in hypertensive animals*

	Normotensive animal Acute effect	Cortexone-hypertension Rat	Metacorticoid-hypertension Rat	Renal hypertension Rat	Renal hypertension Dog	Carotid-sinus denervation Dog
Ganglionic blocking agents	+	∅ *[2]	+ *[3]	(+)	+ *[4]	+ *[6]
Reserpine	+	+	+ *[3]	+	+ *[5]	+ *[6]
Hydralazine	+	+	+ *[3]	+	+	+ *[7]
Guanethidine	+	+	(+) *[3]	+	+	+ *[7]
Isocaramidine	+	+		∅		
α-Methyldopa	∅ (+) *[1]	+	+ *[3]	+		
Hydrochlorothiazide	∅	+	+ *[3]	∅		

* According to data from literature.

[1] STONE et al., 1961. [2] GROSS, 1957. [3] STANTON and WHITE, 1965. [4] HAAS and GOLDBLATT, 1959. [5] GROLLMAN, 1955. [6] MAXWELL et al., 1958. [7] PLUMMER, 1960.

level must, to begin with, remain somewhat arbitrary. In our normotensive rats the blood-pressure levels, recorded in the tail by the plethysmographic method of WILLIAMS et al. (1939), varied between 100 and 130 mm. Hg in the females, the average being 116 ± 9 mm. Hg, and between 95 and 130 mm. Hg in the males (average 112 ± 9 mm. Hg). Levels of 160 mm. Hg or more were regarded as indicative of hypertension (BEIN et al., 1957). Other authors have come to somewhat similar conclusions: STANTON and WHITE (1965), for instance, considered those animals as being hypertensive which exhibited more than the normotensive mean arterial blood pressures plus three standard deviations.

On the other hand, one also has to define the term "antihypertensive", this time in an experimental situation. In our laboratories we distinguish between normalisation of blood pressure, i.e. a return to normotensive pressure (100% effective), and a relatively weak action; this latter category includes compounds which are less than 50% effective; 10% or less is regarded as ineffective. In addition, we only designate a compound as antihypertensive if chronic treatment maintains a lowered blood pressure over a period of at least 12 days, i.e. if no tolerance develops. While there is no doubt that these criteria favour compounds with a long-lasting effect, it should be pointed out in this connection that all the true antihypertensives are compounds which in the experimental animal display a blood-pressure-lowering effect of prolonged duration as one of their most distinctive features (MEIER et al., 1956).

Furthermore, Table 1 shows that some antihypertensives are either particularly active or inactive in the hypertensive animal, depending on the experimental model used. Though we may classify the various experimental forms of hypertension according to the eliciting factors employed, we nevertheless have to realise that the real cause or causes leading to elevated blood pressure are still obscure.

The main effect of all clinically active antihypertensives is the reduction of peripheral resistance. This reduction can be brought about by various mechanisms, one of which consists in blocking the activity of the sympathetic nervous system. Since Dr. CARLSSON has dealt in this symposium with the pharmacology of the sympathetic nerves, we should like to mention only a few aspects:

There seems to be no doubt that reserpine exerts an action on the autonomic nervous system by inducing a loss of neurohumoral transmitter in the sympathetic portion, and that one of its predominant effects is a diminution in sympathetic tone. However, it appears to be extremely difficult to correlate behavioural changes with the changes occurring in the amines in the brain. This conclusion is based not only on experiments comparing behavioural effects with the concentrations of 5-hydroxytryptamine (5-H.T.) and noradrenaline in the brain (BEIN, 1965), but also on results obtained by BENFEY and VARMA (1964) when they investigated the influence of α-methyldopa on certain central effects of reserpine. α-Methyldopa leads to a decrease in the 5-H.T., dopamine, and noradrenaline content of the mouse brain (CARLSSON and LINDQVIST, 1962). It also mimics reserpine in prolonging sleep due to hexobarbitone. If α-methyldopa were to act by depleting the brain amines, one would expect it to potentiate the action of reserpine; instead, however, α-methyldopa antagonises the effect of reserpine on the sleeping time. BENFEY and VARMA think that – with regard to certain effects, at least – there is a direct antagonism between α-methyldopa and reserpine which is not related to changes in the tissue catecholamine levels.

The effect of reserpine on the brain amines has focused attention on this peculiar aspect of its mode of action to such an extent that its effects on other tissue constituents are apt to be neglected.

It should be remembered that reserpine is also reported to change the concentration of glycogen, acetylcholine, γ-aminobutyric acid, nucleic acids, and substance P (for references see BEIN, 1965). In view of the complex pharmacological picture presented by reserpine, the possibility that there may be more than one basic effect should always be borne in mind. Moreover, even so far as only one single basic pharmacological property is concerned, there may still be differences in the pharmacological response from one species to another. Very recently, TRENDELENBURG (1965) reported that the isolated atria of reserpine-pretreated rabbits showed no response to sympathetic stimulation, whereas the atria of reserpine-pretreated guinea-pigs have a compartment in their cardiac noradrenaline stores that is accessible to nerve impulses but not to reserpine. This illustrates the difficulties that arise when one tries to correlate results obtained in one species with those obtained in another, even with respect to such an intimate mode of action as this.

Besides the action of reserpine on the peripheral portion of the sympathetic nervous system, other peripheral sites of attack must also be taken into consideration. TRIPOD and MEIER (1954a, b) showed that reserpine acts in acute experiments as a strong antagonist towards various agents which contract smooth muscle. In the light of views expressed in the literature, one would rather expect hydralazine to be a more powerful agent in this respect. That this is not so, however, is revealed by the data listed in Table 2. In accordance with these findings, KIRPEKAR and LEWIS (1958) showed that reserpine and hydralazine relax strips of horse carotid artery irrespective of the nature of the stimulant used and that both drugs are also capable of causing direct relaxation.

Taking hydralazine as an example, let us examine some further aspects of our problem.

Hydralazine is a strong blood-pressure-lowering agent in the rat, the rabbit, and the cat, but a rather weak one in the dog. In non-anaesthetised rats and dogs it causes tachycardia, but in rats anaesthetised with pentobarbitone it induces bradycardia (Table 3). Obviously, the anaesthesia has a significant influence in this connection. An analysis of the circulatory reactions in the non-anaesthetised dog shows a marked reduction in peripheral resistance; its repercussions on the arterial pressure are to some extent offset by a substantial increase in cardiac output (Fig. 1). Analogous haemodynamic effects have been noted in man. ÅBLAD (1963) put forward the view that the reduction in arterial pressure due to hydralazine would evoke, via the baroceptor reflexes, an increased discharge from the sympathetic nervous system and hence

Table 2. *Antagonism in isolated organs* (According to TRIPOD and MEIER, 1954a, b; MEIER et al., 1958; MEIER et al., 1956)

	Guinea-pig ileum Histamine	Rabbit intestine		Perfused hind quarters of the rabbit			
		Acetylcholine	$BaCl_2$	$BaCl_2$	Histamine	Adrenaline	Angiotensin
Reserpine	$2 \cdot 10^{-7}$ *	$3 \cdot 10^{-7}$	$2 \cdot 10^{-7}$	10^{-6}	$>10^{-5}$	$>10^{-5}$	10^{-6}
Hydralazine	$3 \cdot 10^{-5}$	∅	$3 \cdot 10^{-4}$	$5 \cdot 10^{-6}$	$5 \cdot 10^{-7}$	10^{-4}	$>10^{-4}$

* All concentrations given in g./ml.

Table 3. *Effect of hydralazine on blood pressure and heart rate in dogs and rats* (HEDWALL and MEIER, 1965)

	Mean blood pressure mm. Hg		Heart rate	
	Control	Δ 10—15 min. after hydralazine 1.0 mg./kg. i.v.	Control	Δ 10—15 min. after hydralazine 1.0 mg./kg. i.v.
A) Non-anaesthetised				
Dog	127 ± 4	-13 ± 4	90 ± 12	$+105 \pm 8$
Rat	127 ± 5	-44 ± 3	455 ± 19	$+72 \pm 22$
B) Pentobarbitone anaesthesia				
Dog	154 ± 6	-23 ± 2	190 ± 11	$+18 \pm 7$
Rat	128 ± 7	-67 ± 8	382 ± 28	-97 ± 27

an increase in cardiac output and heart rate. The same hypothesis was also postulated by AHLQUIST et al. (1947) with regard to tolazoline and by MAXWELL et al. (1958) with regard to the ganglionic blocking agent, chlorisondamine. The latter authors analysed in various species, including monkey, dog, rabbit, and rat, the compensatory mechanisms to chlorisondamine. They present evidence indicating that barbiturates interfere with compensatory mechanisms which normally function in the normotensive dog and rat; these mechanisms appear to be less predominant in the monkey and in the rabbit. Another finding which has an important bearing on our theme was made by the same group, namely that in the dog, in the malignant phase of renal hypertension, compensatory mechanisms are more vulnerable to the action of ganglioplegic agents, indicating a difference between normotensive and hypertensive subjects. It is also worth noting that the effect of compensatory reflexes depends upon whether the drug is administered slowly or rapidly (HAAS and GOLDBLATT, 1960).

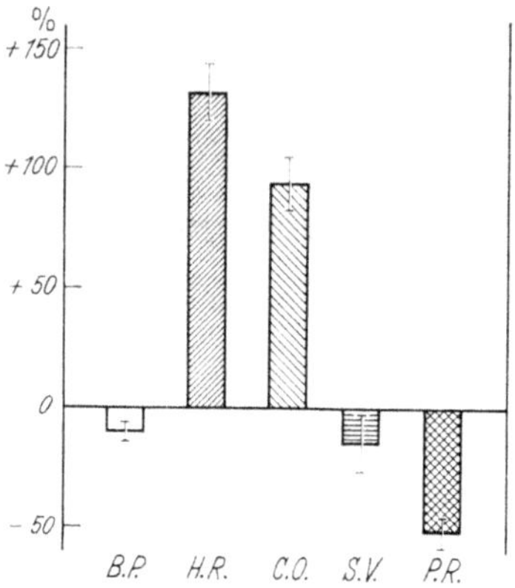

Fig. 1. Non-anaesthetised dog 10 min. after hydralazine 1 mg./kg. i. v. B.P.: blood pressure, H.R.: heart rate, C.O.: cardiac output, S.V.: stroke volume, P.R.: peripheral resistance (MEIER, 1965).

The next question is how hydralazine brings about a decrease in peripheral resistance. There are different opinions as to the extent to which a central effect plays a role in addition to the direct peripheral site of attack (for discussion see ÅBLAD, 1963).

Hydralazine inhibits pressor reactions after stimulation of afferent nerves without interfering to the same extent with the pressor reaction produced by stimulation of an efferent sympathetic nerve. We have therefore postulated a central site of attack (BEIN et al., 1953). In addition, hydralazine is capable of bringing about changes in the concentration of normal brain constituents. It causes a decrease in the adenosine triphosphate concentration which is accompanied by an increase in the adenosine diphosphate concentration. KIRPEKAR and LEWIS (1959) conclude that hydralazine interferes with normal oxidative processes in the brain.

However that may be, a peripheral site of attack undoubtedly plays a major part! It seems unlikely that the adrenolytic activity, which – though certainly present – is relatively weak, can be of decisive importance. Using three different pharmacological agents, hydralazine, phenoxybenzamine, and guanethidine, HENNING et al. (1963) obtained in human subjects an increase in blood flow in the hand which was the same for each of the three substances tested. Hydralazine had only a weak influence on the vasoconstriction produced by cold or by intravenous infusion of noradrenaline, whereas phenoxybenzamine inhibited both types of vasoconstriction, and guanethidine – as was to be expected – inhibited only the vasoconstriction due to cold. When the blood pressure is lowered by hydralazine, reflex vasoconstriction is reported to occur, which, however, can only be demonstrated in a vascular bed that has been excluded from the circulation prior to the administration of hydralazine. It is difficult to understand why the vasoconstriction occurring in the cold pressor test is not inhibited by hydralazine, and why hydralazine nevertheless blocks the adjustment of the circulation to its effect in the periphery.

The antagonistic activity of hydralazine against noradrenaline also shows some peculiarities. The vasoconstrictor action of noradrenaline on the bovine mesenteric artery is – according to ÅBLAD (1963) – only antagonised by hydralazine under aerobic conditions, but is potentiated under anaerobic conditions; this proved to be in contrast to other "spasmolytic" agents, such as papaverine and sodium nitrite.

That hydralazine may be converted from a noradrenaline-antagonist to a noradrenaline-synergist was also found by TRIPOD (1960) in our laboratories. He tested the antagonistic action of hydralazine against various vasoconstrictors in the perfused hind quarters of renal hypertensive rats and in normotensive animals. TRIPOD and BEIN (1960) had observed earlier that adrenaline, histamine, and angiotensin are more active as vasoconstrictors in hypertensive rats than in controls. The vasoconstrictor effect of noradrenaline, however, was rather less pronounced in the hypertensive animals than in the controls. This is in contrast to its effect on blood pressure in hypertensive rats. Hydralazine in a concentration of 10^{-5} does not antagonise but potentiates the vasoconstriction due to noradrenaline – in contrast to its action in normotensive rats (Fig. 2a). The behaviour of adrenaline differs from that of noradrenaline, because the antagonistic effect of hydralazine is enhanced in hypertensive animals as compared with normotensive animals (Fig. 2b).

When interpreting results obtained on perfused vessels one should bear in mind that the activity of pharmacologically active agents — whether they act as agonists or antagonists — depends to a large degree on the "milieu interne". TRIPOD et al. (1958) noted a shift in the activity of hydralazine when the ion composition or the O_2 saturation of the perfusion fluid was altered. Changes in one component, however, do not influence every hypotensive in the same manner and — what is more remarkable — do not

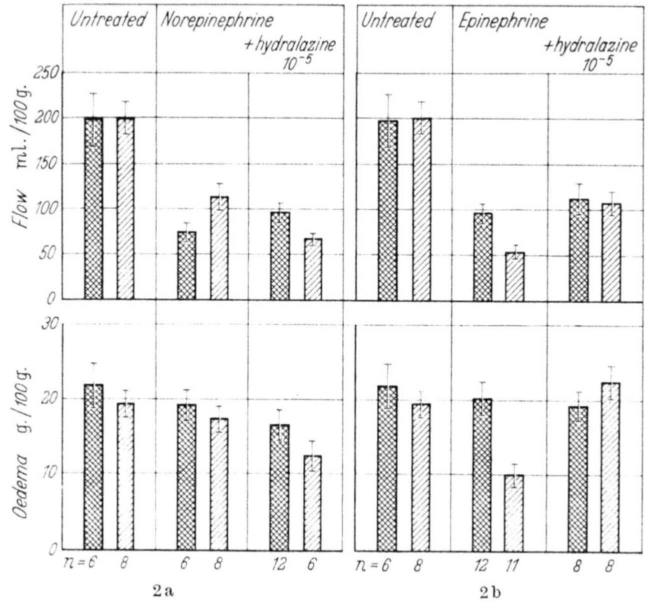

Fig. 2a, b. Changes in flow and in weight of perfused hind quarters. Cross-hatched columns: non-hypertensive animals. Hatched columns: hypertensive animals (TRIPOD, 1960; method see TRIPOD and BEIN, 1960).

necessarily produce the same type of alteration in the spasmolytic activity which one particular hypotensive displays against different spasmogenic agents. When the O_2 saturation of the perfusion fluid is increased, the antagonistic effect of hydralazine towards adrenaline increases, whereas its antagonistic action against histamine is potentiated by a reduction in the O_2 concentration.

The more intimate mechanisms of action underlying the experimentally demonstrable effect of reserpine and hydralazine on peripheral organs have received little attention. It was LEWIS and his team in particular (GILLIS and LEWIS, 1956, 1957) who postulated an influence on the carbohydrate metabolism of smooth muscle, since an antagonistic action by intermediates of the tricarboxylic acid cycle had been demonstrated. It may be of interest to note that reserpine and hydralazine have not been found to influence the respiration of kidney and heart in normotensive animals, but that they do increase the reduced respiration of tissues in cortexone-hypertensive animals (MOORE et al., 1959). JAQUES et al. (1957) and JAQUES and MEIER (1960) drew attention to the complex-forming capacity of hydralazine and to the fact that reserpine, guanethidine, and hydralazine protect mice against lethal doses of x-rays.

We are not aware of any other studies on the more intimate mode of action of antihypertensives in hypertensive subjects. Going through the literature, one is usually confronted with the view that the mode of action of antihypertensives is the same in hypertensives as in normotensives – assuming, of course, that the normotensives show any reduction in blood pressure at all and leaving out of account the fact that, generally speaking, the higher the blood pressure is, the more marked is the hypotensive effect of any given dose, at least within a certain dosage range.

During the very first studies which PELLMONT and MEIER undertook with hydralazine in our laboratories in 1945, attention was focused on the possibility that hydralazine might enhance the vasodilator action of adrenaline. In 1952, BARRETT et al. showed that, in the heart-lung preparation of the dog, hydralazine potentiates the coronary dilator action of adrenaline. The influence of hydralazine on the myocardium and coronary circulation was investigated recently by BARRETT et al. (1965) and BRUNNER et al. (1965a, b). The increase in both myocardial contractility and coronary flow produced by hydralazine could be inhibited by adrenergic β-receptor blockade.

ABBOUD and ECKSTEIN (1962) concluded from experiments on dogs that guanethidine would produce vasodilatation by stimulation of β-adrenergic receptors or other dilator receptors which are blocked by dichloro-isoproterenol.

The antihypertensive action of hydralazine in renal hypertensive rats can in fact be inhibited by propranolol (Fig. 3). The same antagonism is also observed in the case of the antihypertensive effect of reserpine. The same applies to guanethidine (Fig. 4) and to α-methyldopa, the only exception being a monamine-oxidase inhibitor. Incidentally, the antagonism is not confined to the renal hypertensive rat (Table 4). In connection with the findings of Dr. CARLSSON it is of special interest to note that imipramine displays no antagonistic action.

There was no evidence that changes in the concentration of catecholamines in the heart played any part in this phenomenon.

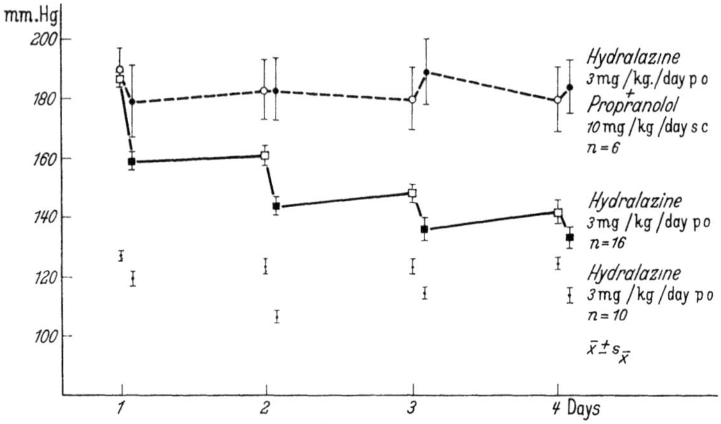

Fig. 3. Blood pressure of rats with renal hypertension, measured before and two hours after daily injection. Administration of hydralazine together with a β-blocker (upper curve), and of hydralazine alone (middle curve). The lower curve shows the effect of hydralazine on normotensive animals.

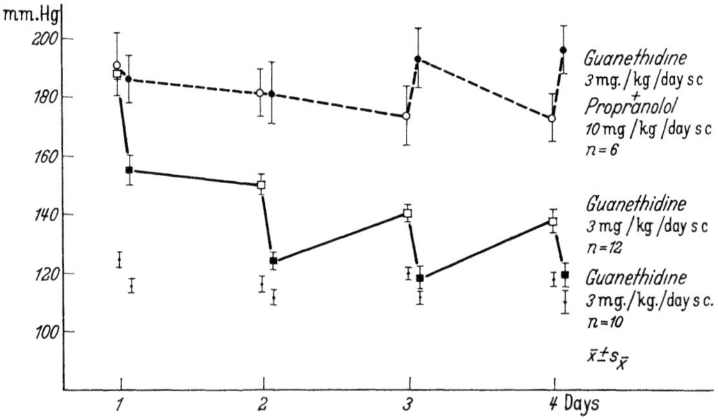

Fig. 4. Blood pressure of rats with renal hypertension, measured before and two hours after daily injection. Administration of guanethidine together with a β-blocker (upper curve), and of guanethidine alone (middle curve). The lower curve shows the effect of guanethidine on normotensive animals.

Moreover, the postganglionic inhibition occurring after guanethidine (nictitating membrane of the cat) cannot be prevented by a β-blocker. The antagonism between the antihypertensive agent and the β-blocker does not therefore involve pharmacological components of the antihypertensives which are considered to be of importance as regards their over-all effect.

Table 4. *Antagonistic effect of propranolol on the blood-pressure-lowering activity of various antihypertensive drugs*

	Renal-hyper-tensive rats	Cortexone-hyper-tensive rats	Renal-hyper-tensive dog
Hydralazine 3 mg./kg./day p.o.	+		
Reserpine 0.3 mg./kg./day s.c.	+		
Guanethidine 3 mg./kg./day s.c..	+	+	+
α-Methyldopa 300 mg./kg./day p.o. . . .	+		
Pargyline 20 mg./kg./day s.c.	∅		

+: Antagonism
∅: No antagonism

Having established that there is an antagonism common to antihypertensives which have different pharmacological modes of action, one is tempted to speculate that the antihypertensive action might conceivably be governed by a common mechanism. What is more, one may even be inclined to wonder whether the mechanism in question has any connection with the sympathetic nervous system at all, or whether the antagonism has anything to do with the β-receptors.

So far we have been dealing chiefly with acute experiments. Whether the mode of action of the antihypertensives changes during prolonged treatment is still a moot point. Here again, there are not many studies to which one can refer. The possibility of a change in the mode of action during chronic treatment has been discussed with particular reference to the saluretics (Freis, 1960; Hoobler, 1960).

When comparing the antagonistic action of various hypotensives against vasoconstrictors in the perfused hind quarters of rabbits, Tripod et al. (1960) noted a change in activity even after treatment of such comparatively short duration as ten days. Reserpine no longer showed any antagonism towards angiotensin, whereas the action of hydralazine against adrenaline, noradrenaline, and angiotensin was now enhanced. In contrast to the findings with catecholamines and angiotensin, hydralazine no longer antagonises vasopressin, but acts synergistically with it. Results obtained in acute experiments do not therefore necessarily apply to the more complex pharmacological situation arising after chronic treatment.

It is difficult to say whether the increases in blood pressure observed in the dog after long-term treatment with ganglionic blocking agents (PARDO and VIDRIO, 1964) — increases which can be counteracted with reserpine, hydrochlorothiazide, and phenoxybenzamine — are of any relevance in this connection. Incidentally, VAN PROOSDIJ-HARTZEMA and DE JONGH (1955) made similar observations in rats.

It is known that the pathological lesions of the blood vessels occurring in hypertensive animals can be influenced by treatment with antihypertensives. In renal hypertensive rats treated with hydralazine, MASSON et al. (1958) observed a close association between blood-pressure levels and the presence and character of the vascular lesions. In addition, they found that the lesions which had developed healed when the blood pressure was restored to normal. Here, however, it is extremely difficult to determine whether the lowering of the elevated blood pressure is causal or incidental and whether pharmacological effects exerted by the antihypertensives outside the circulatory system may be important as well.

Not every antihypertensive has been studied along these lines, but we do at least have a few interesting clues. BEIN et al. (1957) found in renal hypertensive rats that the severity of the typical pathological lesions can be correlated neither with the absolute height of the blood pressure, nor with the duration of the hypertension, nor with the rate at which the hypertension develops. They postulated that clamping the renal artery gives rise to a vascular disease *per se* and that the interference with the renal circulation causes mesenchymal reactions which are not necessarily linked with factors responsible for raising the blood pressure. Besides microscopic examination of the vascular beds, they also attempted to determine the general reactivity of the mesenchyma. For this purpose they resorted to the foreign-body granuloma reaction induced by the subcutaneous implantation of a cotton-wool pellet in the rat. A significant increase in granuloma weight was found in cases where the hypertension was of more than a certain minimum duration and in cases where it had developed comparatively quickly. Furthermore, however, they also noted some increase in the weight of the granuloma in rats which were not hypertensive but clamped, and, last but not least, marked sex differences.

Since renal hypertension involves a variety of connections with the endocrine system — and not only with the gonads — extraordinary difficulties are liable to be encountered in attempting to explain the intimate mode of action in experimentally induced hypertension. As the factors determining blood pressure and mesenchymal reactivity seem to be independent of each other, it hardly seems sufficient to satisfy oneself merely with the statement that a given drug exerts an antihypertensive effect. As far as renal hypertension in the rat is concerned, substances are in fact known which, while admittedly lowering the blood pressure, also make the blood vessels more susceptible to atheromatous lesions; this is the case, for example, with thiouracil and its derivatives. With regard to fat deposition in the large vessels, we find a distinct action with several antihypertensive agents. In rabbits fed on an atherogenic diet, reserpine, hydralazine, and guanethidine each inhibit deposition of cholesterol in the aorta, but without reducing the high concentrations of cholesterol in the blood (SCHULER and ALBRECHT, 1962).

Besides its effect on fat deposition, hydralazine – and to a lesser degree reserpine – also influences mesenchymal inflammatory reactions. It inhibits growth of a foreign-body granuloma as well as local inflammation after mustard oil (MEIER and DESAULLES, 1957) and the formation of exudate in exudative pleurisy in rats (JAQUES, 1965).

It is difficult to assess the precise significance of these experimental results. Our purpose in citing them was merely to illustrate how complex the problem of analysis becomes when anatomopathological lesions have to be considered as well, especially if at the same time one tries to distinguish between the mechanism of action responsible for combating vascular lesions on the one hand and for lowering elevated blood pressure on the other.

References

ABBOUD, F. M., and J. W. ECKSTEIN: Circulation Res. **11**, 788 (1962). — ÅBLAD, B.: Acta pharmacol. et toxicol. **20**, Suppl. 1 (1963). — ABRAMS, W. B., R. A. MOE, H. BATES, R. POCELINKO, E. N. WHITMAN, and I. STARK: Amer. J. Cardiol. **13**, 94 (1964). — AHLQUIST, R. P., R. A. HUGGINS, and R. A. WOODBURY: J. Pharmacol. Exper. Therap. **89**, 271 (1947). — BARRETT, W. E., H. POVALSKI, and R. RUTLEDGE: Fed. Proc. **24**, 712 (1965). — BARRETT, W. E., W. REITZE, A. J. PLUMMER, and F. F. YONKMAN: Fed. Proc. **11**, 320 (1952). — BEIN, H. J.: In: Pharmacology of Oriental Plants. Proc. 2nd Internat. Pharmacol. Meeting, Prague, 1963. Ed. by K. K. CHEN and B. MUKERJI. Pergamon-Czechoslovac Medical Press, Prague, 1965, **7**, p. 87. — BEIN, H. J., P. A. DESAULLES, and P. LOUSTALOT: Experientia **13**, 130 (1957). — BEIN, H. J., F. GROSS, J. TRIPOD, and R. MEIER: Schweiz. med. Wschr. **83**, 336 (1953). — BENFEY, B. G., and D. R. VARMA: Brit. J. Pharmacol. **22**, 366 (1964). — BRUNNER, H., P. R. HEDWALL, and M. MEIER: Experientia **21**, 136 (1965a). — BRUNNER, H., P. R. HEDWALL, and M. MEIER: Experientia **21**, 231 (1965b). — CARLSSON, A., and M. LINDQVIST:

Acta physiol. Scand. **54**, 87 (1962). — FREIS, E. D.: In: Essentielle Hypertonie. Ein internationales Symposion. Ed. K. D. BOCK and P. T. COTTIER. Springer, Berlin, 1960, p. 198. — GILLIS, C. N., and J. J. LEWIS: Nature **178**, 859 (1956). — GILLIS, C. N., and J. J. LEWIS: Nature **179**, 820 (1957). — GROLLMAN, A.: J. Pharmacol. Exper. Therap. **114**, 263 (1955). — GROSS, F.: Arch. exper. Path. Pharmak. **232**, 161 (1957). — HAAS, E., and H. GOLDBLATT: Amer. J. Physiol. **197**, 1303 (1959). — HAAS, E., and H. GOLDBLATT: Amer. J. Physiol. **198**, 1023 (1960). — HEDWALL, P. R., and M. MEIER: To be published (1965). — HENNING, M., G. JOHNSSON, and B. ÅBLAD: quoted by ÅBLAD (1963). — HOOBLER, S. W.: In: Essentielle Hypertonie. Ein internationales Symposion. Ed. K. D. BOCK and P. T. COTTIER. Springer, Berlin, 1960, p. 215. — JAQUES, R.: Helv. Physiol. Acta **23**, 162 (1965). — JAQUES, R., and R. MEIER: Experientia **16**, 75 (1960). — JAQUES, R., J. TRIPOD, and R. MEIER: Arch. exper. Path. Pharmak. **230**, 26 (1957). — KIRPEKAR, S. M., and J. J. LEWIS: J. Pharmacy Pharmacol. **10**, 255 (1958). — KIRPEKAR, S. M., and J. J. LEWIS: Brit. J. Pharmacol. **14**, 40 (1959). — MASSON, G. M. C., L. J. MCCORMACK, H. P. DUSTAN, and A. C. CORCORAN: Amer. J. Path. **34**, 817 (1958). — MAXWELL, R. A., A. J. PLUMMER, S. D. ROSS, A. I. DANIEL, and F. SCHNEIDER: J. Pharmacol. Exper. Therap. **123**, 238 (1958). — MEIER, M.: Unpublished observations (1965). — MEIER, R., H. J. BEIN, F. GROSS, and J. TRIPOD: In: Proc. 3rd Internat. Congress Internal Med., Stockholm, 1954. Acta med. Scand. **154**, Suppl. **312**, 165 (1956). — MEIER, R., and P. A. DESAULLES: J. physiol. **49**, 667 (1957). — MEIER, R., J. TRIPOD, and A. STUDER: Arch. int. Pharmacodyn. **117**, 185 (1958). — MOORE, K. E., J. R. MURRAY, and M. J. HUSTON: Arch. int. Pharmacodyn. **118**, 340 (1959). — PARDO, E. G., and H. VIDRIO: J. Pharmacol. Exper. Therap. **144**, 124 (1964). — PELLMONT, B., and R. MEIER: Unpublished observations (1945). — PLUMMER, A. J.: In: Essentielle Hypertonie. Ein internationales Symposion. Ed. K. D. BOCK and P. T. COTTIER. Springer, Berlin, 1960, p. 262. — VAN PROOSDIJ-HARTZEMA, E. G., and D. K. DE JONGH: Acta physiol. pharmacol. Neerl. **4**, 160 (1955). — SCHULER, W., and W. ALBRECHT: Schweiz. med. Wschr. **92**, 1007 (1962). — STANTON, H. C., and J. B. WHITE, JR.: Arch. int. Pharmacodyn. **154**, 351 (1965). — STONE, C. A., C. C. PORTER, L. S. WATSON, and C. A. ROSS: In: Hypertension, Recent Advances. The Second Hahnemann Symposium on Hypertensive Disease. Ed. by A. N. BREST and J. H. MOYER. Lea and Febiger, Philadelphia, 1961, p. 417. — TRENDELENBURG, U.: J. Pharmacol. Exper. Therap. **147**, 313 (1965). — TRIPOD, J.: Unpublished observations (1960). — TRIPOD, J., and H. J. BEIN: Helv. Physiol. Acta **18**, 394 (1960). — TRIPOD, J., and R. MEIER: Arch. int. Pharmacodyn. **97**, 251 (1954a). — TRIPOD, J., and R. MEIER: Arch. int. Pharmacodyn. **99**, 104 (1954b). — TRIPOD, J., A. STUDER, E. WIRZ, and R. MEIER: Arch. int. Pharmacodyn. **126**, 126 (1960). — TRIPOD, J., E. WIRZ, and R. MEIER: Arch. int. Pharmacodyn. **116**, 464 (1958). — WILLIAMS, J. R., A. GROLLMAN, and T. R. HARRISON: J. Clin. Invest. **18**, 373 (1939).

Discussion

PAGE: I think the two papers illustrate beautifully the complexity that we are facing in the treatment of hypertension. I am always impressed by how much cardiologists contribute to the field of pharmacology. We have really provided these fellows with a steady job of work, and I hope they appreciate it. I should like to raise a question that has always intrigued me, and that is, whether it would be possible to study the relationships among the various humoral agents by using the platelet as a model of what is going on. The platelet, even though we used disparagingly to call it "blood dust", is really a little packet of neurohumours. It has a pump, an "amine pump", if you like to call it that, and in many ways it resembles the synaptic vesicle. I have often wondered whether the platelet and the synaptic vesicle might not be related to each other. If they are, the platelet would provide a very useful model for studying the intermediary metabolism at nerve-terminals.

If I might make another suggestion, I think the use of non-anaesthetised animals with permanently implanted sensors marks the beginning of a new chapter in pharmacology. We measure concurrently blood pressure, cardiac output, heart rate, stroke volume, and calculated peripheral resistance. We have been able to give a continuous infusion for six or more weeks while measuring all of the circulatory aspects. Now we can use animals that are unrestrained and free-moving. We are going to have to re-do most of the study of cardiac drugs by this new method. I was very glad to see that the two assays discussed the problem of chronic treatment as opposed to acute experiments. With our patients it is doubtful whether enough drug is given to elicit the effects seen in acute experiments. For instance, even when ganglionic blocking agents are given over a long period, a break-through occurs and nerve impulses are transmitted, despite the fact that very large amounts of a competitive inhibitor may be present. So I doubt very much whether, even with guanethidine, we have really blocked neural transmission entirely. I have often wondered what would happen to a patient with no neural transmission whatever. I suppose he would be about as irrational as most people. It all adds up to the fact that, although we have very effective antihypertensive agents, we are just beginning to unravel their tremendously complex scheme of intermediary metabolites and their actions, particularly in the brain. In a sense it is ironic that 40 years ago I started as a brain chemist and now, after a long lapse into cardiology, find myself again concerned with cerebral metabolism.

CARLSSON: Dr. PAGE suggested using platelets as a model. Platelets have been used, of course, but I am not sure whether one should concentrate on them. I think one should work on them in parallel. Probably, it will turn out that the platelets are not quite identical with the nerve-endings. I expect there are some differences, and it is possible nowadays, with the methods that have been developed, to study the nerve-endings even *in situ* by means of both biochemical and histochemical techniques. So I think that in order to study the sites of action of these drugs, a combination of a biochemical and a histochemical approach to the question of nerve-endings is the one to concentrate on.

Smirk: Phelan and I[1] have been very interested in the effects of antihypertensive agents in rats and have used in our studies a strain that we have bred selectively over a period of 12 years to develop spontaneous hypertension. This is now a rather good strain, and we have no difficulty in picking out from the colony teams of rats that have developed blood pressures of 160 or 170 mm. Hg spontaneously. Antihypertensive agents that we were proposing to use in man have been administered to these rats. If the drug was soluble, we gave it in the drinking fluid. We fully agree with Dr. Bein that it is possible to produce a very much more striking fall in blood pressure with hypotensive drugs if a hypertensive rat is used instead of a normotensive animal. We do not maintain that these animals are superior for this purpose to rats with experimental renal hypertension, but there is the advantage that the rats in our colony are "production-line" animals; they develop the hypertension spontaneously and they have it at one month of age. In addition to α-methyldopa, guanethidine, and a number of drugs easily given in the drinking fluid, we have used reserpine in the food pellets.

McQueen and Hodge[2] also made observations of the kind that Dr. Bein was referring to on renal hypertensive rats, namely that pathological changes are reduced when the hypertension is decreased by these drugs. There is a considerable reduction in the amount of medial necrosis and periarteritis nodosa, but these changes did not disappear altogether.

I should say that there is a point concerning the pathogenesis of the hypertension in our rat colony that is relevant to the matter of drug testing. Before the rats of our colony had as high pressures as they have now, the elevation in their blood pressure was maintained neurogenically to a large extent. Maximum doses of hexamethonium then reduced their blood pressure to the same level as in normotensive rats[3]. But now as blood pressures in the colony are higher, the rats tend to have a slightly higher hexamethonium floor than the normotensive controls. Chronic renal hypertensives have a distinctly higher hexamethonium floor than genetic hypertensives. Those things can be kept in mind if genetic hypertensives are used for testing.

---

[1] Phelan, E. L., and F. H. Smirk: unpublished.

[2] McQueen, E. G., and I. V. Hodge: Quart. J. Med. New Series **30**, 213 (1961).

[3] Laverty, R., and F. H. Smirk: Circulation Res. **9**, 455 (1961).

Pharmacology of diuretics

By

G. PETERS

A diuretic agent should be redefined for present-day purposes as a drug which increases sodium excretion by direct action on the kidney. A great many drugs – and the number is now growing at the rate of two to five a month – are known or supposed to have this effect. The scope of this paper will be limited to a consideration of some pharmacological aspects of the action of a few major compounds, which are, or at least should be, representative of the drugs currently used in therapeutics.

The benzothiadiazines (Fig. 1), also called thiazide diuretics, are derivatives of chlorothiazide (NOVELLO and SPRAGUE, 1957; BEYER, 1958), which is a very effective diuretic drug when given in fairly high doses. Its low efficacy per unit of weight in man is due

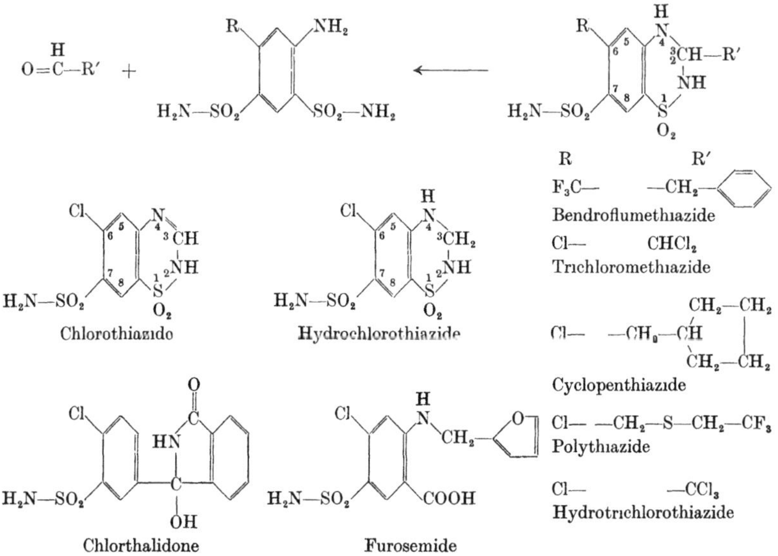

Fig. 1. Constitution of benzothiadiazine diuretics and some related drugs. Bendroflumethiazide and trichloromethiazide have been shown to be hydrolysed and to yield benzene-disulphamoyl compounds. The other diuretics substituted on the same carbon atom may be cleaved in a similar manner.

partly to poor intestinal absorption (YOUNG et al., 1959), but mainly to the fact that it is rapidly excreted by glomerular filtration as well as by active secretion into the proximal renal tubules in all species of mammals. Hydrochlorothiazide and all the newer benzothiadiazines are absorbed more rapidly in man and are cleared more slowly by the kidney, the renal clearance of the drugs being inversely proportional to their diuretic efficacy (BEYER and BAER, 1961; SCRIABINE et al., 1962). The greater liposolubility of the hydrated compound and its derivatives may account for both phenomena. Low renal clearance values probably represent back-diffusion of the liposoluble compounds from tubular fluid in the lower nephron rather than the absence of proximal tubular secretion. Proximal tubular secretion, or at least cellular accumulation of the thiazide diuretics, may be a prerequisite to their diuretic activity.

Hydrochlorothiazide is the most widely used thiazide diuretic and also the most extensively studied. Many derivatives have been synthesised, the main difference between these and the parent compound consisting in substitutions at carbon atom 3, nitrogen atom 2, or the amide nitrogen of the sulphamoyl group in position 7, or in the replacement of chlorine in position 6 by various halogenated alkyls. Compounds involving a substitution at carbon atom 3 are sometimes unstable in solution. Spontaneous hydrolysis within body fluids, which yields the benzene-disulphamoyl derivatives of bendroflumethiazide and trichloromethiazide, may also occur with similar compounds shown in Fig. 1. The diuretic effect of such compounds may be due partly to the resultant benzene-disulphamoyl compounds, since some substituted benzene-disulphamoyl derivatives are quite potent diuretics (DAVID and FELLOWES, 1960; PETROW et al., 1960; TOPLISS et al., 1963).

Quinethazone, chlorthalidone, and furosemide are related, but do not belong chemically, to the benzothiadiazine group. Chlorthalidone is thought to differ from hydrochlorothiazide in having a particularly prolonged action. Furosemide, on the other hand, acts very rapidly, briefly, and intensively (KLEINFELDER, 1963; McILWAINE and SMITH, 1964; MUSCHAWECK and HAJDÚ, 1964; VEREL et al., 1964).

All benzothiadiazines and related diuretics, with the possible exception of furosemide (MUSCHAWECK and HAJDÚ, 1964; KLÜTSCH et al., 1963), have the same effects and the same side effects when given in therapeutically active doses.

Two new classes of diuretics (Fig. 2) bear no chemical or pharmacological resemblance to the benzothiadiazines:

Triamterene (WIEBELHAUS et al., 1961; HERKEN and SENFT, 1961; MIGONE et al., 1963; CROSLEY, 1965) was evidently discovered in an attempt to improve the efficacy and safety of the triazine diuretics (KÜHN, 1957; MEHTA et al., 1960, 1962). Like the triazines, triamterene enhances sodium excretion but depresses urinary potassium excretion. A derivative of triamterene is, however, said to accelerate urinary potassium excretion in the dog, but not in the rat (ROSENTHALE and VAN ARMAN, 1963).

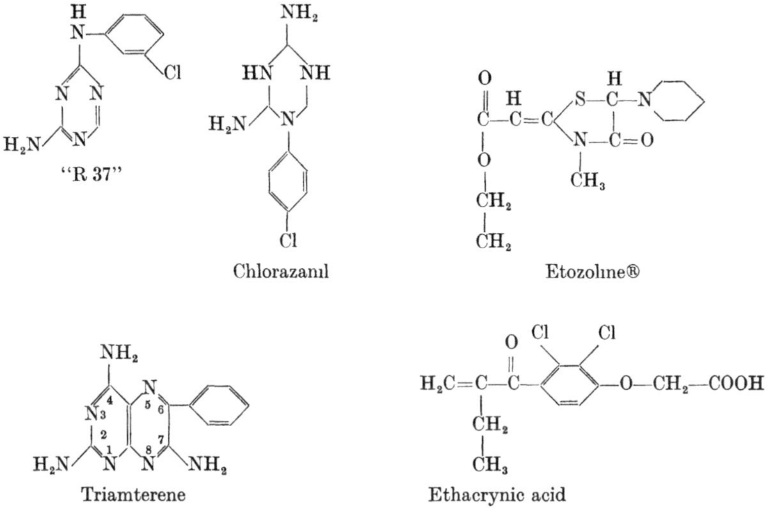

Fig. 2. Constitution of triamterene, some triazines, ethacrynic acid, and Etozoline®.

Ethacrynic acid (Fig. 2) and its congeners (BAER et al., 1964; CANNON et al., 1963; DOLLERY, 1965) constitute an altogether new and original class of diuretic agents. This substance causes particular disturbances of the urinary concentrating mechanism (EARLY and FRIEDLER, 1964; GOLDBERG et al., 1964; MACGAFFEY et al., 1964). It has no renal effect in the rat, and its efficacy in other species may depend on the occurrence of a particular metabolite. An agent remotely related to ethacrynic acid, Etozoline®, is effective in the rat (HEIDENREICH et al., 1964a, b).

Diuretic (natriuretic) effects

Enhanced excretion of sodium may or may not be accompanied by the excretion of sufficient amounts of water to maintain isotonicity of plasma and extracellular fluid. Thus, the benzothiadiazines and their derivatives, again with the possible exception of furosemide (KLÜTSCH et al., 1963), increase salt excretion more than water excretion. This effect is particularly evident in rats receiving brisk intravenous infusions of an isotonic saline solution (PETERS, 1965a). Under the influence of benzothiadiazines, their isotonic urine becomes hypertonic, at least in respect of sodium and potassium concentrations. Provided the mechanism controlling vasopressin release is functional and the kidneys are capable of elaborating a dilute urine, the resulting hyponatraemia will immediately be compensated by water diuresis; if the urine is collected over long periods, this compensation may even mask the initial hypertonicity. In situations where a hypotonic urine cannot be elaborated, a drug which acts on salt excretion more than on water excretion may cause dilutional hyponatraemia.

A drug with the opposite action could be useful in the treatment of dilutional hyponatraemia due to excessive secretion of vasopressin, to the absence of adrenal glucocorticosteroids, or to renal functional disturbances, for instance in patients with heart failure. If their inability to dilute the urine is a result of a low rate of glomerular filtration, mercurial diuretics may, sometimes, help by depressing proximal sodium reabsorption and delivering an increased amount of sodium ions and water to the distal tubule (GROLLMAN, 1965). This is, however, a rather theoretical suggestion, and there are no drugs known to accelerate free water excretion, either directly or by antagonising vasopressin.

Sodium ions excreted under the influence of a diuretic drug must be accompanied by equivalent amounts of anions. If the acid-base composition of the body is to be maintained, the proportions of chloride and bicarbonate in the additional urine must be the same as in extracellular fluid. It is thus evident that carbonic anhydrase inhibitors, such as acetazolamide, which increase excretion of bicarbonate but not of chloride, must induce a metabolic acidosis. This should also be expected to occur with triamterene, which interferes with the tubular secretion of hydrogen ions and, consequently, with the reabsorption of bicarbonate by an as yet unknown mechanism (CROSLEY, 1965; MIGONE et al., 1963). On the other hand, excretion of chloride in preference to bicarbonate results in hypochloraemic alkalosis. This complication used to be seen in patients undergoing long-term treatment with mercurial diuretics. It does not appear to occur often in patients receiving thiazide diuretics, though the newer thiazides may give rise to a urine containing nearly as much chloride as sodium. Hypochloraemic alkalosis has, however, been observed in patients undergoing long-term treatment with polythiazide or chlorthalidone (ROOTH and FURST, 1964), and it has been suggested that it may be responsible for the simultaneous occurrence of hypokalaemia (ROOTH and FURST, 1964; ERBE and WELLER, 1963), although the sequence of events is usually supposed to be the reverse.

Benzothiadiazines usually enhance the renal excretion of potassium, but fortunately not to the same extent as that of sodium. Although every new diuretic drug, given in effective doses, allegedly causes less potassium excretion than its predecessors, there is no sound evidence that any benzothiadiazine diuretic or related drug is less kaliuretic than others in long-term treatment. In experimental potassium depletion in the rat, chlorothiazide does not accelerate potassium excretion, though the natriuretic effect is only slightly decreased (MORRISON, 1963). Accelerated potassium excretion under the influence of thiazide diuretics is usually explained in terms of an increased delivery of sodium ions to a hypothetical distal tubular exchange mechanism in return for potassium or hydrogen ions. The possibility that benzothiadiazine diuretics interfere with active proximal potassium reabsorption in mammals cannot, however, be ruled out at present.

All thiazide diuretics, again with the possible exception of furosemide, depress the glomerular filtration rate (G.F.R.) as measured by the clearance of inulin (C_{In}). The extent to which it is depressed varies considerably from species to species and under different experimental conditions. In rats receiving a continuous infusion of hydrochlorothiazide, depression of G.F.R. appears to be correlated chronologically with the depression of sodium reabsorption (Fig. 3). The mechanism responsible for the decrease in G.F.R. is unknown, but may involve a vasodilator effect on the efferent arteriole. The possibility of an artefact due to diffusional losses of inulin from the lower nephron has been discussed and rejected (PETERS, 1965b; BONJOUR, 1965).

An "escape" phenomenon

When thiazide diuretics are administered repeatedly at short intervals, or continuously, to experimental animals or human subjects, their natriuretic effect gradually diminishes and eventually disappears (BRUNNER, 1959; PETERS, 1963a; GÖRES and JUNG, 1961; LARAGH, 1962). Continued activity in chronic administration may depend on suitable spacing of doses. This loss of natriuretic action may, in some instances, be due to increased aldosterone secretion and enhanced distal exchange for potassium; consequently, the natriuretic effect should be replaced progressively by a kaliuretic effect. An *apparent* escape from the tubular action of benzothiadiazines may also be due to a large decrease in G.F.R. Thus, the disappearance of the diuretic effect of hydrochlorothiazide observed in the contralateral kidney of rats in which one renal artery had been clamped (PETERS, 1965a) was the result of a decrease in G.F.R., while sodium reabsorption was depressed by the drug to the same extent as in a normal kidney. — A *spurious* escape from the action of thiazide diuretics may also be due to increasing dehydration.

There are, however, instances of *true* escape of the renal tubules from the inhibitory action of benzothiadiazines on sodium reabsorption. The results of an experiment on a group of 14 rats receiving an intravenous infusion of isotonic saline at a rate sufficient to maintain a positive sodium and water balance throughout the experiment are shown in Fig. 3. Hydrochlorothiazide was infused at a rate calculated to yield constant, effective plasma

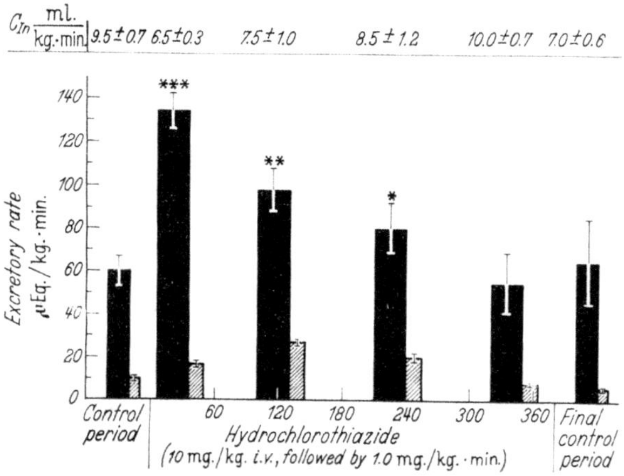

Fig. 3. Escape from the natriuretic effect of hydrochlorothiazide in rats. One treated and one control group, each consisting of 14 rats, received intravenous infusions of 0.15 M NaCl solution at a rate of 0.88 ml./kg.·min. No significant changes in diuretic response or glomerular filtration rate were noted in the control group within 7 hours. After a control period, the treated group received an intravenous injection of 10 mg./kg. hydrochlorothiazide followed by the infusion of 1.0 mg./kg.·min. of the drug for $6^1/_2$ hours. Glomerular filtration rate was measured in terms of inulin clearance. The figures represent the means ± S.E.; the columns the group means ± S.E. ■: renal excretion of sodium; ▨: renal excretion of potassium; both expressed in μEq./kg.·min. The significance of differences between control and treatment periods is shown by the asterisks: *** = $P < 0.001$; ** = $P < 0.01$; * = $P < 0.05$.

concentrations. The diuretic effect gradually diminished during the infusion and disappeared after four hours. The disappearance was neither due to a decrease in G.F.R. nor could it be explained by enhanced excretion of potassium.

An analogous *true* escape phenomenon has not, to my knowledge, been observed with mercurial diuretics. When these drugs cease to act in man or in experimental animals, the cause is usually hypochloraemic alkalosis (which suppresses the diuretic effect of mercurials) or a pronounced fall in G.F.R. Cardiac glycosides, on the other hand, are thought to interfere with all sodium transport by direct inhibition of the cellular "pump". Their diuretic efficacy becomes apparent only when very high doses are given and can therefore be demonstrated only by direct injection into the renal artery or by intravenous infusion in the rat, which is rather insensitive to the cardiac effects of these substances. No escape from the renal effect of ouabain was observed in rats receiving infusions of this drug over a period of eight to ten hours (unpublished results). There are no published data on escape from the diuretic effects of triamterene or ethacrynic acid.

Mechanism of action

Escape from the cellular action of thiazide diuretics may indicate that these drugs act indirectly on tubular sodium reabsorption, whereas organomercurials and cardiac glycosides have a direct effect. Tubular sodium reabsorption depends on active transport of sodium ions through the tubular cells. Transport is accomplished in two steps: first, sodium ions diffuse along an electrochemical gradient into the cells, from which they are then removed by a pumping mechanism analogous to the sodium pump of other body cells (GIEBISCH, 1960; PITTS, 1961; ORLOFF and BURG, 1960). The efficiency of active transport across the contraluminal cell-wall depends on this membrane's being less permeable than the luminal cell-wall to sodium ions. It is possible, though not certain, that sodium extrusion also proceeds across the luminal cell-border (OKEN, 1964), but that its extent does not interfere with sodium reabsorption by the process just outlined.

Interference with sodium reabsorption is probably due to inhibition of the sodium-pumping mechanism. Alternatively, its cause could be an increase in the sodium permeability of the contraluminal cell-wall, which would render the pump ineffective without actually disturbing it. This latter mechanism has been suggested as an explanation of the diuretic effect of organomercurials (KLEINZELLER and CORT, 1957) and may conceivably also contribute to the effects of newer diuretics.

The action of the cellular sodium pump is generally thought to be directly attributable to, or at least closely associated with, a specific enzyme, the sodium-, magnesium-, and potassium-dependent A.T.P.-ase found in cell membranes. A specific sodium-potassium-A.T.P.-ase obtained from rabbit kidneys was found to be inhibited by mersalyl and ouabain in concentrations which did not act on non-specific A.T.P.-ase (TAYLOR, 1963), while inorganic mercuric salts inhibited both A.T.P.-ases. Chlorothiazide had no inhibitory activity on specific membrane A.T.P.-ase.

This observation also seems to suggest that thiazide diuretics have an indirect effect on sodium transport. Such an indirect effect could be due to interference with an energy-providing system or with the transfer of free energy from an energy-providing system to the sodium pump or, alternatively, to inhibition of the synthesis of an enzyme. If it is assumed that an intrarenal regulatory system tends to maintain total sodium transport across tubular cells at a constant level (PETERS, 1963 b), the escape from inhibition by benzothiadiazines could be due to the replacement of one energy- or enzyme-providing mechanism by another. In the same way, escape from the sodium-retaining effect of aldosterone could be due to compensatory suppression of one of these mechanisms, under the influence of the same regulatory system.

It is assumed that both triamterene and ethacrynic acid act on tubular sodium transport rather than on cell permeability.

Although the basic mechanisms of action of the various diuretics are unknown, they are often supposed to differ from one another. When the effect of a diuretic drug cannot be increased by raising the dose, but a supplementary rise in sodium excretion can be induced by adding another drug to the regimen, the second drug is presumed to have a different mechanism of action. This conclusion may be highly fallacious if one neglects to take account of the fact that collecting urine and measuring its salt content is a highly "damped" recording procedure. According to this conventional argument, Figs 4 and 5 show that the mechanism of action of oral hydrochlorothiazide differs from that of intravenous hydrochlorothiazide. In rats receiving an intravenous infusion of isotonic saline, an intravenous dose of 50 mg./kg. hydrochlorothiazide produces maximal sodium excretion within the two hours following the injection. If, however, 10 mg./kg. hydrochlorothiazide are given simultaneously by the oral route, the total amount of sodium excreted within two hours is considerably greater (Fig. 4), though it is not equal to the sum of the effects of the oral and intravenous doses. Since the effect produced by the oral dose of 10 mg./kg. within the two-hour collection period is also maximal, the conclusion must be that oral and intravenous hydrochlorothiazide have different mechanisms of action.

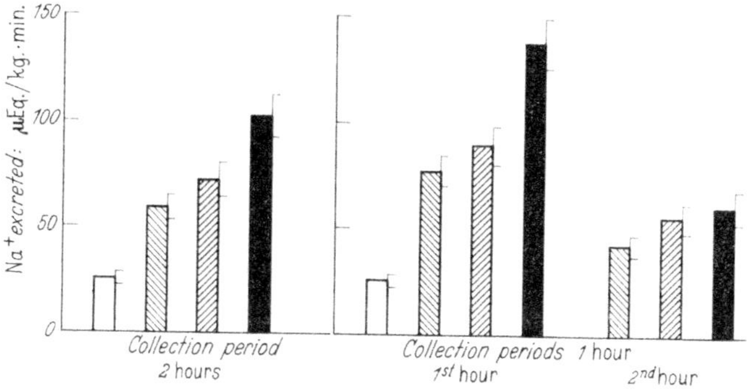

Fig. 4. Increase in the maximal natriuretic response to intravenous hydrochlorothiazide by the administration of an oral dose of hydrochlorothiazide. Four groups of 9-12 rats received intravenous infusions of 0.2 ml./rat · min. of a 0.15 M NaCl solution. One group was treated by an intravenous injection of 50 mg./kg. hydrochlorothiazide (▧), one group by oral administration of 10 mg./kg. hydrochlorothiazide (▨), one group received both 50 mg./kg. intravenous and 10 mg./kg. oral hydrochlorothiazide (■), and one group served as untreated controls (□). The columns show sodium excretion expressed as µEq./kg. · min. (means ± S.E.). The actual collection periods lasted 15 minutes; total sodium excretion for collection periods of one or two hours' duration were calculated from the 15-minute results. Oral hydrochlorothiazide evidently increases the maximal natriuretic effect of intravenous hydrochlorothiazide.

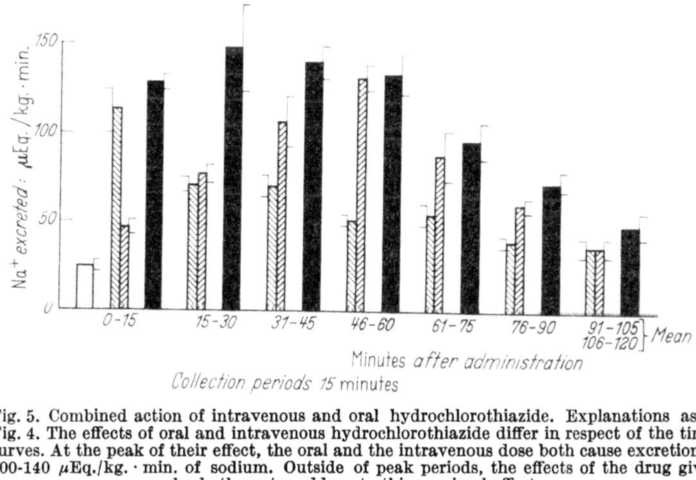

Fig. 5. Combined action of intravenous and oral hydrochlorothiazide. Explanations as in Fig. 4. The effects of oral and intravenous hydrochlorothiazide differ in respect of the time-curves. At the peak of their effect, the oral and the intravenous dose both cause excretion of 100-140 µEq./kg. · min. of sodium. Outside of peak periods, the effects of the drug given by both routes add up to this maximal effect.

A similar, though less obvious, conclusion is reached if the urine-collection period is shortened to one hour (Fig. 4). When the urine is collected every 15 minutes (Fig. 5), it becomes quite evident that the maximal diuretic effect, which, in these conditions, corresponds to the excretion of 100–140 μEq./kg. · min., is never exceeded by combining the oral and the intravenous administration of the drug. Only the chronological course of the diuretic response differs, according to the route of administration. The combination of oral and intravenous administration will therefore result in an apparent supramaximal effect, if the collection periods are long enough to cover an increase or a decrease in the diuretic effect of one of the doses. The *apparent* maximal effect over such a period may, then, become *apparently* supramaximal under the influence of the other dose which, in reality, only extends the duration of the peak effect.

Differences in the *time-course* of the diuretic action of various drugs may thus *erroneously* suggest different mechanisms of action. With short-acting diuretic agents it may not even be possible to detect this source of error.

Even if an increase in the maximum diuretic effect of one drug caused by the addition of another diuretic agent could be demonstrated, it would not prove that the two drugs have different mechanisms of action. Let us imagine, for example, that a brook divides into two branches at some point in its course. One might then try to increase the flow of water in one of these branches by damming the other with a plank of wood. The maximum effect of the plank would depend upon the point at which it breaks under the pressure of the water. If a second barrier, of sturdier material, were set up a little way down-stream, it would withstand a greater pressure and would thus further increase the flow of water in the other branch. One would, however, not be justified in assuming that the mechanism by which, let us say, a sheet of metal would increase the flow of water in the other branch would differ fundamentally from that of the plank of wood.

Site of action

Much thought and experimentation has been spent in attempts to determine the site of action of diuretics within the nephron. Since, under normal circumstances, 60–80% of the sodium filtered by the glomeruli is reabsorbed in the proximal tubules, sodium excretion of more than 20% of the amount filtered must be ascribed to a proximal action. Such large increases in the tubular rejection fraction of sodium are currently observed following administration of furosemide or combinations of several different diuretic agents (MUSCHAWECK and HAJDÚ, 1964; KLÜTSCH et al., 1963; MANN et al., 1964; VORBURGER and HUBER, 1964; VORBURGER, 1964; HEIDENREICH and BAUMEISTER, 1964), and sometimes also after triamterene (LASSEN and NIELSEN, 1963; VESIN et al., 1963; MIGONE et al., 1963) or ethacrynic acid (DOLLERY, 1965). It is often assumed that the maximum effect of hydrochlorothiazide is the excretion of approximately 10% of the filtered sodium, since this was the maximum effect obtained by intravenous injection of chlorothiazide in the dog (PITTS et al., 1958). Experiments in the rat (Table 1) show, however, that the amount of sodium escaping

Table 1. *Effects of the same dose of hydrochlorothiazide in rats infused with isotonic saline solutions at varying rates (lines 1—3) and after ligation of one ureter (line 4).* Figures show means ± S. E. Groups of 7—16 rats. Sodium excretion is expressed as the percentage of filtered sodium escaping tubular reabsorption.

Control periods	Hydrochlorothiazide 50 mg./kg. i.v. or 5 mg./kg. i.v. + 1.0 mg./kg. · min.	Furosemide 40 mg./kg. i.v.	Reference
1.5 ± 0.2	4.8 ± 0.5	17.8 ± 1.3	1
4.0 ± 0.8	7.8 ± 1.1		2
5.9 ± 0.6	16.6 ± 2.5		3
8.8 ± 1.0	26.5 ± 4.3		3

1 BONJOUR and PETERS (unpublished)
2 PETERS (1963c)
3 PETERS (1965a)

tubular reabsorption under the influence of the same dose of hydrochlorothiazide depends on the amount reabsorbed before the drug is given. As the rate of intravenous infusion of isotonic saline solution is increased, sodium reabsorption decreases, whereas the effect of hydrochlorothiazide increases in proportion to the rate of sodium excretion before the administration of the drug. If one kidney is eliminated shortly before the intravenous infusion of saline, the remaining kidney still further restricts its sodium reabsorption (PETERS, 1963b). This state of "compensatory adaptation" also influences the diuretic effect of hydrochlorothiazide (Table 1, last line).

The magnitude of the diuretic effect in this particular condition points to a proximal site of action. Furthermore, it should be remembered that inhibition of even a small fraction of proximal reabsorption must produce a much greater increase in sodium excretion than suppression of large fractions of the total reabsorptive capacity of other segments.

Attempts to locate the site of action of modern diuretics in the dog by "stop-flow" procedures lead to contradictory results: From experimental data it was concluded that the principal site of action of thiazides is the proximal tubule (VANDER et al., 1959; KESSLER et al., 1959) or the distal tubule (CAFRUNY and ROSS, 1962). Similarly, Etozoline® in the dog appears to act mainly on proximal sodium reabsorption and on distal potassium secretion (HEIDENREICH et al., 1964a). The excretion of chlorothiazide as well as of hydrochlorothiazide by the secretory mechanism which transports P.A.H. and is blocked by probenecid (BEYER and BAER, 1961) points to the proximal tubule as site of action. Hydrochlorothiazide labelled with tritium, on the other hand, was found to be concentrated in "either the entire distal or central portion of convoluted tubules" by one group of investigators (DARMADY et al., 1962), while hydrochlorothiazide-3-C^{14} and chlorthalidone-3-C^{14} were excreted and accumulated in the proximal tubule, particularly in the *pars recta*, and at the end of the initial collecting ducts according to autoradiographic results of other investigators (TAUGNER and IRAVANI, 1965).

Micropuncture experiments, which should permit more definite conclusions to be drawn, lead to similar results. Thus, chlorthalidone was found to depress sodium efflux from the proximal tubule (ULLRICH, 1962), and both furosemide and hydrochlorothiazide were found to depress proximal as well as distal sodium reabsorption (HOLZGREVE et al., 1964), while in more recent micropuncture experiments furosemide was found to act only on the proximal tubule and, possibly, on Henle's loop (DEETJEN, 1965). One investigator (MENG, 1965) could not detect any effect of hydrochlorothiazide on proximal sodium and water reabsorption and therefore concluded that the action of this drug was entirely distal. A possible distal effect of the thiazide diuretics has been postulated to contribute to their antidiuretic activity, which will be discussed below.

In the dog and in man, ethacrynic acid in effective diuretic doses completely suppresses the ability of the kidney to elaborate a concentrated urine (EARLY and FRIEDLER, 1964; GOLDBERG et al., 1964; MACGAFFEY et al., 1964). Under the influence of the drug, $T^c_{H_2O}$ falls to zero: an isotonic urine is excreted by the kidneys of dehydrated animals. Although up to now these effects have apparently always proved reversible, a drug with such an action certainly cannot be considered innocuous. Suppression of urinary concentrating ability and even minimal disturbances in the elaboration of a hypotonic urine point to an impairment of the counter-current multiplier system thought to be responsible for the high osmolarity of interstitial fluid in the renal papilla. This impairment is thought, but has not been proved, to be an inhibition of sodium reabsorption in the ascending limb of Henle's loop. Inhibition of proximal tubular sodium reabsorption would decrease urinary osmolarity in dehydrated animals, but would have no influence on $Tm^{c}_{H_2O}$. Inhibition of sodium reabsorption in the ascending limb of Henle's loop certainly does not exclude a simultaneous depression of proximal reabsorption suggested by the high degree of diuretic efficacy of ethacrynic acid.

Triamterene has not been shown to interfere either with urinary concentration or dilution.

The antidiuretic effect of thiazide diuretics

A short time after the introduction of chlorothiazide, it was recognised that this drug, given during water diuresis in normal humans, decreased the clearance of free water (C_{H_2O}) simultaneously with an increase in sodium excretion (HEINEMANN et al., 1959). The same effect is obtained in hydrated rats, in which other diuretic drugs with a purely proximal action either increase or do not influence C_{H_2O} (PETERS, 1964, 1965b). All thiazide diuretics studied possess this antidiuretic effect (DIÈS and RIVERA, 1962).

An analogous effect occurs in rats with experimental (pituitary) diabetes insipidus, as well as in patients with pituitary or nephrogenic diabetes insipidus. More surprisingly, thiazides not only increase urinary osmolarity but subsequently depress urine flow (and water uptake) by a fraction sometimes amounting to 50% (CRAWFORD and KENNEDY, 1959; KENNEDY and CRAWFORD, 1959) in pituitary as well as in vasopressin-resistant (nephrogenic) diabetes insipidus. The efficacy of many different thiazide diuretics in both types of human diabetes insipidus has been repeatedly confirmed in the meantime (for references see EARLY and ORLOFF, 1964).

Interference with sodium reabsorption in the distal tubule without a disturbance of sodium transport in Henle's loop would readily account for the increase in urinary osmolarity in water diuresis (EARLY et al., 1961), but would not result in a depression of urine flow. The decrease in G.F.R. brought about by benzothiadiazines is usually too small to explain the decrease in the rate of urine flow observed. Sodium depletion caused by the diuretic with a contraction of the extracellular volume has therefore been accepted as a possible cause for thiazide antidiuresis in diabetes insipidus (EARLY and ORLOFF, 1962). In support of this conclusion it has been shown that sodium repletion abolishes the antidiuretic effect of thiazide drugs in some patients (CUTLER et al., 1960; EARLY and ORLOFF, 1962), an observation which was, however, not confirmed in other cases (KENNEDY and HILL, 1963). Furthermore, in acute experiments in children with both types of diabetes insipidus, urine flow often decreases before there are any notable losses of sodium (GAUTIER and PETERS, unpublished observations).

Inhibition of distal tubular sodium reabsorption fails to explain the increase in urinary osmolarity observed in isotonic saline diuresis in the rat (PETERS, 1965a) as well as in normal man. It cannot account either for a slight, but consistent increase in $T^c_{H_2O}$ found in dogs receiving a rapid infusion of hypertonic mannitol solution in the absence of exogenous vasopressin (unpublished observations). Finally, it would not explain why furosemide, which otherwise resembles the benzothiadiazine diuretics, does not cause a depression in C_{H_2O} (KLÜTSCH et al., 1963).

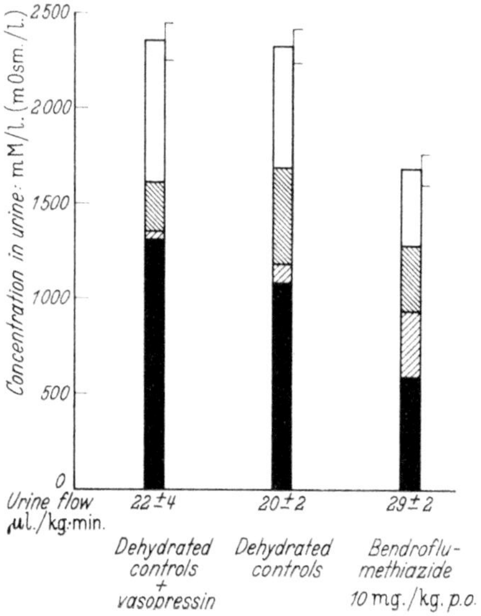

Fig. 6. Urinary osmolarity and urinary urea, sodium, and potassium concentrations in rats dehydrated for 72 hours and given 100 mU./kg. · hour lysine-vasopressin s.c., in dehydrated control rats, and in dehydrated rats given 10 mg./kg. bendroflumethiazide p.o. (▨: 2× [K⁺]; ▨: 2× [Na⁺]; ■: [urea]). Columns represent means ± S.E. Column 1: unpublished data; columns 2 and 3: data from KOBINGER (1965). The decrease in urinary osmolarity caused by bendroflumethiazide is not explained by the increased urine flow; it is due exclusively to the decrease in urinary urea concentration.

All these observations would, however, be explained by the assumption that thiazide diuretics, besides exerting their diuretic activity, increase the water permeability of the distal tubules and the collecting ducts by a mechanism independent of, and supplementary to, the effect of vasopressin (EARLY et al., 1961). Independence of the diuretic and the antidiuretic effects of thiazides is compatible with the discovery of drugs which lack either the one or the other.

That thiazide diuretics influence renal tubular permeability may also be inferred from the results of experiments in dehydrated rats

(KOBINGER, 1965). In these animals, bendroflumethiazide caused a 50% increase in urinary flow, accompanied by a much larger decrease in urinary as well as in papillary tissue-water osmolarity and urea concentration (Figs 6 and 7). The decrease in urea concentration, which was solely responsible for the decrease in urinary osmolarity, was accompanied by a larger decrease in urea excretion than could be accounted for by the 10% decrease in G.F.R. occurring in these circumstances under the influence of benzothiadiazines (unpublished observations). It therefore probably points to enhanced diffusional losses of urea in higher segments of the nephron, which can only be explained by an increase in permeability to urea.

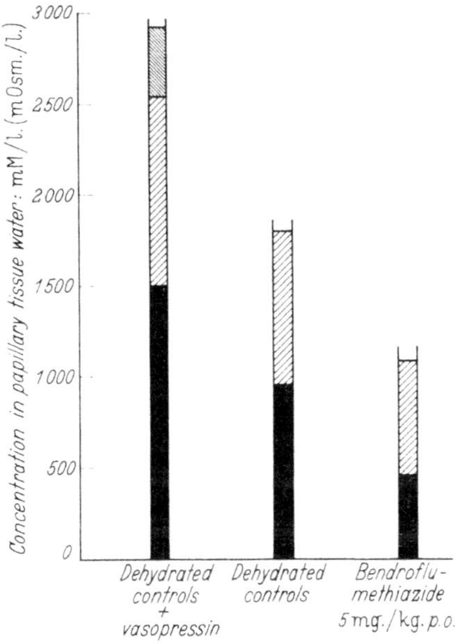

Fig. 7. Urea, sodium, and potassium concentrations in papillary tissue water of dehydrated rats injected with vasopressin, in dehydrated control rats, and in dehydrated rats given bendroflumethiazide. Explanations as in Fig. 6.

Antihypertensive effects

The moderate-to-good efficacy of all modern diuretics in the treatment of many cases of chronic hypertension is practically the most important, though not the most spectacular, effect of these drugs.

There appears to be a close connection between the depression of blood pressure, in animals with experimental hypertension as well as in man with various types of clinical hypertension, and the diuretic effects of the drugs. Thus, benzothiadiazines and related drugs, which are diuretic at very different dose levels, all exert their antihypertensive effects at the doses needed to enhance sodium excretion (BARENBERG and GIFFORD, 1963; BORHANI, 1960; CIER, 1964; DANIEL, 1962; FRANK et al., 1960; KLAPPER, 1962; McQUEEN and MORRISON, 1960; SPIEKERMAN et al., 1963; SIMPSON,

1964; SELLER, 1965). Furthermore, diuretics which differ so widely from the thiazides as triamterene and ethacrynic acid apparently share their antihypertensive effect (HEATH and FREIS, 1963; GROWE et al., 1962; SPERBER and DEGRAFF, 1965; CONWAY and LEONETTI, 1965; DOLLERY et al., 1964). The discovery of diazoxide, a non-sulphonamide derivative of the benzothiadiazines, which has a strong sodium-retaining action as well as antihypertensive activity, at one time suggested that the antihypertensive and diuretic properties of these drugs were independent. It was, however, found that the pattern of the antihypertensive effect of diazoxide differs widely from that of the thiazide diuretics (RUBIN et al., 1962; CARMINATI, 1963; WILSON and OKUN, 1963).

Although the relationship between diuretic and antihypertensive efficacy seems to be established, it is still uncertain why diuretic agents lower blood pressure. It is generally agreed that effective doses of the diuretics are purely antihypertensive and have no influence on normal blood pressure. If the thiazide diuretics alone were antihypertensive, one would be tempted to believe that some type of dilutional hyponatraemia played a role. The contrary, however, seems to apply: in rats with experimental hypertension, in which blood pressure had been lowered by treatment with thiazide diuretics, the infusion of a hypotonic fluid sometimes caused an increase in blood pressure, whereas injections of a hypertonic solution did not interfere with the antihypertensive action of the diuretic (FRIEDMAN et al., 1960; DANIEL, 1962).

There is little doubt that treatment with diuretics in hypertensive patients initially leads to a contraction of extracellular and intravascular space and a secondary decrease in cardiac output. With continued treatment, and probably with partial or total escape from the diuretic action of the drug, the fluid volumes revert to normal, but the blood pressure remains low or at least lowered. In this second phase, a decrease in peripheral resistance accounts for the hypotensive effect, which, however, remains reversible upon withdrawal of the drug.

It is highly doubtful whether this decrease in peripheral resistance bears any relationship to the numerous acute cardiovascular effects observed after large single doses of thiazide diuretics in man and in experimental animals (CROSLEY et al., 1960; GREENE et al., 1961; MAXWELL and McLUSKY, 1964; PREZIOSI et al., 1961).

In animals with experimental hypertension, thiazide diuretics have been found to cause changes in the water and electrolyte content of arterial walls (CAVALCA et al., 1961) or of muscular tissue (TAQUINI, 1962). These changes were generally the opposite of those induced by experimental hypertension. They were described either as a decrease in water, sodium, and potassium concentration in fresh tissue, or else as a decrease in sodium and water accompanied by an increase in potassium concentration. Both types of change are probably secondary to the initial depletion of extracellular fluid induced by the diuretics and have not been shown as yet to persist into the second phase of decreased peripheral resistance. In nephrectomised experimental animals, chlorothiazide has no influence on tissue water and electrolytes (ORBISON, 1962). There is thus no reason to assume that diuretics influence tissue electrolytes by a direct extrarenal effect. The inhibition of trans-membrane sodium transport by diuretic agents appears to be restricted to the kidney, presumably because these drugs are concentrated in renal tissue.

A number of investigators found that acute as well as chronic treatment with thiazide diuretics depresses or abolishes the vascular responsiveness to the vasoconstrictor action of various sympathomimetic amines (ALEKSANDROW et al., 1959; BOCK and GROSS, 1960; ECKSTEIN et al., 1962, 1964; FEISAL et al., 1961; GREENE et al., 1963; SILAH et al., 1965). Cardiac as well as vascular responses to adrenaline, noradrenaline, and phenylephrine are abolished as a consequence of the diuretic action of the drugs. Since this inhibitory effect occurs after acute short-term as well as after long-term treatment (ECKSTEIN et al., 1964), it bears a closer relationship to the antihypertensive effect than other changes observed. If one considers, furthermore, the antihypertensive efficacy of drugs such as guanethidine or reserpine, which act by depressing the endogenous catecholamine discharges, one may very well conclude that the antihypertensive effect of diuretics is mainly due to a decrease in vascular response to endogenous sympathomimetic amines. The data available on the influence of diuretics on tissue catecholamine stores are still contradictory.

In contrast to the pressor effect of sympathomimetics, the vasoconstrictor action of angiotensin is not inhibited by treatment with thiazide diuretics (SILAH et al., 1965; BOCK and GROSS, 1960).

Chlorthalidone has been reported to cause an increase in plasma renin activity in man, presumably as a consequence of salt depletion (VEYRAT et al., 1964). No data are available on the influence of thiazide diuretics on renin activity in kidney tissue. Hydrochlorothiazide has no direct effect on the velocity of angiotensin production from angiotensinogen *in vitro* (unpublished observations).

The antihypertensive effect of modern diuretics thus seems to be a consequence of their diuretic effect and of a temporary salt (and water) depletion. It is maintained as long as it is not annihilated by another temporary phase of salt retention, which occurs, for instance, upon cessation of diuretic therapy. One may thus speculate that a transient decrease in body sodium triggers off an as yet unknown change in vascular and/or cardiac tissue, which results in a decrease in blood pressure to normal levels. This unknown change may produce its effect mainly by decreasing responsiveness to sympathomimetic amines. An opposite, also unknown, change may be the triggering mechanism responsible for some types of experimental hypertension, such as hypertension caused by salt, by aldosterone, or by desoxycorticosterone, in which there are reasons to assume that a temporary increase in body-sodium stores takes place, and in which the hypertensive process is also interrupted by the occurrence of a phase of sodium loss.

The "diabetogenic" effect

To speak of a "diabetogenic" effect of thiazide diuretics is a considerable exaggeration. There is no sound evidence to show that any initially normal human being or experimental animal ever acquired permanent diabetes as a result of treatment with a diuretic drug (FAIRBAIRN, 1965; *Editorial*, 1964). The term is used to designate increases in fasting blood-sugar values as well as elevations of the blood-sugar concentrations after an oral glucose load (CARLINER et al., 1965). These changes, which, furthermore, are usually reversible in normal subjects and animals when the diuretic is withdrawn, may amount to a worsening of the metabolic state in patients with diabetes at the onset of treatment (WILKINS, 1959; GOLDNER et al., 1960; FAIRBAIRN, 1965; *Editorial*, 1964). Actual diabetes may occur when patients with latent diabetes are treated with benzothiadiazines (SHAPIRO et al., 1960; LYON and DE GRAFF, 1964); otherwise it is so rare that coincidence appears much more probable than a causal relationship (WOLFF et al., 1963a, b).

An increase in blood-glucose concentration after an oral glucose load is, however, observed in the majority of normal subjects treated with benzothiadiazines and related diuretic drugs (CARLINER et al., 1965). Elevations of fasting blood sugar occur more rarely.

It is quite uncertain whether the "diabetogenic" effect of the diuretics is related to their diuretic efficacy. On the one hand, the non-diuretic benzothiadiazine derivative, diazoxide, has a much more pronounced diabetogenic activity in humans and in experimental animals than any known thiazide or non-thiazide diuretic (Dollery, 1962; Wilson et al., 1964; Wolff et al., 1963a; Wolff and Parmley, 1964); on the other hand, more or less pronounced "diabetogenic" effects are also said to have been observed in subjects treated with triamterene or ethacrynic acid (Lasagna, 1965).

Diazoxide diabetes in dogs or rats, like thiazide hyperglycaemia in man, is reversible in most instances. It can be induced in hypophysectomised and adrenalectomised rats (Wolff and Parmley, 1964). A direct pancreatic action of the drug could only amount to a temporary inhibition of insulin release: the fact that the diabetogenic activity of diazoxide can be fully antagonised by effective doses of tolbutamide shows that insulin production cannot be depressed. Although diazoxide does not cause potassium losses, its diabetogenic action in the rat can apparently be suppressed by simultaneous administration of high doses of potassium.

Table 2. *Influence of chronic treatment with hydrochlorothiazide on fasting blood-glucose concentrations in normal and partially pancreatectomised rats treated with hydrochlorothiazide.* Groups of 7—14 rats. Figures are means ± S. E. Increases in blood sugar after an oral glucose load were determined 90 minutes after 3 g./kg. of glucose given in a 20% solution by stomach tube. Blood glucose was measured by the glucose oxydase method. Hydrochlorothiazide was dissolved in dilute NaOH immediately before administration (from R. Guidoux: unpublished data).

	Blood glucose: mg./100 ml.			
	Sham-operated		Partially pancreatectomised	
	Fasting[1]	Glucose load[2]	Fasting[1]	Glucose load[2]
Control	79 ± 2	+ 34 ± 3	76 ± 3	+ 43 ± 4
Hydrochlorothiazide 100 mg./kg. · day p.o.				
2 weeks	75 ± 5	+ 38 ± 4	78 ± 4	+ 40 ± 6
4 weeks	81 ± 7	+ 33 ± 5	69 ± 4	+ 39 ± 7

[1] After 14-16 hours of food deprivation
[2] 90 minutes after 3 g./kg. glucose by stomach tube

The diabetogenic activity of diazoxide in rats can be increased by the simultaneous administration of some, but not all, thiazide diuretics in doses slightly higher than the diuretic doses (Wolff and Parmley, 1964). It is highly doubtful whether this adjuvant diabetogenic activity contributes anything to the explanation of the "diabetogenic" effects of the thiazide diuretics when these drugs are given by themselves.

Table 3. *Absence of a hyperglycaemic effect of single oral doses of hydrochlorothiazide in rats.* Groups of 7-10 rats. 50 mg./kg. hydrochlorothiazide (freshly dissolved in dilute NaOH), given by stomach tube, did not induce any rise in blood sugar either in normal or in partially pancreatectomised rats. Treatment with hydrochlorothiazide for 16-20 days did not reveal any acute hyperglycaemic effect (from R. GUIDOUX: unpublished data).

	Blood glucose: mg./100 ml.							
	Sham-operated controls				Partially pancreatectomised			
	Fasting[1]	2 hours	5 hours	8 hours[2]	Fasting[1]	2 hours	5 hours	8 hours[2]
Untreated	77 ± 5	−5 ± 5	−0.2 ± 5	−4 ± 5	80 ± 5	−1 ± 2	−8 ± 4	−11 ± 4
After 16-20 days' treatment (hydrochlorothiazide 100 mg./kg. · day p.o.)	90 ± 6	+9 ± 6	−9 ± 2	−9 ± 3	83 ± 5	+2 ± 4	−4 ± 3	−7 ± 3

[1] 14-16 hours of food deprivation
[2] After a single dose of 50 mg./kg. hydrochlorothiazide by stomach tube

Like diazoxide, many benzothiadiazine diuretics were found to have an acute hyperglycaemic effect following oral administration of single doses, an effect which must be distinguished from the diabetogenic activity after chronic administration (WOLFF and PARMLEY, 1964).

In normal rats, two groups of investigators (MENG and KRONEBERG, 1964; LOSERT et al., 1965) observed slight-to-pronounced increases in fasting blood sugar after treatment over a period of five to 15 days with hydrochlorothiazide in high diuretic doses. We could not confirm this result (Table 2). No change occurred in the fasting blood sugar of normal rats within two to four weeks as a consequence of the oral administration of 100 mg./kg. daily of hydrochlorothiazide, nor after a single dose of 50 mg. (Table 3). Partial pancreatectomy, which is known to sensitise rats to the diabetogenic activity of drugs as well as of high carbohydrate diets, did not induce the appearance of "hydrochlorothiazide-diabetes". Similarly, WATSON et al. (1964) failed to induce a rise in fasting blood sugar in rats given extremely high doses of chlorothiadiazide or hydrochlorothiazide for short or long periods. Since potassium depletion is sometimes thought to be responsible for the diabetogenic effect of thiazide diuretics, chlorothiazide or hydrochlorothiazide administration was combined with a low-potassium diet; even under these conditions, no increase in blood sugar was obtained (WATSON et al., 1964). These contradictory results may be due to the use of different solvents.

In human patients, thiazide diuretics were found to depress the so-called typical insulin-like activity of plasma, thought to be identical with insulin secreted from the pancreas. This finding was confirmed in some, though not in all, instances of diazoxide hyperglycaemia in man and in animals (WOLFF, 1965). It would thus be an attractive hypothesis to speculate that thiazide diuretics may cause a specific block to insulin release in response to the physiological stimulus of hyperglycaemia, but not to the insulin-liberating activity of pharmacological agents like tolbutamide.

A direct pancreatic action of the thiazides would seem to be in keeping with occasional observations of acute pancreatitis or pancreatic atrophy in patients treated with thiazide diuretics (SHANKLIN, 1962; JOHNSTON and CORNISH, 1959). It should, however, be pointed out that diabetogenic agents known to affect the pancreatic islets have not been reported to cause pancreatitis or pancreatic atrophy.

There are, however, some observations which seem to indicate the occurrence of a peripheral block to the action of insulin in thiazide-treated animals. While benzothiadiazines *in vitro* may (WELLER and BORONDY, 1965) or may not (FIELD and MANDELL, 1964) inhibit glucose uptake by adipose tissue from the rat, it seems to be an established fact that pretreatment of rats with benzothiadiazines depresses the effect of insulin on the glucose uptake of their adipose tissue *in vitro*. One is, however, somewhat disturbed by this finding in a species in which the drugs apparently do not exert a constant diabetogenic effect.

The scope of this report does not allow discussion of the many other renal and extrarenal side effects of modern diuretics. Though some of these side effects may occasionally cause severe illness and even death, their occurrence does not, as yet, weigh very heavily in the balance of therapeutic judgement. Thiazide and other modern diuretics are important drugs in the treatment of salt retention as well as of hypertension.

Undoubtedly, a better understanding of the basic mechanism of action of these drugs would be desirable and might facilitate their application in other conditions or in complicated situations. It might also be helpful in the development of new and more effective drugs for the treatment of hypertension.

Summary

The diuretic, antidiuretic, antihypertensive, and diabetogenic effects of benzothiadiazines and related drugs, and some effects of triamterene and triazines and of ethacrynic acid are discussed.

Although there are major differences in the pattern of the diuretic effects of benzothiadiazines and related drugs on the one hand and the other two groups of diuretics on the other, different benzothiadiazines, benzene-sulphamoyl compounds, benzene-disulphamoyl compounds, and chlorthalidone, given in maximum effective doses, cause practically the same changes in renal and extrarenal functions and differ only in their duration of action. Furosemide may differ more fundamentally from the thiazide diuretics.

The basic mechanism of the natriuretic action of the modern diuretics is not yet known. The thiazides are thought to inhibit the active transport of sodium ions from the tubular fluid to renal interstitial tissue and the blood stream. This inhibition does not appear to affect the sodium pump itself: it may have a bearing on energy-providing or enzyme-synthesising mechanisms.

These diuretics act on proximal as well as on distal tubular sodium transport. While the proximal effect is more important from the quantitative standpoint, a possible distal effect has been thought to explain the decrease in the clearance of free water during water diuresis. The antidiuretic effect, which is used in the drug therapy of human diabetes insipidus, appears, however, to be due to a direct action of the thiazide diuretics on water permeability of the distal tubule and the collecting duct rather than on their effect on distal sodium reabsorption.

While benzothiadiazines and related drugs interfere mainly with the elaboration of a hypotonic urine, ethacrynic acid abolishes the concentrating ability of the kidney, presumably by acting on the ascending limb of Henle's loop.

The antihypertensive effect of all modern diuretics is a consequence of their diuretic effect. It does not seem to be due to any extrarenal action of the drugs. The occurrence of temporary sodium losses induced by the diuretic drugs seems to trigger off an as yet unknown change in vascular reactivity. Decreased responses of the heart and blood vessels to the action of sympathomimetic amines may be an expression of this unknown change. Neither reactivity to angiotensin nor the renin-angiotensin system is influenced directly by diuretic drugs.

The diabetogenic effect of benzothiadiazine diuretics, though clinically rather unimportant, has interesting theoretical implications. The diuretics do not cause permanent diabetes. They are not diabetogenic in normal or partially pancreatectomised rats, but induce increased responses to oral glucose loads in normal humans. These changes in carbohydrate tolerance may be due to a block of the secretory response of pancreatic islets to stimulation by hyperglycaemia.

Zusammenfassung

Die diuretischen, antidiuretischen, antihypertensiven und diabetogenen Wirkungen der Benzothiadiazine und chemisch verwandter Substanzen, von Triamteren und Triazinen, sowie einzelne Wirkungen von Äthacrynsäure werden besprochen.

Während stärkere Unterschiede im Typus der diuretischen Wirkung von Benzothiadiazinen und verwandten Stoffen einerseits und demjenigen der beiden anderen Gruppen andererseits bestehen, rufen die verschiedenen Benzothiadiazine, Benzolsulphamyl-Verbindungen, Benzoldisulphamyl-Verbindungen und Chlorthalidon in maximal wirksamen Dosen praktisch gleiche Veränderungen renaler und extrarenaler Funktionen hervor und weichen lediglich in ihrer Wirkungsdauer voneinander ab. Furosemid dürfte sich grundsätzlich von den Thiazid-Diuretika unterscheiden.

Der Mechanismus der natriuretischen Wirkung der modernen Diuretika ist noch nicht bekannt. Man nimmt an, daß die Thiazide den aktiven Transport von Natriumionen aus der Tubulusflüssigkeit in das interstitielle Nierengewebe und das Blut hemmen. Diese Hemmung scheint nicht die Natriumpumpe selbst zu betreffen: sie könnte über eine Beeinflussung energieliefernder oder fermentsynthetisierender Prozesse gehen.

Die genannten Diuretika beeinflussen sowohl den proximalen als auch den distalen tubulären Natriumtransport. Während die proximale Wirkung in quantitativer Hinsicht die wichtigere ist, wurde ein möglicher distaler Effekt zur Erklärung der Abnahme der freien Wasserclearance bei der Wasserdiurese herangezogen. Der antidiuretische Effekt der Thiazid-Diuretika, der für die Behandlung des Diabetes insipidus beim Menschen ausgenutzt wird, scheint jedoch auf der direkten Wirkung auf die Wasserpermeabilität des distalen Tubulus und der Sammelrohre zu beruhen und weniger auf einem Effekt auf die distale Natriumrückresorption.

Während Benzothiadiazine und verwandte Substanzen vor allem die Produktion eines hypotonischen Urins beeinträchtigen, setzt die Äthacrynsäure die Konzentrationsfähigkeit der Niere herab, möglicherweise durch Hemmung des Natriumtransportes aus dem aufsteigenden Schenkel der Henle'schen Schleife.

Der antihypertensive Effekt aller modernen Diuretika ist eine Folge ihrer diuretischen Wirkung und scheint nicht von irgendeiner extrarenalen Wirkung abzuhängen. Das Auftreten eines vorübergehenden Natriumverlustes durch die Diuretika scheint eine bis jetzt unbekannte Veränderung in der Ansprechbarkeit der Gefäße auszulösen. Die verminderte Reaktion des Herzens und der Gefäße auf die Wirkung sympathikomimetischer Amine kann ein Ausdruck dieser Veränderung sein. Weder die Ansprechbarkeit auf Angiotensin noch das Renin-Angiotensin-System werden direkt durch die Diuretika beeinflußt.

Der diabetogene Effekt der Benzothiadiazin-Diuretika bietet interessante theoretische Aspekte, spielt jedoch klinisch keine wesentliche Rolle. Die Diuretika rufen keinen permanenten Diabetes hervor. Sie sind nicht diabetogen bei normalen oder partiell pankreatektomierten Ratten, führen aber beim normalen Menschen zur Verminderung der Glukosetoleranz. Diese Änderung der Glukosetoleranz könnte auf einer Hemmung der sekretorischen Antwort der Inselzellen auf einen hyperglykämischen Reiz beruhen.

Résumé

Les effets diurétique, antidiurétique, antihypertenseur et diabétogène des benzothiadiazines et des substances apparentées, du triamtérène et des triazines, ainsi que quelques particularités de l'acide éthacrynique sont discutés.

Il y a des différences essentielles entre les modalités de l'action diurétique d'une part des benzothiadiazines et des substances apparentées, d'autre part des deux autres groupes de diurétiques. Les différentes benzothiadiazines, les composés benzène-sulphamoyl, benzène-disulphamoyl et la chlorthalidone, administrés à des doses donnant une réponse maximum, provoquent cependant des modifications pratiquement identiques des fonctions rénales et extrarénales et ne diffèrent que par leur durée d'action. La furosémide se distingue probablement des thiazides diurétiques d'une façon plus fondamentale.

Le mécanisme à la base de l'action natriurétique des diurétiques modernes n'est pas encore connu. On pense que les thiazides inhibent le transport actif des ions sodium du liquide intratubulaire vers le tissu rénal interstitiel et le sang. Il ne semble pas que cette inhibition affecte la pompe à sodium elle-même: il est possible qu'il s'agisse d'une influence sur des mécanismes de la production d'énergie ou de la synthèse des enzymes.

Ces diurétiques agissent sur le transport du sodium aussi bien au niveau du tube proximal qu'au niveau du tube distal. Alors que l'effet proximal est plus important du point de vue quantitatif, on a pensé pouvoir expliquer la diminution de la clearance de l'eau libre au cours de la diurèse aqueuse par un effet distal. L'action antidiurétique, qui est mise à profit dans le traitement du diabète insipide chez l'homme, semble cependant être due à une action directe des diurétiques thiazidiques sur la perméabilité à l'eau du tube distal et du canal collecteur plutôt qu'à une action sur la résorption distale du sodium.

Alors que les benzothiadiazines et les substances apparentées interviennent surtout dans le cas de l'élaboration d'une urine hypotonique, l'acide éthacrynique abolit la faculté de concentration du rein, probablement en agissant sur la branche ascendante de l'anse de Henlé.

L'effet antihypertenseur de tous les diurétiques modernes est une conséquence de leur effet diurétique. Il n'est pas dû à une action extrarénale. Il semble que les pertes temporaires de sodium provoquées par les diurétiques déclenchent une modification, de nature encore inconnue, de la réactivité vasculaire. La diminution de l'action des amines sympathomimétiques sur le coeur et les vaisseaux peut être l'expression de cette modification inconnue. Ni la réactivité à l'angiotensine ni le système rénine-angiotensine ne sont modifiés directement par les agents diurétiques.

L'effet diabétogène des benzothiadiazines diurétiques, bien que de peu d'importance en clinique, conduit à d'intéressantes considérations théoriques. Les diurétiques ne provoquent pas de diabète permanent. Ils ne sont pas diabétogènes chez le rat normal ou ayant subi une pancréatectomie partielle, mais ils renforcent les réponses aux charges orales de glucose chez l'homme normal. Ces modifications de la tolérance aux hydrates de carbone peuvent être dues à une inhibition de la réponse sécrétoire des ilôts du pancréas à la stimulation par l'hyperglycémie.

Acknowledgements

I am indebted to my collaborators Dr. F. ROCH-RAMEL, Dr. G. SCHAECHTELIN, Dr. R. GUIDOUX, and Dr. J. P. BONJOUR for their help in the preparation of this text and for the permission to quote from their unpublished results. I wish to thank Miss C. SCHWENTER and Miss H. AMSTUTZ for their expert technical assistance, and Dr. G. SCHAECHTELIN, Dr. P. RIEDEL, Miss C. SCHWENTER, and Mr. K. BREITENFELD for preparing the figures.

The experimental work discussed in this review was supported by the Fonds National Suisse de la Recherche Scientifique (grant No. 2966) and by a research grant from CIBA Limited, Basle.

References

ALEKSANDROW, D., W. WYSZNACKA, and J. GAJEWSKI: N. England J. Med. **261**, 1052 (1959). — BAER, J. E., J. K. MICHAELSON, D. N. MCKINSTRY, and K. H. BEYER: Proc. Soc. Exper. Biol. Med. **115**, 87 (1964). — BARENBERG, R. L., and R. W. GIFFORD: Ohio Med. J. **59**, 805 (1963). — BEYER, K. H.: Ann. N. Y. Acad. Sc. **71**, 363 (1958). — BEYER, K. H., and J. E. BAER: Pharmacol. Rev. **13**, 517 (1961). — BOCK, K. D., and F. GROSS: Arch. exper. Path. Pharmak. **238**, 339 (1960). — BONJOUR, J. P.: Paper read at the 33rd Meeting of the Association des Physiologistes Français, Louvain, 1965. — BORHANI, N. O.: Ann. Int. Med. **53**, 342 (1960). — BRUNNER, H.: Arch. exper. Path. Pharmak. **236**, 559 (1959). — CAFRUNY, E. J., and C. J. ROSS: J. Pharmacol. Exper. Therap. **137**, 324 (1962). — CANNON, P. J., R. P. AMES, and J. H. LARAGH: J. Amer. Med. Ass. **185**, 854 (1963). — CARLINER, N. H., J. L. SCHELLING, P. RUSSELL, R. OKUN, and M. DAVIS: J. Amer. Med. Ass. **191**, 535 (1965). — CARMINATI, G. M.: Arch. internat. pharmacodyn. thérap. **143**, 446 (1963). — CAVALCA, L., F. F. GILARDI, V. MARINI, and R. BERETTA: Fol. endocr. **14**, 558 (1961). — CIER, J. F.: Actualités Pharmacol. **17**, 41 (1964). — CONWAY, B., and G. LEONETTI: Circulation **31**, 661 (1965). — CRAWFORD, J. D., and G. C. KENNEDY: Nature **183**, 891 (1959). — CROSLEY, A. P., Jr.: In: Cardiovascular Drug Therapy. The 11th Hahnemann Symposium. Ed. by A. N. BREST and J. H. MOYER. Grune and Stratton, New York, 1965, p. 184. — CROSLEY, A. P., Jr., R. C. CULLEN, D. WHITE, J. J. FREEMAN, C. A. CASTILLO, and G. C. ROWE: J. Laborat. Clin. Med. **55**, 191 (1960). — CUTLER, R., C. R. KLEEMAN, J. T. DOWLING, and M. H. MAXWELL: J. Clin. Invest. **39**, 980 (1960). — DANIEL, E. E.: Circulation Res. **11**, 941 (1962). — DARMADY, E. M., T. T. MOWLES, A. A. RENZI, M. SHEPPARD, and F. STRANACK: Clin. Sc. **22**, 295 (1962). — DAVID, A., and K. P. FELLOWES: J. Pharmacy Pharmacol. **12**, 65 (1960). — DEETJEN, P.: Arch. Physiol. **284**, 184 (1965). — DIÈS, A., and A. RIVERA: Clin. Pharmacol. Therap. **3**, 172 (1962). — DOLLERY, C. T.: Brit. Med. J. 1962/II, 337. — DOLLERY, C. T.: Practitioner **194**, 286 (1965). — DOLLERY, C. T., E. H. PERRY, and D. S. YOUNG: Lancet 1964/I, 947. — EARLY, L. E., and R. M. FRIEDLER: J. Clin. Invest. **43**, 1495 (1964). — EARLY, L. E., M. KAHN, and J. ORLOFF: J. Clin. Invest. **40**, 857 (1961). — EARLY, L. E., and J. ORLOFF: J. Clin. Invest. **41**, 1988 (1962). — EARLY, L. E., and J. ORLOFF: Annual. Rev. Med. **15**, 149 (1964). — ECKSTEIN, J. W., F. M. ABBOUD, and S. A. PEREDA: J. Clin. Invest. **41**, 1578 (1962). — ECKSTEIN, J. W., M. G. WENDLING, and F. M. ABBOUD: J. Laborat. Clin. Med. **64**, 853 (1964). — *Editorial*: Ned. tschr. geneesk. **108**, 2224 (1964). — ERBE, R. W., and J. M. WELLER: Clin. Res. **11**, 240 (1963). — FAIRBAIRN, J. H., II: In: Cardiovascular Drug Therapy. The 11th Hahnemann Symposium. Ed. by A. N. BREST and J. H. MOYER: Grune and Stratton, New York, 1965, p. 24. — FEISAL, K. A., J. W. ECKSTEIN, A. W. HORSLEY, and H. M. KEASLING: J. Appl. Physiol. **16**, 549 (1961). — FIELD, J. B., and S. MANDELL: Metabolism **13**, 959 (1964). — FRANK, H., H. DENTLER, F. EBERLEIN, and E. SCHMID: Arzneimittel-Forsch. **10**, 434 (1960). —

FRIEDMAN, S. M., M. NAKASHIMA, and C. C. FRIEDMAN: Amer. J. Physiol. **198**, 148 (1960). — GIEBISCH, G.: Circulation **21**, 879 (1960). — GOLDBERG, M., D. K. MCCURDY, E. L. FOLTZ, and L. W. BLUEMLE, Jr.: J. Clin. Invest. **43**, 201 (1964). — GOLDNER, M. G., H. ZAROWITZ, and S. AKGUN: N. England J. Med. **262**, 403 (1960). — GÖRES, E., and F. JUNG: Acta Biol. Med. Germ. **6**, 35 (1961). — GREENE, M. A., A. J. BOLTAX, M. NIV, and E. ROGOW: Amer. J. Med. Sc. **246**, 578 (1963). — GREENE, M. A., A. J. BOLTAX, and E. S. SCHERR: Amer. Heart J. **62**, 659 (1961). — GROLLMAN, A.: In: Cardiovascular Drug Therapy. The 11th Hahnemann Symposium. Ed. by A. N. BREST and J. H. MOYER. Grune and Stratton, New York, 1965, p. 179. — GROWE, G., S. ALFONSO, C. A. CASTILLO, W. C. LOWE, and C. W. CRUMPTON: Proc. Soc. Exper. Biol. Med. **110**, 27 (1962). — HEATH, W. C., and E. D. FREIS: J. Amer. Med. Ass. **186**, 119 (1963). — HEIDENREICH, O., and L. BAUMEISTER: Klin. Wschr. **42**, 1236 (1964). — HEIDENREICH, O., G. FULLGRAFF, L. BAUMEISTER, and K. SCHMIZ: Arch. exper. Path. Pharmak. **249**, 432 (1964a). — HEIDENREICH, O., G. GHAREMANI, P. KELLER, Y. KOOK, and K. SCHMIZ: Arzneimittel-Forsch. **14**, 1242 (1964b). — HEINEMANN, H. O., F. E. DEMARTINI, and J. H. LARAGH: Amer. J. Med. **26**, 853 (1959). — HERKEN, H., and G. SENFT: Klin. Wschr. **39**, 1205 (1961). — HOLZGREVE, H., A. FRICK, G. RUMRICH, M. WIEDERHOLT, and K. J. ULLRICH: Paper read at the 3rd Symposium of the Gesellschaft für Nephrologie, Berlin, 1964. — JOHNSTON, D. H., and A. L. CORNISH: J. Amer. Med. Ass. **170**, 2054 (1959). — KENNEDY, G. C., and J. D. CRAWFORD: Lancet 1959/I, 866. — KENNEDY, G. C., and L. E. HILL: Quart. J. Exper. Physiol. **48**, 248 (1963). — KESSLER, R. H., K. HIERHOLZER, R. S. GURD, and R. F. PITTS: Amer. J. Physiol. **196**, 1346 (1959). — KLAPPER, M. S.: South. Med. J. **55**, 297 (1962). — KLEINFELDER, M.: Dtsch. med. Wschr. **88**, 1695 (1963). — KLEINZELLER, A., and J. H. CORT: Biochem. J. **67**, 15 (1957). — KLÜTSCH, K., A. HEIDLAND, and F. SUZUKI: Atti Accad. med. lombarda **18**, 1255 (1963). — KOBINGER, W.: Arch. exper. Path. Pharmak. **249**, 501 (1965). — KÜHN, G.: Klin. Wschr. **35**, 346 (1957). — LARAGH, J. H.: Circulation **26**, 121 (1962). — LASAGNA, L.: Personal communication (1965). — LASSEN, J. B., and O. E. NIELSEN: Acta pharmac. tox. **20**, 309 (1963). — LOSERT, W., G. SENFT, and R. SITT: Arch. exper. Path. Pharmak. **251**, 120 (1965). — LYON, A. F., and A. C. DEGRAFF: Amer. Heart J. **68**, 710 (1964). — MACGAFFEY, K., L. A. LEZOTTE, Jr., J. H. SNYDER, E. W. MOORE, and H. JICK: Proc. Soc. Exper. Biol. Med. **116**, 11 (1964). — MANN, M., J. GFELLER, and W. SIEGENTHALER: Zschr. klin. Chem. **2**, 123 (1964). — MAXWELL, D. R., and J. M. MCLUSKY: Nature **202**, 300 (1964). — MCILWAINE, C. L. K., and D. H. K. SMITH: Brit. Med. J. 1964/II, 1265. — MCQUEEN, E. G., and R. B. I. MORRISON: Lancet 1960/I, 1209. — MEHTA, D. J., C. V. DELIWALA, M. H. SHAH, V. K. SHETH, R. VALADARES, and S. B. MARATHE: Arch. internat. pharmacodyn. thérap. **138**, 480 (1962). — MEHTA, D. J., V. K. SHETH, and C. V. DELIWALA: Nature **187**, 1034 (1960). — MENG, K.: Arch. exper. Path. Pharmak. **251**, 170 (1965). — MENG, K., and G. KRONEBERG: Arch. exper. Path. Pharmak. **247**, 351 (1964). — MIGONE, L., S. AMBROSOLI, and V. FERIOLI: Minerva nefrol. **10**, 79 (1963). — MORRISON, A. B.: Amer. J. Physiol. **205**, 494 (1963). — MUSCHAWECK, R., and P. HAJDÚ: Arzneimittel-Forsch. **14**, 44 (1964). — NOVELLO, F. C., and J. M. SPRAGUE: J. Amer. Chem. Soc. **79**, 2028 (1957). — OKEN, D. E.: Nephron **1**, 31 (1964). — ORBISON, J. L.: Proc. Soc. Exper. Biol. Med. **110**, 161 (1962). — ORLOFF, J., and M. BURG: Amer. J. Physiol. **199**, 49 (1960). — PETERS, G.: Atti Accad. med. lombarda **18**, 931 (1963a). — PETERS, G.: Amer. J. Physiol. **205**, 1042 (1963b). — PETERS, G.:

Proc. Soc. Exper. Biol. Med. 112, 771 (1963c). — PETERS, G.: Helvet. physiol. pharmacol. acta 22, C34 (1964). — PETERS, G.: Nephron 2, 95 (1965a). — PETERS, G.: Proc. Europ. Soc. Study Drug Toxic. 5, 18 (1965b). — PETROW, V., O. STEPHENSON, and A. M. WILD: J. Pharmacy Pharmacol. 12, 37 (1960). — PITTS, R. F.: Progr. Cardiovascular Diseases 3, 537 (1961). — PITTS, R. F., F. KRÜCK, R. LOZANO, D. W. TAYLOR, P. A. HEIDENREICH, and R. H. KESSLER: J. Pharmacol. Exper. Therap. 123, 89 (1958). — PREZIOSI, A., A. F. DE SHAEPDRIJVER, E. MARMO, and E. MIELE: Arch. internat. pharmacodyn. thérap. 131, 209 (1961). — ROOTH, G., and C. FURST: Acta med. Scand. 176, 51 (1964). — ROSENTHALE, M. E., and C. C. VAN ARMAN: J. Pharmacol. Exper. Therap. 142, 111 (1963). — RUBIN, A. A., F. E. ROTH, R. M. TAYLOR, and H. ROSENKILDE: J. Pharmacol. Exper. Therap. 136, 344 (1962). — SCRIABINE, A., E. C. SCHREIBER, M. YÜ, and E. H. WISEMAN: Proc. Soc. Exper. Biol. Med. 110, 872 (1962). — SELLER, R. M.: Cardiovascular Drug Therapy. The 11th Hahnemann Symposium. Ed. by. A. N. BREST and J. H. MOYER. Grune and Stratton, New York, 1965, p. 172. — SHANKLIN, D. R.: N. England J. Med. 266, 1093 (1962). — SHAPIRO, A. P., T. G. BENEDEK, and J. L. SMALL: N. England J. Med. 265, 1028 (1960). — SILAH, J. G., R. E. JONES, F. A. BASHOUR, and N. M. KAPLAN: Amer. Heart J. 69, 301 (1965). — SIMPSON F. O.: Curr. Ther. Res. 6, 21 (1964). — SPERBER, R. J., and A. C. DEGRAFF: Amer. Heart J. 69, 134 (1965). — SPIEKERMANN, R. E., R. W. P. ACHOR, K. G. BERGE, and W. F. MCGUCKIN: J. Amer. Med. Ass. 184, 191 (1963). — TAQUINI, A. C.: Arch. internat. pharmacodyn. thérap. 140, 549 (1962). — TAUGNER, R., and I. IRAVANI: Arzneimittel-Forsch. 15, 538 (1965). — TAYLOR, C. B : Biochem. Pharmacol. 12, 539 (1963). — TOPLISS, J. G., M. C. DALY, A. LIPSKI, P. SHAPIRO, and N. SPERBER: J. Med. Chem. 6, 312 (1963). — ULLRICH, K. J.: Biochem. Pharmacol. 9, 181 (1962). — VANDER, A. J., R. L. MALVIN, W. S. WILDE, and L. P. SULLIVAN: J. Pharmacol. Exper. Therap. 125, 19 (1959). — VEREL, D., N. M. STENTIFORD, F. RAMMAN, and R. SAYNOR: Lancet 1964/II, 1088. — VESIN, P., B. RUEFF, H. TRAVERSO, H. HIRSCH-MARIE, and R. CATTAN: Bull. Mém. Soc. Méd. Hôp. Paris 114, 47 (1963). — VEYRAT, R., J. DE CHAMPLAIN, R. BOUCHER, J. GENEST, and A. F. MULLER: Helvet. med. acta, 31, 432 (1964). — VORBURGER, C.: Rev. méd. Suisse rom. 84, 277 (1964). — VORBURGER, C., and A. HUBER: Therap.-woche 14, 708 (1964). — WATSON, L. S., S. M. VAN PELT, and C. A. WINTER: Fed. Proc. 23, 438 (1964). — WELLER, J. M., and P. E. BORONDY: Metabolism 14, 708 (1965). — WIEBELHAUS, V. D., J. WEINSTOCK, F. T. BRENNAN, G. SOSNOWSKI, and T. J. LARSEN: Fed. Proc. 20, 409 (1961). — WILKINS, R. W.: Ann. Int. Med. 50, 1 (1959). — WILSON, W. R., and R. OKUN: Circulation 28, 89 (1963). — WILSON, W. R., D. B. STOWE, R. OKUN, and R. P. RUSSEL: Ann. Int. Med. 60, 317 (1964). — WOLFF, F. W.: personal communication (1965). — WOLFF, F. W., R. G. LANGDON, B. H. RUEBNER, C. HOLLANDER, and R. D. SKOGLUND: Diabetes 12, 335 (1963a). — WOLFF, F. W., and W. W. PARMLEY: Diabetes 13, 115 (1964). — WOLFF, F. W., W. W. PARMLEY, and R. OKUN: Clin. Res. 11, 231 (1963b). — YOUNG, D. S., T. M. FORRESTER, and T. N. MORGAN: Lancet 1959/II, 765.

Discussion

HOOD: Dr. PETERS, have you any information on whether the thiazides have an effect on the tubular transport of phosphate, creatine, and some of the amino acids? I am thinking particularly of glycine and alanine. The reason for asking this question is that in a few experiments in diabetes insipidus, after an acute injection of chlorothiazide followed by a sustained infusion, we observed the same percentage increase in phosphate excretion as in sodium and chloride excretion. We have not followed this up — and we measured the amino acids mentioned and creatine only in one single experiment — but if it is true, this would certainly suggest a type of mechanism other than the sodium pump itself, and it would be more in accordance with an effect on the energy-providing mechanisms.

PETERS: I am glad to hear that somebody has observed a consistent effect of thiazides on renal phosphate excretion. The data in the literature on this topic are scarce and contradictory. No study seems to have been done under conditions that would exclude the possibility of an enhanced secretion of parathyroid hormone, which could account for temporary increases in phosphaturia observed sometimes. In other studies, the drugs had no effect on phosphate excretion in normal animals[1], with the possible exception of a small, initial, wash-out effect. I am not aware of any evidence of a possible depression of phosphate reabsorption.

It should be mentioned at this point that thiazide diuretics depress the renal excretion of calcium[1–4] and apparently also of citrate[4]. The mechanism of this calcium-retaining effect is unknown. Though it is accompanied by temporary hypercalcaemia in man, it may be due to extrarenal changes.

No investigation of the effects of diuretics on the reabsorption of amino acids has come to my knowledge. Since the plasma concentration of amino nitrogen is not primarily regulated by renal reabsorption, indirect influences are possible. Creatine may be reabsorbed, in the dog, by the same mechanism as that responsible for the reabsorption of glycine and alanine[5]. The influence of diuretics on this mechanism or on the depression of phosphate reabsorption by alanine[6] does not seem to have been investigated.

The clearance of exogenous creatinine is depressed by hydrochlorothiazide to a larger extent than the clearance of inulin in the rat.

---

1 LAMBERG, B. A., and B. KOHLBÄCK: Scand. J. Clin. Laborat. Invest. **11**, 351 (1959).

2 LICHTWITZ, A.: Pathol. Biol. (Sem. hôp.) **8**, 1873 (1960).

3 POUTSIAKA, J. W., H. MADISSOO, L. G. MILLSTEIN, and J. KIRPAN: Toxicol. Appl. Pharmacol. **3**, 455 (1961).

4 SEITZ, H., and Z. F. JAWORSKI: Canad. Med. Ass. J. **90**, 414 (1964).

5 PITTS, R. F.: Amer. J. Physiol. **109**, 532 (1934).

6 PITTS, R. F., and R. S. ALEXANDER: Amer. J. Physiol. **142**, 648 (1944).

Functional, biochemical, and morphological changes produced by hypotensive drugs

By

Eleanor Zaimis

It was over 15 years ago that hexamethonium was introduced in the treatment of hypertension. Since then we have seen the introduction of other and more effective hypotensive drugs. On the clinical side, there is a certain satisfaction in knowing that the clinician has new and valuable weapons at his disposal. On the other hand, if we are not content to accept the magic, but wish instead to have an intimate picture of the way in which hypotension is brought about by these newer drugs, then we, as pharmacologists, must admit that in spite of the tremendous amount of work devoted to the study of this aspect, their mechanism of action is still veiled in mystery.

Our failure to solve this problem may have two main causes. On the one hand, the mode of action of these drugs may be too complex for our present knowledge of events at cellular level to cope with. Alternatively, and this is my strong suspicion, we may have been following up the wrong clues.

The discovery that reserpine can influence the storage and uptake of the catecholamines has quite understandably aroused a great deal of interest; but there is now an almost compulsive desire to demonstrate, for all drugs that affect structures innervated by sympathetic nerve fibres, a drug effect in terms of uptake, or storage, or metabolism, of adrenergic transmitter substance. Moreover, there has been a growing tendency to represent the pharmacological effects of these drugs as if they took place exclusively at the nerve-endings – in other words, as if the effector cells played a minor role or none at all. This approach is, to my mind, unrealistic. If a drug, by virtue of its chemical structure or other specific properties, affects structures innervated by sympathetic nerves, it has as much chance of acting upon effector cells as upon the nerve-endings, especially as most of these drugs penetrate cell membranes with great ease.

Pharmacological studies on cholinergic synapses, our knowledge of which is much more complete than our knowledge of adrenergic ones, have taught us that drugs produce, as a rule, a wealth of effects by acting on the effector cells themselves, and that only very rarely do we come across drugs that act exclusively on the nerve-ending. It is also useful to remember that both cardiac and smooth muscles exhibit spontaneous rhythmic activity, which is an intrinsic property of the muscle and is not due to external stimulation. Autonomic nerves, therefore, unlike motor nerves, are not essential for the contraction of either cardiac or smooth muscle. Local mechanisms become prominent after the normal nervous control is interrupted; a few weeks after the surgical removal of the sympathetic nervous system, the peripheral vessels regain a measure of control, which permits rapid adaptation and fairly normal activity. This does not mean that the sympathetic nervous system is not important, but indicates that additional mechanisms in the effector cells themselves can take over much of its function. One would, therefore, expect pharmacological actions that are restricted to the nerve-endings to be more uniform and less severe than those in fact produced by drugs such as reserpine, guanethidine, and α-methyldopa.

α-Methyldopa

α-Methyldopa is an inhibitor of dopa decarboxylase, but the significance of this inhibition in the reduction of blood pressure is uncertain. There is also experimental evidence to show that the administration of α-methyldopa is followed by a decrease in the catecholamine content of the heart and other tissues. However, there are great doubts as to the significance of catecholamine depletion in the hypotensive action of α-methyldopa. Finally, direct actions of the metabolites of α-methyldopa have been considered as an alternative explanation of the lowering of blood pressure, but there are a variety of experimental results which do not fit in with this "false transmitter" theory (for references see PARDO et al., 1965).

Guanethidine

A great number of workers have shown that guanethidine can reduce the noradrenaline content of peripheral tissues. However, significant depletion occurs only with large doses of guanethidine and, even then, only after two or more hours. In contrast, similar doses of guanethidine abolish the effects elicited by stimulation of sympathetic nerves within a few minutes. Moreover, SANAN and VOGT (1962) have found that in both rabbits and cats, even after large doses of guanethidine (15—20 mg./kg.), the loss of transmitter substance in sympathetic ganglia was too small and too slow to explain the failure of sympathetically innervated tissue to respond to electrical stimulation of its nerves; only about half of the noradrenaline in the ganglion was lost in the course of two to four hours – a loss which is not sufficient to cause functional failure (MUSCHOLL and VOGT, 1958).

Reserpine

The powerful capacity of reserpine to deplete the heart and other tissues of their catecholamine content has often been proposed as the primary cause of its pharmacological action. It is true that almost complete depletion can be caused by daily doses as small as 5 μg./kg. (for references see ZAIMIS, 1964a). Nevertheless, as the doses are progressively increased beyond this level, or as they are extended in time, the myocardium and other tissues show even more marked functional and histological changes. This interrelation of dose level and exposure period has been consistently evident throughout our studies based either on long-term administration of the drug to animals in doses more closely approximate to those used in therapeutics, or on short-term treatment with larger doses.

For example, in cats receiving daily doses of 10 μg./kg. reserpine, the resting values of both blood pressure and heart rate at the end of periods ranging from 5 to 6, 8 to 15, and 24 to 26 weeks were significantly lower than those of the control animals. These effects increased progressively with the duration of treatment, although catecholamine depletion was almost complete at the end of the first two weeks (WITHRINGTON and ZAIMIS, in preparation).

In collaboration with M. SCOTT, we found that reserpine can produce a variety of degenerative alterations in the myocardium and, once more, that the morphological changes increased progressively as the treatment was extended in time or as the dose was raised. Histological specimens removed from the hearts of cats treated with 10 μg./kg. daily for six months showed only localised alterations of the myocardial tissue (ZAIMIS, 1964b). With larger doses, the degenerative changes in both cats and guinea-pigs spread throughout the myocardium and were more severe; the amount of stainable sarcoplasm was reduced, and lipochrome granules were numerous.

Histochemical investigations carried out by SOPHIA KAKARI, on specimens removed from the hearts of guinea-pigs treated with reserpine, have also demonstrated considerable changes, which progressed either with the prolongation of the treatment or with an increase in the dose administered. The effects were as follows: –

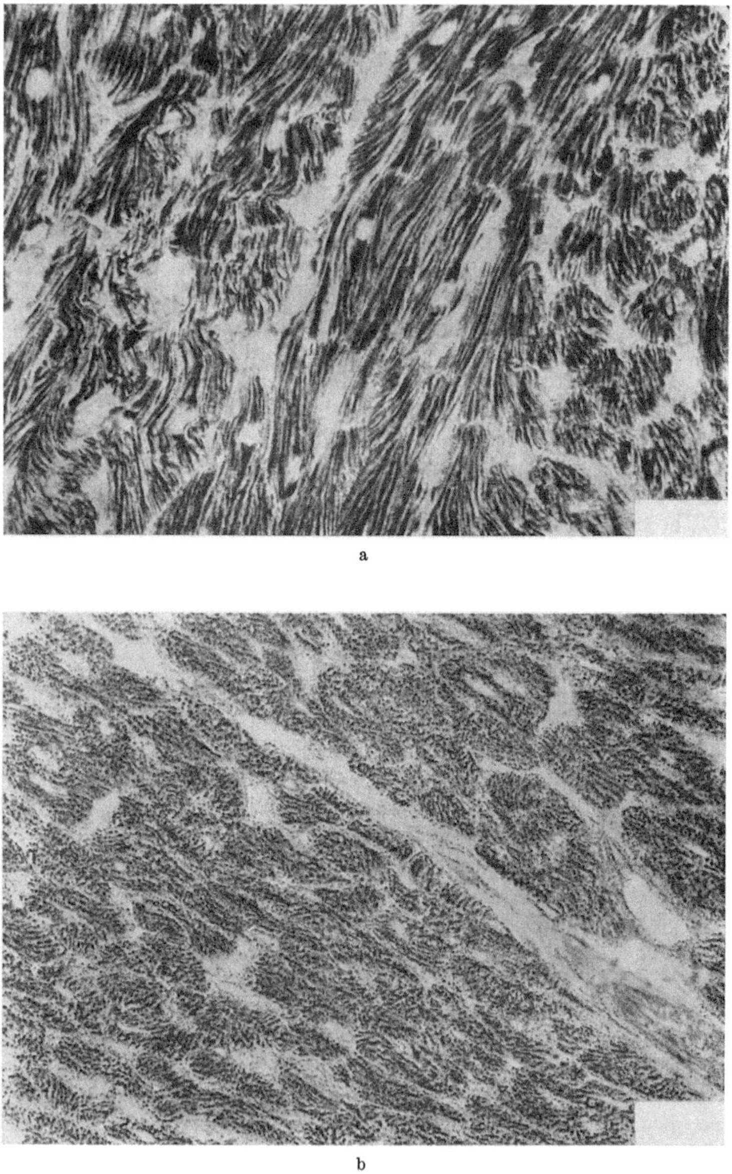

a

b

Fig. 1. Guinea-pig: microphotographs of ventricular muscle showing succinic dehydrogenase localisation in a control (a) and a reserpine-treated (b) animal (1 mg./kg. for two days) (× 317).

First, the reaction for the oxidative enzyme, succinic dehydrogenase, which in the untreated animals was predominantly "myofibrillar", appeared granular in the treated animal. Typical changes are shown in Fig. 1. The cytochemical localisation of this enzyme was carried out on fresh cryostat sections by using the nitro-blue tetrazolium salt as an electron acceptor. Second, good histochemical evidence was also obtained of a parallel increase in the lipid content of the heart in the reserpine-treated animals.

My colleagues M. CYMBALIST and R. SOARES DE MOURA found that the oxygen uptake of cardiac tissue removed from guinea-pigs pretreated with reserpine was depressed and, in addition, that there was a high degree of correlation between the depression of oxygen uptake and (a) the dose of reserpine administered, (b) the length of treatment, and (c) the decrease in heart rate. Moreover, both bradycardia and depression of oxygen uptake went on increasing as the treatment was extended in time, and long after the various tissues were almost entirely depleted of their catecholamine content.

Lack of correlation between catecholamine depletion and pharmacological effects was also shown in the results of a further study in cats, in which reserpine was compared with guanethidine and α-methyldopa (ZAIMIS, 1965a). The results showed that, of the three drugs, reserpine (20 μg./kg. for 14 days) produced the most pronounced depletion and that there was no apparent difference in the ability of α-methyldopa (100 mg./kg. for 14 days) and guanethidine (2 mg./kg. for 14 days) to lower tissue noradrenaline. Although α-methyldopa and guanethidine were almost equipotent in decreasing catecholamine levels in the heart and other tissues, the pattern of cardiovascular responses elicited by adrenaline and noradrenaline was markedly different. In the animals treated with guanethidine, adrenaline and noradrenaline produced positive chronotropic and inotropic responses and marked rises in blood pressure – effects similar to those found in the reserpine-treated animals. By far the most obvious change was the prolongation of the responses. In contrast, in the animals pretreated with α-methyldopa the responses were either similar to those of the control group or reduced. Thus, whereas in the animals treated with guanethidine and reserpine any rise in blood pressure was uniformly associated with an increase in both the force of heart contraction and the heart rate, in the animals treated with α-methyldopa, adrenaline and noradrenaline failed to produce significant inotropic and chronotropic responses. Moreover, after phenoxybenzamine, the percentage reduction in the pressor responses to both adrenaline and noradrenaline was larger in the controls and in the animals pretreated with α-methyldopa than in those treated with guanethidine and reserpine. It was concluded therefore that the large and especially prolonged pressor responses observed in the guanethidine- and reserpine-treated animals were the result of an increased cardiac output and not of an increased sensitivity of the peripheral vessels.

If all these results are taken into consideration, it seems unlikely that the pharmacological and toxic effects of drugs such as reserpine, guanethidine, and α-methyldopa are merely secondary to catecholamine depletion.

The immunosympathectomised animal

While this work was developing, we became aware of the startling discovery made by LEVI-MONTALCINI and her co-workers (for references see LEVI-MONTALCINI, 1964) that more than 90% of the population of sympathetic nerve cells can be increased up to sixfold, or conversely wiped out, by supplying a protein or its antiserum to the new-born mammal. This protein, known as nerve-growth factor (N.G.F.), is isolated at present from mouse salivary glands. The so-called "immunosympathectomised" animals provide an ideal experimental tool on which to test current theories concerning the way in which structures innervated by the sympathetic nervous system can be affected by drugs. We therefore included this type of animal in our studies concerned with the mode of action of hypotensive drugs.

Using a generous supply of N.G.F. antiserum provided by LEVI-MONTALCINI and ANGELETTI, we were able to treat a reasonable number of new-born rats. This treatment resulted in almost complete destruction of the paravertebral ganglia and a 75% atrophy of the coeliac ganglion. Only the mesenteric ganglion escaped this massive destruction. The reduction in volume and in nerve-cell density of the paravertebral ganglia was greater than 90% (Fig. 2); moreover, the few surviving cells were, as a rule, reduced in size and did not stain as deeply with basic dyes as those of the control rats (BERK et al., 1964).

In the treated animals, there was a good correlation between the degree of destruction of the sympathetic ganglia and the biochemical changes in tissues supplied with adrenergic neurones by these ganglia. For example, the noradrenaline content of the heart and spleen was almost zero, that of the small intestine about 25%, and that of the vas deferens 65% of the control levels. In contrast, the total catecholamine levels in the adrenals were not significantly

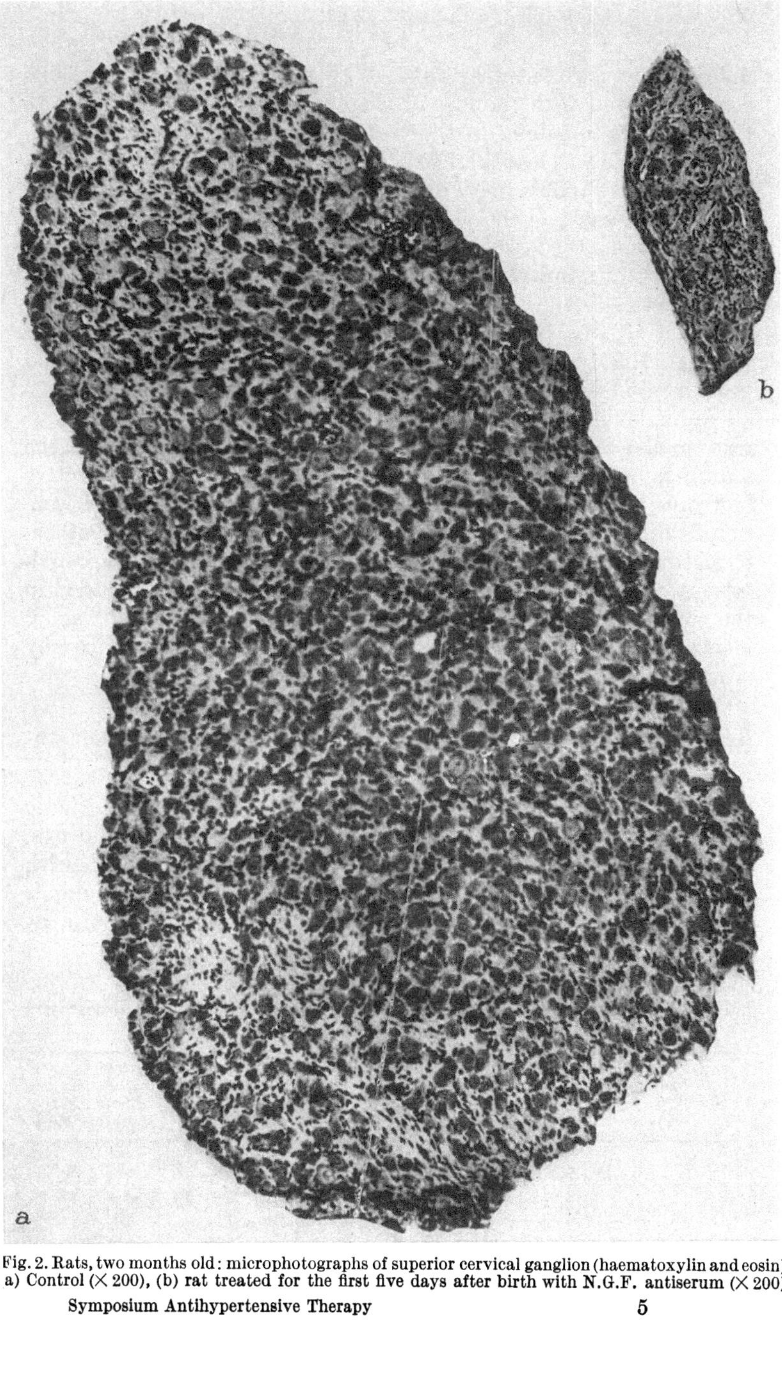

Fig. 2. Rats, two months old: microphotographs of superior cervical ganglion (haematoxylin and eosin). a) Control (× 200), (b) rat treated for the first five days after birth with N.G.F. antiserum (× 200).

different from those in the controls (Fig. 4). Finally, these results correlated well with the loss of the capacity of various tissues to take up noradrenaline. In the treated animals, the uptake of ^{3}H-noradrenaline was less than 14% of the control value in the heart, spleen, lungs, and kidney, about 30% in the small intestine and colon, unchanged in the uterus, and increased in the vas deferens (ZAIMIS et al., 1965).

The body temperature of the immunosympathectomised rats was practically the same as that of the controls. Moreover, they were active, ate, drank, cleaned themselves, and bred normally (ZAIMIS, 1965b). In the conscious treated rat, the average blood pressure and heart rate were very similar to those of the untreated animals. After chloralose anaesthesia, however, the average resting blood pressure, but not the heart rate, was lower in the immunosympathectomised rats. Both the pressor and the positive inotropic responses to injected adrenaline and noradrenaline were significantly greater and more prolonged in the immunosympathectomised rat, and tyramine, before as well as after bilateral adrenalectomy, caused pressor responses comparable to those recorded in the controls. The essential feature of the tyramine action was an increase in heart rate significantly greater than that produced by either adrenaline or noradrenaline.

Reserpine, guanethidine, and α-methyldopa in immunosympathectomised rats

In order to find out to what degree the absence of sympathetic innervation alters the effects produced by hypotensive drugs, immunosympathectomised and normal rats were treated with reserpine, guanethidine, and α-methyldopa. The number of animals used, the range of daily doses, and the duration of the treatment are shown in Table 1.

Table 1. *Number of animals, doses, and duration of treatment with hypotensive substances in immunosympathectomised animals*

	Number of rats	
	Control	Immunosympathectomised
Saline 0.4 ml./day for 30—48 days	3	4
α-Methyldopa 150 mg./kg./day for 28—48 days	3	3
Guanethidine 8 mg./kg./day for 35—44 days	4	3
Reserpine 90 μg./kg./day for 26—39 days . .	6	4

In both groups of animals, observations were made of: a) the growth rate; b) the resting blood pressure and heart rate; c) the catecholamine content of the heart, spleen, intestine, and adrenals; d) the blood-pressure and heart-rate responses to adrenaline (30 ng.), noradrenaline (30 ng.), and tyramine (30 μg.) injected intravenously.

The *growth rate* of both control and immunosympathectomised animals was not affected by either α-methyldopa or guanethidine. All the rats receiving reserpine, however, lost weight during the last two weeks of treatment, and the percentage loss was almost the same in both control and immunosympathectomised animals.

At the end of the chosen period, the animals were anaesthetised with chloralose, both vagi were cut, and the systemic *blood pressure* and *heart rate* were recorded simultaneously on a Grass polygraph. In the normal and immunosympathectomised rats, treated with guanethidine and reserpine, there was a significant decrease in the resting heart rate and blood pressure. The heart-rate decrease was almost the same in the two groups of animals. The over-all decrease in blood pressure, however, was smaller in the immunosympathectomised animals, possibly because their resting blood pressure,

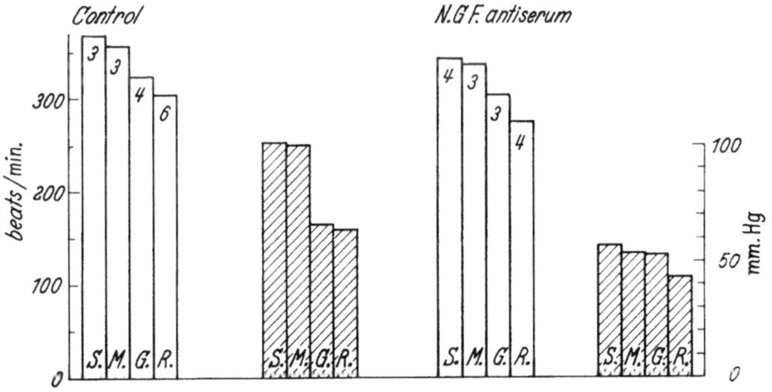

Fig. 3. Effect of saline (S.), α-methyldopa (M.), guanethidine (G.), and reserpine (R.) on the heart rate (□) and systemic blood pressure (▨) of control and immunosympathectomised (N.G.F. antiserum) rats. Number of experiments indicated in each column.

under anaesthesia, is always lower than that of normal rats. Treatment with α-methyldopa made little difference to the resting blood pressure and heart rate in either normal or immunosympathectomised rats (Fig. 3).

Assays of *catecholamine content* in peripheral tissues were carried out by my colleague Lucienne Berk. The results, illustrated in

Fig. 4, showed that in the control animals guanethidine produced a marked reduction in the noradrenaline content of the heart, spleen, and intestine, and reserpine an almost complete depletion. On the other hand, the over-all reduction in the animals treated with α-methyldopa was only about 50%. Finally, the catecholamine content of the adrenals in both normal and immunosympathectomised animals was little affected by any of the three drugs.

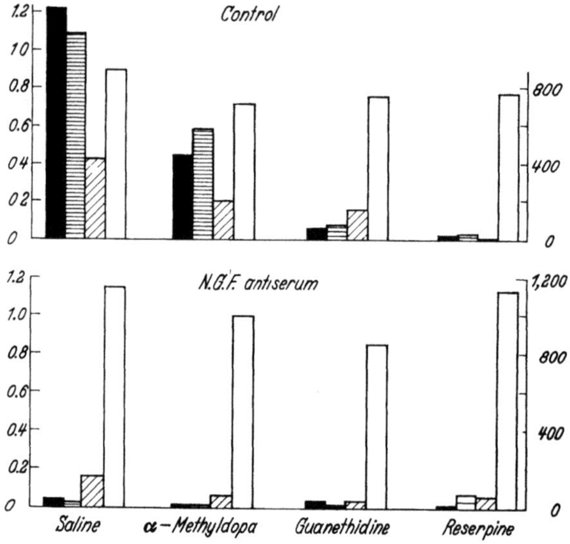

Fig. 4. Catecholamine content (μg./g.) of the heart (■), spleen (▤), intestine (▨), and adrenals (□) of control and immunosympathectomised (N.G.F. antiserum) rats.

A comparison of changes in blood pressure and heart rate in response to adrenaline (30 ng.), noradrenaline (30 ng.) and tyramine (30 μg.) in both control and immunosympathectomised animals is shown in Fig. 5. For the calculation of percentage changes in blood pressure and heart rate, measurements of areas in the tracing were made. In this way, both duration and magnitude of the effect were taken into account. The results show that the responses to the three pressor agents were significantly altered by reserpine-, guanethidine-, and α-methyldopa-treatment, but that the recorded changes were very similar in both control and immunosympathectomised animals. For example, noradrenaline and especially adrenaline produced larger rises in blood pressure in all the animals treated with any of the three drugs. The pressor response to tyramine was significantly increased in the rats treated with α-methyldopa, both normal and immunosympathectomised. On the other hand, the chronotropic response to tyramine was increased in all the animals treated with guanethidine. A comparison between the groups of animals treated with saline and those given reserpine shows that, in both normal and immunosympathectomised rats, the pressor responses to adrenaline and noradrenaline were potentiated, whereas the pressor responses to tyramine remained the same or were slightly reduced.

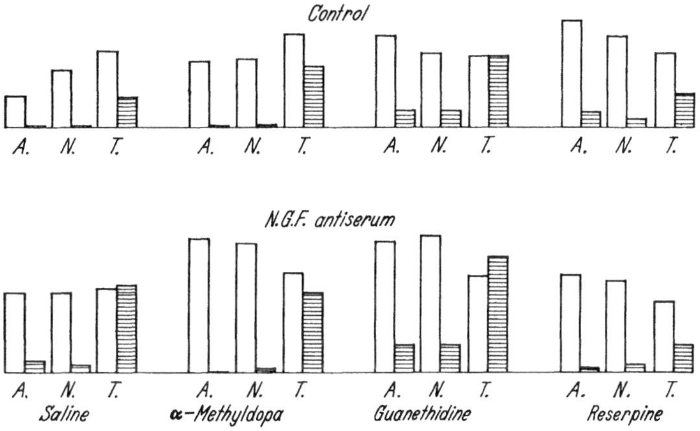

Fig. 5. Over-all comparison of changes in blood pressure (□) and heart rate (▤) in control and immunosympathectomised (N.G.F. antiserum) rats in response to total doses of 30 ng. adrenaline (A.), 30 ng. noradrenaline (N.), and 30 μg. tyramine (T.), administered intravenously.

From these results it is obvious that the peripheral adrenergic neurone is not the only point of attack of reserpine, guanethidine, and α-methyldopa. The fact that the three hypotensive drugs produced very similar effects in both normal and immunosympathectomised animals strongly suggests a direct action on the effector cells themselves. Therefore it may be justifiable to say that a great many of the "therapeutic" and "toxic" effects of reserpine, guanethidine, and α-methyldopa result from their ability to affect and alter important processes located in the heart and smooth-muscle cells. Clearly, a great deal of work remains to be done before the precise mode of action of these drugs is fully understood. All I can say at this stage is that it seems worth while to shift our efforts and attention from the nerve-ending to the effector cell.

Summary

Current theories on the mode of action of reserpine, guanethidine, and α-methyldopa are briefly reviewed and their inadequacies discussed. Experimental results obtained from normal and immunosympathectomised animals are presented and strongly suggest: a) that the adrenergic neurone is not the only point of attack of the three hypotensive drugs and b) that the cardiovascular changes produced by reserpine, guanethidine, and α-methyldopa are, to a large degree, the result of a direct action on the effector cells themselves.

Zusammenfassung

Die heute geltenden Auffassungen über den Wirkungsmechanismus von Reserpin, Guanethidin und α-Methyldopa werden kurz geschildert und ihre Unzulänglichkeiten besprochen. Experimentelle Befunde bei normalen und immunosympathektomierten Tieren werden mitgeteilt, aus denen hervorgeht, daß a) das adrenergische Neuron nicht der einzige Angriffsort der drei genannten Antihypertensiva ist und daß b) die cardiovaskulären Veränderungen, die durch Reserpin, Guanethidin und α-Methyldopa hervorgerufen werden, in einem erheblichen Maße das Ergebnis einer direkten Wirkung auf die Effektorzellen selbst sind.

Résumé

Les théories actuelles sur le mode d'action de la réserpine, de la guanéthidine et de l'α-méthyldopa sont brièvement passées en revue et leurs insuffisances sont discutées. Des résultats expérimentaux obtenus chez l'animal normal ou ayant subi une "sympathectomie immunologique" suggèrent fortement que: a) le neurone adrénergique n'est pas le seul point d'attaque de ces trois agents hypotenseurs, b) les modifications cardio-vasculaires produites par la réserpine, la guanéthidine et l'α-méthyldopa sont dans une large mesure le résultat d'une action directe sur les cellules effectrices elles-mêmes.

Acknowledgement

I should like to thank the Honorary Editors of the Royal Society of Medicine (London) for their permission to make use in this chapter of some of the material presented in a Presidential Address (May, 1965).

References

BERK, L., I. FILIPE, and E. ZAIMIS: J. Physiol. **177**, 1P (1965). — LEVI-MONTALCINI, R.: Science **143**, 105 (1964). — MUSCHOLL, E., and M. VOGT: J. Physiol. **141**, 132 (1958). — PARDO, E. G., R. VARGAS, and H. VIDRIO: Annual Rev. Pharmacol. **5**, 77 (1965). — SANAN, S., and M. VOGT: Brit. J. Pharmacol. **18**, 109 (1962). — WITHRINGTON, P., and E. ZAIMIS: in preparation. — ZAIMIS, E.: Annual Rev. Pharmacol. **4**, 365 (1964a). — ZAIMIS, E.: In: Cardiomyopathies. Ciba Foundation Symposium. Ed. by G. E. W. WOLSTENHOLME and M. O'CONNOR. Churchill Ltd., London, 1964b, p. 214. — ZAIMIS, E.: In: Evaluation of New Drugs in Man. Proc. 2nd Internat. Pharmacol. Meeting, Prague, 1963. Ed. by E. ZAIMIS. Pergamon Press, Oxford, 1965a, p. 57. — ZAIMIS, E.: J. Physiol. **177**, 35P (1965b). — ZAIMIS, E., L. BERK, and B. A. CALLINGHAM: Nature **206**, 1220 (1965).

Discussion

PAGE: I think the last sentence was very interesting and important. The question is: are these animals completely sympathectomised? I am frankly a little dubious, although I recognise many of the signs of sympathetic denervation. It makes one wonder whether the sympathetic system is of any real use to the body. So far, the evidence from the clinical point of view is that it mostly causes a lot of trouble. Maybe we should have a prophylactic sympathectomy along with circumcision.

ZAIMIS: As far as the cardiovascular system is concerned, the answer is "yes". I think I can say this with almost 100% certainty. With two of Dr. WILSON's colleagues, Dr. J. M. LEDINGHAM and Dr. M. A. FLOYER, we have attempted to produce hypertension in some of our immunosympathectomised rats. The results obtained support our belief that these animals, as far as the cardiovascular system is concerned, are truly sympathectomised.

WILSON: Dr. ZAIMIS very kindly supplied us with a group of immunosympathectomised rats to enable us to investigate the effects of renal artery constriction. Fig. 1 summarises the results obtained by Dr. FLOYER in our laboratory. It is apparent that in all cases the blood pressure rises very steeply

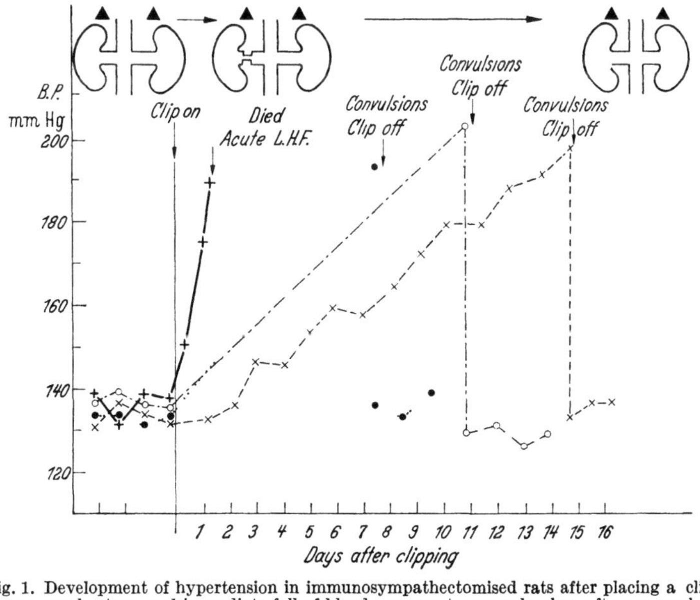

Fig. 1. Development of hypertension in immunosympathectomised rats after placing a clip on one renal artery, and immediate fall of blood pressure to normal values after removal of the clip (by kind permission of Dr. M. A. FLOYER).

after renal artery clipping. The first rat died within 24 hours in acute heart failure; the others, with less tight clipping, all developed acute hypertensive encephalopathy, which was immediately relieved when the clip was released, the blood pressure dropping abruptly to normal. This accelerated rise and fall in blood pressure is presumably due to absence of the damping effect of the baroceptor mechanism and supports Dr. ZAIMIS' suggestion that the cardiovascular component of the sympathetic nervous system is in abeyance. These observations also provide further evidence that this form of renal hypertension is not dependent on the integrity of the sympathetic nervous system.

GROSS: Do these immunosympathectomised rats show a similar increase in sensitivity to angiotensin and to renin as to adrenaline and noradrenaline?

ZAIMIS: I won't say it is enhanced, but the response to angiotensin in the immunosympathectomised rats is still there, even after adrenalectomy.

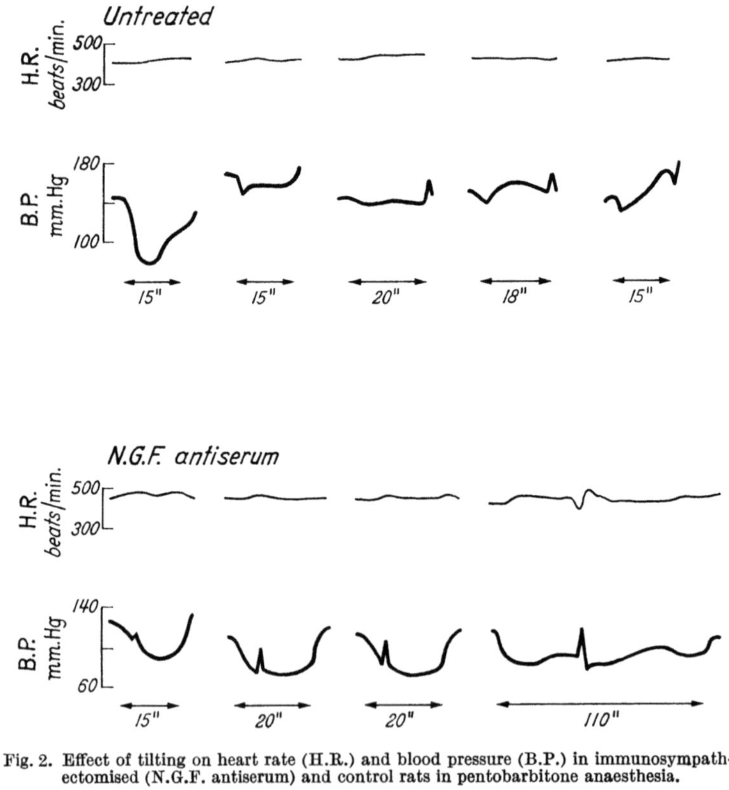

Fig. 2. Effect of tilting on heart rate (H.R.) and blood pressure (B.P.) in immunosympathectomised (N.G.F. antiserum) and control rats in pentobarbitone anaesthesia.

DOLLERY: In Dr. WILSON's slide (Fig. 1) it seemed that the resting blood pressure was normal before the clip was applied. I thought Dr. ZAIMIS said it was low.

ZAIMIS: I think I said that in the non-anaesthetised rats the blood pressure was between 130 and 145 mm. Hg, almost exactly the same as that of the controls, but was very labile. After anaesthesia, however, the average resting blood pressure in the immunosympathectomised animals was 70 mm. Hg, whereas that of the controls was 100 mm. Hg. Moreover, it became very steady.

CARLSSON: Dr. ZAIMIS, could you qualify your statement that the cardiovascular system is free of noradrenaline? I think you showed that the intestine contained some 30% of the normal value. What about the intestinal vessels; did you look at them?

ZAIMIS: They don't appear to play any significant role.

CARLSSON: I think the vessels of the splanchnic area are very important.

ZAIMIS: They aren't. The results we have obtained by tilting the animals were quite impressive in comparison with those obtained in the control rats. Fig. 2 illustrates results of experiments in which tilting was applied to control and immunosympathectomised animals. Pentobarbitone anaesthesia was used. The top tracing shows that in the control animals, while anaesthesia was deep, tilting induced a significant fall in blood pressure. As anaesthesia became lighter, however, tilting became less and less effective because of the return of the vasoconstrictor reflexes. In contrast, in the immunosympathectomised animals, tilting continued to produce a significant fall in blood pressure even during light anaesthesia.

Influence of sleep on circulation in normal and hypertensive animals

By

A. Zanchetti, M. Guazzi, and G. Baccelli

1. Introduction

Until recently, the difficulty of simulating in the laboratory the conditions prevailing in the human body in health or disease has been an obstacle to the study of normal body functions. It is obvious that however much the information obtained by research on perfused organs, eviscerated preparations, and even on intact but anaesthetised animals may contribute towards our understanding of the basic mechanisms and functional relationships, it does not necessarily explain what happens in the intact non-anaesthetised animal or the human subject.

Recent technical developments have made it much easier to study circulatory events in the free-moving animal. Although, in the long run, a deeper knowledge of circulatory functions as they occur under normal conditions of life may help us to discover the whys and the hows of several cardiovascular diseases, including arterial hypertension, there is no doubt that studies on intact animals can be of more immediate value to the pharmacologist as a means of assessing the properties and the efficacy of drugs that may subsequently be given to human beings; and they can also help the clinician to judge the significance of his cruder measurements on the patient.

The study of circulation in the normal, unrestrained animal during sleep seemed likely to provide a suitable first approach to the investigation of circulatory events under normal conditions, not only because sleep occupies such a large part of our daily life, but more particularly because in recent years the mechanisms of wakefulness and sleep have been intensively investigated, and, in many respects, elucidated (*34, 39, 47*). As the mechanisms of sleep are fundamentally neural in character, sleep may well be an ideal condition in which to study the scope of neural control of the circulation, both in naturally occurring physiological situations and situations where the normal circulatory patterns are disrupted by experimentally induced alterations.

Before talking about circulation, we shall briefly summarise the recent additions to our knowledge of the mechanisms of sleep. Both in the lower mammals and in man, sleep is made up of two rather different conditions, or stages, which alternate regularly. The stage which occupies the longer portion of the time devoted to sleep was, until a few years ago, considered to be the only type of physiological sleep. It is characterised by the appearance of slow waves and spindle bursts in the electro-encephalogram (E.E.G.) recorded from the neocortex, irregular activity in the hippocampus, and a decrease in, though not the disappearance of, electrical activity in the posterior cervical muscles, marking a decrease in, but, once again, not the complete disappearance of, postural tonus. During this stage, the cat is commonly in a relaxed, curled position, with closed eyes. This condition is regularly interrupted, at intervals of 30–60 minutes or more, by shorter periods (ranging in duration from less than one minute to 10–15 minutes), during which the E.E.G. changes to fast, low-voltage activity, indistinguishable from that typical of the waking state. From the hippocampus a regular 4–5/sec. rhythm, known as a "theta" rhythm, is recorded, and intermittent spiky waves can be picked up from the pontine tegmentum. At the beginning of each of these episodes of sleep, the electrical activity recorded from the neck muscles completely disappears. This coincides with the loss of postural tonus and the slow fall of the animal's head. Simultaneously, the otherwise quiet behaviour is frequently interrupted by bursts of clonic movements of the eyeballs, face, and limbs. Curiously enough, although associated with an activated E.E.G., this type of sleep is, at least in the cat, deeper than that characterised by slow waves and spindles. since the threshold for sensory or reticularly induced arousal is remarkably raised. This stage of sleep has been given various names, such as "activated", "paradoxical", and "rapid-eye-movement" (R.E.M.) sleep, but we shall refer to it simply as "deep" sleep and call the other type of sleep, in which the E.E.G. shows synchronous waves, "light" sleep.

It has been known for several years that arterial pressure decreases to some extent during sleep, both in experimental animals and in man (*23*, *27*, *46*). Quite recently, Rossi's group in Italy (*5*, *8*) as well as Kanzow and co-workers (*24*) in Germany carried out a more thorough study of blood-pressure changes during sleep. Both groups of investigators agree that only a slight decrease in arterial blood pressure occurs in cats during light sleep, when the E.E.G. shows synchronous, slow waves and electromyographic activity in the neck indicates persistence of postural tone. A more marked fall, of 20—30 and sometimes 40 mm. Hg, is observed only during the recurrent episodes of deep sleep, when the E.E.G. is desynchronised, the cervical electromyogram is flattened, and bursts of rapid eye movements occur. During this kind of sleep, marked fluctuations in arterial pressure and heart rate are often recorded (*13*), such as have also been observed in normal human subjects (*43*).

All the above-mentioned observations, however interesting and stimulating they may be, are rather incomplete, since most of them are derived from studies carried out to investigate neurophysiological rather than circulatory problems. Consequently, we set out to achieve a better, and more detailed, quantitative assessment of the circulatory changes occurring throughout the wakefulness-sleep cycle in intact, normotensive animals (*18*, *19*) and in animals rendered hypertensive either by constriction of the renal arteries (Guazzi et al., in preparation) or by bilateral sino-aortic deafferentation (*18*, *19*).

All our investigations were performed in free-moving cats, and blood pressure was recorded by means of a thin polyethylene tube with an inner diameter of 1.5 mm. which was permanently implanted in a femoral artery and connected to a variable-inductance transducer (Sanborn 267 B) located a short distance from the animal. Injections of heparin (25 mg. twice daily) were administered to prevent clotting of the blood. In this way we were able to obtain a faithful record of systolic and diastolic blood pressures throughout the experiment. The cats were placed in a sound-attenuating, electrically insulated and illuminated cage, and their behaviour was observed through a large unidirectional glass window. To enable us to identify the various stages throughout the wakefulness-sleep cycle, each animal had screw-type electrodes implanted and cemented in place in the skull and in the floor of both frontal sinuses; electrical activity in the right and left cerebral cortices, and eye movements, could thus be regularly recorded. The electromyogram from the neck was obtained by means of two needles, permanently inserted into the paravertebral musculature.

2. Arterial pressure during sleep in intact, normotensive cats

Our observations in intact cats have basically confirmed the previous reports by Candia et al. (*8*) and Kanzow et al. (*24*). Light sleep was accompanied by a slight decrease in arterial pressure, whereas more consistent falls occurred only during episodes of deep sleep, at the end of which blood pressure reverted to levels similar to those recorded before the onset of deep sleep. An example of hypotension and increased blood-pressure variability during an episode of deep sleep is given in Fig. 1.

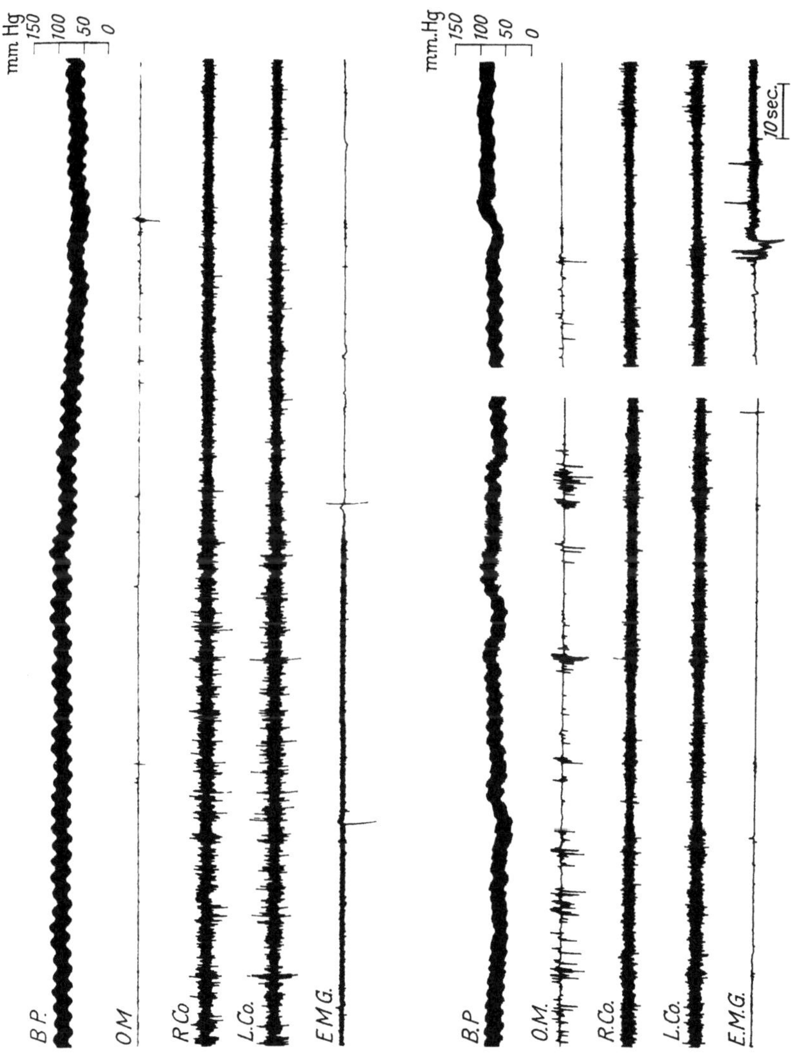

Fig. 1. Arterial-pressure fall during deep sleep in an intact, normotensive cat. Here, as in Figs 4, 5, and 7, the following abbreviations have been used: B.P.: femoral arterial pressure; O.M.: ocular movements; R.Co. and L.Co.: activity of right and left cerebral cortices; E.M.G.: electromyogram of the neck [by courtesy of Arch. ital. biol. (19)].

Less anecdotal information was obtained, however, by statistical analysis of all the data gathered, providing a detailed quantitative assessment of blood-pressure changes in sleep. Up to now, no such assessment has been available. Means and standard errors of the mean of systolic and diastolic arterial pressure during different stages of the wakefulness-sleep cycle have been calculated from pooled observations in normotensive cats and are shown in Table 1. Blood-pressure differences at the various stages of sleep

Table 1. *Arterial pressure during sleep: intact, normotensive animals*

	n.	Mean (mm. Hg)	S.E. (mm. Hg)	P.
Systolic B.P.				
Waking	22	118.0	4.8	<0.005
Light sleep lowest . .	82	102.0	2.4	<N. S.
Light sleep final . . .	82	106.5	2.5	<N. S.
Deep sleep initial. . .	82	110.3	2.4	<0.001
Deep sleep lowest . .	82	85.5	2.1	<0.001
Deep sleep arousal . .	82	108.4	2.5	N. S.
After deep sleep . . .	82	104.9	2.2	
Light sleep range. . .	82	8.9	0.8	<0.001
Deep sleep range . . .	82	20.6	1.4	
Diastolic B.P.				
Waking.	22	67.2	2.6	<0.05
Light sleep lowest . .	82	59.5	1.5	<N. S.
Light sleep final . . .	82	62.7	1.6	<N. S.
Deep sleep initial. . .	82	65.4	1.7	<0.001
Deep sleep lowest . .	82	46.8	1.7	<0.001
Deep sleep arousal . .	82	65.7	1.6	N. S.
After deep sleep . . .	82	62.8	1.5	
Light sleep range. . .	82	5.7	0.6	<0.001
Deep sleep range . . .	82	17.4	1.3	

N. S.: not significant

have been evaluated by analysis of variance, and the results reported as probability in the last column of Table 1. The following measurements have been entered in the tables: 1) blood pressures during quiet wakefulness at the beginning of each recording session (*Waking*); 2) lowest blood pressures recorded during each period of light sleep (*Light sleep lowest*); 3) blood pressures occurring during light sleep, two minutes before the overt beginning of each episode of deep sleep (*Light sleep final*); 4) blood pressures at the exact moment when electro-encephalographic desynchronisation and electromyographic flattening appeared (*Deep sleep initial*); 5) lowest blood pressures recorded during each episode of deep sleep (*Deep sleep lowest*); 6) blood pressures at the moment of arousal from deep sleep (*Deep sleep arousal*); 7) blood pressures two minutes after the end of each episode of deep sleep (*After deep sleep*). The last two measurements in Table 1 (*Light sleep range* and *Deep sleep range*) have been used as criteria for assessing blood-pressure variability during the conditions of light and deep sleep, and represent the difference between the highest and the lowest blood pressures recorded during each period of light and deep sleep respectively.

It will be seen from Table 1 that in normotensive animals, when light sleep supervened, both systolic and diastolic blood pressures decreased slightly as compared with the values observed during quiet wakefulness. Towards the end of light sleep and at the very beginning of each episode of deep sleep, systolic and diastolic pressures tended to rise, but the increases were too small and inconstant to be statistically significant. On the other hand, the fall in blood pressure during deep sleep was definite, though never

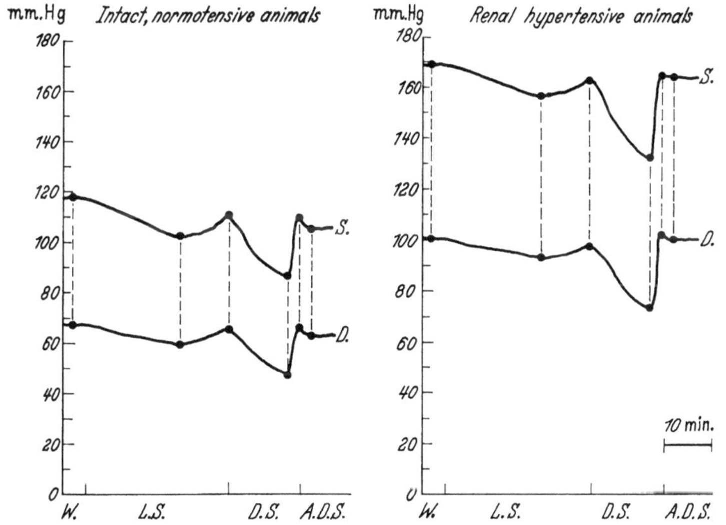

Fig. 2. Schematic representation of systolic (upper lines) and diastolic (lower lines) blood pressure during the wakefulness-sleep cycle in intact, normotensive (left) and renal hypertensive (right) cats. Here, as in Figs 3 and 6, W. denotes wakefulness, L.S. light sleep, D.S. deep sleep, and A.D.S. after deep sleep (from GUAZZI et al., in preparation).

dramatic: on the average, systolic and diastolic pressures fell by 24.8 and 18.6 mm. Hg respectively. At the end of each episode of deep sleep, blood pressure rose again; the levels recorded two minutes later were still about the same and not significantly different from those measured during light sleep, just before the onset of the deep-sleep episode. Blood-pressure variability was not marked during light sleep, but was more pronounced during deep sleep.

The changes in systolic and diastolic arterial pressure occurring during the various stages of sleep in intact, normotensive cats are shown graphically in the left half of Fig. 2, in which the mean values contained in Table 1 have been plotted.

3. Arterial pressure during sleep in renal hypertensive cats

Arterial pressure during sleep has so far been studied in five cats rendered hypertensive by constriction of both renal arteries with Goldblatt's clamps. Polyethylene catheters were implanted in the femoral arteries, and arterial-pressure changes during wakefulness and sleep recorded for a total of 31 cycles, from three to four weeks after clamping of the renal arteries. At that time, systolic and diastolic arterial pressures during quiet wakefulness at the beginning of each recording session varied respectively between 156 and 200 mm. Hg and 96 and 108 mm. Hg, the corresponding mean values being 169.4 and 100.8 mm. Hg.

The results of a quantitative assessment of blood-pressure changes occurring during sleep in renal hypertensive cats, as compared with changes observed in intact, normotensive cats under similar conditions, are summarised in Table 2. Comparison between the two groups of animals was made by analysis of variance. A slight decrease in both systolic and diastolic blood pressures was also observed in renal hypertensive cats; but blood pressure remained at hypertensive levels throughout light sleep and, furthermore, rose slightly at the very beginning of each episode of deep sleep. A marked fall in systolic and diastolic blood pressures also occurred during deep sleep in renal hypertensive cats, but this was not significantly greater than in the normotensive group: the average fall in systolic pressure was 31.5 mm. Hg in hypertensive, and 24.8 mm. Hg in normotensive cats, whereas the corresponding falls in diastolic pressure were, on the average, 24.4 mm. Hg and 18.6 mm. Hg. Consequently, even the lowest pressures measured during deep sleep in renal hypertensive cats were not only considerably higher than those measured in normotensive cats during comparable episodes of deep sleep, but also slightly higher than the blood-pressure values shown by normotensive cats during quiet wakefulness.

At the end of each episode of deep sleep, blood pressure reverted to the higher values recorded before the onset of deep sleep in renal hypertensive animals also. Pressure variability was no greater in renal hypertensive cats than in intact ones, during either light or deep sleep.

Table 2. *Blood pressure during sleep in normotensive and renal hypertensive cats*

	Intact animals			Renal hypertension			P.
	n.	Mean (mm. Hg)	S.E. (mm. Hg)	n.	Mean (mm. Hg)	S.E. (mm. Hg)	
Systolic B.P.							
Waking	22	118.0	4.8	5	169.4	—	—
Light sleep lowest .	82	102.0	2.4	31	157.1	2.3	<0.001
Deep sleep initial .	82	110.3	2.4	31	162.6	2.5	<0.001
Deep sleep lowest .	82	85.5	2.1	31	131.5	2.5	<0.001
Deep sleep arousal.	82	108.4	2.5	31	163.4	2.0	<0.001
After deep sleep. .	82	104.9	2.2	31	163.0	2.0	<0.001
Light sleep range .	82	8.9	0.8	31	9.5	1.2	N. S.
Deep sleep range .	82	20.6	1.4	31	23.2	2.4	N. S.
Diastolic B.P.							
Waking	22	67.2	2.6	5	100.8	—	—
Light sleep lowest .	82	59.5	1.5	31	92.5	1.1	<0.001
Deep sleep initial .	82	65.4	1.7	31	97.0	1.2	<0.001
Deep sleep lowest .	82	46.8	1.3	31	72.6	1.9	<0.001
Deep sleep arousal.	82	65.7	1.6	31	101.2	1.6	<0.001
After deep sleep. .	82	62.8	1.5	31	99.4	1.7	<0.001
Light sleep range .	82	5.7	0.6	31	7.8	1.3	N. S.
Deep sleep range .	82	17.4	1.3	31	24.7	2.6	<0.01

N. S.: not significant

The data reported in Table 2 have been summarised in Fig. 2. It will be seen that in renal hypertensive animals both systolic and diastolic blood pressures fell slightly during light sleep and more markedly during deep sleep, but always remained at much higher levels than in intact animals under comparable conditions.

4. Arterial pressure during sleep in cats subjected to sino-aortic deafferentation

The effects of sino-aortic deafferentation on arterial-pressure changes during sleep were investigated in 14 otherwise intact cats; six were studied both before and after deafferentation, and eight after deafferentation only. The latter procedure was performed under pentobarbitone anaesthesia (30 mg./kg. intraperitoneally) and consisted in cutting both carotid sinus nerves and in carefully stripping the carotid sinus walls. The aortic nerves were isolated from the cervical vagal trunks and bilaterally severed. Cardiopulmonary afferents in the vagi were left intact to avoid the adverse effects of bilateral vagotomy. All of the animals were studied from three to 11 days after sino-aortic deafferentation.

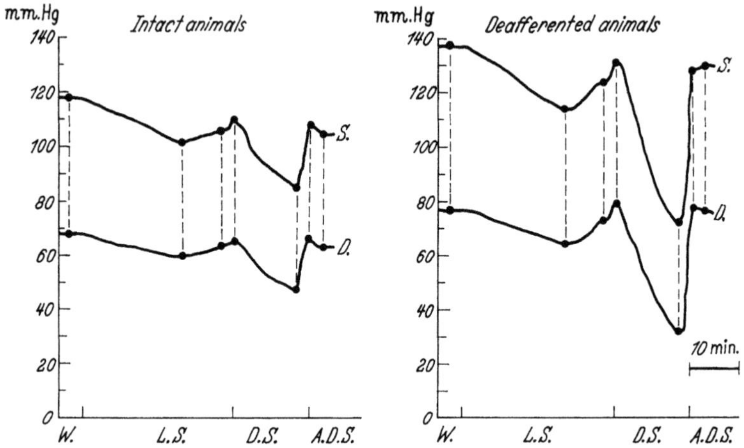

Fig. 3. Schematic representation of systolic (upper lines) and diastolic (lower lines) blood pressure during the wakefulness-sleep cycle in cats with intact sino-aortic reflexes (left) and in cats after sino-aortic deafferentation (right) [by courtesy of Arch. ital. biol. (*19*)].

A glance at Fig. 3 will suffice to show the main differences in the blood-pressure behaviour during sleep between cats with intact sino-aortic reflexes and cats in which these reflexes had been eliminated. Systolic and diastolic blood pressures were slightly, but significantly, higher in deafferented than in intact animals, both during quiet wakefulness (W.) and throughout light sleep (L.S.), although in the latter condition a consistent decrease in pressure usually occurred in deafferented animals also. In spite of the fact that higher pressures were still observed in deafferented cats at the end of light sleep and at the beginning of deep sleep (D.S.), such surprisingly large falls were recorded during the course of deep-sleep episodes that arterial pressure finally attained much lower absolute levels in deafferented than in intact animals. At the end of deep-sleep episodes, the blood pressure usually reverted to levels significantly, though moderately, higher than those recorded in intact animals under similar conditions.

In Table 3, the means and standard errors of the mean of arterial pressure during various stages of the wakefulness-sleep cycle have been compared in cats with intact sino-aortic reflexes and in cats subjected to sino-aortic deafferentation. The last column on the right shows the results of an analysis of variance. Throughout quiet wakefulness and light sleep, as well as at, and after, the end of episodes of deep sleep, both systolic and diastolic

Table 3. *Arterial pressure during sleep in intact and deafferented cats*

	Intact			Deafferented			P.
	n.	Mean (mm. Hg)	S.E. (mm. Hg)	n.	Mean (mm. Hg)	S.E. (mm. Hg)	
Systolic B.P.							
Waking	22	118.0	4.8	18	138.1	5.0	<0.01
Light sleep lowest .	82	102.0	2.4	142	114.1	1.9	<0.001
Light sleep final . .	82	106.5	2.5	142	124.4	2.2	<0.001
Deep sleep initial .	82	110.3	2.4	145	131.2	2.6	<0.001
Deep sleep lowest .	82	85.5	2.1	145	71.8	1.9	<0.001
Deep sleep arousal .	82	108.4	2.5	145	128.6	2.3	<0.001
After deep sleep . .	82	104.9	2.2	143	129.9	2.4	<0.001
Light sleep range .	82	8.9	0.8	142	18.0	1.5	<0.005
Deep sleep range .	82	20.6	1.4	145	40.5	2.6	<0.001
Diastolic B.P.							
Waking	22	67.2	2.6	18	76.1	3.5	<0.05
Light sleep lowest .	82	59.5	1.5	142	63.6	1.5	N. S.
Light sleep final . .	82	62.7	1.6	142	71.9	1.7	<0.001
Deep sleep initial .	82	65.4	1.7	145	78.4	2.1	<0.001
Deep sleep lowest .	82	46.8	1.7	145	30.9	1.3	<0.001
Deep sleep arousal .	82	65.7	1.6	145	77.3	2.0	<0.001
After deep sleep . .	82	62.8	1.5	143	76.3	2.0	<0.001
Light sleep range .	82	5.7	0.6	142	14.9	1.2	<0.001
Deep sleep range .	82	17.4	1.3	145	34.1	2.3	<0.001

N. S.: not significant

pressures are slightly but consistently higher in deafferented than in intact animals. Differences between the means range from 12 to 25 mm. Hg. Only during the course of deep sleep do systolic and diastolic pressures reach definitely lower levels in deafferented than in intact cats. The differences between the two groups become particularly striking when we compare the magnitude of the blood-pressure falls recorded during deep sleep (computed by subtracting Deep-sleep-lowest from Deep-sleep-initial values): the respective average falls in systolic and diastolic pressure are 24.8 and 18.6 mm. Hg in intact, and 59.4 and 47.5 mm. Hg in deafferented cats. In the latter group — as shown in Table 3 — variability of blood-pressure values is markedly increased, both in light and in deep sleep, the mean values of the ranges being at least twice as large as in intact animals.

Actual recordings made in one cat before and after sino-aortic deafferentation are shown in Fig. 4. These conform to the pattern illustrated in Fig. 3.

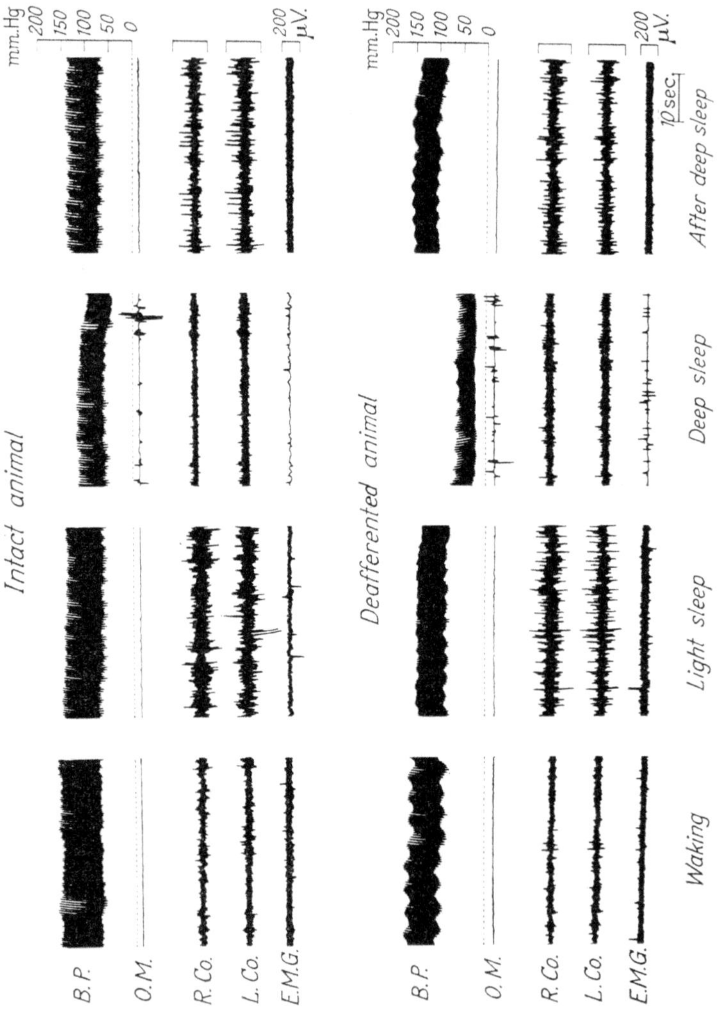

Fig. 4. Blood pressure during various stages of the wakefulness-sleep cycle before and after sino-aortic deafferentation. Recordings in both upper and lower halves are taken from the same cat [by courtesy of Arch. ital. biol. (*19*)].

Not infrequently, the blood-pressure values recorded in deafferented cats during deep sleep were low enough to endanger their lives. In several instances, when the lowest blood-pressure levels were recorded and, particularly, whenever diastolic blood pressure approached or attained 0 mm. Hg, signs of cerebral ischaemia became manifest. Fig. 5 shows the records of a deafferented cat in which the beginning of an episode of deep sleep, characterised by cortical desynchronisation, electromyographic flattening, and rapid eye movements, was associated with a decrease in

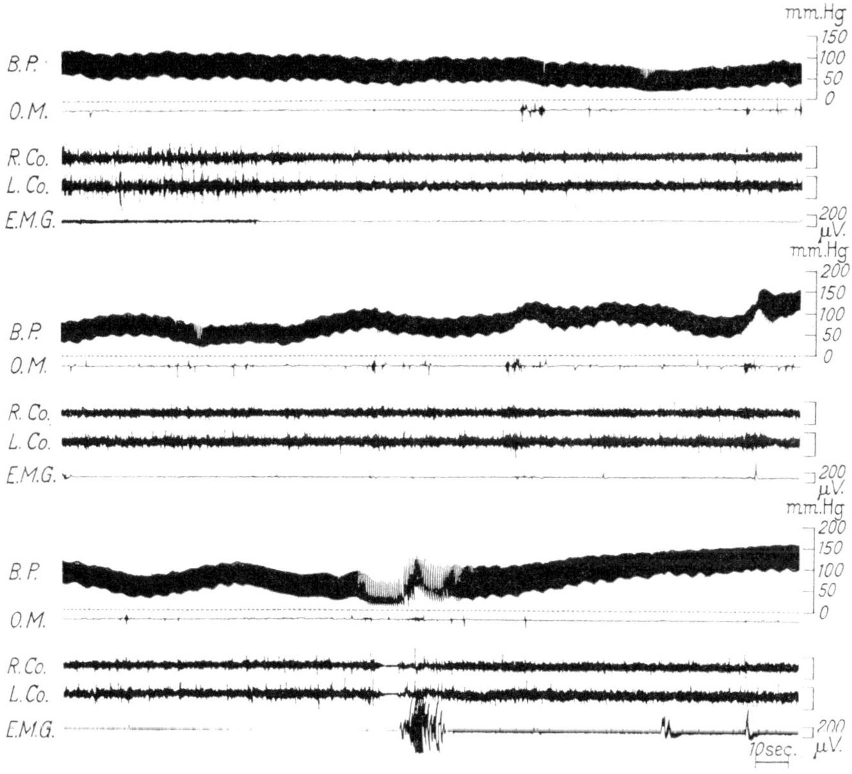

Fig. 5. Episode of transient cerebral ischaemia during deep sleep in a cat with sino-aortic deafferentation [by courtesy of Arch. ital. biol. (*19*)].

systolic and diastolic blood pressures from initial values of 115 and 60 mm. Hg respectively. Blood pressure soon became conspicuously irregular and fluctuated markedly throughout the eight-minute duration of this episode, systolic and diastolic levels as low as 70 and 25 mm. Hg, and as high as 160 and 120 mm. Hg being observed. Finally, when diastolic blood pressure had fallen to levels of only 10–15 mm. Hg, the electrocorticogram rapidly flattened, and generalised seizures ensued (note the large artefact in the E.M.G. lead); suddenly, the arterial pressure showed a prolonged, hypertensive rebound, and the animal awoke in fright, the electro-encephalogram promptly resuming its normal "waking" appearance. The slow, persistent increase in blood pressure after arousal from deep sleep might, in this instance, result from adrenaline secretion.

It should be emphasised that these dramatic signs of transient cerebral ischaemia, though observed only in a few deafferented cats (and in these animals during only a few episodes of deep sleep), never occurred either in our group of intact cats or in several hundred normal cats whose behaviour during sleep was recently studied in our laboratory.

5. Effects of sino-aortic deafferentation on arterial pressure in renal hypertensive cats during sleep

Some of the renal hypertensive cats were subsequently subjected to sino-aortic deafferentation, which was found to cause a further marked increase in both systolic and diastolic pressures, thus confirming previous reports by other authors (*25, 26, 30*).

Table 4. *Arterial pressure during sleep in a renal hypertensive cat before and after sino-aortic deafferentation*

Cat 52	Intact			Deafferented			P.
	n.	Mean (mm. Hg)	S.E. (mm. Hg)	n.	Mean (mm. Hg)	S.E. (mm. Hg)	
Systolic B.P.							
Waking	1	175.0	—	3	217.0	—	—
Light sleep lowest .	8	155.5	3.0	15	144.5	3.9	N. S.
Deep sleep initial .	8	160.6	1.6	15	183.1	3.7	<0.001
Deep sleep lowest .	8	124.0	2.6	15	78.8	3.8	<0.001
Deep sleep arousal .	8	165.1	2.6	15	177.8	6.7	<N. S.
Light sleep range .	8	16.1	2.3	15	40.4	3.1	<0.001
Deep sleep range .	8	29.4	3.7	15	54.9	8.9	N. S.
Diastolic B.P.							
Waking	1	105.0	—	3	153.0	—	—
Light sleep lowest .	8	95.4	2.2	15	94.0	2.5	N. S.
Deep sleep initial .	8	100.9	2.1	15	128.1	3.0	<0.001
Deep sleep lowest .	8	73.6	1.9	15	39.7	3.4	<0.001
Deep sleep arousal .	8	112.0	2.1	15	131.1	5.2	<0.05
Light sleep range .	8	14.5	3.2	15	35.5	2.4	<0.001
Deep sleep range .	8	28.1	2.4	15	52.8	8.7	N. S.

N. S.: not significant

Table 4 exemplifies what happened in one of these animals. The increase in blood pressure was clear-cut under the conditions of quiet wakefulness taken as the starting point of our recording session, but was even more conspicuous when the animal explored its environment or was excited by some novel stimulus. No significant change in the level to which arterial pressure fell during light sleep was noted after deafferentation, but the levels of blood pressure recorded at the beginning of deep sleep were higher after deafferentation than before. The moderate fall in systolic and diastolic pressures observed in the renal hypertensive cat with intact sino-aortic reflexes (36.6 and 27.3 mm. Hg) changed to a conspicuous, often precipitous, fall after sino-aortic deafferentation: on the average, systolic pressure was reduced by 104.3 mm. Hg,

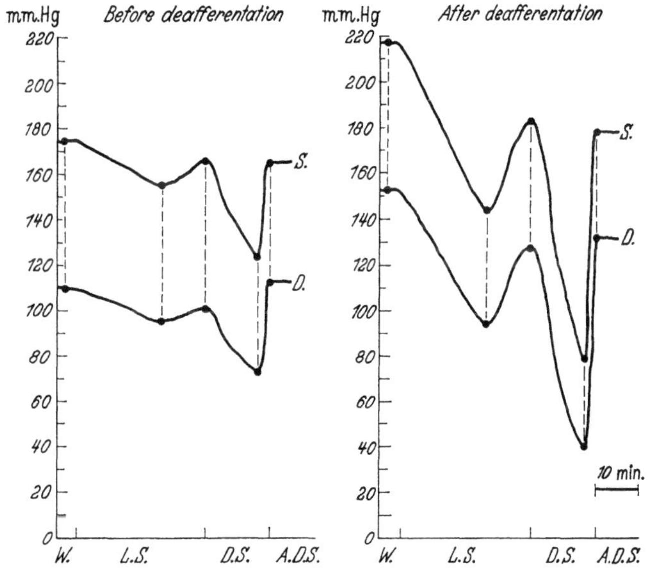

Fig. 6. Schematic representation of systolic (upper lines) and diastolic (lower lines) blood pressure during the wakefulness-sleep cycle in a renal hypertensive cat before (left) and after (right) sino-aortic deafferentation (from GUAZZI et al., in preparation).

and diastolic pressure by 88.4 mm. Hg. Thus, in renal hypertensive animals, as in cats without interference to the renal circulation, blood pressure during deep sleep reaches much lower absolute levels after deafferentation than before, hypertensive levels being promptly restored at the very end of each episode of deep sleep.

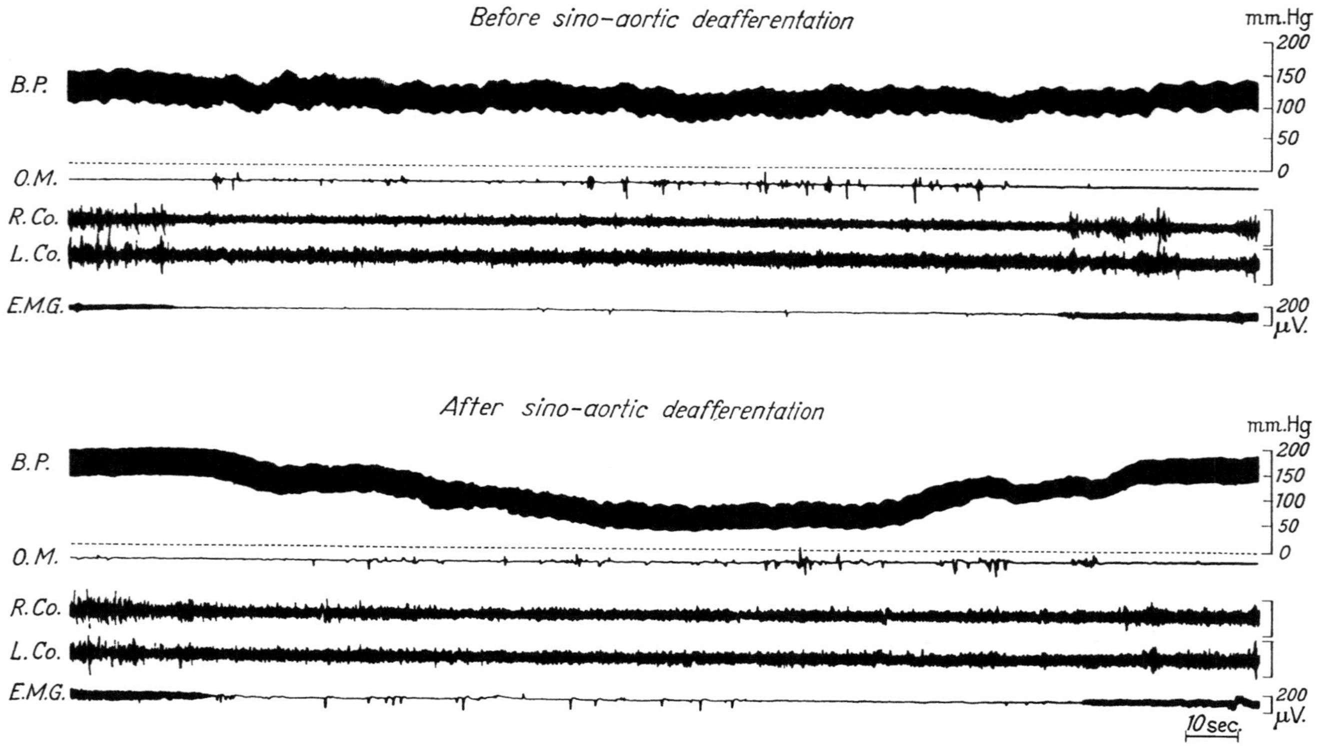

Fig. 7. Blood-pressure fall during deep sleep in a renal hypertensive cat before (upper half) and after (lower half) sino-aortic deafferentation (from GUAZZI et al., in preparation).

The effects of sino-aortic deafferentation on the arterial pressure of renal hypertensive animals during sleep have been summarised in Fig. 6, using the mean values contained in Table 4. The blood-pressure changes during two episodes of deep sleep of comparable durations (slightly less than three minutes) are illustrated in Fig. 7, the former having been observed before sino-aortic deafferentation and the latter after interruption of these reflexes in the same renal hypertensive cat. Both systolic and diastolic pressures fell slightly (from 155 to 115 and from 100 to 70 mm. Hg respectively) when the sino-aortic reflexes were intact, whereas a dramatic drop (from 185 to 75 and from 130 to 35 mm. Hg respectively) was observed after deafferentation.

6. Discussion

The fact that arterial pressure decreases during sleep, and particularly during deep sleep, in the intact, normotensive cat, indicates that the neural mechanisms of sleep also involve cardiovascular regulation, and that sleep is one of the behavioural conditions in which neural regulation of circulation plays an important role. A complete haemodynamic picture of what happens during deep sleep is not yet available: we do not know whether the conspicuous decrease in systolic and diastolic arterial pressures is due more to peripheral vasodilatation than to a decrease in cardiac output. The latter effect is likely to occur, at least in some degree, since a marked bradycardia is always apparent and pulse pressure is often reduced; but it is impossible to say to what extent the probable fall in cardiac output is due to a direct effect upon the heart rather than to a decreased venous return. Until the results of current studies using implanted electromagnetic flow-meters and cardiac-denervation techniques are available, this important point will remain unsettled.

It is impossible to say at present whether the neurogenic mechanisms affecting circulation during deep sleep merely remove a tonic facilitating influence acting on pressor centres, such as the medullary vasomotor centre, or whether they actively inhibit the vasomotor centre, the spinal preganglionic neurones, or other structures which have pressor effects. However, the latter hypothesis seems to be the more likely, by analogy with the recent findings of Pompeiano and co-workers (*14*, *15*, *16*), who have shown that active inhibition of spinal somatic reflexes occurs during deep sleep.

In renal hypertensive cats, three to four weeks after bilateral constriction of the renal arteries, arterial-pressure changes during sleep were found to be quite similar, both in direction and in magnitude, to those recorded in intact cats. Therefore blood pressure, though variable during the wakefulness-sleep cycle, was continuously higher than in normotensive animals.

The effects of sino-aortic deafferentation on blood pressure during quiet wakefulness and sleep require a somewhat longer commentary. Our extensive studies on non-anaesthetised, unrestrained cats carrying an implanted arterial cannula have shown that a consistent increase in both systolic and diastolic blood pressures occurs during quiet wakefulness after sino-aortic deafferentation. However, this increase was quite moderate in our animals, measuring about 20 mm. Hg. We do not know whether the moderate degree of this rise is attributable to the fact that deafferentation was incomplete, as we have never cut the afferent vagal fibres from the heart and lungs which exert a tonic reflex inhibition on cardiovascular centres similar to that produced by fibres from the carotid sinus and the aortic area (*6*, *17*, *28*, *29*). Alternatively, one might suppose that the pressor effects of chronic sino-aortic deafferentation can be seen to a marked degree only in those conditions of excited wakefulness in which they have mostly been tested in the past, when the arterial pressure of the chronically studied animal was usually measured soon after direct arterial puncture (*21*, *22*).

Our observations in cats have shown that arterial pressure is not found to be steadily increased after deafferentation; it diminishes to some degree during light sleep, although the values recorded then are still moderately, but significantly, higher than in normotensive animals with intact reflexes under similar conditions of sleep. This agrees with what was reported by Samaan (*40*) on the heart rate of chronically deafferented dogs. Whether a similar decrease in arterial pressure in sleeping deafferented dogs was observed, or simply inferred, by Samaan (*40*) and Heymans and Bouckaert (*20*) is not clear from the papers published by these authors. Quantitative analysis of our data, however, indicates that such a fall definitely takes place.

The instability of the pressure rise following sino-aortic deafferentation is further emphasised by our observation that, in deafferented animals, blood pressure falls during deep sleep to levels which are considerably lower than those found in animals with intact reflexes and are often near to, and sometimes beyond, the threshold value for cerebral anoxia. Since section of the carotid sinus and aortic nerves interrupts both pressoreceptor and chemoreceptor fibres, we cannot conclude that abolition of the pressoreceptor rather than the chemoreceptor reflexes is responsible for the falls in systolic and diastolic pressure to such dramatically low levels. However, it is obviously difficult to explain the occurrence of lower pressures in deafferented than in intact animals, by reference either to the classical conception that pressoreceptor inactivation releases pressor centres from a tonic inhibitory inflow or to the current opinion that the role of chemoreceptors in circulatory regulation is limited to such emergencies as acute anoxia or shock.

This brings us to our preliminary observations on the effect of sino-aortic deafferentation in renal hypertensive animals. There has been a lot of talk about the persistence or reappearance of neurogenic control of circulation during early or late stages of experimental renal hypertension. Obviously, no definitive conclusions could be arrived at by such crude means of abolishing neural tone as pithing (*9*, *44*, *45*) or the administration of ganglionic blocking and other drugs (*1*, *35*, *36*, *37*, *41*). Even more delicate methods, such as cocainisation of the fourth ventricle floor combined with upright tilting of the animal, which we employed several years ago (*1*, *2*), or chemical (*31*) or electrical (*4*) stimulation of the carotid sinuses, are quite artificial and do not permit one to draw quantitative conclusions.

On the other hand, the conspicuous depressor influence which is active during deep sleep and greatly exaggerated after sino-aortic deafferentation provides an invaluable means of testing, even quantitatively, the importance of the neural regulation of circulation in a completely physiological state and during a common physiological event.

In renal hypertension, the marked fall in blood pressure to normotensive, or even hypotensive, levels during deep sleep, when sino-aortic reflexes are interrupted, demonstrates that — at least, three or four weeks after clamping of the renal arteries — neural control of the circulation is functioning with great efficiency or is re-established to a marked degree, although its activity is largely obscured by homoeostatic mechanisms when the sino-aortic reflexes are intact.

The persistence of a normally effective neurogenic tone simultaneously with increased production of a peripherally acting substance like angiotensin can perhaps be explained by one of the two following hypotheses. According to the recent work of McCubbin and Page (*32*) and to data of Benelli et al. (*3*), angiotensin would act at the peripheral nerve-endings by promoting a greater output of endogenous neurotransmitter, thus intensifying the effectiveness of neurogenic vasomotor activity. Although this suggestive hypothesis may well explain at least part of the maintained neurogenic vasoconstriction in renal hypertension, other alternative mechanisms should be given careful consideration. One of the facts emerging from the mass of interesting information accumulated in FOLKOW's laboratory (see *11*) is that in any given vascular circuit the capacitance vessels have a much lower threshold to vasoconstrictor-fibre activity than the resistance vessels (*33*). Moreover, venous control is almost entirely dominated by its extrinsic nervous supply, while other types of control, such as autoregulation and local accumulation of metabolites, are essentially confined to the precapillary resistance vessels (*12*). Finally, in contrast with the action of noradrenaline, when angiotensin is given in such concentrations as may be expected to occur in certain types of hypertensive disease, its vasoconstrictor activity is practically confined to resistance vessels, the effects on the venous side being negligible (*10*). That both pressoreceptor and chemoreceptor reflexes play an important role in the regulation of venous tone is also clearly established (*7*). It is therefore conceivable that in the renal hypertensive animal, while resistance vessels are continuously under the direct control of angiotensin, overriding the neurogenic arteriolar constriction, capacitance vessels are still subject to neurogenic control only. Therefore, whenever the neural depressor influence of deep sleep is fully released as a result of sino-aortic deafferentation and practically abolishes vasoconstrictor tone, blood is pooled in the dilated capacitance vessels. Consequently, cardiac output is dramatically reduced and blood pressure falls to very low levels, in spite of the persisting arteriolar constriction due to angiotensin.

There is no time now to discuss the extent to which these data relating to cats may be compared with preliminary observations of blood-pressure changes during sleep in normal human subjects and in hypertensive patients (*38, 42, 43*). This may be a good subject for subsequent discussion. However, in spite of the fact that this symposium bears the sub-title "*Principles and Practice*", we are well aware of Dr. JOHNSON's observation that "nature has taken sufficient care that theory shall have little influence upon practice" — a wise comment which makes one doubt whether there will be much to compare between our present data on cats and what we know now of human hypertension.

Summary

1. Blood-pressure changes during quiet wakefulness and sleep have been studied in non-anaesthetised, unrestrained cats carrying an implanted polyethylene cannula in a femoral artery and various electrodes fixed to the skull and neck to permit electro-encephalographic, electro-oculographic, and electromyographic recordings to be made.

2. In intact, normotensive cats, both systolic and diastolic blood pressures decreased slightly, but significantly, during light sleep (i.e. sleep characterised by synchronous E.E.G. waves), while a much larger fall was only observed during deep sleep (i.e. sleep characterised by a desynchronised E.E.G. and rapid eye movements).

3. In cats rendered hypertensive by bilateral renal artery stenosis, systolic and diastolic blood pressures, although subject to some decrease during light and particularly during deep sleep, always remained at much higher levels than those recorded in intact cats under comparable conditions.

4. In cats subjected to sino-aortic deafferentation but otherwise intact, blood pressure was slightly higher than in intact cats, both during quiet wakefulness and throughout light sleep. However, in deafferented animals, such surprisingly large falls were recorded during episodes of deep sleep that arterial pressure finally attained much lower absolute levels than in intact animals. In a few instances, when the lowest blood-pressure levels were recorded, signs of cerebral ischaemia (electro-encephalographic flattening and seizures) became manifest.

5. Some of the renal hypertensive animals were also subjected to sino-aortic deafferentation. In these cats, too, the moderate fall in systolic and diastolic blood pressures observed during deep sleep before sino-aortic deafferantation changed to a dramatic fall when the sino-aortic reflexes were interrupted.

6. It is suggested that sleep may be a very convenient experimental condition for studying the importance of neural regulation of the circulation in normotensive and hypertensive animals.

Zusammenfassung

1. Im ruhigen Wachzustand und während des Schlafes wurden Blutdruckveränderungen an nicht narkotisierten, in ihrer Bewegung nicht eingeschränkten Katzen untersucht, denen eine Polyäthylenkanüle in eine Femoralarterie implantiert war, und bei denen verschiedene Elektroden auf der Schädeldecke und am Hals fixiert waren. Auf diese Weise ließen sich elektroenzephalographische, elektrookulographische und elektromyographische Aufzeichnungen vornehmen.

2. An intakten, normotonen Katzen nimmt im leichten Schlafzustand (charakterisiert durch synchrone EEG-Wellen) sowohl der systolische als auch der diastolische Blutdruck mäßig, aber signifikant ab. Ein wesentlich stärkerer Blutdruckabfall wird nur im tiefen Schlaf (charakterisiert durch ein desynchronisiertes EEG und rasche Augenbewegungen) beobachtet.

3. Bei Katzen mit Hochdruck nach doppelseitiger Nierenarterienstenose fiel der Blutdruck während leichtem und besonders während tiefem Schlaf zwar ebenfalls etwas ab, blieb jedoch immer auf wesentlich höheren Werten als bei intakten Katzen unter vergleichbaren Bedingungen.

4. Nach Durchschneidung der vom Sinus caroticus und Aortenbogen ausgehenden afferenten Nerven fand sich sowohl im ruhigen Wachzustand als auch während leichtem Schlaf ein etwas höherer Blutdruck als bei intakten Katzen. Bei deafferentierten Tieren war jedoch ein auffallend starker Blutdruckabfall im tiefen Schlafzustand zu beobachten, wobei der Druck wesentlich niedrigere absolute Werte erreichte als bei intakten Tieren. In einigen wenigen Fällen zeigten sich, wenn die tiefsten Blutdruckwerte registriert wurden, Zeichen zerebraler Ischämie (elektroenzephalographische Abflachung und Krämpfe).

5. Auch einige der renal-hypertonen Tiere wurden einer sino-aortalen Deafferentierung unterworfen. Bei ihnen ließ sich vor der Durchtrennung der Nerven ebenfalls ein mäßiger Abfall des systolischen und diastolischen Blutdrucks im tiefen Schlaf beobachten, dagegen ein dramatischer Abfall, wenn die sino-aortalen Reflexbahnen unterbrochen waren.

6. Die Befunde zeigen, daß der Schlafzustand eine sehr zweckmäßige experimentelle Bedingung darstellt, um die Bedeutung der nervösen Regulation des Kreislaufes beim normotonen und hypertonen Tier zu untersuchen.

Résumé

1. Les modifications de la tension artérielle au cours de l'état de veille tranquille et au cours du sommeil ont été étudiées chez le chat non anesthésié, n'étant soumis à aucune contrainte et portant un cathéter en polyéthylène dans l'artère fémorale, ainsi que différentes électrodes fixées au crâne et au cou aux fins d'enregistrements électro-encéphalographiques, électro-oculographiques et électro-myographiques.

2. Chez le chat intact, normotendu, à la fois la diastolique et la systolique s'abaissent de façon discrète mais significative au cours du sommeil léger (c'est-à-dire le sommeil caractérisé par des ondes lentes à l'E.E.G.), alors qu'une chute beaucoup plus importante n'a été observée qu'au cours du sommeil profond (c'est-à-dire caractérisé par des ondes rapides à l'E.E.G. et des mouvements rapides des yeux).

3. Chez le chat chez lequel on a provoqué une hypertension par sténose bilatérale des artères rénales, les pressions systolique et diastolique, bien que présentant également une certaine baisse au cours du sommeil léger et surtout du sommeil profond, restent toujours à des niveaux beaucoup plus élevés que ceux enregistrés chez le chat intact dans les mêmes conditions.

4. Chez le chat chez lequel on a pratiqué une dénervation sino-aortique, la pression artérielle s'est montrée légèrement plus élevée que chez le chat normal, à la fois au cours de l'état de veille tranquille et au cours du sommeil léger. Cependant, chez les animaux ainsi dénervés, on a observé au cours des épisodes de sommeil profond des chutes si importantes que la pression artérielle atteignait finalement des niveaux absolus beaucoup plus bas que chez l'animal intact. Dans quelques cas, lorsque les plus basses valeurs tensionnelles ont été enregistrées, sont apparus des signes manifestes d'ischémie cérébrale (aplatissement des ondes à l'E.E.G., convulsions).

5. Quelques-uns des animaux porteurs d'une hypertension rénale ont été aussi soumis à une dénervation sino-aortique. Chez ces animaux également la baisse modérée des pressions systolique et diastolique observée durant le sommeil profond avant la dénervation s'est transformée en des chutes impressionnantes lorsque les réflexes sino-aortiques ont été interrompus.

6. L'état de sommeil peut constituer une condition expérimentale très appropriée pour l'étude de l'importance de la régulation nerveuse de la circulation chez l'animal normo et hypertendu.

Acknowledgements

This research has been sponsored by the Air Force Office of Scientific Research under Grant AF EOAR 64-41 through the European Office of Aerospace Research (OAR), United States Air Force, and the Consiglio Nazionale delle Ricerche (Electrophysiology Group).

References

1. BARTORELLI, C., G. FOLLI, and A. ZANCHETTI: Fol. cardiol. **11**, 3 (1952). — 2. BARTORELLI, C., and A. ZANCHETTI: Compt. rend. Congr. Internat. Cardiol., Paris **2**, 263 (1950). — 3. BENELLI, G., D. DELLA BELLA, and A. GANDINI: Brit. J. Pharmacol. **22**, 211 (1964). — 4. BILGUTAY, A. M., and C. W. LILLEHEI: J. Amer. Med. Ass. **191**, 649 (1965). — 5. BONAMINI, F., V. DE CAROLIS, P. PASTORINO, and G. F. ROSSI: Riv. neurobiol. **8**, 394 (1962). — 6. BOYD, J. D., and G. P. MCCULLAGH: Quart. J. Exper. Physiol. **27**, 293 (1938). — 7. BRAUNWALD, E., J. ROSS, Jr., R. L. KAHLER, T. E. GAFFNEY, A. GOLDBLATT, and D. T. MASON: Circulation Res. **12**, 539 (1963). — 8. CANDIA, O., E. FAVALE, A. GIUSSANI, and G. F. ROSSI: Arch. ital. biol. **100**, 216 (1962). — 9. DOCK, W.: Amer. J. Physiol. **130**, 1 (1940). — 10. FOLKOW, B., B. JOHANSSON, and S. MELLANDER: Acta. physiol. Scand. **53**, 99 (1961). — 11. FOLKOW, B., and S. MELLANDER: Amer. Heart J. **68**, 397 (1964). — 12. FOLKOW, B., and B. ÖBERG: Acta physiol. Scand. **53**, 105 (1961). — 13. GASSEL, M. M., B. GHELARDUCCI, P. L. MARCHIAFAVA, and O. POMPEIANO: Arch. ital. biol. **102**, 545 (1964). — 14. GASSEL, M. M., P. L. MARCHIAFAVA, and O. POMPEIANO: Arch. ital. biol. **102**, 471 (1964). — 15. GIAQUINTO, S., O. POMPEIANO, and I. SOMOGYI: Arch. ital. biol. **102**, 245 (1964). — 16. GIAQUINTO, S., O. POMPEIANO, and I. SOMOGYI: Arch. ital. biol. **102**, 282 (1964). — 17. GUAZZI, M., A. LIBRETTI, and A. ZANCHETTI: Circulation Res. **11**, 7 (1962). — 18. GUAZZI, M., and A. ZANCHETTI: Science **148**, 397 (1965). — 19. GUAZZI, M., and A. ZANCHETTI: Arch. ital. biol. in press. — 20. HEYMANS, C., and J.-J. BOUCKAERT: Compt. rend. Soc. biol., Paris **117**, 252 (1943). — 21. HEYMANS, C., J.-J. BOUCKAERT, and P. REGNIERS: Le sinus carotidien et la zone homologue cardio-aortique. Physiologie-pathologie-clinique. Doin, Paris, 1933. — 22. HEYMANS, C., and E. NEIL: Reflexogenic Areas of the Cardiovascular System. Churchill Ltd., London, 1958. — 23. HILL, L.: Lancet 1898/I, 282. — 24. KANZOW, E., D. KRAUSE, and H. KÜHNEL: Pflügers Arch. Physiol. **274**, 593 (1962). — 25. KEZDI, P.: Circulation Res. **8**, 934 (1960). — 26. KEZDI, P.: Circulation Res. **11**, 145 (1962). — 27. KLEITMAN, N.: Sleep and Wakefulness. University of Chicago Press, Chicago, 1963. — 28. KOCH, E., and K. MATTONET: Zschr. exper. Med. **94**, 105 (1934). — 29. KOCH, E., and H. MIES: Krkh.forschung **7**, 241 (1929). — 30. LAWRENCE, J. R., and C. J. DICKINSON: Clin. Sc. **27**, 381 (1964). — 31. MATTON, G.: Arch. internat. pharmacodyn. thérap. **110**, 471 (1957). — 32. MCCUBBIN, J. W., and I. H. PAGE: Circulation Res. **12**, 553 (1963). — 33. MELLANDER, S.: Acta physiol. Scand. **50**, Suppl. **176** (1960). — 34. MORUZZI, G.: Harvey Lectures **58**, 233 (1963). — 35. MOSS, W. G., and G. E. WAKERLIN: Amer. J. Physiol. **161**, 435 (1950). — 36. OGDEN, E.: Bull. N. Y. Acad. Med. **23**, 643 (1947). — 37. REED, R. K., L. A. SAPIRSTEIN, F. D. SOUTHARD, Jr., and E. OGDEN: Amer. J. Physiol. **141**, 707 (1944). — 38. RICHARDSON, D. W., A. J. HONOUR, G. W. FENTON, F. H. STOTT, and G. W. PICKERING: Clin. Sc. **26**, 445 (1964). — 39. ROSSI, G. F., and A. ZANCHETTI: Arch. ital. biol. **95**, 199 (1957). — 40. SAMAAN, A.: Compt. rend. Soc. biol., Paris **115**, 1383 (1934). — 41. SAPIRSTEIN, L. A., and R. K. REED: Proc. Soc. Exper. Biol. Med. **57**, 135 (1944). — 42. SHAW, D. B., M. S. KNAPP, and D. H. DAVIS: Lancet 1963/I, 797. — 43. SNYDER, F., J. A. HOBSON, D. F. MORRISON, and F. GOLDFRANK: J. Appl. Physiol. **19**, 417 (1964). — 44. TAQUINI, A. C., Jr.: Circulation Res. **12**, 562 (1963). — 45. TAQUINI, A. C., Jr., P. C. BLAQUIER, and D. F. BOHR: Amer. J. Physiol. **201**, 1173 (1961). — 46. TARCHANOFF, J.: Arch. ital. biol. **21**, 318 (1894). — 47. ZANCHETTI, A.: Annual Rev. Physiol. **24**, 287 (1962).

Discussion

Pickering: May I show you what happens in man? Blood pressures, recorded on our automatic machine which inflates a Gallivardin double cuff on the upper arm, in this instance every five minutes, are shown in Fig. 1; they are the pressure records of Dr. D. Richardson, who is the Professor of

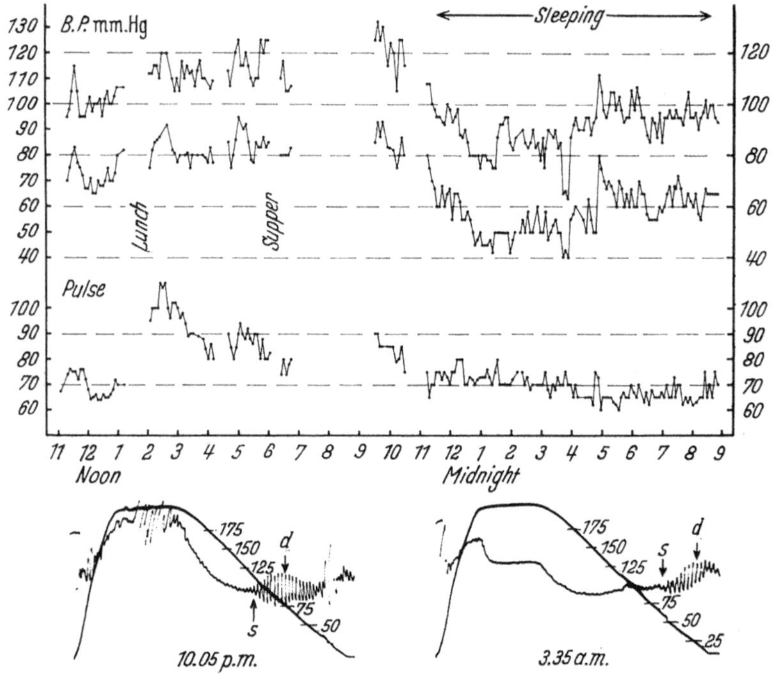

Fig. 1. Variation in blood pressure throughout 24 hours in a subject with normal blood pressure. Below: Specimen records from a subject with normal blood pressure at two different hours [from Richardson, D. W., A. J. Honour, G. W. Fenton, F. H. Stott, and G. W. Pickering: Clin. Sc. *26*, 445 (1964)].

Cardiology in the Medical School of Virginia. During his ordinary day, his systolic pressure varied between about 98 and 130 mm. Hg. About midnight, he fell asleep, and during sleep his systolic and diastolic both fell, the lowest points being about 64 mm. systolic and 40 mm. diastolic. If you don't believe it, the record at 3.35 a.m. is given in the lower part of the figure. You can also notice that the pulse rate, on the whole, was not very different from when he was quietly awake.

The patient whose record is given in Fig. 2 was in hospital for episodes of forgetfulness, and you can see that he had a raised arterial pressure; he had lunch, and after lunch he fell asleep. He was awakened from sleep by a neurologist who was expressing the opinion that he had organic brain

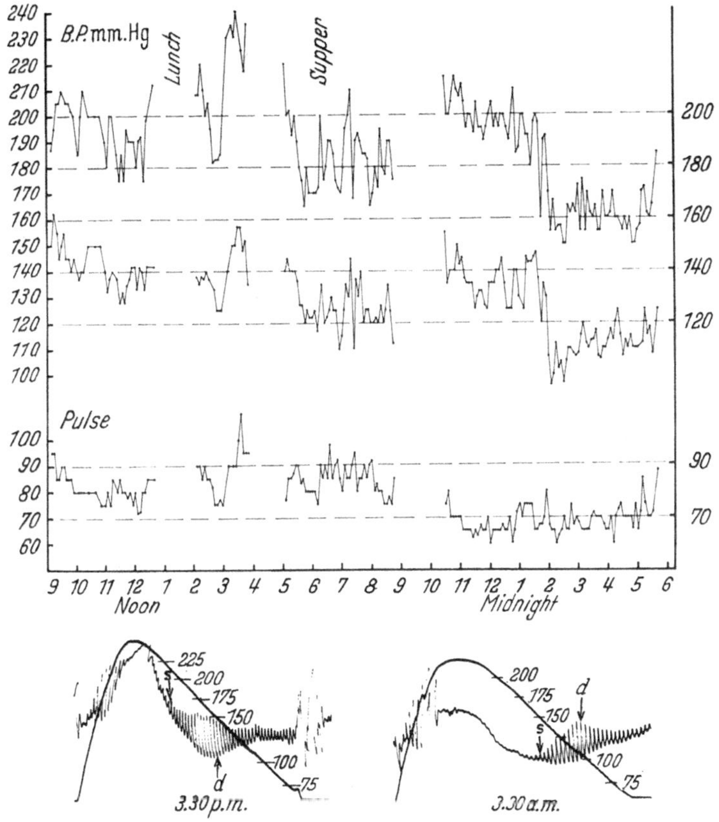

Fig. 2. Variation in blood pressure throughout 24 hours in a hypertensive subject. Below: Specimen records from a hypertensive subject at two different hours [from Richardson, D. W., A. J. Honour, G. W. Fenton, F. H. Stott, and G. W. Pickering: Clin. Sc. *26*, 445 (1964)].

damage, and his arterial pressure rose to 245 mm. Hg systolic and 158 mm. diastolic. Later, much later, he fell asleep again, and during sleep his systolic fell to about 150 mm. Hg and his diastolic to about 100 mm. Hg. There was a slowing of the pulse, on the whole.

Fig. 3 shows the range that we found in normal subjects, subjects with elevated arterial pressure of unascertained cause, commonly called essential hypertension, and patients with renal disease, and there isn't really any systematic difference.

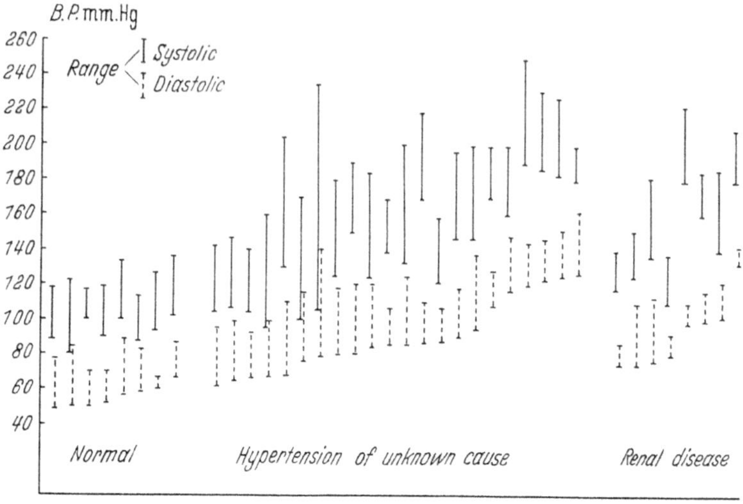

Fig. 3. Ranges of blood pressure in 8 normals, 22 patients with essential hypertension, and 8 subjects with renal disease. Top bar of each range represents average pressure during highest hour of a 24-hour record. The bottom bar represents the average during the lowest hour [from RICHARDSON, D. W., A. J. HONOUR, G. W. FENTON, F. H. STOTT, and G. W. PICKERING: Clin. Sc. *26*, 445 (1964)].

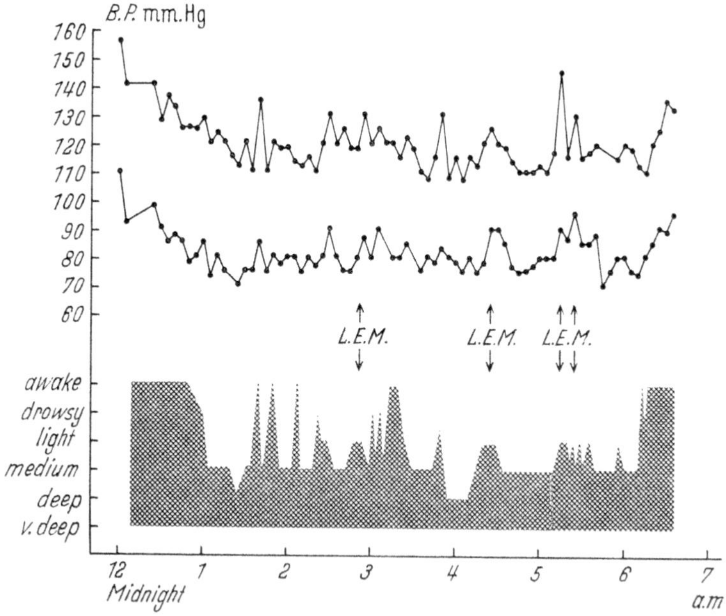

Fig. 4. Correlation between the level of blood pressure and depth of sleep, the depth of sleep determined from electro-encephalographic record. L.E.M.: lateral eye movement [from RICHARDSON, D. W., A. J. HONOUR, G. W. FENTON, F. H. STOTT, and G. W. PICKERING: Clin. Sc. *26*, 445 (1964)].

Fig. 4 gives the record of one of the workers, in fact Dr. A. J. HONOUR; the hatched area at the bottom shows the depth of sleep as judged by the E.E.G., and some of the spikes were associated with rapid eye movements. Now they have done this rather better. This automatic recorder is not very good during sleep, because it records too infrequently. They have therefore done direct observations on themselves with a catheter in the brachial artery, recording the pressures continuously on a strain gauge. In deep sleep, the blood pressure is pretty level at quite a low value; the pulse rate is about the same as it is in waking. If, however, there is a K complex in the E.E.G., that is followed very very quickly indeed by a rise in pulse pressure, in systolic and diastolic pressure, and in heart rate.

BOCK: We have also done these studies in human beings and in a larger number of hypertensives. In principle, there is no difference with regard to the nocturnal drop in pressure in hypertensives and in normotensives, but the more severe the hypertension, the less the nocturnal drop in pressure, and in the most severe cases, in malignant hypertension, a nocturnal drop in pressure is often completely lacking.

SMIRK: I have been most interested in this paper. We have also been recording the blood pressure during sleep[1]. The cuff round an arm is automatically inflated at appropriate intervals and we tape-record the sounds over the corresponding brachial artery. Moreover, we simultaneously record electromyograms of eye movements, E.E.G., E.C.G., body movements, and posture in bed (on back, left or right lateral). The patient is also asked to operate a signal if he is awake when the cuff is inflated. The results we obtained are really very similar to those which have been described in animals by Dr. ZANCHETTI and in man by Dr. BOCK. We have noted the E.E.G. changes associated with rapid heart rate — a heart-rate change of extraordinarily rapid onset. Indeed, it may be of some clinical interest, because in addition to our young, healthy subjects in whom the phenomenon occurs, we had a patient who was suffering from angina of decubitus, in the sense that he developed spontaneous angina when he was apparently completely at rest and emotionally undisturbed; these anginal attacks would sometimes awaken him from sleep. We made an all-night recording in this case. While the patient was asleep, he developed some of the complexes which Dr. PICKERING was describing; his heart rate increased, his blood pressure increased, there was no movement in bed, his S.T. segment became depressed, and shortly afterwards he was awakened from sleep by pain and pressed the signal button which indicated the presence of pain.

There is one thing I should like to ask: Dr. PICKERING, would you say whether in these experiments body posture was monitored? Was the posture of the patients at any given moment during sleep known?

PICKERING: There were some observations in which this was done, but naturally RICHARDSON was in bed at home, and I don't think he had any insight into himself when he was asleep. As regards the patients, there was no monitory guard asleep in the ward, and the automatic recorder was at their bedside. So there was no way of telling the position.

SMIRK: I think this is very important, and it probably explains the considerable discrepancy between the very low levels of blood pressure which you sometimes recorded and the levels which we obtained. We have done ten

---

[1] SMIRK, F. H., and A. T. WALLIS: unpublished observations.

observations on healthy normotensives. The lowest blood pressure recorded during sleep among these was approximately 79 mm. Hg systolic. The basal blood pressure on the same person, taken on the machine, was 84 mm. Hg. On the average, there has been a comparatively small difference (less than 10 mm. systolic, 10 mm. diastolic) in our measurements between the basal pressure and the lowest sleeping pressure. Now I am quite sure in hypertensives there will be a bigger difference.

Referring again to posture, this is very important, because whether you study a patient awake or asleep, deliberately turning, or turning inadvertently during sleep, the difference between the systolic and diastolic pressures with the cuff arm upwards (above heart level) and with the patient lying on his back (with the cuff arm at heart level) is somewhere about 15 mm. systolic and 15 mm. diastolic. We also noticed that the patients were quite unaware of their movements during sleep, but in our experiments, the posture changes were recorded automatically. The very low blood pressures which you obtained may possibly have been due to the subject's lying on one side with the cuff arm upwards.

Introduction to the General Discussion

By

A. C. Taquini

Before entering into the general discussion of this morning's papers, I should like to review rapidly some experimental data collected in our laboratory.

Haemodynamically, arterial hypertension is accepted to be the result of an increase in peripheral resistance. However, although this is so in experimental and clinical nephrogenic hypertension, in human essential hypertension several investigators have frequently found an elevated cardiac output. In addition, we have observed (*1*) that in patients with essential hypertension, especially in those with an unstable blood pressure, cardiac output varies at successive determinations, even when these are made under the strictest experimental conditions, involving, for instance, previous training of the patient in the procedure to be carried out, suitable ambient conditions, prolonged rest, etc. There seems to be no reasonable explanation for this lability in cardiac output. It has no relation to the basic state evaluated in terms of oxygen consumption or to any other apparent cause. To what extent the sympathetic blocking agents, including especially guanethidine sulphate, which has an intensive cardiac stimulating effect owing to the local liberation of noradrenaline, or the β-adrenergic blocking agents, nethalide or Inderal, may act differently in patients with a labile cardiac output is a point that might be taken into consideration.

There is clinical and experimental evidence revealing that the nervous system is primarily responsible for the maintenance of vascular tone in hypertension (*2*); but there is no experimental or clinical evidence to prove that sympathetic tone is augmented in hypertension.

If one considers that the excretion of catecholamines reflects sympathetic activity, this may suggest differences in the case of hypertensive patients. In fact, however, 24-hour catecholamine excretion in a group of 166 hypertensive subjects was found to be of the order of $78.7 \pm 48\ \mu g$. – which is not significantly different from that measured in normal subjects, whose total catecholamine excretion in 24 hours was 63.4 $\pm$ 18.6 μg. A more detailed analysis made it possible to separate two groups of hypertensives: one comprising approximately 75% of the cases, in which the daily excretion was 59.3 $\pm$ 20.7 μg., and the other – the remaining 25% – with an excretion of 159.4 $\pm$ 33.2 μg. in 24 hours. The difference between these two groups, as well as the difference between the last group and the normal population, was statistically significant (P $<$0.0001) (*3*).

Whether this observation sheds any light on the mode of action of the sympathetic blocking agents is another point that could be considered.

In relation to the sympathetic blocking agents, I should like to comment briefly on the pharmacological properties of D.M.I. (desmethylimipramine) studied in our laboratory (*4*). D.M.I. is an antidepressive drug in current use. It possesses two fundamental actions: a moderate sympathetic blocking effect (Fig. 1) and an

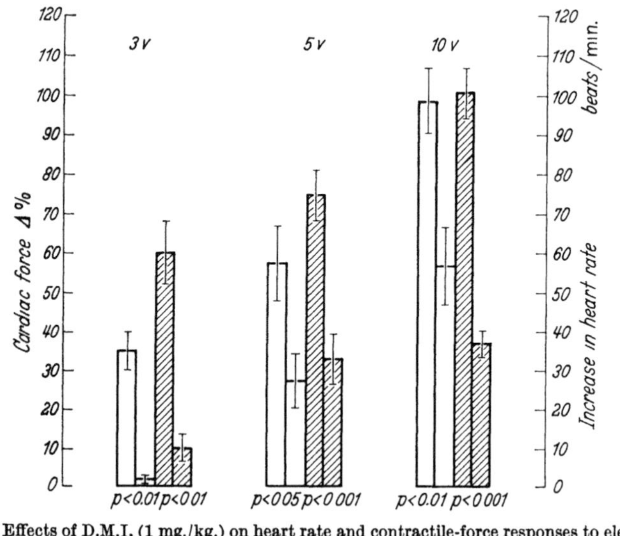

Fig. 1. Effects of D.M.I. (1 mg./kg.) on heart rate and contractile-force responses to electrical stimulation of the right stellate ganglion. Blank columns: contractile force. Hatched columns: heart rate. The vertical lines in the columns represent the standard error of the mean. In each pair of columns, the left-hand column represents controls and the right-hand column D.M.I.-treated animals.

adrenergic cardio-stimulant effect. As in the case of guanethidine, the cardio-stimulant action is independent of the nervous system. Although the action of these two drugs is similar in many respects, administration of D.M.I. antagonises the action of guanethidine for two reasons: firstly, D.M.I. interferes with the depletion of noradrenaline produced by guanethidine (Fig. 2); secondly, although D.M.I. displays a much weaker sympathetic blocking activity than guanethidine, it has a stronger affinity for the postganglionic noradrenaline-transporting mechanisms. It may therefore competitively inhibit the blocking action of guanethidine, in which case the simultaneous use of these two drugs would be contra-indicated.

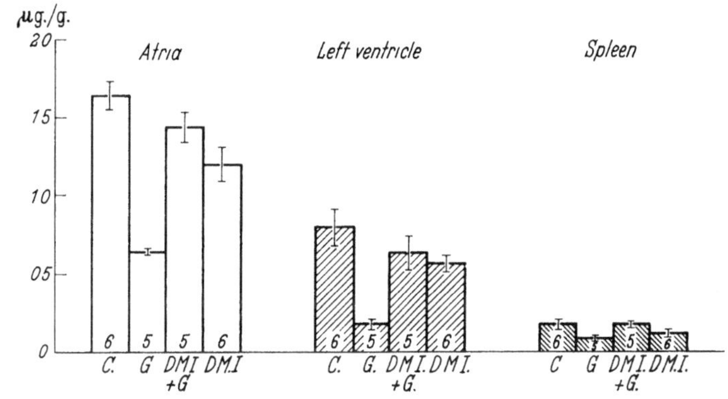

Fig. 2. Noradrenaline content in rabbits expressed in μg./g. wet tissue. The columns represent mean values ± standard error. The number of experiments carried out is shown in each column. C.: control; G.: guanethidine depletion; D.M.I. + G.: blocking effect of D.M.I. on the depleting effect of guanethidine; D.M.I.: effects of D.M.I. on noradrenaline content.

The pharmacological action of saluretics, in both the short-term and prolonged treatment of hypertension, now seems to be understood. Nevertheless, any study concerned with the properties of vaso-active drugs — the effects of which are probably mediated by internal ionic shifts — should take into consideration the fact that the investigation of the distribution of Na^+ in the different compartments of the arterial wall still involves appreciable methodological difficulties.

To solve this problem, studies have been started in our laboratory, in which effluxes of Na^{22} (*5*) are used in addition to conventional techniques. At 17° C two exponentials can be detected: a very fast one, which exchanges by diffusion and comprises about 90 mM/kg. wet weight, and a slower and metabolically dependent one, comprising about 15 mM/kg. (Fig. 3). This latter phase is assigned to smooth muscle because of its relatively low half-life and because this tissue constitutes the bulk of the cellular mass of the artery. Using a value of 362 ± 5 ml./kg. wet weight for the inulin space, and a total tissue water of 736 $\pm$ 4 ml., the value obtained for Na is about 40 mM/l. of intracellular water. This value is lower than those reported in visceral muscle, calculated from total sodium content and inulin space. This suggests the possibility that, using conventional methods, not only the "bound" fraction is allotted to the intracellular space, but also a fraction dissolved in a third compartment not penetrable by inulin. This

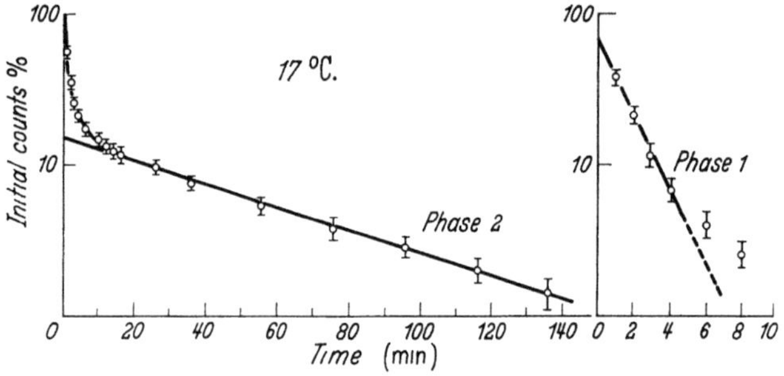

Fig. 3. Na^{22} effluxes in the arterial wall at 17° C. Mean values with standard error. The right-hand curve is an amplification of the rapid phase (Phase 1).

hypothesis is supported by the finding of an "excess" of sodium (sodium exchanging by diffusion – sodium dissolved in the inulin space) of about 40 mM which cannot be fully accounted for by the "bound" fraction. In fact, by studying the sodium distribution and Cl^{36} effluxes in media with normal and high sodium concentrations, a fixed fraction of about 10 mM, probably bound to mucopolysaccharides, was detected. The remaining 30 mM would be dissolved in a third compartment of uncertain location, having a volume (calculated from the space of "fast-moving" chloride) of about 200 ml./kg. wet weight.

With reference to the change in the Na content or in the ionic distribution as the causes of either an increase or a decrease in blood pressure, one also has to bear in mind the possibility that changes in ionic content could, at least in part, be the result and not the cause of changes in blood pressure. In fact, in experiments carried out in normal dogs, in which the blood pressure was raised to 50 mm. Hg above the control level by means of a 15-minute infusion of noradrenaline, we have observed the following modifications in the arterial wall (*6*): a) a decrease in the extracellular space (Fig. 4); b) a rise in the Na content and Na concentration in the intracellular and bound fraction (Fig. 5); c) a significant reduction in the content and concentration of intracellular K (Fig. 6).

These results, which are in agreement with FRIEDMAN's experiments (7), may signify that the pharmacological action of the drugs can be potentiated by the ionic variations, depending on the blood pressure which is determined by them.

Finally, I should like to refer to the central nervous system. There is much experimental evidence to indicate that the activity of the vasomotor centre is modified not only by the pressoreceptors but also by excitatory and inhibitory influences from the cerebral cortex. Recent research carried out by ZANCHETTI's group (8) shows that stimulation of the aortic nerve has a predominantly cardiovascular excitatory effect in decorticated animals and an inhibitory effect in decerebrate ones. TAQUINI et al. (9) studied the neuronal responses of the posterior hypothalamus in those zones in which previous stimuli produced a rise in blood pressure, induced by experimental modification of the blood pressure achieved by the administration of adrenaline or by clamping the abdominal aorta. Their re-

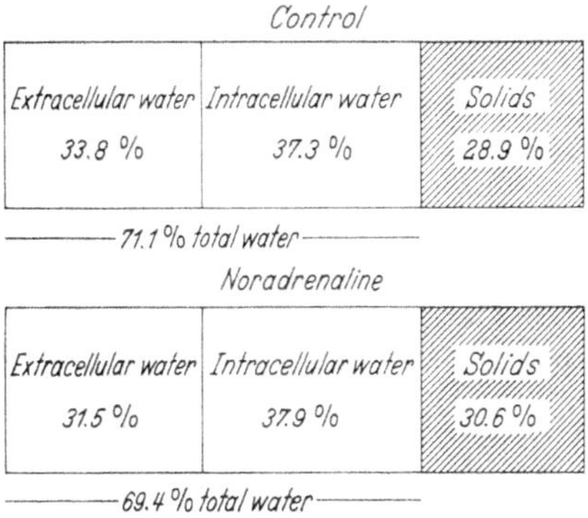

Fig. 4. Changes in the relationship between water and solids produced in the arterial wall after a 15-minute infusion of noradrenaline in order to keep the blood pressure 50 mm. higher than in the control period.

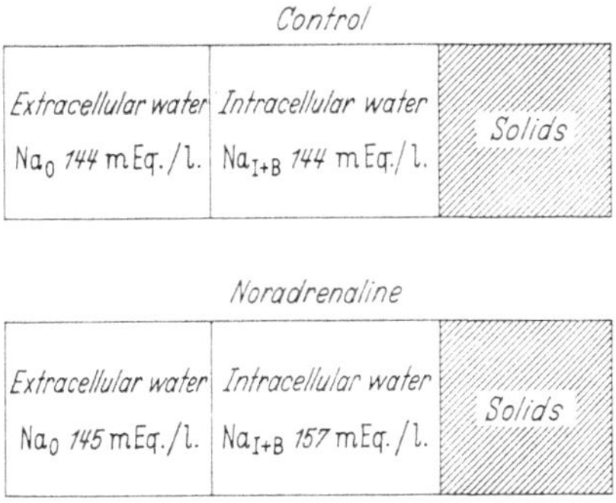

Fig. 5. Concentration of extracellular Na and intracellular + bound Na (Na_0 and Na_{I+B}) in the arterial wall in the control period and after a 15-minute infusion of noradrenaline.

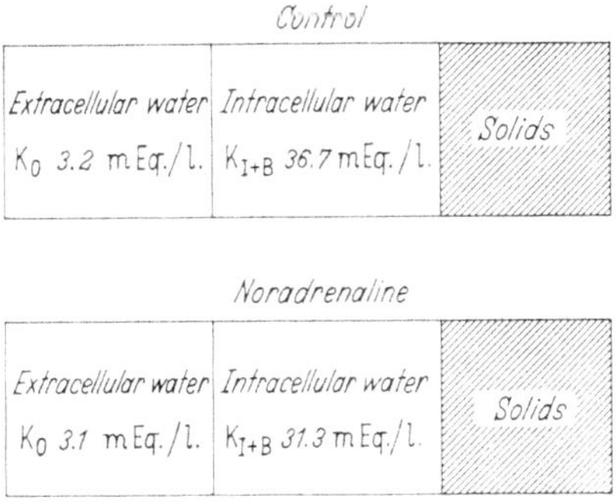

Fig. 6. Concentration of extracellular K and intracellular + bound K (K_0 and K_{I+B}) in the arterial wall in the control period and after a 15-minute infusion of noradrenaline.

sults show the existence of two groups of neurones which change the rate of discharge in opposite directions when the blood pressure rises. It is also known that stimulation of the hypothalamus can increase its catecholamine content.

These experiments, like many others which are beyond the scope of this discussion, demonstrate a complex integration in the regulation of arterial pressure, which opens up an extensive field of speculation from both the physiological and the pharmacological points of view.

References

1. TAQUINI, A. C., Jr., J. D. FERMOSO, C. M. TAQUINI, and A. C. TAQUINI: Acta physiol. Latinoamer. **13**, 367 (1963). — 2. TAQUINI, A. C., Jr.: Circulation Res. **12**, 562 (1963). — 3. BASSO, N., A. C. TAQUINI, Jr., and A. C. TAQUINI: Medicina **25**, 60 (1965). — 4. KAUMANN, A., N. BASSO, and P. ARAMENDIA: J. Pharmacol. Exper. Therap. **147**, 54 (1964). — 5. VILLAMIL, M. F., and N. YEYATI: Medicina **25**, 117 (1965). — 6. DE LA RIVA, I. J., P. BLAQUIER, N. BASSO, and A. C. TAQUINI: Medicina **25**, 59 (1965). — 7. FRIEDMAN, S. M., M. NAKASHIMA, and C. L. FRIEDMAN: Circulation Res. **13**, 223 (1963). — 8. BACCELLI, G., M. GUAZZI, A. LIBRETTI, and A. ZANCHETTI: Amer. J. Physiol. **208**, 708 (1965). — 9. TAQUINI, C. M., D. T. BRAZIER, L. L. BOYARSKY, and F. WILSON: To be published.

General Discussion

BRUNNER: There are two points mentioned by Dr. BEIN in his paper that I should like to discuss further: firstly, the inhibition of the action of hydralazine by adrenergic β-receptor blockade and, secondly, the differences in the action of hydralazine in conscious and anaesthetised animals.

The left side of Fig. 1 shows the effect of 1.0 mg./kg. hydralazine i.v. in the conscious dog. Total peripheral resistance was decreased by 50%, but, owing to the marked increase in heart rate and cardiac output, blood pressure fell only slightly. A second group of conscious dogs was pretreated with 1 mg./kg. propranolol i.v. (right side of Fig. 1), a dose which blocks the vasodepressor and positive chronotropic effects of 0.5 μg./kg. isoprenaline i.v. completely. In these animals, adrenergic β-receptor blockade produced a partial inhibition of all the effects of hydralazine, including the decrease in total peripheral resistance. In pentobarbitone-anaesthetised dogs, however, the action of hydralazine was not influenced by β-blockade.

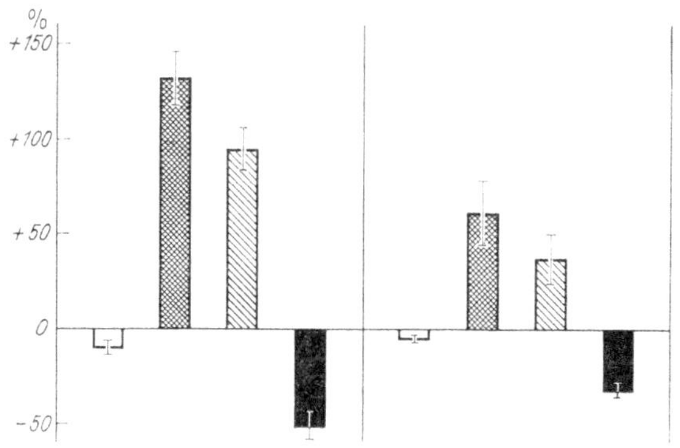

Fig. 1. Changes in blood pressure □, heart rate ▨, cardiac output ▨, and total peripheral resistance ■ 10 minutes after the intravenous injection of 1.0 mg./kg. hydralazine in conscious dogs without (left side) and with (right side) pretreatment with propranolol (1.0 mg./kg. i.v.).

In the conscious dog, pretreated with propranolol, and in the anaesthetised dog, with or without pretreatment with propranolol, hydralazine decreased the total peripheral resistance to the same extent. In the conscious, non-pretreated dog, however, the decrease in total peripheral resistance was more pronounced (Fig. 2).

These observations can be explained as follows: hydralazine dilates peripheral vessels — mainly resistance vessels — by a more or less direct action. In the conscious dog, this vasodilatation produces a fall in blood pressure, which stimulates a reflex cardiovascular mechanism. This reflex adjustment is mediated principally by activation of the sympathetic nervous system, other mechanisms being less important, as was shown by Glick and Braunwald[1]. In a normal, non-pretreated dog, which has not received hydralazine but in which vasodilatation has been produced by other means,

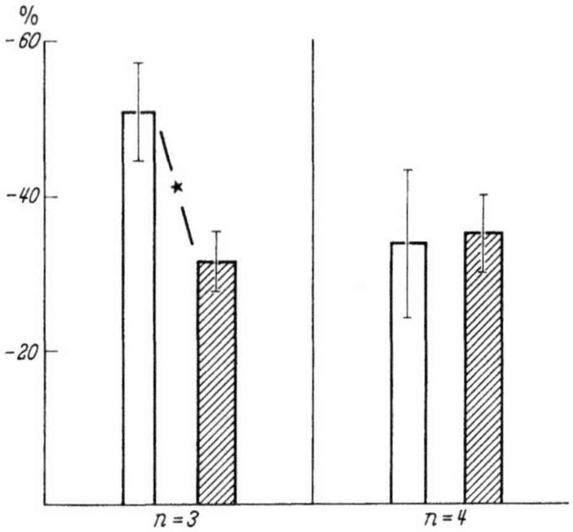

Fig. 2. Changes in the total peripheral resistance after intravenous injection of 1.0 mg./kg. hydralazine in conscious (left side) and pentobarbitone-anaesthetised (right side) dogs with (▨) or without (□) pretreatment with propranolol (1.0 mg./kg. i.v.). $\bar{x} \pm s_{\bar{x}}$, initial control values = 100%. * = $p < 0.05$.

the increased sympathetic discharge would lead — by stimulation of α-receptors — to vasoconstriction and — by stimulation of β-receptors — to tachycardia, increased cardiac output, and additional peripheral vasodilatation (Table 1).

Table 1. *Scheme of blood-pressure adjustment*

Peripheral vasodilatation

↓

Blood-pressure fall

↓

Reflex adjustment:

1.) **Sympathetic activation**
α-receptors: vasoconstriction
β-receptors: tachycardia, increase in cardiac output, additional peripheral vasodilatation

2.) **Other mechanisms (e. g. parasympathetic inhibition)**

The reflex constriction mediated by α-receptors is, however, inhibited by hydralazine, as shown by Åblad[2] in man, and the stimulation of β-receptors becomes prevalent. Thus, the decrease in total peripheral resistance is more pronounced in the conscious, non-pretreated dog than after anaesthesia

[1] Glick, G., and E. Braunwald: Circulation Res. **16**, 363 (1965).
[2] Åblad, B.: Acta pharmac. tox. **20**, Suppl. **1** (1963).

or β-blockade, as is the tachycardia and the increase in cardiac output. In the anaesthetised dog, the reflex adjustment is more or less suppressed, depending on the anaesthetic used. In the conscious animal, the effects of reflex β-receptor stimulation can be inhibited by propranolol, whereas it is not possible to demonstrate such an effect in the anaesthetised dog. It seems, therefore, that the primary effect of hydralazine is not mediated by a direct stimulation of adrenergic β-receptors.

As postulated by KRONEBERG[1], an effective antihypertensive agent must not only produce vasodilatation, but also inhibit the reflex adjustment to the fall in blood pressure. The results of our experiments with hydralazine show that a partial (only α) inhibition of this reflex is sufficient. After vasodilatation and partial inhibition, tachycardia results; but, since a reflex adjustment by stimulation of the heart is possible within certain limits, orthostatic side effects are rare. On the other hand, after a complete sympathetic blockade, heart rate is not increased, but orthostatic symptoms are more frequent.

BEIN: The morphological changes in the myocardium in response to high doses of reserpine reported by Dr. ZAIMIS were not observed by us when we carried out similar experiments in the cat. The pathological evaluation was done by Dr. HESS, who is an experimental pathologist and a histochemist of quite long experience. He found an apparently progressive fatty infiltration of the fibres which can be ascribed to inanition. Fatty infiltration can also be observed with hexamethonium. The reaction for mitochondrial function (cytochrome oxidase) was the same as in the controls. No elevation of serum transaminase levels was noted. Dr. ZAIMIS, you showed in your lecture histological pictures of the guinea-pig heart. Incidentally, TRENDELENBURG[2] very recently published a paper about the functional characteristics of the guinea-pig atrium when compared with the rabbit heart after treatment with reserpine. He found a depletion of noradrenaline in the guinea-pig heart, but he also observed that the guinea-pig heart still responded to sympathetic stimulation, contrary to the findings in rabbits and in other animal species. He concluded that the guinea-pig has a compartment of catecholamines in the heart that is not accessible to reserpine, but accessible to sympathetic nerve stimulation. Therefore I am wondering, Dr. ZAIMIS, whether the conclusions you have given us are based on findings in several animal species and whether you have observed species differences.

In the histological picture that you showed, the possibility that the technique used was inadequate — resulting, for example, in a fixation artefact — cannot be ruled out. I should therefore like to ask you how many blocks per heart you have investigated histologically and how you standardised your histological technique. The "centres of necrosis" you found in the myocardium after long-term treatment need not necessarily have been due to the effect of the substance administered. Focal necrosis of this kind is very common in experimental animals and seems to be due to septic metastasis. We are therefore wondering about the incidence of focal inflammatory necrosis in a fairly large selection of control animals.

ZAIMIS: My answer is very simple, Dr. BEIN. I am not a histologist, nor a histochemist either. All I can say is that the evidence was provided by

[1] KRONEBERG, H. G.: Verh. Dtsch. Ges. Kreisl.-forsch. 28. Tagg., 172 (1962).

[2] TRENDELENBURG, U.: J. Pharmacol. Exper. Therap. **147**, 313 (1965).

workers in these fields whose reputation is well established and whose findings I have no reason to doubt. Dr. M. SCOTT, who studied the histological changes, is Senior Lecturer at the Royal Veterinary College, London, and the histochemical work was carried out by Miss SOPHIA KAKARI under the supervision of Dr. A. G. E. PEARSE of the Postgraduate Medical School of London.

The action of reserpine was studied in cats, dogs, guinea-pigs, and rats. The myocardium of cats and dogs proved to be the most sensitive, that of the guinea-pig followed, and the rat's myocardium was the most resistant. Wide-spread changes were produced only by large doses of reserpine of the order of 1 mg./kg. Doses of 10 μg./kg., administered daily to cats for several months, produced localised changes only. While receiving this daily dose of reserpine, the cats appeared healthy.

PICKERING: May I suggest that it might be an awfully good idea if Dr. BEIN and Dr. ZAIMIS actually visited each other's laboratories and looked down the microscope together. I am sure that we shall not clear up this controversy here today.

CARLSSON: I have a suggestion that might solve this problem. It could be that owing to the different temperatures you probably have in your laboratories — in England temperature is low, and ...

ZAIMIS: Our laboratories and our animal-houses are well heated, Dr. CARLSSON. We are not so under-developed.

CARLSSON: But did you measure body temperatures?

ZAIMIS: Yes. In our department we are very temperature-conscious.

CARLSSON: It goes down, doesn't it, after reserpine.

ZAIMIS: Body temperature goes down with larger doses of reserpine, but not with 10—20 μg./kg.

CARLSSON: These are not single doses, are they. I think you are treating your cats for a long time in order to produce the pathological changes.

ZAIMIS: Yes. This was daily administration for long periods of time, but the body temperature of these animals, because of the relatively low dose of reserpine, was maintained at normal levels.

CARLSSON: And do the animals still maintain their health — drink and eat, *et cetera*?

ZAIMIS: Yes. With the exception of occasional diarrhoea and mild sedation, cats receiving 10 μg./kg./day of reserpine look healthy, and their appetite is good. After all, this dose is very similar to that administered to man. In this series, in only three of the 12 treated cats was there a 10—15% loss in body weight over a period of eight weeks. The remaining nine cats gained in weight, and their growth rate was just below that accepted as normal.

Hypertension and vascular disease

Experimental atherosclerosis and hypertension

By

Q. B. Deming

Our studies have consisted of an experimental exploration of the relationship between hypertension and atherosclerosis and the metabolism of cholesterol.

After reviewing some clinical data and our findings in the rat, which indicate that hypertension intensifies dietary atherogenesis and that pharmacological control of the blood pressure reverses this effect, I shall present evidence that hypertension increases the amount of cholesterol in the arterial wall prior to the development of visible atherosclerosis, that the amount of cholesterol in the arterial wall is more closely dependent on blood pressure than on diet or serum cholesterol, and, finally, that hypertension increases the rate of synthesis of cholesterol in the arteries and the liver.

The background for this work is clinical. It is the known but ill-understood relationship between hypertension and atherosclerosis.

There are many possible *causes* of hypertension, but the *effects* seem to be the same whatever the cause. The final common pathway, except in that small group who develop necrotizing arteritis or progressive nephrosclerosis, the final common pathway for the vast majority of hypertensives is via atherosclerosis and ischemic disease of heart, brain, or other organs. If it is important to lower an elevated blood pressure, not associated with necrotizing arteritis, it must be to slow atherogenesis.

The vast collection of data gathered in 1959 for the Society of Actuaries by Lew (*1*) on *4 million* lives and 102,000 deaths (of insurable individuals) established the following facts: Life expectancy in *both sexes*, at *all ages* varies inversely with arterial blood pressure (whether measured as *systolic* or *diastolic*) through *all* blood-pressure ranges which are high enough to sustain adequate flow.

If we look specifically at the relationship between hypertension and ischemic heart disease, we find:

There have been many retrospective studies giving the percentage of patients with cardiac infarction who had antecedent hypertension. In five series in males and three series in females, the percentages with antecedent hypertension were given as 58, 54, 64, 57, 41, 52, 60, and 71 (*16*).

In 1953, MASTER (*2*), in a study which he interpreted differently, presented data showing ten times the expected incidence of hypertension in the infarct group.

A number of convincing prospective studies have been conducted. The most beautiful data are those of DAWBER and KANNEL (*3*) who, at Framingham, demonstrated a consistent correlation between systolic blood pressure at entry to the study and the incidence of new coronary arterial disease in the next eight years. Again, this correlation is evident at all blood-pressure levels down to the subaverage.

If we look specifically at the relationship between hypertension and ischemic brain disease, we find fewer studies, but probably an even closer correlation.

In 1960, PATERSON et al. (*4*) dissected out and extracted the lipid from various arteries of 184 consecutive fatalities in a group of patients who had been permanently hospitalized. They demonstrated a significant correlation between the amount of lipid in the arteries of both the brain and the heart and the blood pressure measured during life.

It can be accepted that hypertension intensifies atherogenesis. It is not the only contributing factor. The roles played by the serum cholesterol concentration and various diets have received justified attention both in clinical and in experimental studies. In DAWBER's (*5*) reports, it is shown that blood pressure and serum cholesterol are *independently* related to the development of coronary artery disease.

Serum cholesterol would appear to be a stimulus acting uniformly throughout the vasculature, yet many observations indicate that not all arterial beds are equally affected.

GUBNER (*6*) showed from LEW's data that a blood-pressure level which increased a young man's chance of having a cardiac infarct three and a half times, increased his chance of having a cerebral infarct fifteen times.

Studies (*7*, *8*, *9*) of the Japanese in Japan, of Yemenite Jews in Israel, and of Negroes in Jamaica have indicated that conditions (believed to be dietary) characterized by unusually low concentrations of cholesterol in the serum result in a much greater decrease in *cardiac* ischemic disease than in *cerebral* or *aortic* ischemic disease. Yet the serum cholesterol must be the same in the heart as in the head.

Our first work in rats was begun in the hope of learning whether the lowering of elevated blood-pressure levels by pharmacological means would slow the pathological rate of atherogenesis.

In 1958 (*10*) we demonstrated in the rat – as others had before us in the dog and rabbit – first, that hypercholesteremia and atherosclerosis can be produced by feeding a diet containing cholesterol, cholic acid, and thiouracil, and second, that if the rat was made hypertensive, either by endocrine or renal vascular techniques, this atherosclerosis developed more rapidly and more severely and sometimes led to ischemic damage and cardiac infarction.

In 1960 (*11*) we reported on experiments involving two matched groups of hypertensive CFN rats kept on such a diet for four months. Blood pressure in one group was maintained at near normal levels by pharmacological means. In this treated group, atheroma formation was much less marked than in the untreated group – indeed it approached the mild degree of atheroma found in normotensive controls. The intensification of dietary atherosclerosis produced by hypertension can be reduced by pharmacological control of the blood pressure.

In the course of our early experiments, we made the unanticipated observation that in Wistar rats on the cholesterol and thiouracil regimen, elevation of blood pressure induced an increase in cholesterol in the serum, in the liver, and in the whole animal. The serum cholesterol of the Wistar rat is not very labile, and a correlation with blood pressure is readily shown only when the animal is fed this highly atherogenic diet.

The reverse was seen in experiments involving the more labile Carworth Nelson strain. In these animals a diet of cholesterol and thiouracil produced extremely high serum cholesterols, regardless of blood pressure. However, when they were fed on a less abnormal diet – either 2% cholesterol or a chow diet with no added sterol – a correlation between blood pressure and the serum cholesterol level was evident.

Thus, if dietary conditions appropriate to the sensitivity of the strain are selected, it is possible to show an effect of blood pressure on serum cholesterol in rats. Conceivably, the lack of consistency in clinical reports may reflect a similar variability, both in individual sensitivity and in dietary conditions.

The existence in the rat of this correlation between blood pressure and serum cholesterol raised the possibility that the effect of blood pressure on atherogenesis might have been merely a secondary manifestation of its effect on serum cholesterol. This seemed unlikely, since in the treatment experiment dissimilar degrees of atherosclerosis had developed in the presence of similarly elevated serum cholesterols.

However, to test the possibility further, parabiotic pairs were established with one member of each pair rendered hypertensive (in the manner described by Floyer and Richardson (*12*). These pairs were then maintained on a regimen of cholesterol and thiouracil. While the blood pressures were dissimilar, the cross circulation kept serum cholesterol the same.

Fig. 1 demonstrates the four-month course of one such pair. The systolic blood pressures (solid lines) were consistently different. The serum cholesterols, rising in response to the diet, remained closely similar throughout. At sacrifice, the hypertensive animal showed cardiac infarcts and 6(+) atheromatous lesions around the valves; the normotensive animal showed no infarcts and 3(+) lesions[1].

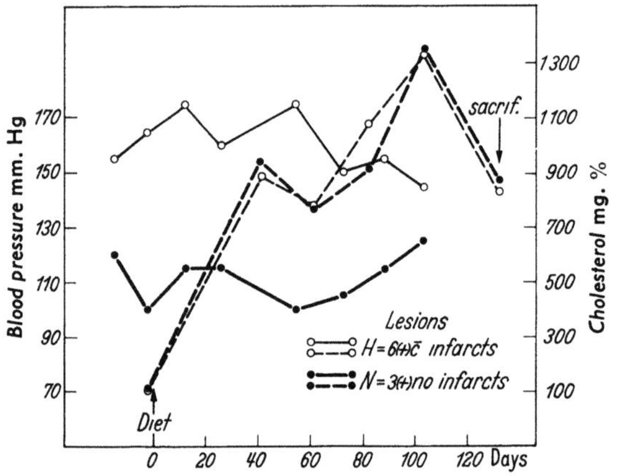

Fig. 1. Course of blood pressure (solid lines) and serum cholesterol (dashed lines) of the two members of a parabiotic pair of rats. Although the blood pressures were consistently different, the serum cholesterols were consistently similar.

Thirteen pairs were studied which satisfied the following arbitrary criteria:

a) A difference of more than 25 mm. Hg in the average systolic blood pressures of the two animals.

b) A difference of less than 15% in the average serum cholesterol of the two animals.

[1] + Gross lesions graded by an arbitrary system 1—3 on size of individual lesions and the grading of all lesions in one animal added.

c) Evidence of atherosclerosis in at least one animal of the pair at sacrifice.

On analysis of the data for each pair, it was found that the hypertensive animal showed more extensive atherosclerosis than the normotensive in 12 of 13 instances. The probability that this would occur by chance is less than 1%. Therefore the effect of blood pressure on atherogenesis is not dependent on the effect of blood pressure on serum cholesterol.

The earlier experiment had demonstrated that in Wistars on cholesterol, cholate, thiouracil feeding, not only *serum* cholesterol, but also *liver* and *carcass* cholesterol were higher in the hypertensive animal.

Our principal interest, however, is in vessels. DALY et al. (*13*) have examined the relationship of the cholesterol content in the nonatherosclerotic aortic wall to both blood pressure and serum cholesterol content. The cholesterol was measured in the aortas of seven parabiotic pairs. Although the serum cholesterols were similar, the cholesterol concentration in the aortic wall was higher in the hypertensive ("clipped") animal (Table 1). There was a clear-cut difference in aortic cholesterol in the first five pairs, in which the blood pressures were different, but not in the last two, in which they were not.

Table 1. *Comparison of cholesterol concentrations in aortas of parabiotic pairs in which serum cholesterol concentrations are similar but blood pressures differ. The effect of blood pressure on aorta cholesterol concentration is shown to be independent of serum cholesterol concentration* [modified from DALY et al. (*13*)]

Rat	Systolic blood pressure	Serum cholesterol mg./100 ml.	Aortic cholesterol μg./mg. nitrogen
Clipped	141	1000	96.7
Control	94	888	38.3
Clipped	160	871	89.8
Control	112	873	33.3
Clipped	158	674	74.6
Control	108	643	35.3
Clipped	150	1209	135
Control	112	1028	52.2
Clipped	142	1154	99.7
Control	105	1047	35.4
Clipped	114	663	35.8
Control	92	682	31.8
Clipped	111	493	33.2
Control	101	482	22.2

In another experiment, a different approach was taken. The concentrations of cholesterol in aorta and serum were compared in groups of normotensive and hypertensive rats, on either a standard chow diet without added sterol or the cholesterol, cholate, and thiouracil diet.

The results obtained in the four groups are summarized as group averages (Table 2). The two shown on the left side were on a

Table 2. *The serum and aorta cholesterol values on the left are from rats on a normal diet. The values on the right are from rats on a diet with added cholesterol 4%, cholic acid 1%, and thiouracil 0.5%. Hypertension increases aorta cholesterol in both groups. Dietary hypercholesteremia increases aorta cholesterol only in the presence of hypertension*

	Serum mg./100 ml.	Aorta μg./mg. N	Aorta μg./mg. N	Serum mg./100 ml.
Normotensive .	82	35	31	1257
Hypertensive .	135	46	67	1206

standard chow diet and had modest serum cholesterols. The two on the right were on a cholesterol, cholate, and thiouracil diet; in these animals the serum cholesterol levels were astronomical. The two top groups were normotensive and the two lower groups hypertensive. The figures within the square are the *aortic* cholesterol concentrations.

Within the 14-week period of this experiment, hypertension increased aorta cholesterol significantly, whether the animals were on a normal diet with low serum cholesterols or were on an atherogenic diet with high serum cholesterols.

The diet, however, and hypercholesteremia did not increase aorta cholesterol unless there was also hypertension. Diet increased the effect of hypertension markedly, but diet alone had no effect. While this is only cholesterol concentration and is *not* atheroma, there is a possible parallel here with the observations in humans of the apparent difference in response of different arterial beds to the dietary vagaries and serum cholesterol differences of different societies.

The Japanese and Yemenite with their spare diets and low serum cholesterol still get atheroma and vascular accidents in the brain when they are hypertensive. The cerebral arteries are exposed to the full arterial pressure (see the rat group in the lower left). But with their low cholesterol they do not get atheroma in those vessels, like the coronaries, which are not exposed to the full systemic pressure during systole and are supported from outside by the cardiac pressure (see the rat group in the upper left).

On the other hand, in the overfed, hypercholesteremic populations (for which I am a spokesman) the dietary stimulus, in conjunction with the modest increase in blood pressure which does occur in coronaries of hypertensives, leads (cf. Table 2, lower right) to atheroma and heart disease.

The observation that elevation of the blood pressure in the rat could, under suitable circumstances, increase the amount of cholesterol in the serum, liver, aorta, and even the total carcass, required explanation. If the hypertensive animal eventually contains more cholesterol than the normotensive animal, one must assume either that hypertension increases ingestion or absorption of cholesterol, or that hypertension decreases metabolism or excretion of cholesterol, or that hypertension increases synthesis of cholesterol. It must do at least one of these three. We therefore tried to examine each of these possibilities.

1. Our data on absorption are still inconclusive. However, an experiment based on the method of MORRIS et al. (*14*) failed to support this hypothesis.

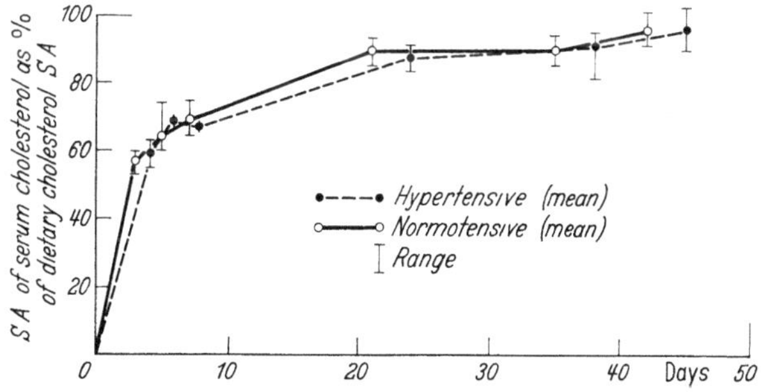

Fig. 2. The identical rise in specific activity (S.A.) of serum cholesterol of hypertensive and normotensive rats, fed a diet containing 2% cholesterol 2-C^{14}, shows no difference in absorbtion of dietary cholesterol.

A diet containing 2% cholesterol 2-C^{14} was fed to 12 normotensive and 12 hypertensive animals, and the specific activity (S.A.) of the serum cholesterols was determined at frequent intervals. If one group absorbed a higher proportion of the labelled dietary cholesterol than the other, the S.A. of its serum cholesterol might be expected to rise faster. No difference was observed between the hypertensive and the normotensive animals (Fig. 2). This experiment is not conclusive. We can only say that so far we have not been able to demonstrate an increased rate of absorption.

2. In order to determine whether hypertension decreases the metabolism or excretion of cholesterol, 1 ml. of pooled, highly labelled, hypercholesteremic rat serum (407 mg.% cholesterol and 94,000 cholesterol counts/min./ml.) was injected intravenously into each of six normotensive and six hypertensive rats which had been paired according to weight. Feces were collected daily for 14 days, and the excretion of counts (representing carbon derived from lipoprotein cholesterol) by normotensive and hypertensive animals was compared. As Fig. 3 shows, there was no difference.

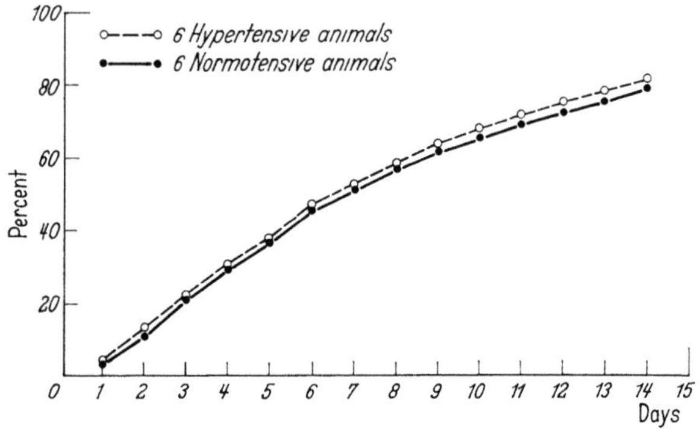

Fig. 3. Mean cumulative fecal excretion of radioactivity after intravenous administration of C^{14}-labelled rat lipoprotein cholesterol expressed as percent of total counts injected on day 0. No difference is shown between normotensive and hypertensive rats.

Cholesterol is not metabolized and excreted more slowly by the hypertensive animal than by the normotensive.

The tentative exclusion of increased absorption and the definite exclusion of decreased excretion imply that a difference in rate of synthesis of cholesterol between normotensive and hypertensive must exist – it does.

3. In order to compare the rate of synthesis of cholesterol in normotensive and hypertensive rats, ADEL et al. (*15*) measured incorporation of labelled precursor into cholesterol, both in living animals and in isolated tissues (liver slices and arterial segments). Acetate 1-C^{14} was given intraperitoneally to 24 matched pairs of hypertensive and normotensive rats, fed on a standard chow diet, and the extent of its incorporation into cholesterol in serum, liver, and carcass was determined after two hours.

The total counts (i.e. acetate) incorporated into cholesterol found in the liver were higher in the hypertensive group (Fig. 4, on the right, indicated by crosses) than in the normotensive group. Exactly similar data were obtained for serum cholesterol and total carcass cholesterol. This is good evidence of an over-all increase in synthesis of cholesterol in the whole animal, but in what organs does it occur?

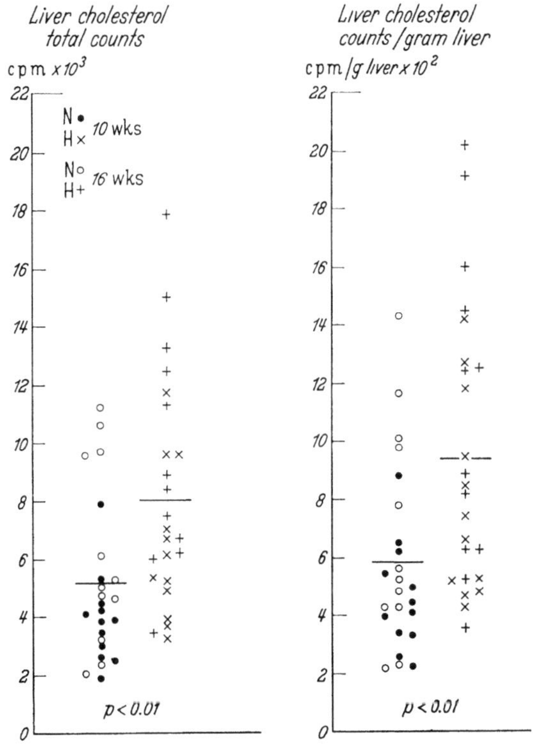

Fig. 4. Hepatic cholesterol synthesis as measured by incorporation of intraperitoneally injected acetate 1-C^{14} is more rapid in hypertensive than in normotensive rats [from Adel et al. (*15*)].

Slices of liver from hypertensive and normotensive rats were incubated with labelled acetate. The incorporation of acetate into cholesterol was more rapid in livers derived from hypertensive animals than in livers derived from normotensive animals.

Daly et al. (*13*) incubated opened, cleaned thoracic aortas from normotensive and hypertensive rats with labelled acetate. The results obtained in nine matched incubations are presented in Table 3. The cholesterol counts were calculated from the counts remaining after serial purification through bromination until constant S.A. was reached.

The incorporation of acetate into cholesterol, whether expressed as counts/min./aorta or as counts/min./mg. aorta nitrogen, was higher in the aortas of hypertensive rats. The average increase was about twentyfold.

Table 3. *Paired incubations show increased incorporation of acetate into cholesterol by aortas from hypertensive rats* [modified from DALY et al. (*13*)]

Rats	c.p.m./aorta	c.p.m./mg. nitrogen
N (5)	1.6	0.8
H (5)	14.4	4.9
N (2)	3	1.3
H (2)	41.5	13.5
N (4)	6.8	4.7
H (3)	20	9.5
N (1)	14	6.7
H (1)	21	7.2
N (1)	5	2.6
H (1)	53	27.2
N (1)	47	21.0
H (1)	157	53.0
N (1)	8	2.6
H (1)	116	39.5
N (1)	3	1.6
H (1)	300	101
N (1)	2	1.3
H (1)	300	68.2

The implication of these studies is clear. It is that hypertension does something which increases the rate of cholesterol synthesis in arterial wall and in liver. The incubation experiments demonstrate that this effect is still operative after the vessel has been removed from the immediate stimulus of blood pressure and placed in a flask.

Incubation experiments always leave a question, since the conditions cannot be described as physiological. Under normal circumstances does the aorta of a hypertensive rat synthesize cholesterol faster than that of a normotensive rat? Indeed, can synthesis in the aorta *in vivo* be demonstrated at all? There is convincing evidence of exchange of cholesterol between plasma and the arterial wall. Most studies have suggested that the cholesterol in plaques at least is derived from plasma.

Because there is exchange between vessel and plasma and because synthesis of cholesterol in the liver and the intestine is rapid, studies with labelled acetate could not be used to answer this question. Instead, the reverse approach was used. A large group of Carworth Nelson rats (average weight 53 g.) was taken at weaning. Eleven were killed immediately and the cholesterol content of their aortas measured. The remaining animals were then placed on a diet containing 2% cholesterol 2-C^{14} of constant S.A. The serum cholesterol of all rats therefore soon approached the S.A. of the dietary cholesterol. It was monitored monthly and averaged 545. Half the rats were made hypertensive by renal artery compression. At sacrifice after 138 days on this diet and 116 days after arterial constriction, the aortic cholesterol content was measured and the counts/min. of aortic cholesterol were determined.

The amount of cholesterol in the aorta closely correlated with the average blood pressure of the animal (Fig. 5). The shaded segment on the left side of the figure represents the amount of

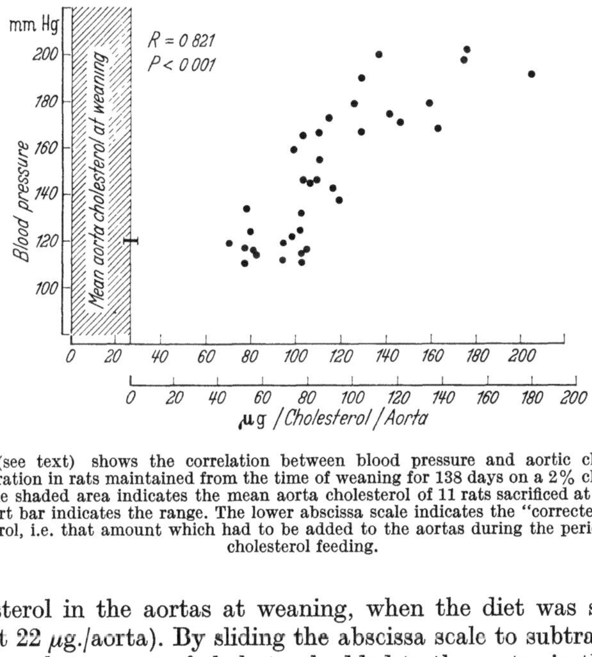

Fig. 5 (see text) shows the correlation between blood pressure and aortic cholesterol concentration in rats maintained from the time of weaning for 138 days on a 2% cholesterol diet. The shaded area indicates the mean aorta cholesterol of 11 rats sacrificed at weaning. The short bar indicates the range. The lower abscissa scale indicates the "corrected" aortic cholesterol, i.e. that amount which had to be added to the aortas during the period of 2% cholesterol feeding.

cholesterol in the aortas at weaning, when the diet was started (about 22 μg./aorta). By sliding the abscissa scale to subtract this amount, the amount of cholesterol added to the aortas in the diet period, during which serum cholesterol was labelled, can be seen. We shall call this the "corrected" aorta cholesterol.

If all the cholesterol in aortas is derived from the plasma and the plasma cholesterol is labelled, the aorta cholesterol must be equally labelled. If, on the other hand, the cholesterol in the aorta is synthesized locally from cold precursors, the S.A. of aorta cholesterol should be lower than that of plasma cholesterol. The known exchange between plasma and aorta will tend so obscure this difference.

We found that the S.A. of the aortic cholesterol (calculated after correction for the amount present at weaning) is lower in the hypertensive than in the normotensive animals (Fig. 6); in the latter, it approaches the S.A. of the plasma cholesterol.

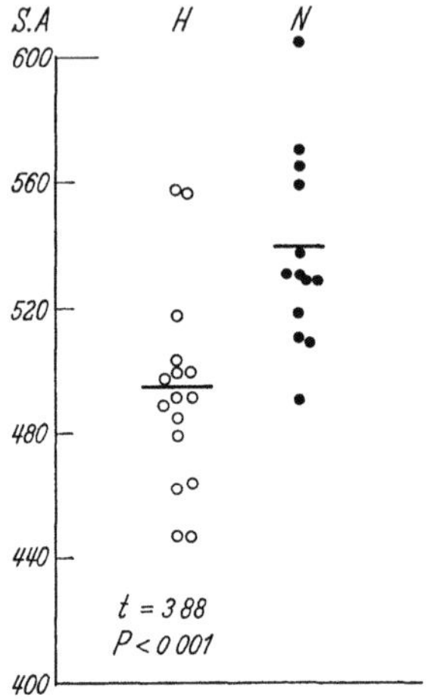

Fig. 6. The "corrected specific activity" (see text) of cholesterol in aortas of hypertensive and normotensive rats maintained at constant serum cholesterol specific activity (S.A.) from time of weaning. The lower specific activity in the aortas of the hypertensive rats implies a greater local synthesis of cholesterol from non-labelled precursors.

If the amount of unlabelled cholesterol in the aorta which cannot be accounted for by the initial pool at weaning is calculated for each animal, it is found that this minimum amount of cholesterol which must have been synthesized (even if there were no exchange with plasma) is proportional to the blood pressure of the animal. This is true whether the calculation is made on the basis of the total aortic cholesterol or, as in Fig. 7, on the basis of cholesterol per mg. of aorta nitrogen. These are minimum figures. Since we know that cholesterol exchange between artery and plasma is rather rapid, it is reasonable to assume that much more was actually synthesized locally.

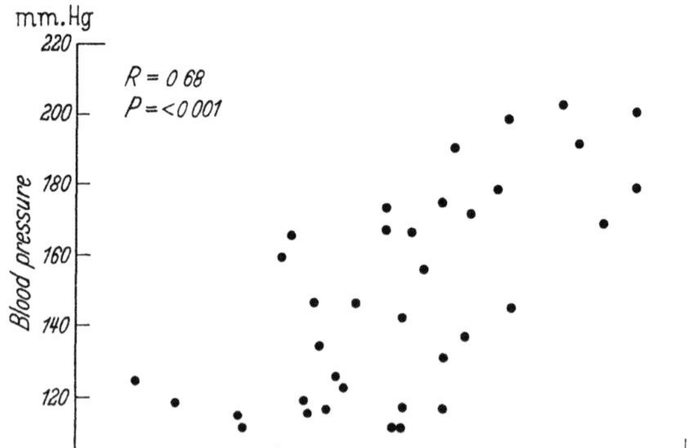

Fig. 7. The minimum amount of cholesterol (in µg./mg. aorta N) synthesized locally in aorta wall is shown to be proportional to the blood pressure of the animal (see text).

Summary

It has been demonstrated in rats that

1. hypertension intensifies dietary atherogenesis,
2. pharmacological control of blood pressure reverses this effect,
3. hypertension increases the amount of cholesterol in artery wall prior to visible atherosclerosis development,
4. this increase in artery cholesterol and the increased rate of atherogenesis are not dependent on increased plasma cholesterol,
5. hypertension increases the rate of synthesis of cholesterol in arteries and in liver, an effect demonstrable both *in vitro* and *in vivo.*

Zusammenfassung

An Ratten ließ sich zeigen, daß

1. Hochdruck die diätetisch hervorgerufene Atherogenese verstärkt,
2. dieser Effekt durch medikamentöse Blutdrucksenkung rückgängig zu machen ist,
3. beim Hochdruck der Cholesteringehalt der Arterienwand vermehrt ist, ehe es zur Entwicklung einer sichtbaren Atherosklerose kommt,
4. diese Zunahme des Cholesterins in den Arterien und die größere Häufigkeit der Atherogenese nicht von einer gesteigerten Cholesterinkonzentration im Plasma abhängen,
5. der Hochdruck die Geschwindigkeit der Cholesterinsynthese in den Arterien und der Leber beschleunigt, ein Effekt, der sowohl *in vitro* als auch *in vivo* nachweisbar ist.

Résumé

On a démontré chez le rat que:

1. l'hypertension renforce le processus athéromateux provoqué par un régime approprié,
2. la réduction pharmacologique de l'élévation tensionnelle supprime cet effet,
3. l'hypertension augmente le taux de cholestérol dans la paroi artérielle avant l'apparition des lésions visibles d'athérosclérose,
4. cet accroissement du taux de cholestérol dans la paroi artérielle et l'augmentation de l'athérogénèse sont indépendants de l'élévation du taux de cholestérol dans le plasma,
5. l'hypertension accélère la synthèse du cholestérol dans les artères et le foie, phénomène qu'il est possible de démontrer à la fois *in vitro* et *in vivo.*

Acknowledgement

The work and thoughts I have presented are not, of course, exclusively my own. They are the results of studies made by a group which currently includes Dr. Marie M. Daly, Dr. H. N. Adel, Dr. Aida Baltazar, Mrs. L. M. Brun, and Mrs. V. M. Raeff at the Albert Einstein College of Medicine and which formerly included Dr. E. H. Mosbach, Dr. Margaret Bevans, Dr. J. Edreira, and Miss R. Kaplan at Columbia University.

References

1. LEW: Build and Blood Pressure Study. Society of Actuaries. Chicago, 1959. — 2. MASTER, A. H.: Circulation 8, 170 (1953). — 3. DAWBER, T. R., and W. B. KANNEL: Mod. Concepts Cardiovasc. Dis. **30**, 674 (1961). — 4. PATERSON, J. C., J. MILLS, and C. H. LOCKWOOD: Canad. Med. Ass. J. **82**, 65 (1960). — 5. KANNELL, W. B., T. R. DAWBER, A. KAGAN, N. REVOTSKIE, and J. STOKES: Ann. Int. Med. **55**, 33 (1961). — 6. GUBNER, R. S.: In: Hypertension. Recent Advances. The Second Hahnemann Symposium on Hypertensive Disease. Ed. by A. N. BREST and J. H. MOYER. Lea and Febiger, Philadelphia, 1961, p. 21. — 7. Annual Epidemiologic and Vital Statistics (1957). World Health Organization, Geneva, 1960. — 8. UNGAR, H., and G. KALLNER: In: Israel. Ethnic Laboratory, Roche Medical Image **3**, No. 3, 1961. — 9. ROBERTSON, W. B.: J. Atherosclerosis Res. **2**, 79 (1962), and Lancet 1959/I, **444**. — 10. DEMING, Q. B., E. H. MOSBACH, M. BEVANS, M. M. DALY, L. L. ABELL, E. MARTIN, L. M. BRUN, E. HALPERN, and R. KAPLAN: J. Exper. Med. **107**, 581 (1958). — 11. DEMING, Q. B., L. M. BRUN, R. KAPLAN, M. M. DALY, J. BLOOM, and M. SCHECHTER: In: Hypertension. Recent Advances. The Second Hahnemann Symposium on Hypertensive Disease. Ed. by A. N. BREST and J. H. MOYER. Lea and Febiger, Philadelphia, 1961, p. 160. — 12. FLOYER, M. A., and P. C. RICHARDSON: Lancet 1961/I, 253. — 13. DALY, M. M., Q. B. DEMING, V. M. RAEFF, and L. M. BRUN: J. Clin. Invest. **42**, 1606 (1963). — 14. MORRIS, M. D., I. L. CHAIKOFF, J. M. FELTS, S. ABRAHAM, and N. O. FANSAH: J. Biol. Chem. **224**, 1039 (1957). — 15. ADEL, H. N., Q. B. DEMING, M. M. DALY, V. M. RAEFF, and L. M. BRUN: J. Laborat. Clin. Med. **66**, 571 (1965). — 16. a) WARTMAN, W. B., and H. K. HELLERSTEIN: Ann. Int. Med. **28**, 41 (1948); — b) ZINN, W. J., and R. S. COSBY: Amer. J. Med. 8, 169 (1950); — c) GREISMAN, H., and S. Z. ROSENFIELD: N. Y. State J. Med. **48**, 1277 (1948); — d) BILLING, T. E., Jr., B. M. KALSTONE, J. L. SPENCER, C. O. T. BALL, and G. R. MENEELY: Amer. J. Med. **7**, 356 (1949); — e) WRIGHT, I. S., C. D. MARPLE, and D. F. BECK: In: Myocardial Infarction. Report of Committee on Anticoagulants. Published for Amer. Heart Ass. Grune and Stratton, New York, 1954, p. 46; — f) WEINREB, H. L., E. GERMAN, and B. ROSENBERG: Ann. Int. Med. **46**, 285 (1957); — g) JAMES, T. N., H. W. POST, and F. J. SMITH: Ann. Int. Med. **43**, 153 (1955); — h) MASTER, A. H.: Circulation **8**, 170 (1953).

The vascular crisis in hypertension

By

F. B. Byrom*

The hypertensive vascular crisis may be defined as a phase of hypertension in which some terminal arteries and arterioles are unable to respond physiologically to excessive filling tension. It can be conveniently studied in the rat with a solitary kidney, the artery to which has been constricted by a simplified Goldblatt clamp devised by Wilson (*1*). This clamp consists of a staple made from pure silver tape, with a gap of 0.02 to 0.025 cm.; it is easily applied and almost as easily removed. The clip protects the single kidney against secondary hypertensive damage (*2*), and when it is removed the blood pressure invariably returns to normal within two to four hours (*3*). It is therefore possible to make observations before, during, and after the hypertension – the proof and counter-proof of Claude Bernard.

In rats so treated, blood pressure rises gradually over a period of days, weeks, or months, to reach a fairly constant level, and when this level is very high, that is to say 200 mm. Hg systolic or more as measured by tail-cuff and microphone, an acute vascular crisis may occur, sometimes at once, often only after many weeks (*4*). The underlying vascular disturbance, though focal, is wide-spread, but the signs are usually cerebral. They include coma, generalised epileptiform convulsions which normally start with twitching of one limb, rhythmical spasmodic contractions of groups of muscles, and disorientation. Left to itself, the rat will sometimes recover but will usually relapse. More often, death occurs in coma within three days. If the clip is removed, however, convulsions will have ceased by the time the rat has recovered from the anaesthetic, and other symptoms will have disappeared by the following day, unless the animal is moribund at the time of operation.

The causation of the symptoms

In extreme or malignant hypertension, focal necrotic or proliferative lesions and small haemorrhages are common in or around

* Member of the External Staff of the Medical Research Council

terminal arteries. Identical lesions are found in the brain and elsewhere in rats with encephalopathy, but not often enough to account for the signs. Moreover, signs which disappear within minutes or hours of the correction of the hypertension cannot be ascribed to lesions which require days or weeks to heal, but clearly indicate a more labile abnormality which may or may not be severe enough to destroy tissue. The coma suggests oedema

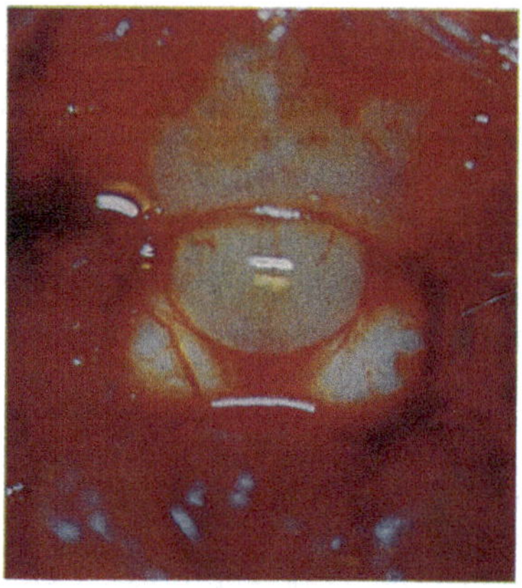

Fig. 1. Post-mortem dissection of the dorsal aspect of the neck in a rat with fatal encephalopathy, showing a bulbous protrusion of the vermis of the cerebellum through the foramen magnum [from F. B. BYROM: Lectures on the Scientific Basis of Medicine. Athlone Press, London, 8, 256 (1958/59)].

of the brain, and this suspicion is borne out by a progressive rise in the water content of the brain and the presence of a cerebellar pressure cone in fatal cases (Fig. 1). If trypan blue is injected intravenously shortly before the animal is killed, multiple blue spots are regularly found in the cerebral cortex (Fig. 2). These sometimes coincide with structural lesions, but in four out of five blue areas no histological abnormality can be detected, at any rate in single sections. The water content of the blue areas, however, is markedly increased, whereas that of the unstained areas is normal in early encephalopathy, but moderately increased if the symptoms persist. It is therefore clear that the oedema springs from a finite number of points in the cerebral vascular tree and spreads widely in fatal cases. Localised oedema is also found in the pancreas and occasionally in the retina, which may become detached (Fig. 3).

The focal oedema is accompanied by the following changes in the arteries and arterioles of the brain, as observed through permanent acrylic cranial windows, and in the arterioles of the retina,

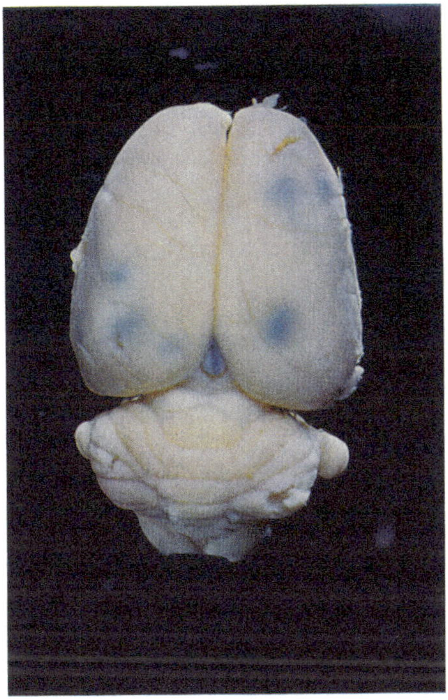

Fig. 2. Brain of a rat with encephalopathy killed soon after an intravenous injection of trypan blue, showing rounded areas of stain on the surface of the cerebral cortex [from F. B. Byrom (*4*)].

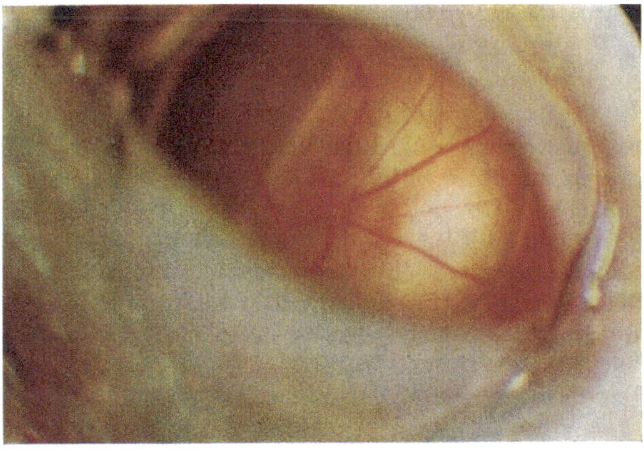

Fig. 3. Retina of a rat during a vascular crisis showing a) detachment of one half of the retina by focal oedema and b) obliterative spasm of arterioles in the other half.

as seen through a cover-slip over a drop of mydriatic solution in the conjunctival sac: 1. slight dilatation, tortuosity, and unevenness in calibre of large arteries, 2. intense constriction, occasionally with zones of dilatation, of terminal arteries, and 3. an irregular pattern of constriction and dilatation of intermediate vessels. The over-all appearance is one of constriction and pallor; the pallor may be secondary to the oedema.

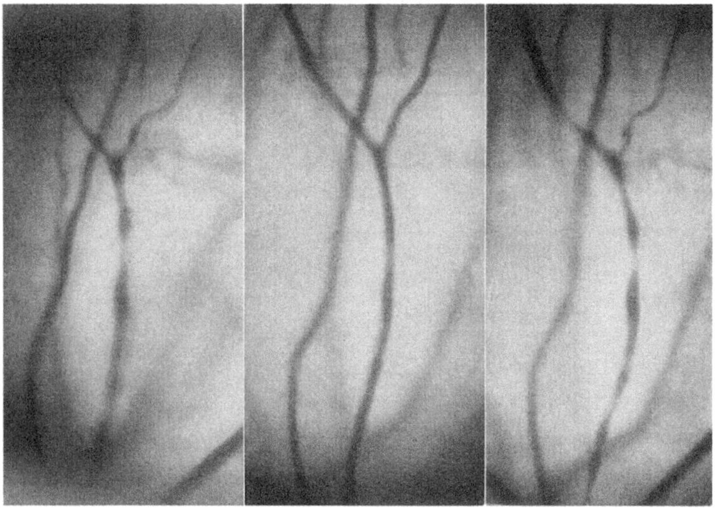

4 5 6

Figs 4—6. Reversible focal spasm of the retinal arterioles in a rat with a vascular crisis. Fig. 4. Light ether anaesthesia. The arteriole shows alternating zones of constriction and dilatation. Fig. 5. Five minutes later, deep ether anaesthesia. The calibre of the arteriole is almost uniform. Fig. 6. Ten minutes after suspending ether. Constrictions and dilatations have reappeared in the same places [from F. B. Byrom (*5*)].

These changes in calibre develop gradually before the onset of symptoms, are fixed in pattern and remarkably persistent, and strongly suggest irreversible changes in structure (Fig. 4). Nevertheless, the calibre of the vessels can almost always be restored to normal, in the early stages by deep ether anaesthesia (Figs 5 and 6), and later by removing the clip from the renal artery (*5*) (Figs 7—9).

It remains to consider the causes of the change in calibre and relate them to the various features of the vascular crisis. During the development of renal hypertension, the cardiac output rises and provokes a compensatory, probably myogenic, increase in tone in the resistance vessels; in early or moderate hypertension this is covered by the normal physiological reserves of tone and perhaps, given time, by compensatory hyperplasia. If the severity of the hypertension increases, however, the blood pressure may reach critical levels, at which *even* contraction of the resistance vessels

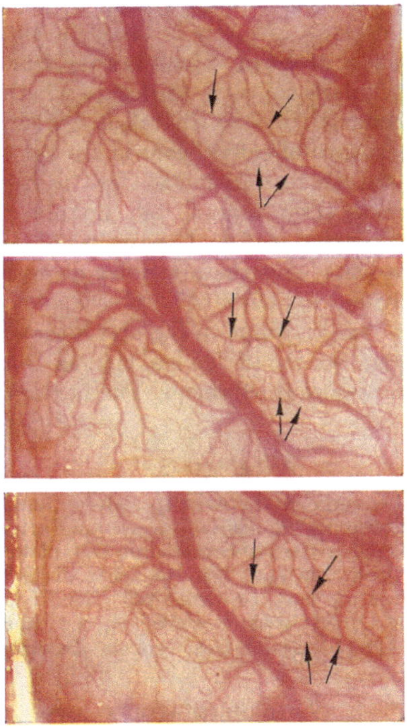

Figs 7—9. Focal spasm in the branches of the middle cerebral artery in encephalopathy, as seen through a permanent cranial window. Fig. 7. Oct. 20th. Blood pressure 170. No symptoms. Artery even and dilated. Fig. 8. Dec. 1st. Blood pressure 230. Early encephalopathy, showing localised arterial narrowing, one branch being barely visible. Fig. 9. Dec. 4th. Three days after removing clip from renal artery. Blood pressure 140. Vessels normal [from F. B. Byrom (*4*)].

would be possible only if the distribution of muscle fibres along the course of the artery were uniform. If the distribution of fibres in the cerebral vessels is only slightly uneven when the critical range of pressure is reached, the more muscular parts of the vessel can contract. In doing so, they relieve the strain on the wall by reducing its radius, while the weaker regions dilate and so become more vulnerable. In this way, the characteristics of the disorderly contraction can be plausibly explained, and it is not surprising to find disturbed circulation in tissues irrigated by vessels which cannot counteract filling tension by even contraction. Nevertheless, the exact nature of the disturbance is still far from clear. Since PAL (*6*) first described vascular crises, they have been attributed by some workers to excessive vasoconstriction (spasm) and by others to overdilatation of resistance vessels. It now seems true to say that both changes are present, not only in the same subject, but in the same vessels. The real problem, which is crucial to an understanding of malignant hypertension, is to decide whether the vascular crisis is caused by constriction, by dilatation, by both, or by neither. The rapid disappearance of convulsions in the rat upon removal of the clip and the sudden restoration of sight in human encephalopathy during venesection suggest, but do not prove, that the observed vasoconstriction is in fact spasm which causes the symptoms, the focal oedema, and the arteriolar necrosis. On the other hand, there is clear-cut evidence of local escape of plasma into the tissues, both in the rat and in man (*7*), and it may well be that the dilated zones are the source of the leakage, as DOLLERY suggests, and that the leakage does the damage. Further work in this field is clearly needed.

Summary

In some cases of experimental renal hypertension, uniform physiological contraction of some terminal branches of the systemic arterial tree gradually gives way to an irregular pattern of constriction and dilatation. In some way that is not quite clear, this may lead to acute disturbance of function (encephalopathy), focal oedema, or structural lesions typical of malignant hypertension. If the hypertension is abolished, the calibre of the vessels returns to normal, symptoms and focal oedema disappear, and structural lesions heal.

Zusammenfassung

Beim experimentell-renalen Hochdruck an der Ratte läßt sich gelegentlich beobachten, daß in einigen arteriellen Endverzweigungen die gleichmäßige physiologische Kontraktion allmählich einer unregelmäßigen Verteilung von Konstriktion und Dilatation Platz macht. Dies kann in einer bisher noch nicht völlig geklärten Weise zu akuten Funktionsstorungen (Enzephalopathie), fokalem Ödem oder strukturellen Schädigungen führen, wie sie für die maligne Hypertension typisch sind. Wird der Druck zur Norm gesenkt, so normalisiert sich der Gefäßdurchmesser, die Symptome und das fokale Ödem verschwinden, und die Läsionen können ausheilen.

Résumé

Dans quelques cas d'hypertension expérimentale rénale du rat, la contraction physiologique uniforme de certaines branches terminales de l'arbre artériel fait graduellement place à des aspects irréguliers de constriction et de dilatation. D'une manière qui n'est pas tout à fait claire, ce phénomène peut aller jusqu'à des perturbations fonctionnelles aiguës (encéphalopathie), des foyers d'oedème ou des aspects lésionnels typiques d'hypertension maligne. Si on supprime l'hypertension, le calibre des vaisseaux redevient normal, les symptômes et les foyers d'oedème disparaissent, les lésions organiques guérissent.

Acknowledgement

I am indebted to Prof. CLIFFORD WILSON and the Board of Governors of the London Hospital, London, for temporary laboratory accommodation.

References

1. WILSON, C., and F. B. BYROM: Lancet 1939/I, 136. — 2. WILSON, C., and G. W. PICKERING: Clin. Sc. **3**, 343 (1938). — 3. BYROM, F. B., and L. F. DODSON: Clin. Sc. 8, 1 (1949). — 4. BYROM, F. B.: Lancet 1954/II, 201. — 5. BYROM, F. B.: Lancet 1963/I, 516. — 6. PAL, J.: Die Gefaßkrisen. Hirzel, Leipzig, 1905. — 7. DOLLERY, C. T., and J. V. HODGE: Transact. Ophth. Soc. Unit. Kingdom **83**, 115 (1963).

Discussion

Pickering: I think I told Dr. Byrom before that when I was a student at Cambridge, Joseph Barcroft said that Newton Richards had introduced a new principle into physiology, which was that if you wanted to find out what was happening, you should look and see. This, I think, is the great virtue of these lovely experiments. Now I am extremely curious about this effect of anaesthesia, and I should like to ask Dr. Byrom one or two questions: 1) Has he ever denervated any of the arteries, such as the intestinal arteries, which I think share the same phenomenon ? 2) Has he ever infused renin into rats, and do they show the same kind of changes ? Prinzmetal and I[1] found that ether, amongst other anaesthetics, interfered with the action of renin in the rabbit.

Byrom: Cervical sympathectomy neither prevents nor abolishes calibre changes in the cerebral arteries. — I have not tried renin. I have tried infusing angiotensin and found nothing but a very fleeting vasoconstriction. I think that infusing angiotensin for several days might possibly cause changes in calibre.

Carlsson: With regard to the question of denervation, it may be of interest to note that the intraretinal vessels lack adrenergic innervation[2]. Do these changes occur even if there is no anaesthesia ?

Byrom: I cannot see the unanaesthetised rat's retina, but others[3] have reported marked changes.

Carlsson: I asked the question because it may be that in light ether anaesthesia adrenalinaemia occurs. Did you try adrenaline to see whether you could produce the changes in deep ether anaesthesia ?

Byrom: Yes, but ether only works in the very early stages of the experiment.

Carlsson: Yes, but perhaps adrenalinaemia occurs early in light ether anaesthesia, whereas in deep ether the plasma adrenaline concentration probably goes down.

Byrom: You can reverse this change with the aid of ether in the early days or weeks. If the change persists for many weeks or months, as it may, it will no longer react to ether, but will still usually disappear if the clip is removed.

Hood: I'd like to turn to Dr. Deming's paper. I think he left us with a very strong impression that the rate of cholesterol synthesis goes up in his hypertensive animals. However, not knowing the specific activity of the immediate intra-tissue precursor pool, there might still be some slight doubt. Now it is interesting that the whole carcass cholesterol, liver cholesterol, and aortic cholesterol were all high. In man, for instance, we found no relation

[1] Pickering, G. W., and M. Prinzmetal: Clin. Sc. **3**, 211 (1937—1938).
[2] Malmfors, T.: Acta physiol. Scand. to be published (1965).
[3] Abt, von, and K., R. Brückner: Ophthalmologica **119**, 17 (1951).

whatsoever between muscle, liver, red cell, and serum cholesterol in the 50 subjects we have measured. Can you pin-point the possible defect? Did you study the incorporation of C^{14} in CO_2 or in long-chain fatty acids or both?

Deming: We have not done these studies in the Warburg apparatus; we used a Dubnoff incubator-shaker. I don't think that there is any doubt in this instance, because we have obtained consistent results both *in vitro* and *in vivo*. That is, in the last experiment, we were working with a labelled cholesterol environment and in the end we found in the tissue unlabelled cholesterol which must have been synthesised. In the former experiment, we started with a labelled precursor and, both in the whole animal and in incubation studies, we ended up with more label in the cholesterol of the tissue from the hypertensive rats. But we have not measured the carbon dioxide radio-activity.

Gross: I should like to ask Dr. Byrom what effect deep ether anaesthesia had on the height of blood pressure. Did blood pressure in the hypertensive animal fall substantially or even become normal?

Byrom: Between light and deep ether anaesthesia in these experiments the mean carotid pressure falls by at least 30—40 mm. Hg.

Bein: In experiments of eight weeks' duration, Wanner, a student of mine, studied in rats the influence of renal hypertension on the fatty infiltration of the aorta caused by an atherogenic diet. He, too, found that renal hypertension enhances lipid infiltration. Furthermore, he discovered that some animals, despite clamping, did not develop high blood pressure and reacted with an enhanced lipid infiltration. However, this was the case only in gonadectomised females and in thyroidectomised animals. In gonadectomised males, clamping *per se* did not lead to enhanced lipid deposition; an enforced lipoidosis was connected with elevated blood pressure in this group.

Deming: There is no doubt that, even without hypertension, you can get lipid infiltration and, in fact, frank atheroma. They are not in a one-to-one relationship. The only point I was trying to make is that the higher the blood pressure, the more readily and the more rapidly it develops; but certainly from human data we know that you don't have to have hypertension to have atherosclerosis. The artery does not draw a line between normal and abnormal pressures, but the rate of damage is affected by the pressure.

Peart: I wonder if Dr. Byrom tried the effect of increasing the amounts of CO_2 in these rats. A high CO_2 concentration is one of the things one would expect to occur in deep ether anaesthesia, and it may be that dilatation of the vessels would remove these areas of vasoconstriction. Further, have you sectioned these areas where you pin-point the lesion and found any organic change histologically at that area subsequently?

Byrom: CO_2 may be concerned. I use an ether-oxygen mixture, but the respiration becomes very slow, and there may be a build-up of CO_2. However, ether becomes ineffective in chronic experiments. — As for pin-pointing the lesions in relation to the dilatations and constrictions, I am afraid my histological technique is not good enough.

Dollery: I should like to raise two points, Dr. Byrom. The first concerns the uneven distribution of muscle down the retinal arterioles. I am not familiar with the rat, but using the digestion technique in the rhesus monkey, the dog, and the cat, you can see the musculature very clearly, and it is evenly distributed in these species. It used to be said that there was no smooth muscle in the retinal arterioles, but this is not true. — The other point is that in man, if you infuse noradrenaline or angiotensin intravenously and so raise the blood pressure in a normotensive, you can cause retinal arteriolar constriction; but it's not a focal constriction, it is uniform.

Byrom: Perhaps I might add that this is very often the case in the rat. It is only the isolated rat with an excessively high pressure, a really very bad case of renal hypertension, that shows these focal changes. The diffuse changes are very much commoner.

Dengler: Dr. Deming, do you have any evidence whether these changes in cholesterol synthesis are due to adaptive enzyme formation?

Deming: No, we don't.

Byrom: Dr. Deming, have you tried or thought of the possibility of producing hypertension by constricting the aorta and using the lower part as a control in these atheroma studies?

Deming: We have not done this, because the upper and lower aorta are quite different from each other without constriction; in fact, as we go along, there is a progressive change in the concentration of almost any element you pick; whether it's the muscle or connective tissue or lipid or anything else, they all change as you go down the arterial tree.

Page: I think we all recognise that the next great phase in the treatment of hypertension will be the treatment and prevention of atherosclerosis. So we are in business for a long, long time. I assure you we are not working ourselves out of an occupation by treating hypertension. And it is clear that a reduction in mortality is going to result from the reduction in blood pressure which will in turn prevent "atheropoiesis", if I may use this term as an alternative to "atherogenesis".

Vascular disease and hypertension

By

G. W. Pickering

There are many kinds of vascular disease, and they are each related differently to raised arterial pressure. In this communication the diseases will be reviewed in terms of arterial size. Only the commonest conditions can be considered.

It should be pointed out at the beginning that this subject has been utterly confused by the use of the terms "arteriosclerosis" and "atherosclerosis" either to include all non-inflammatory diseases of every coat of every artery, ranging in size from aorta to retinal arteries, or for a specific disease, at the whim of the writer. Atherosclerosis is a particularly ridiculous term. It means literally "hardening by means of porridge".

Diseases of large arteries

1. Nodular arteriosclerosis or atheroma. This is essentially an intimal disease in which raised plaques or nodules project into the lumen; the media is thinned over them, and the adventitia is thickened and vascular. The fatty-fibrous intimal plaques are chiefly important because of the tendency of thrombi to form on them. The thrombi, which are composed of platelet masses fringed with leucocytes and interspersed with fibrin strands, may occupy a segment of the wall, where they may organise into fibrous plaques, from which they may become detached as emboli (producing transient ischaemia in retina and brain); or they may occlude the lumen completely, producing arrest of blood flow until this is re-established through collateral channels.

The disease is thus a cause of two of the important complications of hypertension — stroke and myocardial infarct. It is not the only cause of stroke, nor — as we shall see — is it the disease which is responsible for the very close relationship between stroke and elevated arterial pressure. It is virtually the sole cause of myocardial infarction.

It is still uncertain whether the atheromatous part of the plaque or nodule and the thrombus represent different processes or whether the disease is a thrombotic disease throughout (Pickering, 1964).

The frequency of the development of coronary heart disease in the Framingham survey in relation to serum cholesterol and diastolic arterial pressure is shown in Fig. 1. Other factors known to affect the prevalence of myocardial infarction are the smoking of cigarettes and lack of physical exercise. This disease has thus a

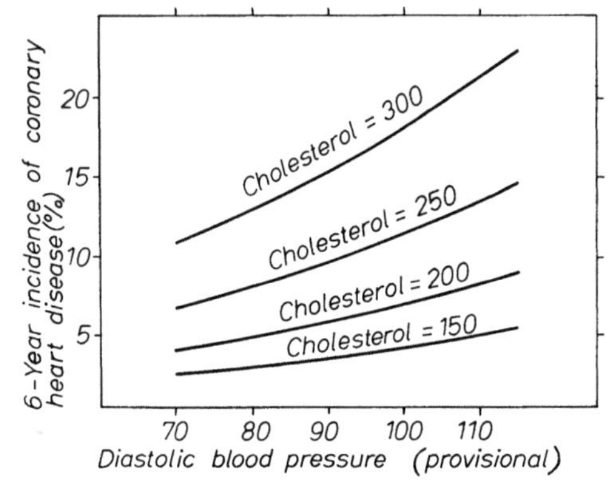

Fig. 1. Risk of coronary heart disease according to level of diastolic blood pressure, Framingham men, aged 45-62, with various serum cholesterol levels.

definite but low correlation with arterial pressure. That it is so lowly correlated led ALLBUTT to recognise this disease, which he termed "decrescent arteriosclerosis", as being different from his "hyperpiesia" or essential hypertension.

2. Senile ectasia. This degenerative disease of the media is symptomless apart from aneurysm and dissection. Its relationship to raised arterial pressure is not clear, though it is generally supposed to be associated with systolic hypertension.

3. Moenckeberg's medial calcification. This is a symptomless disease. Its relationship to raised arterial pressure is not known for certain.

Diseases of small arteries and arterioles

Diseases affecting the intima

1. Elastosis. Fragmentation and reduplication of internal elastic lamina with intimal thickening.

2. Cellular intimal thickening. Thick layers of cells between internal elastic lamella and intima.

3. Fatty hyaline intimal thickening. A layer of hyaline and fatty material between intimal elastic lamella and intima.

These conditions, affecting progressively smaller arteries, are particularly frequent in the kidneys of patients with essential hypertension. Their severity is proportional to the height of arterial pressure (Table 1, Fig. 2). These conditions are difficult to produce experimentally, and our knowledge of them is based on human material. It is generally assumed that they are the result in part of raised arterial pressure.

Table 1. *The relation between the severity of hypertension, as gauged by the diastolic blood pressure, and renal vascular disease* (from SMITHWICK and CASTLEMAN, 1951)

Severity of hypertension	Percentage having renal vascular disease	
	None to mild	Moderate to severe
Intermittent	75	25
Persistent:		
Diastolic blood pressure 90—109 mm. Hg.	61	39
Diastolic blood pressure 110—139 mm. Hg.	37	63
Diastolic blood pressure 140+ mm. Hg	29	71

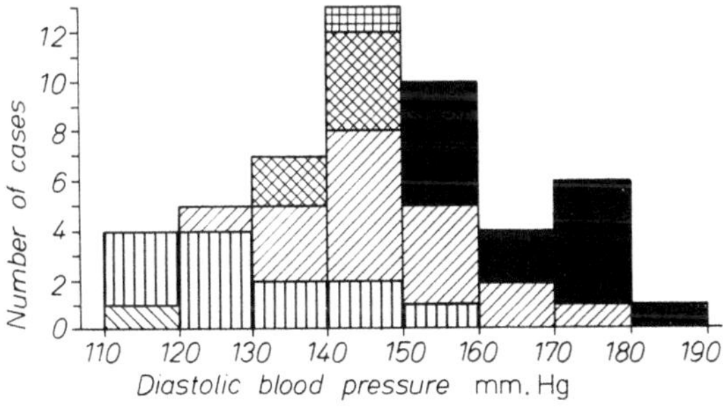

Fig. 2. Relationship of the grade of change in the small arteries and arterioles of the kidney to the diastolic arterial pressure in 50 patients with high blood pressure in whom renal biopsies were performed at operation for sympathectomy. The degree of change is graded 0 to IV, N. represents fibrinoid necrosis. 0: ▧, I: ▥, II: ▨, III: ▩, IV ▦, N.: ■ [from R. H. HEPTINSTALL: Brit. Heart J. *16*, 133 (1954)].

Diseases affecting the media

1. Cerebral micro-aneurysms. These are the most important for our present purpose. CHARCOT and BOUCHARD, in 1868, demonstrated that there was a close association between micro-aneurysm of small cerebral arteries and death from cerebral haemorrhage. The arteries affected were, particularly, the small perforating arteries, such as the lenticulostriate artery. CHARCOT and BOUCHARD used an unconventional technique: they allowed the brains to decompose in running water. The arteries rotted more slowly and were left behind when the brain had disintegrated; the swellings on the small arteries were then clearly visible. These small aneurysms were not well revealed by the conventional pathological methods. They were rediscovered in 1963 by ROSS RUSSELL, who injected a barium sulphate gelatin mass into the brains of 54 subjects freshly coming to autopsy in Boston City Hospital. In the hypertensive group the state of the brain was as follows:

four normal,
five multiple small infarctions,
five massive recent haemorrhages,
three massive recent infarctions,
four small old haemorrhages.

RUSSELL found (a) that atheromatous stenosis of the basal arteries was increased with age and with elevated arterial pressure; (b) that the walls of the small arteries were thickened and their lumens diminished in patients with hypertension; and (c) that

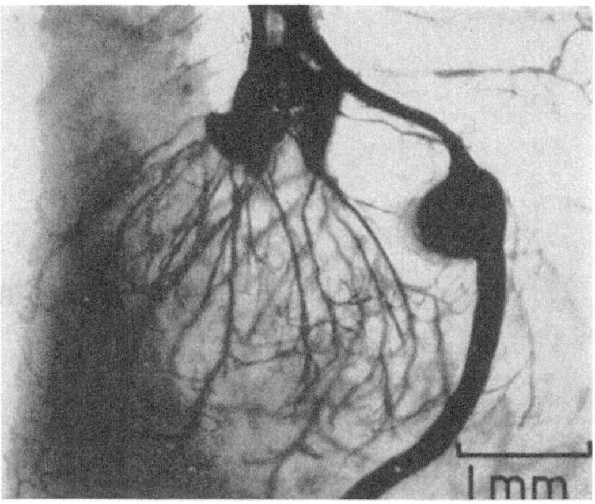

Fig. 3. Aneurysm 800 μ. in diameter on long penetrating artery from parietal cortex of a 71-year-old man dying of cerebral haemorrhage. Note dissection of the injection mass within the aneurysm wall (from ROSS RUSSELL, 1963).

aneurysms were present on small arteries in well-defined areas of the brain, particularly in the regions of the basal ganglia. These aneurysms were found on small arteries 100–300 μ. in diameter, particularly on lateral branches of the striate arteries or on penetrating vessels from the cortex (Fig. 3). The muscular tissue of the parent vessel terminated abruptly at the point of origin of the aneurysm and the remnants of elastica could be seen to extend for a short distance into the aneurysm before disappearing. The wall of the aneurysm was composed of connective tissue only, an inner hyaline layer derived from the intima fusing with an outer collagenous layer continuous with the adventitia of the parent vessel. Such aneurysms were present in all but one of the brains of the hypertensive group and in ten of the brains of the normotensive group. Frequently the aneurysms showed evidence of leaking and of thrombosis.

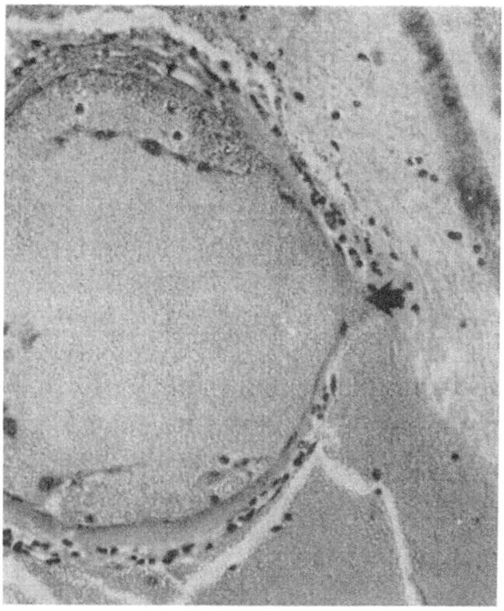

Fig. 4. High-power view of aneurysm wall. Stained haematoxylin and eosin. There is a small break in the wall (arrow), and injection mass communicates with the Virchow-Robin space (from Ross Russell, 1963).

Russell's observations suggest that such aneurysms form quickly and continuously in patients with elevated pressure as they grow

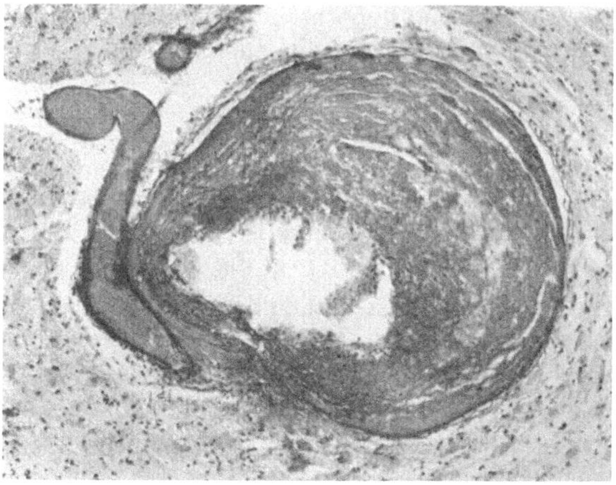

Fig. 5. Elderly hypertensive subject. Aneurysm on small striate artery showing evidence of thrombosis. Stained elastica (van Gieson; × 125). Serial sections confirmed that this structure was an aneurysm and not a portion of a larger artery (from Ross Russell, 1963).

older. They can produce small haemorrhages (Fig. 4) and small thromboses (Fig. 5) with local softening which would resemble the miliary infarcts described by ROSENBERG (1940). When the thromboses extend proximally into larger arteries, larger areas of softening may result. Finally, there may be massive rupture with massive intracerebral haemorrhage. It would seem likely that these intracerebral aneurysms are the missing link between raised arterial pressure and cerebral vascular disease.

2. Fibrinoid necrosis. This is the most important, though not the only, lesion of small arteries and arterioles in the malignant phase. There seem to be three processes involved: the destruction of muscle fibres of the media, the deposition in both intima and media of "fibrinoid", i. e. material staining like fibrin, and the reaction (more or less inflammatory) accompanying these changes. Fibrinoid necrosis is not only diagnostic of the malignant phase; it largely determines its course and progress.

There are two broadly opposing views of the relationship of fibrinoid necrosis to raised arterial pressure: one is that there is no, or at most a negligible, relationship between the two, fibrinoid necrosis being due to a humoral agent which may or may not be associated with hypertension; the other is that there is a close relationship, fibrinoid necrosis and the malignant phase being the results of a very severe hypertension. Now, the first of these is not a true scientific hypothesis, because it is incapable of refutation; it can always be argued that the substance has not yet been isolated or extracted. The second hypothesis is capable of refutation, both in man and in animals. Let us take man first.

The evidence in man

(i) If this second hypothesis is correct, there should be a relationship between arterial pressure and both the fibrinoid and the malignant phase. In fact there is (PICKERING, 1961), though there is naturally much overlap (e.g. Fig. 2).

(ii) The malignant phase should occur in any sufficiently severe form of hypertension. DEROW and ALTSCHULE pointed out in 1934 that this was so, but were unable to put forward an explanation.

(iii) If the arterial pressure can be reduced and kept down, then the malignant hypertension should revert to the benign phase and the patient should have an extended life-span. There is now abundant evidence that this is so. To take one example, HARINGTON et al. (1959) judged that the expectation of life of those with early malignant hypertension was increased six to eight times by therapy that effectively reduced arterial pressure.

(iv) The reversal of the malignant phase. In 1952, WRIGHT, HEPTINSTALL, and I published details of three patients in whom the malignant phase was reversed to the benign, by nephrectomy in one case, by sympathectomy and adrenalectomy in the second, and by adrenalectomy in the third. These three patients were unique in my experience, since the diagnosis depended not only on clinical findings, but also on the demonstration of fibrinoid necrosis of small arteries in adrenals and kidneys. When we published the paper, the patients had survived for at least six years. Subsequently, Case 1 died of a cerebral haemorrhage nine years after operation. Cases 2 and 3 are both alive. Case 2, who was 11 years old at the onset of the disease and had a diastolic pressure of 240/170, underwent bilateral sympathectomy and subtotal adrenalectomy in 1946. Fibrinoid necrosis was found in both adrenals and the left kidney. The patient was last seen on June 26th, 1965, when her blood pressure was 170/110. Her urine contained no more than a trace of protein and no excess of red cells. Her pyelonephritis is inactive.

Case 3 was aged 13 when first seen and had a blood pressure of 255/180. She had pyelonephritis. Despite the removal of the smaller, left kidney in July, 1946, her arterial pressure and signs remained unaffected. Subsequently, she underwent subtotal adrenalectomy, after which her arterial pressure varied between 250/150 and 220/115. However, her retinopathy improved and in 1951 nothing remained but scars. She had fibrinoid necrosis and pyelonephritis in the left kidney and in both adrenals. The extent of these lesions is shown in Fig. 6. This girl was subsequently treated with ganglion blockers and is at present under the care of Professor PEART. She married and was delivered of a baby in March, 1965, after a somewhat stormy pregnancy.

The remarkable things about these cases are the extent to which the malignant phase has been reversed and the illustration of how chronic pyelonephritis may be cured or arrested. The extent to which the deposits of fibrinoid material have reduced the arterial lumen makes one wonder what happens to it when the arterial pressure falls. This will be referred to again.

(v) The objections to the theory that severe hypertension is a major factor in the pathogenesis of the malignant phase. — Three sets of facts have been alleged to be inconsistent with this hypothesis concerning the pathogenesis of fibrinoid necrosis and the malignant phase:

In the first place, there is no hint of a dividing line between the pressures of benign and malignant hypertension. I cannot believe seriously that anyone familiar with the variability of arterial

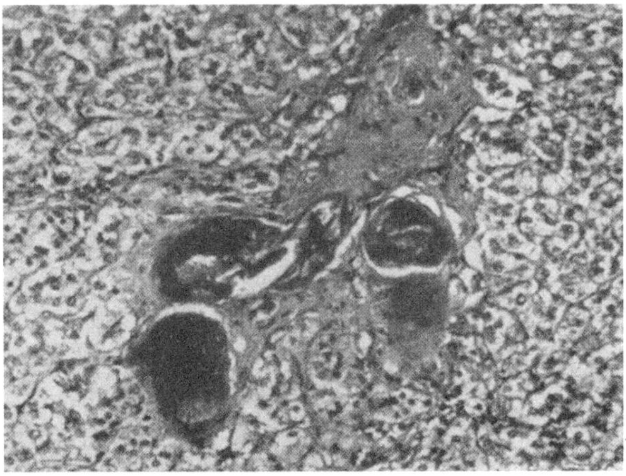

Fig. 6. Case 3. Necrotic vessels in substance of right adrenal. Solid appearance of one of these is due to tangential cutting of its wall.

pressure and its dependence on the circumstances of measurement would have expected this. Moreover, biological variability is characteristic of heterogenous collections of individuals such as laboratory animals and, *a fortiori*, human beings. Finally, I know of no phenomenon which has a single causation uninfluenced by any other factor. Nevertheless, it is notable that the phenomena of the malignant phase occur at much lower pressures in some diseases, e.g. acute nephritis and toxaemia of pregnancy, than in others, e.g. essential hypertension. Whether this is owing to the rate of the rise in pressure or to other factors, e.g. anaemia (PICKERING, 1952), is not known, but it demonstrates that the arterial factor is not the only factor involved – which, indeed, I for one have never considered it to be. Secondly, in a few patients, retinopathy may clear up without a marked lowering of blood pressure. This is an exceptionally rare event and it usually occurs following treatment designed to lower arterial pressure (e.g. Case 3 above). It seems much more likely to me that the isolated readings made in these patients have, through chance factors, obscured a real lowering which more continuous measurement would have disclosed. Thirdly, malignant hypertension has been described without hypertension. Unfortunately, collagen diseases were not excluded. In them, neuroretinopathy, closely mimicking that of the malignant phase, is frequently found.

The evidence from animals

The evidence obtained in animals is of a similar nature. WILSON and I (1938) found in the rabbit, as GOLDBLATT (1938) did in the dog, that, after constriction of the renal artery, fibrinoid necrosis occurred in some animals in the same distribution as in the malignant phase in man, except that the kidney distal to the clamp was spared. In our rabbits, there was pronounced association between the severity of hypertension and that of the arterial lesions. WILSON and BYROM (1939) showed that in the rat constriction of one renal artery, the other kidney being intact, could produce severe hypertension. In such animals, arterial lesions were found in the unclamped kidney but not in the early stages in the clamped kidney. BYROM and DODSON (1948) showed that abrupt raising of the aortic pressure in rats produced acute arteriolar lesions in the kidney which could be prevented by occluding the renal artery during the rise of pressure.

To test the hypothesis that arterial pressure is a major factor in producing fibrinoid necrosis and to see what happens to the lesions when they resolve, we decided to take serial biopsies of the small intestine from rabbits with severe hypertension before and after removing the clamp from the renal artery. This proved an exhausting exercise, perhaps because I have lost my cunning with the renal artery clamp. Of 164 animals which had the right kidney removed and the left renal artery clamped, only 12 developed arterial pressures persistently over 130 mm. Hg. Of these 12 animals, 11 showed fibrinoid necrosis in the arterioles of the gut. When two readings of over 130 mm. Hg had been obtained, a time for operation was agreed. At operation, my colleague, Professor ALLISON, resected a segment of small intestine while I removed the clamp from the renal artery. In only five of these animals was this achieved successfully; the other seven died while the operation was being arranged, during the operation, or immediately afterwards. Of the five rabbits operated on successfully, four had fibrinoid changes at the first biopsy.

The course of the arterial pressure in one of these rabbits is shown in Fig. 7, and a section through a small artery in the wall of the small gut at the first biopsy in Fig. 8. It will be noted that

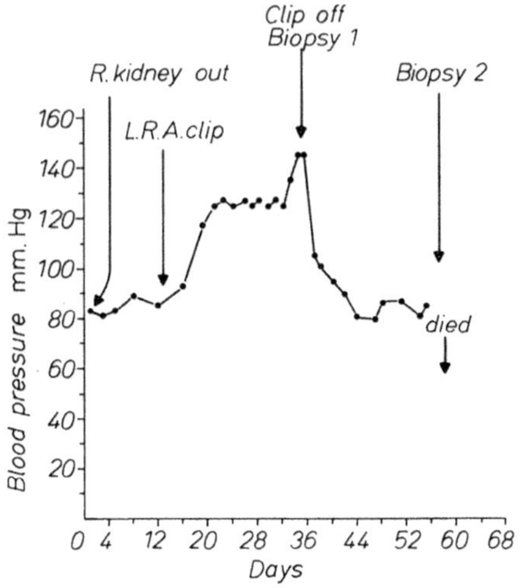

Fig. 7. The procedures and arterial pressures in rabbit 91. The animal died of intestinal obstruction after the second gut biopsy.

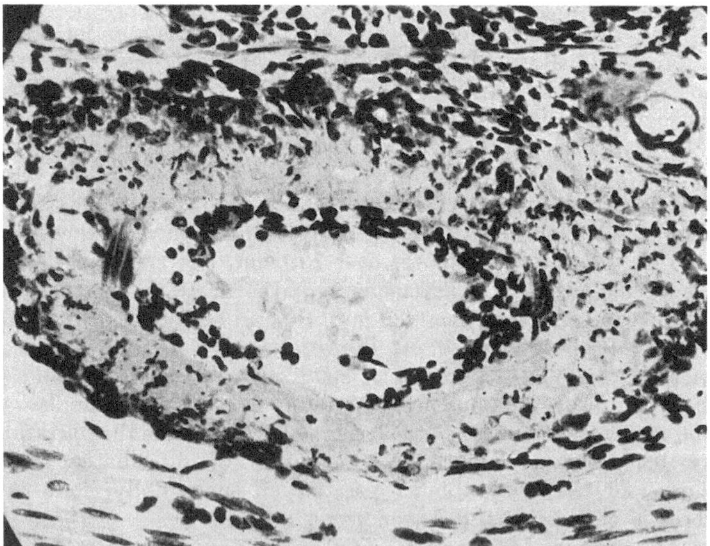

Fig. 8. Rabbit 91. A small artery in the wall of the small intestine obtained at the first biopsy. This artery was typical of the others.

the whole of the media is involved by fibrinoid necrosis, with only an occasional muscle cell surviving. The arterial wall is being invaded by inflammatory cells from the adventitia, and endothelial cells and polymorphs are grouped around the endothelial lining. A corresponding artery from the small intestine at the second biopsy, three weeks after the removal of the renal artery clamp and the consequent fall in the arterial pressure, can be seen in Fig. 9.

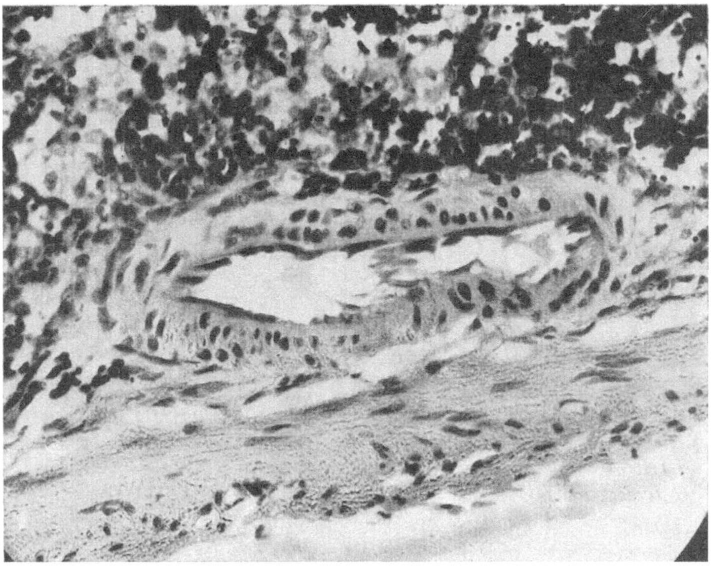

Fig. 9. An artery similar in size and position to that shown in Fig. 8, but obtained at second biopsy in rabbit 91. This artery, again, was typical.

The smooth-muscle cells in the media are still quite irregular and the endothelial cells of the intima are unduly prominent. Nevertheless, the fibrinoid material has entirely disappeared and the inflammatory cells almost entirely. These changes are representative of what we have observed in these rabbits. The fibrinoid material is clearly something which can disappear from the artery wall very quickly, as it can probably arrive very quickly. We have also, so far, found endothelial thickening to be less conspicuous at subsequent biopsies after the first.

The hypothesis that a grossly raised arterial pressure is one of the chief factors in producing fibrinoid necrosis of small arteries and arterioles in the malignant phase of hypertension has so far not been refuted by observation and experiment. That this represents the nature of the malignant phase is thus reasonable as a working hypothesis. In fact, this hypothesis is completely in conformity with therapeutic experience. That fibrinoid can appear and disappear so quickly from the arterial wall emphasises the urgency of early and effective reduction of arterial pressure.

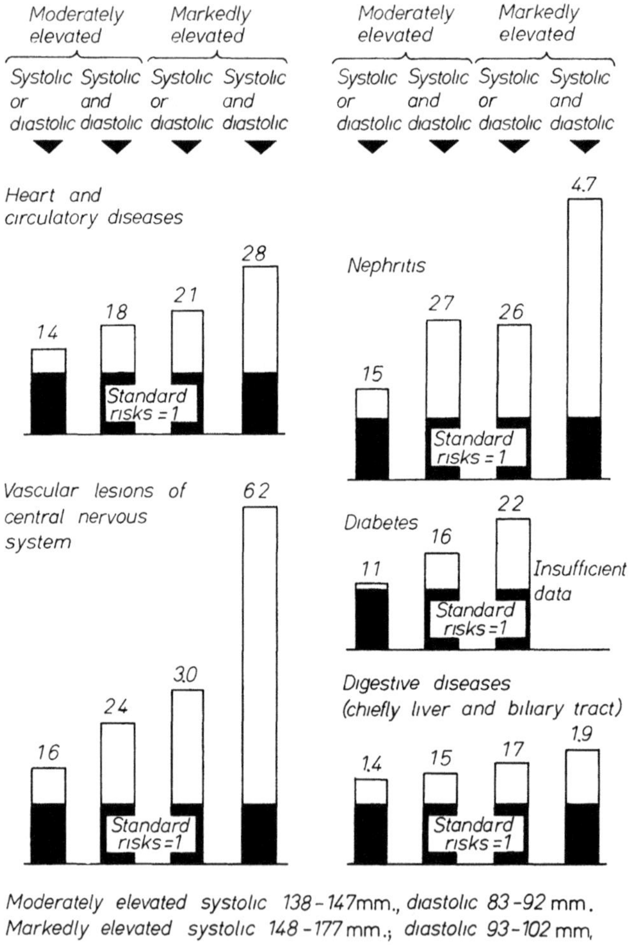

Fig. 10. Relationship between degree of elevation of arterial pressure at the time of examination for life insurance and subsequent mortality from various diseases. (The experience of 26 companies in 1935-54. Computations by the Metropolitan Life Assurance Company.)

Finally, let us see whether we have got our dimensions right. Fig. 10 shows the relationship between different degrees of elevation of arterial pressure as recorded at first examinations by insurance companies and the subsequent mortality. It is to be noted that there is a quantitative relationship between the two, and this is one of the many pieces of evidence which support the quantitative hypothesis concerning the nature of essential hypertension (PICKERING, 1961). It is also to be noted that the steepest rise in the mortality rates based on arterial pressure is associated with vascular lesions of the central nervous system. The contrast with heart disease is quite striking. The difference is due to the appearance of a totally different vascular disease in the cerebral vessels – the micro-aneurysms of CHARCOT (1868) and ROSS RUSSELL (1963). This is a new factor in our understanding of vascular disease and hypertension – a new factor which is effectively obscured by the out-moded term "atherosclerosis".

Summary

There are a number of quite separate vascular diseases affecting different coats of different sizes of arteries and having different relationships to elevated arterial pressure. Unfortunately, the prevalent addiction to the term "atherosclerosis" (literally "hardening through the agency of porridge") confuses these diseases and makes what should be a simple series of problems a hopeless morass.

From the clinical point of view there are three diseases of arteries which are of outstanding importance in patients with elevated pressure. First, nodular arteriosclerosis, which affects the intima of large arteries, producing plaque formation; it is the chief cause of myocardial infarction and a chief cause of stroke; it is lowly correlated with raised arterial pressure. Second, micro-aneurysms of the small cerebral arteries, which is a totally different disease. It affects arteries about one tenth of a millimetre in diameter; the muscular part of the media gives way with ballooning out into aneurysms, which may thrombose or rupture. These aneurysms are probably one cause of the small yellow pits so frequently found in the brains of patients with hypertension, one cause of little strokes, and the chief cause of cerebral haemorrhage. These lesions probably account for the high correlation between raised arterial pressure and death from cerebral vascular disease. The third arterial disease is fibrinoid necrosis of the arterioles and is due to a variety of factors, of which by far the most important is a grossly raised arterial pressure. This lesion is responsible for the phenomena of the malignant phase. Clinical and experimental evidence strongly suggests that when arterial pressure is reduced, the fibrinoid is quickly removed, thus allowing the lumina of the arteries to increase in diameter.

Zusammenfassung

Es gibt eine Anzahl gesonderter Gefäßerkrankungen, die verschiedene Schichten von Arterien verschiedener Größe betreffen und ganz verschiedene

Beziehungen zum erhöhten Arteriendruck haben. Bedauerlicherweise verwirrt die derzeitige Vorliebe für den Ausdruck „Atherosklerose“ (wörtlich: Verhärtung durch Brei) die Abgrenzung zwischen diesen Krankheiten und verwandelt eine an sich einfache Reihe von Problemen in einen hoffnungslosen Morast.

Vom klinischen Gesichtspunkt aus stechen drei Erkrankungen der Arterien bei Patienten mit erhöhtem Blutdruck hervor. Erstens, die noduläre Arteriosklerose, welche die Intima der großen Arterien befällt und dort zur Bildung von "plaques" führt; sie ist die hauptsächliche Ursache für den Myokardinfarkt und eine der Ursachen für die Apoplexie; sie ist nur in geringem Maße mit erhöhtem Arteriendruck korreliert. Zweitens, Mikroaneurysmen der kleinen Hirnarterien, die eine völlig andere Erkrankung darstellen und Arterien von etwa 0,1 mm Durchmesser befallen. Der muskuläre Anteil der Media gibt unter Aufblähungen nach, und es bilden sich Aneurysmen, die thrombosieren oder platzen. Diese Aneursymen sind wahrscheinlich eine Ursache der kleinen, gelben Grübchen, die sich häufig in den Gehirnen von Patienten mit Hochdruck finden, eine Ursache der leichten Schlaganfälle und die Hauptursache für die zerebrale Hämorrhagie. Diese Schädigungen dürften verantwortlich sein für die hohe Korrelation zwischen erhohtem Arteriendruck und Tod infolge Erkrankung der Hirnarterien. Die dritte Arterienerkrankung ist die fibrinoide Nekrose der Arteriolen, für die verschiedene Faktoren verantwortlich zu machen sind, von denen der wichtigste ein stark erhöhter arterieller Druck ist. Die Erscheinungen der malignen Verlaufsphase sind auf diese Schädigungen zurückzuführen. Klinische und experimentelle Befunde lassen vermuten, daß nach Senkung des Arteriendruckes das Fibrinoid rasch zurückgeht, und daß als Folge davon der Durchmesser der Arterienlumina wieder zunehmen kann.

Résumé

Il existe un certain nombre d'affections vasculaires tout à fait distinctes intéressant les différentes tuniques des artères de différent calibre et dont la relation avec l'élévation de la pression artérielle est de degré variable. Malheureusement, l'attachement actuel au terme "athérosclérose" (étymologiquement: "durcissement par l'action d'une bouillie") fait régner la confusion parmi ces maladies et transforme ce qui devrait être une simple série de problèmes en un marécage sans espoir.

Du point de vue clinique il existe trois affections artérielles présentant une grande importance chez les hypertendus. Premièrement, l'artériosclérose nodulaire, qui affecte l'intima des grosses artères et aboutit à la formation de plaques; c'est la cause principale de l'infarctus du myocarde et une des causes de l'ictus cérébral; ses rapports ne sont que lointains avec l'élévation de la pression artérielle. Deuxièmement, les micro-anévrismes des petites artères cérébrales, qui représentent une maladie totalement différente. Ils affectent les artères d'environ 0,1 mm de diamètre. La tunique musculaire de la média cède, d'où saillie arrondie, aboutissant à l'anévrisme qui peut se thromboser ou se rompre. Ces anévrismes sont probablement une des causes des petites lacunes jaunes si fréquemment rencontrées dans le cerveau des hypertendus, l'une des causes des petites attaques cérébrales et la cause principale de l'hémorragie cérébrale. Ces lésions expliquent sans doute la haute corrélation entre une tension artérielle élevée et la mort par affection vasculaire cérébrale. La troisième maladie artérielle est la nécrose fibrinoïde des artérioles; elle est due à une série de facteurs, parmi lesquels le plus important de beaucoup est l'élévation manifeste de la pression artérielle. C'est cette lésion qui est responsable des manifestations de la phase maligne. Des faits cliniques expérimentaux suggèrent fortement que lorsque la pression artérielle est abaissée, la substance fibrinoïde disparaît rapidement, ce qui permet ainsi l'accroissement du diamètre de la lumière des artères.

References

BYROM, F. B., and L. F. DODSON: J. Path. Bact. **60**, 357 (1948). — CHARCOT, J. M., and C. BOUCHARD: Arch. physiol. **1**, 110, 643, and 725 (1868). — DEROW, H. A., and M. D. ALTSCHULE: N. England J. Med. **213**, 951 (1935). — GOLDBLATT, H.: Bull. N. Y. Acad. Med. **14**, 523 (1938). — HARINGTON, M. ,P. KINCAID-SMITH, and J. MCMICHAEL: Brit. Med. J. 1959/II, 969. — PICKERING, G. W.: Circulation **6**, 599 (1952). — PICKERING, G. W.: The Nature of Essential Hypertension. Churchill Ltd., London, 1961. — PICKERING, G. W.: Brit. Med. J. 1964/I, 517. — PICKERING, G. W., A. D. WRIGHT, and R. H. HEPTINSTALL: Lancet 1952/II, 952. — ROSENBERG, E. F.: Arch. Int. Med. **65**, 545 (1940). — ROSS RUSSELL, R.: Brain **86**, 425 (1963). — SMITHWICK, R. H., and B. CASTLEMAN: In: Hypertension. Ed. by E. T. BELL. University of Minnesota Press, Minneapolis, 1951, p. 199. — WILSON, C., and G. W. PICKERING: Clin. Sc. **3**, 343 (1938). — WILSON, C., and F. B. BYROM: Lancet 1939/I, 136.

Discussion

COTTIER: I should like to ask Dr. PICKERING to comment further on the pathogenesis of Charcot's aneurysms. Is the development of these vascular changes related to the duration or severity of hypertension, or are there other factors involved? I am thinking of the aneurysms in diabetics which, apparently, do not merely correlate with the severity of the disturbance in carbohydrate metabolism.

PICKERING: The aneurysms in diabetics are on the venules. These aneurysms are arterial, more precisely, on small arteries. CHARCOT[1], of course, discovered them in 1868, before the blood pressure was measured in life. ROSS RUSSEL's[2] observations were made on 50 patients dying in the Boston City Hospital. He found that there were two relevant factors: one was age and the other was arterial pressure. As far as I know, these are the only two sets of observations on these aneurysms. Their rediscovery is so recent that practically nothing is known of them except the relatively high correlation of arterial pressure with vascular lesions of the central nervous system which cannot be accounted for by that other disease causing strokes — this disease of the intima of large arteries which I think is best called nodular arteriosclerosis.

SMIRK: Dr. PICKERING, could you elaborate a little more on the relationship between nodular atherosclerosis and coronary artery disease? My particular reason for asking the question is that with the decrease in the mortality from congestive heart failure and from cerebral vascular accidents HODGE and I[3] have found in the last six years that 42% of deaths in our patients are now due to coronary disease or are sudden deaths, probably, but not proved to be, due to coronary disease; if we cut out the persons who died from irrelevant causes, 51% are in the coronary field.

PICKERING: As far as I know, this intimal disease of large arteries is *the* cause of coronary artery disease; there is virtually no other. That, I would say, is 90% true, which I think is a very high rate of truth for medical science. — The relationship, I think, was quite clearly shown in Fig. 1 of my paper. The higher your pressure, the more likely you are to get coronary artery disease. But you can get it, as I think Dr. DEMING said, at pressures that nobody would call abnormal. This was pointed out years ago by CLIFFORD ALLBUTT, who said that Bright's disease really comprises three kinds of disease. Firstly, there is Bright's disease proper; secondly, there is a disease which he called hyperpiesis, in which the blood pressure rises excessively in middle age; and thirdly, there is a quite different disease, not usually associated with elevated pressure, which he called decrescent arteriosclerosis. In broad outline, ALLBUTT's classic treatment was right.

PAGE: Dr. MASON SONES has done cinecoronary angiography on Dr. DUSTAN's and my hypertensive patients, and we find a very high incidence

[1] CHARCOT, J. M., and C. BOUCHARD: Arch. physiol. **1**, 110, 643, and 725 (1868).

[2] ROSS RUSSELL, R.: Brain **86**, 425 (1963).

[3] HODGE, J. V., and F. H. SMIRK: unpublished.

of coronary disease. This emphasises what I said before, that the next great phase in the management of hypertension will be prevention of atherosclerosis.

SMIRK: May I refer to the work of SMITH[1] from the Mayo Clinic? He had a very interesting pathological series. In his series of hypertensives, 9.8% of deaths were due to manifest coronary disease, but autopsies showed pathological evidence of coronary artery disease in 55—65% of those hypertensives who died from other conditions. The position within this range depended on the retinal grade.

KIRKENDALL: I wonder, Dr. PICKERING, if you found the emboli in other circulations, such as the end arterioles of the nail beds.

PICKERING: I don't think you would, because I think the extraordinary thing about the brain and the retina is that if you disturb their blood supply, in 20 seconds you get ischaemic symptoms. I don't think you get anything in the heart or limb in that time. I am quite sure you get emboli from these atheromatous plaques. I have never seen these emboli in the retina, except in patients who have been complaining of lost vision, usually transient.

KIRKENDALL: The reason I asked is that I think there is a great increase in the number of splinter haemorrhages in the nailbeds of older persons. There are so many possible factors involved and I don't know the cause. They may represent micro-emboli from atherosclerotic lesions central to the circulation of the nailbed.

KINCAID-SMITH: If I understood Dr. PICKERING correctly, he suggested that the intimal proliferation in the vessels which he showed disappears after lowering the blood pressure, as well as the fibrinoid necrosis. Our experience, based on renal biopsies in patients with severe hypertension, suggests that, whereas the fibrinoid necrosis disappears quite rapidly, within a period of days, the narrowing of the vessel by intimal proliferation does not disappear, but changes over to a form of intimal fibrosis. I wonder whether I understood correctly and whether these animals do show different changes from those which we have observed in humans.

PICKERING: You did understand me correctly. I am not sure that I believe it, and my pathological colleague must look at some more sections.

PAGE: In other words, you think that rabbits and human beings are different.

PICKERING: Of course rabbits and men differ, but I am not sure whether they differ in this way. I don't think that we have looked at enough material from our biopsy specimens.

DUSTAN: Dr. PICKERING, we, also, agree with you that the rabbit is different from man. In a pathological study of kidneys of patients who died following reversal of malignant hypertension, MCCORMACK from the Cleveland Clinic[2] has described what he calls "healed malignant nephrosclerosis". These patients do in fact have residual arteriolar disease, and this raises the question whether the renal vascular bed isn't quite different from the intestinal vascular bed.

---

[1] SMITH, D. E., H. M. ODEL, and J. W. KERNOHAN: Amer. J. Med. **9**, 516 (1950).

[2] MCCORMACK, L. J., J. E. BÉLAND, R. E. SCHNECKLOTH, and A. C. CORCORAN: Amer. J. Path. **34**, 1011 (1958).

Retinal vascular alterations in hypertension

By

C. T. Dollery, P. S. Ramalho*, and J. W. Paterson

Keith et al. (*8*) divided hypertensive retinopathy into four degrees of severity and showed that these correlated closely with the prognosis in the untreated patient. The diagnosis of the two most severe categories (Grades III and IV) depends on the presence of exudative changes, such as flame-shaped haemorrhages, cotton-wool spots, hard exudates, and papilloedema. The two milder grades (Grades I and II) are diagnosed by the presence of narrowing and irregularity of arterioles, thickening of the walls with increase in light reflex, and nipping of the vein at arteriovenous crossings.

As many of the consequences of severe hypertension depend upon damage to small blood vessels, it is clearly important to try to understand the pathogenesis and natural history of the retinal lesions. The exudative changes and the changes in the visible arterioles will be considered separately.

1. Exudative retinopathy

The appearance of cotton-wool spots and flame-shaped haemorrhages in the retina is one of the most important clinical signs that benign hypertension is entering an accelerated phase. The pathogenesis of the lesions has occasioned much controversy since their first clinical description soon after the invention of the ophthalmoscope nearly 100 years ago. Recently, we have made a further study of these lesions, using photographic methods to document the visible lesions and a fluorescence angiographic technique to visualise the flow disturbances and changes in the capillary circulation (*7*) .

Natural history of the cotton-wool spot. The visible cotton-wool spot passes through a characteristic cycle of changes. At the start, there is a greyish discoloration of the retina which, in the course of 24–48 hours, develops into a shiny white patch with ill-defined, frayed edges. As it increases in size, the lesion may displace larger veins, which return to their initial position as it disappears. Over

* In receipt of a Fellowship from the Gulbenkian Foundation

the next 6–12 weeks, the patch becomes dull and takes on a fragmented, granular appearance. At this stage it may be confused with hard exudate, although the localised collection of fine granular material is characteristic. The individual segments of hard exudate are usually larger and shinier in appearance. As the dull white

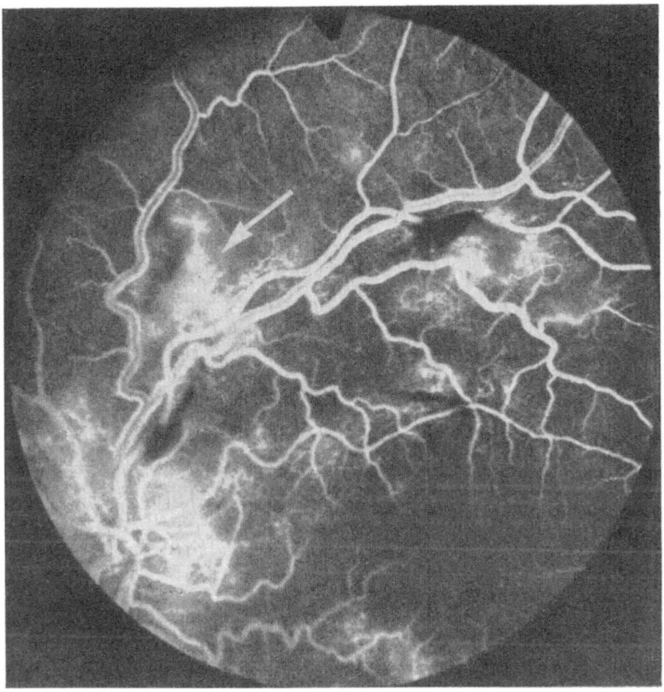

Fig. 1. Fluorescence angiogram of the retina of a man aged 21 with untreated malignant hypertension. There are several prominent areas of vascular leakage (arrow).

fragments of the cotton-wool spot fade, the remaining area of retina is usually normal. Occasionally, a small micro-aneurysm or abnormal vessel may be seen in the base of the lesion as it fades.

Fluorescence angiography of the cotton-wool spot. Vascular abnormalities which can be detected by fluorescence angiography often precede the formation of the visible cotton-wool spot. These abnormalities are of two kinds: in untreated malignant hypertension there are often ill-defined points of leakage from small arterioles; later, a cotton-wool spot may appear in the vicinity of such a leaking point. In other patients, the site of the lesion may be revealed by one or two micro-aneurysms. When the cotton-wool spot is fully developed, the central region often appears dark on the fluorescence angiogram, suggesting that the capillary bed in that area may not be perfused. Around the edge of the cotton-wool spot there are small aneurysms that may form an almost complete

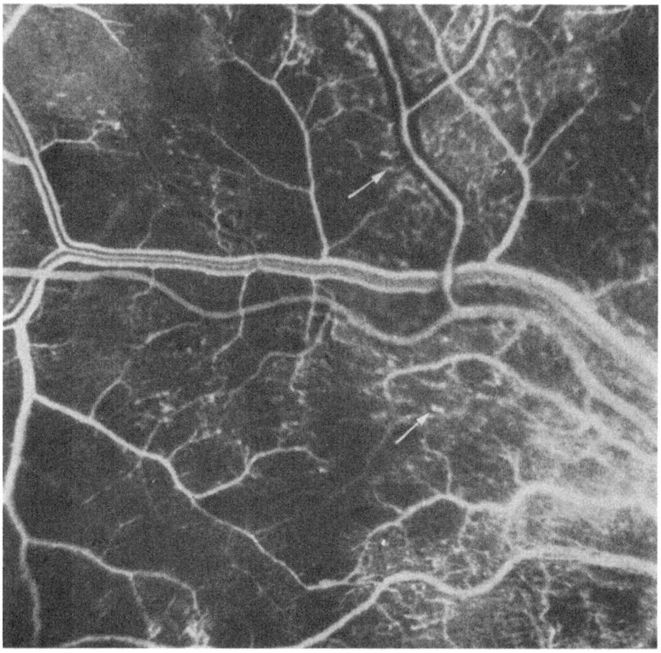

Fig. 2. Fluorescence angiogram of the retina of a woman aged 34 with malignant hypertension that had remained untreated for six months. Many capillaries are dilated and show saccular or fusiform aneurysms (arrows). There were no soft exudates in this area of the retina.

ring. These aneurysms usually cannot be seen with the ophthalmoscope, but they have been demonstrated by injecting Indian ink into the eye after death (*1*). Cotton-wool spots usually become diffusely fluorescent within a few minutes of intravenous injection of the fluorescent dye. The fluorescence spreads outwards from the points of leakage on arterioles and from the dilated capillaries and aneurysms surrounding the white area (Fig. 1).

Effective reduction of blood pressure speedily corrects focal leakage from points on small arterioles. As the cotton-wool spot fades, the surrounding aneurysms slowly resolve, sometimes faster and sometimes more slowly than the visible lesion. After 10–12 weeks, when the last trace of the cotton-wool spot has faded, the vascular bed in the region appears normal, and it is rare for capillary abnormalities to be visible at this stage.

In some patients with long-standing malignant hypertension, the fluorescence angiogram may reveal severe and wide-spread capillary abnormalities, even when there are no cotton-wool spots in the vicinity. These changes include saccular and fusiform dilatations of capillaries (Fig. 2) and sheets of abnormal capillaries cascading off the swollen optic disc (*4*).

The pathogenesis of the cotton-wool spot has given rise to controversy, and some recent experimental observations may throw light on the interpretation of the phenomena demonstrated in clinical investigations. In these experiments, the retinae of pigs were embolised by intracarotid injections of glass microspheres, $20-60\ \mu$. in diameter (*5*). Following embolisation, the arterioles containing the glass microspheres are completely occluded. A few minutes after embolisation, an area of greyish discoloration appears in the retina downstream to the block, and 24 hours later, there is often a creamy-white spot indistinguishable from a cotton-wool spot in the human retina. The lesion fades quickly, and within two weeks, no more than a faint white granularity in the retina remains. Thus, the experimental cotton-wool spot passes through all the stages seen in the human eye, but does so more rapidly.

One point of interest is that profuse local leakage of dye from the arteriole often occurs in the vicinity of the embolus, particularly when the ball has moved slowly down a segment of the vessel. Electron microscopy of two such areas has revealed local damage or destruction of the vascular endothelium (*10*). Despite the leakage, the capillary bed in the immediate vicinity of the leaking area is perfused normally, although further downstream flow takes place only through collaterals. In these experimental studies, micro-aneurysms and dilated capillaries have not been found around the edge of the visible cotton-wool spot and there was little or no fluorescence within the lesion.

Comment

The most probable explanation of the leaking areas observed in patients with untreated malignant hypertension is that they, too, represent sites of damage to the arteriolar wall. One of the most characteristic pathological features of malignant hypertension is arteriolar necrosis, and it is possible that the leaking areas are the sites of local necroses of the arteriolar wall. The cotton-wool spot downstream probably results from obstruction of the arteriole following the damage to its wall. The aetiology of the surrounding micro-aneurysms and abnormal capillaries in man remains obscure, and it has not been possible to reproduce them experimentally. It seems more likely that they are a reaction to the presence of the cotton-wool spot than that they are related to its cause. However, in man the cotton-wool spot or soft exudate shows much more vascular leakage and diffuse fluorescence than the lesions produced experimentally by emboli. Until cotton-wool spots can be produced in experimental hypertension, a full explanation of their pathogenesis must remain somewhat speculative.

2. Changes in retinal arterioles

Calibre irregularity. Irregularity of calibre with focal narrowing is one of the most common features of the retinal arterioles in the hypertensive patient. Focal narrowing of retinal vessels is sometimes considered to be evidence of active vasospasm. We have sought an answer to this question by observing the changes that occur in narrow segments of arterioles when the blood pressure is reduced by drugs or renal surgery. Scrutiny of sequential colour photographs of about 100 major or minor areas of narrowing in retinal arterioles shows that the great majority of these areas remained unchanged, even if hypertension was apparently cured by renal surgery. There were four instances in which narrow areas regressed over a period of time, but in other patients narrow areas appeared despite good control of the blood pressure. In some cases, pathological observations were made and the structure correlated with the photographs taken during life (*2*). Evidence was obtained that some, at least, of the narrow areas show structural changes in the vessel wall with gross narrowing of the lumen.

The pathogenesis of the narrow segments remains a problem, but the lesions seen in the eye of a patient with established hypertension appear to be fixed and represent structural changes in the vessel wall.

Vessel narrowing. The retinal arterioles of patients with severe hypertension are often diffusely narrowed. Some clinical observers record the degree of narrowing by reference to a ratio relating the calibre of the artery to that of the accompanying vein, but such ratios are difficult to estimate accurately with the ophthalmoscope and can be seriously misleading. If papilloedema is present, the retinal veins are often dilated, and in response to antihypertensive treatment, which relieves the papilloedema, they return to a normal calibre. It may appear that the arterioles have increased in size in relation to the vein, when in fact they are unchanged but the veins are smaller.

It has proved difficult to make a quantitative estimate of the degree of vessel narrowing, because the branching pattern of the retinal vessels is so variable. In six normal subjects and six with severe hypertension, we measured the diameters of all arterioles and veins as they leave the disc; we then found the respective sums of all the venous and arteriolar diameters in each case and compared the ratios thus obtained. In the normal subjects the range was from 1.24 to 0.81, whereas in the hypertensive subjects it was from 0.90 to 0.61. Thus, there was considerable overlap between the two groups. One source of difficulty may have been the decision to measure the vessels at the edge of the optic disc, as hypertensive arterioles often become attenuated beyond this point. However, it is difficult to find a fixed point further out in the retina at which to make measurements.

3. The calibre of retinal arterioles after blood-pressure reduction

If good-quality colour photographs of the retina are taken, it is possible to measure the calibre of retinal arterioles by using a low-power microscope and screw micrometer eye-piece (*3*). The sites for measurements are marked on an accurate drawing and are identified on the transparencies by reference to vessel crossings and branches. The largest arterioles near the optic disc are normally about 110 μ. in diameter, and it is possible to measure vessels as small as 30 μ. in diameter under favourable circumstances. During measurement, the date and time at which the individual transparencies were taken is usually concealed by the use of a code number.

Effects of renal surgery. Few forms of hypertension can be cured. The nearest approach to a cure is a successful operation on the kidney. We were able to measure retinal vessels in ten patients who had undergone renal surgery; in seven of these, the operation was successful in that blood pressure fell to less than 160/100 mm. Hg and remained below that level for at least a year. In the patients whose blood pressure was unaffected by the operation, no systematic change could be found in the calibre of the retinal arterioles. The seven patients whose blood pressure was reduced to near normal levels all showed the same pattern (*6*). The large retinal arterioles (70–100 μ.) near the optic disc were either unchanged or had become slightly narrowed after the operation; small retinal arterioles (30–60 μ.) had increased in diameter by a relatively large amount (Fig. 3). Although the degree of change varied in different individual vessels, almost all conformed to the general pattern in the direction in which they moved. These changes suggested that the smallest retinal vessels might have been under an active vasoconstrictor influence that had been removed as a

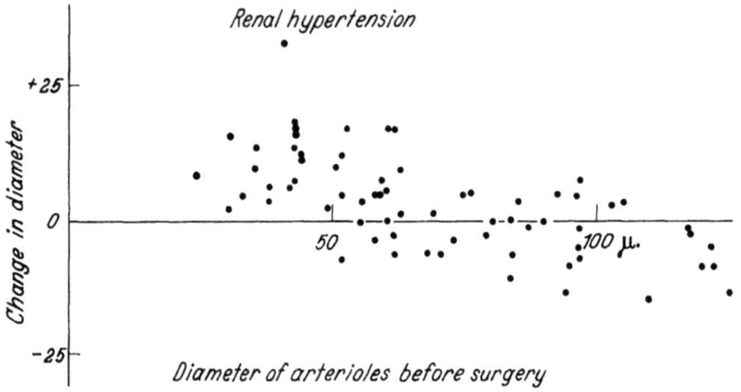

Fig. 3. A plot of the diameter of the retinal arterioles in seven patients with severe hypertension. The diameter before treatment was plotted against the change in diameter at each site after the blood pressure had been reduced to less than 160/100 mm. Hg by successful renal surgery. In six instances nephrectomy was performed and in the other an endarterectomy.

result of surgery. The changes in the large arterioles were difficult to explain, but it appeared that they might have been due to structural changes in the vessel wall which had rendered them unresponsive to vasoconstrictor influences.

Effect of sympathetic blocking drugs. When a patient under treatment with a sympathetic blocking drug (guanethidine or bethanidine) changes from the upright to the recumbent position, there is often a substantial change in blood pressure. We selected patients who had a particularly large postural swing, took retinal photographs, and measured the blood pressure in five of them in both postures (Table 1). To our surprise, the same type of pattern was found as that observed in the patients who had undergone successful renal surgery. The increase in size of the smallest vessels was less striking than in the surgical patients, but it was nevertheless highly significant (Fig. 4).

This observation made interpretation of the results obtained by surgery more difficult. The drug-treated patients were under the influence of the drug in both body positions, and the main difference was the large reduction in the level of the blood pressure on standing. It is possible that dilatation of the smallest arterioles on standing is a local adjustment to the reduction in the perfusion pressure. The change in the larger arterioles, both in the patients given drugs and in those who had undergone surgery, may be purely passive,

Table 1. *Mean supine and standing blood pressure in hypertensive patients treated with various drugs*

Patient	Age (years)	Mean B.P. lying flat (mm. Hg)	Mean B.P. standing (mm. Hg)	Drug and dose (by mouth)
217638	35	155	117	Guanethidine 200 mg. daily
298222	41	143	123	Bethanidine 60 mg. daily
291246	52	139	106	Guanethidine 250 mg. daily Hydrochlorothiazide 50 mg. daily
210154	54	166	125	Pempidine 22.5 mg. daily Reserpine 0.3 mg. daily
291004	57	160	140	α-Methyldopa 3 g. daily Hydrochlorothiazide 50 mg. daily

reflecting an alteration in the transmural pressure in vessels which have lost their smooth muscle. To test this hypothesis we decided to observe the effects of a vasodilator drug.

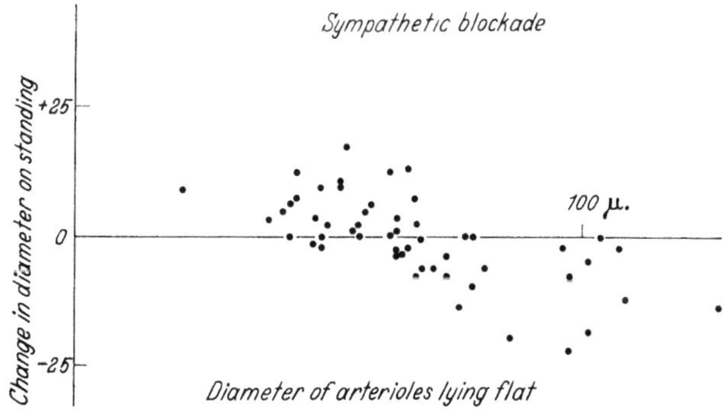

Fig. 4. A plot of the diameter of retinal arterioles in five patients with severe hypertension receiving treatment with sympathetic blocking drugs (guanethidine or bethanidine). The initial diameter is plotted against the change in diameter which took place at each site when the patient was upright. The average blood pressure in the standing position was less than 160/100 mm. Hg, but in recumbency it was much higher.

Effect of hydralazine. Five patients were studied in the recumbent position before and after slow intravenous administration of 20–40 mg. hydralazine. In four of the five the drug produced a tachycardia, and in all there was a substantial reduction of the blood pressure. The retinal arterioles of all sizes dilated, but the increase in diameter was much greater in the smallest vessels. Even so, some of the main arterioles still appeared relatively narrow after the blood pressure had been reduced to near normal levels with hydralazine. The increase in diameter of the larger vessels, although small, suggests that these arterioles still have the ability to react to the drug.

Other effects. Therapeutically, the most encouraging change in the retinal arterioles of a hypertensive patient would be a general increase in diameter which restored their calibre to normal. A response of this type was observed only once, in a 21-year-old man with a short history of malignant hypertension who was treated with guanethidine; yet the results obtained with hydralazine suggest that a response of this kind would have been possible in other patients. The larger arterioles are not entirely incapable of vasomotion. Recent observations of the vasoconstrictor effects of oxygen (*9*) suggest that even the most severely narrowed arterioles in the hypertensive retina retain some reactivity, although it is much less than normal.

Thus, the differential effect on large and small arterioles observed in patients whose blood pressure was lowered with drugs or by surgery still presents a problem. One explanation may be that there is a fundamentally different response by the different vascular segments. However, when normal subjects are rendered hypertensive by intravenous infusions of angiotensin and noradrenaline, all segments of the arteriole constrict (*3*).

Comment

The most reactive vessels of the retinal vascular tree in hypertensive patients are the small arterioles below 60 μ. in diameter. These vessels dilate in response to various stimuli which lower the systemic blood pressure. It is still uncertain whether they are narrowed because of the local activity of sympathetic nerves or vasoconstrictor substances, or possibly as a direct reaction to the level of the blood pressure. The reaction of the larger arterioles also presents problems of interpretation. These vessels are less reactive than they are under normal conditions and have probably suffered hypertensive damage. However, the changes in diameter under different circumstances cannot be purely passive.

The pattern that emerges is one of larger arterioles damaged by the hypertensive process, narrowed diffusely or locally, and relatively unresponsive to alterations in blood pressure or the action of drugs. The small arterioles remain reactive and are able to change their diameter over a wide range, despite the severity of the hypertensive process to which they have been exposed.

Summary

The appearance of soft exudates and haemorrhages in the fundus of a patient with hypertension is a sign that the disease is entering an accelerated phase. Fluorescence angiography of the retina at this stage reveals ill-defined points of leakage on minute arterioles and non-perfused areas of capillary bed surrounded by capillary dilatations and aneurysms in the vicinity of soft exudates. Similar leaking points can be demonstrated experimentally after local damage to the vascular endothelium. The evidence suggests that the leaking spots represent areas of arteriolar necrosis. Impairment of the circulation beyond these spots leads to formation of the exudate. Thus, retinal soft exudates in hypertensive patients are a clinical indication of the presence of arteriolar necrosis.

Lowering the blood pressure to normal, either by renal surgery or by administration of sympathetic blocking drugs, does not usually bring about any dramatic change in the focal or general narrowing of the larger arterioles. Careful measurement of these vessels reveals that there is often a substantial increase in calibre of the smallest vessels, accompanied by a small decrease in size of the largest arterioles near the optic disc. The vasodilator antihypertensive drug, hydralazine, produces a general increase in vascular diameter, but, even so, the arterioles do not return to a normal calibre.

The larger arterioles in the retina are damaged by the hypertensive process and become narrowed diffusely or locally. They are then relatively unresponsive to alterations in blood pressure or to the action of drugs. The small arterioles are more reactive and undergo calibre changes in response to changes in blood pressure or the use of drugs. These small arterioles are damaged in accelerated hypertension and develop local areas of arteriolar necrosis.

Zusammenfassung

Das Auftreten von weichen Exsudaten und Hämorrhagien im Augenhintergrund eines Patienten mit Hochdruck ist ein Zeichen dafür, daß die Erkrankung begonnen hat, einen beschleunigten Verlauf zu nehmen. Fluoreszenzangiographie der Retina zeigt in diesem Stadium schlecht definierbare Flüssigkeitsaustritte aus kleinen Arteriolen und nicht durchströmten Kapillargebieten, die von Kapillarerweiterungen und Aneurysmen in der Nachbarschaft der Exsudate umgeben sind. Ähnliche Lecks lassen sich experimentell nach örtlicher Schädigung des Gefäßendothels nachweisen. Es ist anzunehmen, daß die Arteriolen an diesen undichten Stellen nekrotisch sind. Verschlechterung der Zirkulation jenseits dieser Partien führt zur Bildung von Exsudaten. Daher sind die weichen Retina-Exsudate bei hypertonischen Patienten ein klinischer Hinweis für die Anwesenheit von Arteriolen-Nekrosen.

Senkung des Blutdruckes zur Norm, entweder durch chirurgische Eingriffe an der Niere oder durch Gabe von sympathikusblockierenden Pharmaka, führt im allgemeinen nicht zu dramatischen Änderungen der herdförmigen oder allgemeinen Verengerungen der großen Arteriolen. Sorgfältige Messung dieser Gefäße ergibt, daß oft eine erhebliche Zunahme des Durchmessers der kleinsten Gefäße vorliegt, die von einer geringen Abnahme des Durchmessers der größten Arteriolen in der Nähe der Papille begleitet ist. Das vasodilatatorisch und blutdrucksenkend wirkende Hydralazin ruft eine allgemeine Zunahme des Gefäßdurchmessers hervor, aber auch dabei erreichen die Arteriolen nicht ihre normale Weite.

Die größeren Arteriolen in der Retina werden durch den Hochdruck geschädigt und allgemein oder lokal verengt. Sie reagieren dann relativ schlecht auf Änderungen des Blutdruckes oder auf Pharmaka. Die kleinen Arteriolen sprechen besser auf Senkungen des Blutdruckes oder auf die Gabe von Pharmaka mit Kaliberänderungen an. Diese kleinen Arteriolen sind bei rasch verlaufendem Hochdruck geschädigt und weisen örtliche Nekrosen auf.

Résumé

L'apparition d'exsudats flous et d'hémorragies au fond d'oeil d'un hypertendu indique que la maladie est entrée dans une phase d'évolution rapide. A ce stade, l'angiographie de la rétine par fluorescence montre des points mal limités de suffusion hémorragique au niveau des toutes petites artérioles et des zones du réseau capillaire non irriguées, entourées de capillaires dilatés et d'anévrysmes au voisinage des exsudats. On peut provoquer expérimentalement de semblables points de suffusion hémorragique par lésion locale de l'endothélium vasculaire. Il est probable que ces taches de suffusion correspondent à des zones de nécrose artériolaire. Les troubles circulatoires au-delà de ces taches entraînent la formation d'exsudats. Ainsi, l'existence d'exsudats rétiniens chez un malade hypertendu est un signe clinique de nécrose artériolaire.

Si l'on ramène la tension artérielle à des chiffres normaux, soit par la chirurgie rénale, soit par l'administration d'inhibiteurs du sympathique, on n'observe habituellement aucune modification importante du rétrécissement soit focal soit généralisé des artérioles de gros calibre. La mensuration soigneuse de ces vaisseaux montre qu'il existe souvent une augmentation notable du calibre des plus petits d'entre eux, accompagnée d'une légère diminution du calibre des plus volumineux au voisinage du disque optique. L'hydralazine, substance vasodilatatrice antihypertensive, qui provoque une augmentation générale du diamètre vasculaire, ne ramène pas ces artérioles à leur calibre normal.

Les grosses artérioles de la rétine sont lésées par le processus hypertenseur et présentent des rétrécissements diffus ou localisés. Elles sont alors relativement insensibles aux modifications de la pression artérielle ou à l'action des médicaments. Les petites artérioles sont plus sensibles et subissent des modifications de calibre sous l'influence des variations de la pression artérielle ou sous l'action des médicaments. Ces petites artérioles sont lésées dans les hypertensions à évolution rapide et présentent des zones localisées de nécrose artériolaire.

Acknowledgement

This work was supported by the Medical Research Council.

References

1. ASHTON, N.: Brit. J. Ophthalm. **35**, 189 (1951). — 2. ASHTON, N., and J. HARRY: Transact. Ophth. Soc. Unit. Kingdom **83**, 91 (1963). — 3. DOLLERY, C. T., D. W. HILL, and J. V. HODGE: J. Physiol. **165**, 500 (1963). — 4. DOLLERY, C. T., C. M. MAILER, and J. V. HODGE: J. Neurol. Neurosurg. Psychiat. **28**, 241 (1965). — 5. DOLLERY, C. T., J. W. PATERSON, P. S. RAMALHO, D. W. HILL, P. HENKIND, M. SHAKIB, and N. ASHTON: Lancet 1965/I, 1303. — 6. HILL, D. W., and C. T. DOLLERY: Transact. Ophth. Soc. Unit. Kingdom **83**, 61 (1963). — 7. HODGE, J. V., and C. T. DOLLERY: Quart. J. Med. **33**, 117 (1964). — 8. KEITH, N. M., H. P. WAGENER, and N. W. BARKER: Amer. J. Med. Sc. **197**, 332 (1939). — 9. RAMALHO, P. S.: unpublished. — 10. SHAKIB, M., and N. ASHTON: unpublished.

Discussion

BROD: Dr. DOLLERY, what do you think is the reason for the fact that, given the same degree of severe increase in blood pressure, malignant changes in the eyegrounds are seen only quite occasionally? There are many patients with diastolic blood pressures of 140 or 150 mm. Hg, who have none of the symptoms you have shown to occur in some patients with a diastolic blood pressure of 130 mm. Hg. — My second question concerns the relationship between these malignant changes in the eyegrounds and the cerebrospinal pressure. I think Dr. PICKERING did some studies on this relationship many years ago, and we have also seen that malignant eyeground changes usually do not occur unless cerebrospinal pressure is very high. — Finally, are the eyeground changes you noticed in malignant hypertension the same as those found in normotensive patients with intracranial hypertension, which look ophthalmologically identical?

DOLLERY: Regarding your first question, malignant hypertension is common in young patients who have a high level of pressure, and, although hypertension becomes more common in older people, the malignant phase becomes less common, particularly after the age of 65. LEISHMAN[1], a Glasgow ophthalmologist who has done distinguished work on the retinal vessels, speculated that ageing changes in arterioles protect them against the bursting effects of a high transmural pressure. He put forward the term "defence by sclerosis". This seems a reasonable hypothesis, but I know of no way of proving it. — As to the cerebrospinal-fluid pressure, we have not measured it in any of these studies. I leave it to Dr. PICKERING, who has made observations on this point, to answer that question. — Concerning the third question, exudative retinal changes appear in the eyegrounds in other conditions, such as gastro-intestinal haemorrhage or severe anaemia. The exudates are similar to those we have observed in hypertension. We have studied a few anaemic patients, but have not seen leaking points on arterioles such as we have seen in malignant hypertension. However, our opportunities for studying such patients have been few, and usually the patients were not at the most acute stage. Nevertheless, I have some support in thinking that the observation may be correct, because our colleague N. ASHTON[2], at the Institute of Ophthalmology in London, has made pathological studies of exudates caused by anaemia. He has shown fatty changes in the wall of the arterioles feeding cotton-wool-spot areas in malignant hypertension, but has not found any change of this kind in relation to cotton-wool spots in anaemia.

BROD: What about brain tumours?

DOLLERY: In brain tumour you get papilloedema, which closely resembles the papilloedema of malignant hypertension, but you don't usually see cotton-wool spots away from the optic disc.

---

[1] LEISHMAN, R.: Brit. J. Ophthalm. **41**, 641 (1957).

[2] HARRY, J., and N. ASHTON: Transact. Ophth. Soc. Unit. Kingdom **83**, 71 (1963).

COTTIER: May I ask Dr. DOLLERY whether hypertensives retaining salt and water are perhaps more prone to develop exudates than hypertensives with increased diuresis and natriuresis?

DOLLERY: There is the bad old term "albuminuric retinopathy" — a very bad term, because normotensive people with albuminuria do not get retinal exudates. But there is more than a hint that a patient who is uraemic and has hypertension may develop more extensive exudative retinopathy than a patient who is not uraemic but has the same degree of hypertension. However, I don't think anybody has ever treated this question on a quantitative basis.

PICKERING: I have got some pictures of these anaemic fundi. Fig. 1 refers to a woman of 32 years of age with gastro-intestinal bleeding. Fig. 2 shows the eyeground of a man of 56 years of age who fell downstairs after a

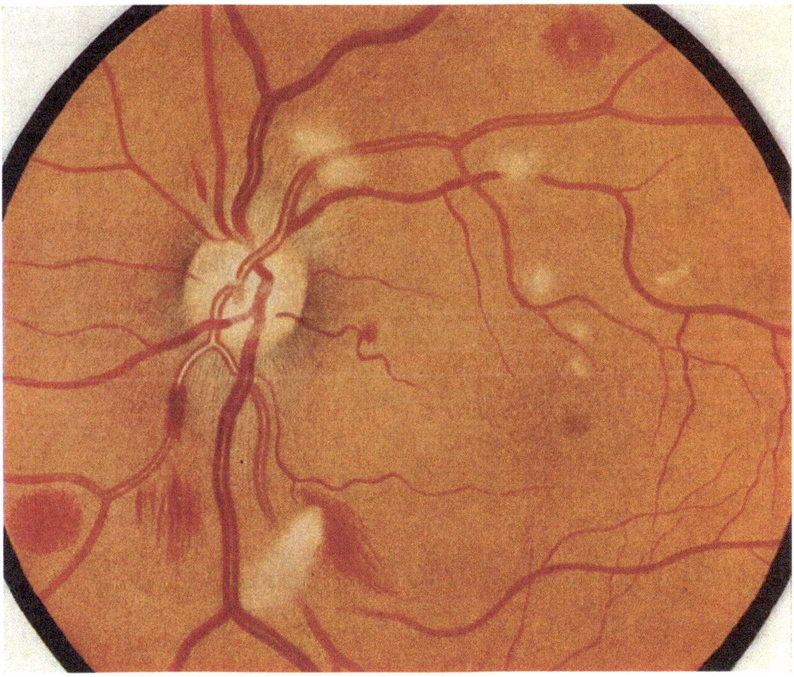

Fig. 1. Left fundus of a woman aged 32 who had bled from a duodenal ulcer for 21 days and required 42 pints of blood. The lesions disappeared after 23 days [from M. A. PEARS and G. W. PICKERING: Quart. J. Med. *29*, 153 (1960)].

Christmas party, recovered consciousness the next day, but then lost consciousness again after an intestinal haemorrhage and became anaemic. I heard about it, because they wanted to open his skull. He was transfused, and Fig. 3 shows his eyeground a few weeks later. Fig. 4 is his picture a few

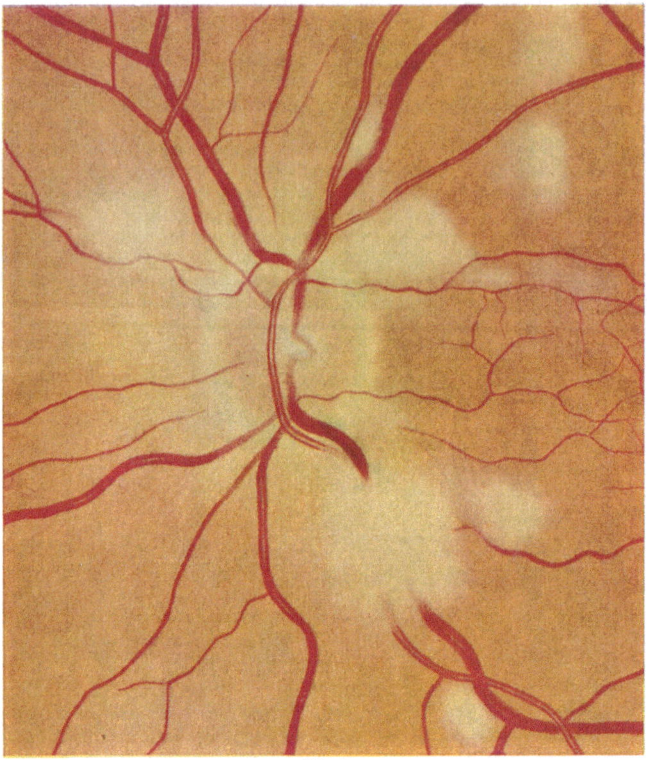

Fig. 2

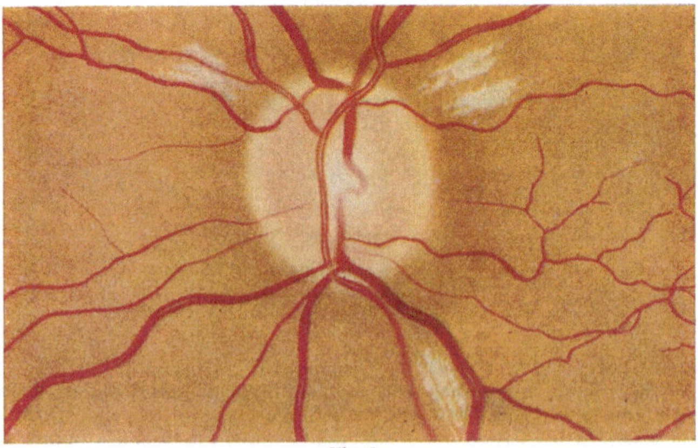

Fig. 3

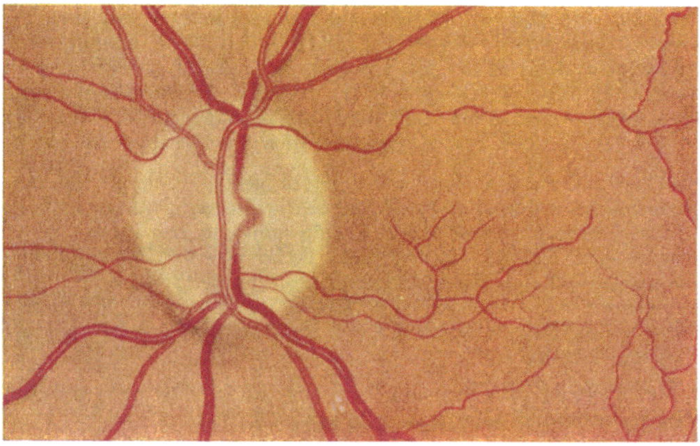

Fig. 4

Figs 2, 3, and 4. The left fundus of a man of 56 who had a gastro-intestinal haemorrhage producing hypotension and anaemia. The fundus is shown on 11. 1. 55, when his haemoglobin was 25%, on 7. 2. 55, and on 6. 9. 55 [from M. A. PEARS and G. W. PICKERING: Quart. J. Med. *29*, 153 (1960)].

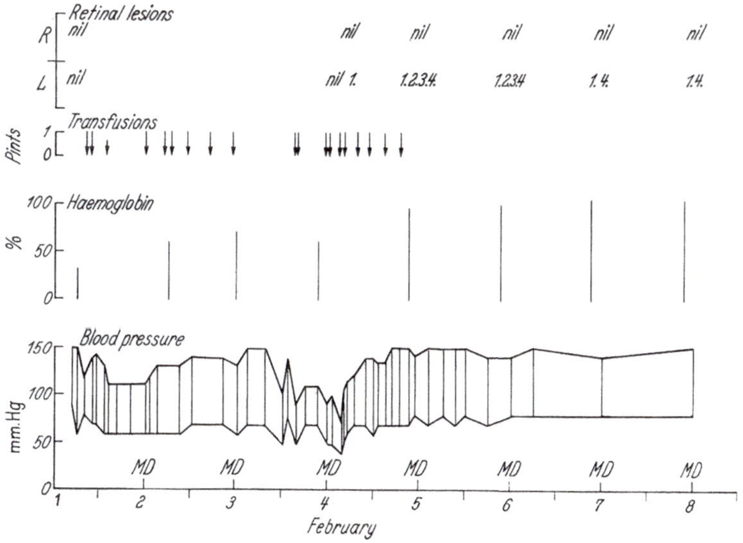

Fig. 5. Relationship between arterial pressure, haemoglobin, transfusions, and the development of retinal lesions in gastro-intestinal haemorrhage. The lesions are numbered in order of their appearance [from M. A. PEARS and G. W. PICKERING. Quart. J. Med. *29*, 153 (1960)].

months later, and you can see that the exudate has entirely disappeared. Fig. 5 shows the interval between the falls in blood pressure and the appearance of the exudates. As you see, the exudates did not appear until quite a few days after the big fall in arterial pressure. I understood from your colleague ASHTON that, after embolisation of retinal arteries, exudates don't come out for some time. Is this true, and what is the explanation?

DOLLERY: We have observed a latent period between the stimulus which causes the cotton-wool spots and their appearance, both experimentally and in humans. In the pig, following embolisation, a fully developed cotton-wool spot did not appear until 24 hours later, although electron microscopy showed changes in the neurones after only one hour. In hypertensive patients we have observed cotton-wool spots developing up to three days after we have demonstrated a leaking point, presumably betraying a region of arteriolar necrosis.

BYROM: Would you consider the suggestion that the oedema, the arteriolar necrosis, and the cotton-wool exudates are all due to leaky vessels?

DOLLERY: I think that is possible, though I can't say more.

GROSS: I should like to ask Dr. DOLLERY about the dilatation of the small arterioles. Is this effect as acute as the one Dr. BYROM showed under ether anaesthesia? Are there any comparable effects if, for example, hydralazine or guanethidine is given intravenously, leading to a prompt decrease in blood pressure? — In your patients in whom you lowered blood pressure by giving hydralazine, did changing position have an effect similar to that which you saw under the influence of sympathetic inhibitors?

DOLLERY: Perhaps I wasn't very clear when I gave the paper. Our observations with hydralazine and posture were acute. With hydralazine the observations were made within an hour of the intravenous administration of the drug, and in the postural studies, there was an even shorter interval between the two sets of observations. We have also observed this pattern of changes, i.e. dilatation of small arterioles and constriction of the larger ones, in patients who have been treated with drugs for an extended period. I think our observations on small arterioles fit in very well with Dr. BYROM's observations, except that we have not observed focal narrowing, but a uniform narrowing.

PAGE: Have you ever used CO_2 or drugs like Doryl (carbamoylcholinium-chloride) or acetyl-β-methyl-choline?

DOLLERY: No, I haven't. We have made many observations of the effect of changes in respiratory gases, because these vessels are very sensitive to changes in inspired-oxygen pressure. High CO_2 concentrations at normal oxygen pressure have little effect on the calibre of the human retinal arteriole.

TAQUINI: What is the diameter of the vessels you are dealing with?

DOLLERY: The largest vessels near the disc in the human eye are about 110 μ. in diameter, the smallest we can visualise on our best pictures are about 30 μ. in diameter.

PEART: Wouldn't perhaps the explanation of the observation on the variable diameter be that the larger arterioles are following passively the course of the blood pressure, whereas the resistance vessels, which are the smaller ones, are the ones that are reacting and contributing to the maintenance of blood flow through the particular organ at the lower pressures? You, of course, had the supreme opportunity of following what happens to the actual resistance vessels as opposed to the others.

DOLLERY: I think that is probably correct. The difficulty is that with hydralazine the larger arterioles did dilate a little.

PEART: But that is hydralazine, which may have its own action on all these blood vessels.

The heart and hypertension

By

W. M. Kirkendall

No physician needs to be reminded that the heart participates in the vascular disease associated with hypertension. Concentric hypertrophy of the left ventricle, left axis deviation, and left ventricular hypertrophy are important signs of hypertensive damage. The syndrome of congestive heart failure associated with hypertensive disease (usually with coronary atherosclerosis) is one of the two major causes of death in the patient with hypertension. I will not be concerned with these clinical aspects of the heart in hypertension, but, rather, with less well recognized or controversial relationships. Two major points of interest are the significance of the myocardial hypertrophy seen in patients with hypertension and the role of the heart in the production of essential and renal hypertension.

Linzbach (*1*) recently reviewed quantitative aspects of cardiac hypertrophy and revealed that the uncomplicated hypertensive heart was associated with concentric hypertrophy of the myocardium and with normal volume of the ventricle. When dilatation occurred with hypertrophy, as, for instance, in primary myocardial disease or valvular regurgitation, the enlargement was described as eccentric hypertrophy associated with cardiac-chamber dilatation and with disruption of some muscle fibers and fibrosis. The wall of the dilated chamber was thinner than that of the heart with concentric enlargement which showed an actual increase in the number of fibers and only moderate thickening of cells; indeed, the number of fiber layers in the wall was markedly increased in some instances of hypertrophy. Obviously, in some patients, concentric hypertrophy appeared first, followed by dilatation and eccentric changes.

Under the stimulation of chronic systemic arterial hypertension, the heart hypertrophies and the force of contraction increases, which means that greater pressures develop in the lumen of the heart to maintain normal outflow against increased resistance. It appears that the force per unit area ("stress") remains unchanged in this situation. Sandler and Dodge (*2*) noted that left ventricular stress in patients with cardiac hypertrophy was not different from that in patients with normal left ventricular thickness, which one would expect if the greater contractile force developed because of greater myocardial mass.

In contrast, patients with acute increases in volume or in peripheral resistance show increases in the force per unit of cross-sectional area and in oxygen uptake of the myocardium (*3*). The heart apparently shifts to a different ventricular-function curve as a result of, firstly, increased cardiac sympathetic activity, secondly, increase in circulating catecholamines, or, thirdly, other stimuli.

There is little question that the heart responds to increase in circulating volume and systemic arterial pressure with left ventricular hypertrophy. A major unanswered question is whether concentric left ventricular hypertrophy, developed in response to increased peripheral resistance or increased filling pressure, actually increases the work capacity of the heart. Experimental studies by DIECKHOFF (*4*), HASENFELD and ROMBERG (*5*), and BEZNAK (*6*) all suggest that maximal cardiac output and mean arterial pressure are somewhat greater in laboratory animals with uncomplicated cardiac hypertrophy than in normal controls.

On the other hand, YURCHAK et al. (*7*) studied mean left ventricular ejection rates in hypertensive patients and found that, with exercise, pressure rose more and ejection rate less in hypertensive than in normotensive subjects. Lowering the systemic pressure to normal with a ganglion blocker shifted the exercise response toward a more normal pattern, but absolute performance levels during exercise were the same before and after the ganglion blocker. Although this study suggests that force and velocity of ejection are impaired in hypertension, and more particularly with cardiac hypertrophy, the conclusion remains in doubt, because it is distinctly possible that the subjects had other, undetected heart diseases and dilatation.

I am not aware of any clinical evidence which proves that hypertrophy alone decreases cardiac function. Indeed, in the absence of valvular disease, coronary artery atherosclerosis, or primary myocardial disease, the hypertrophied heart maintains the circulation quite well until it outstrips its nutrition, when dilatation begins and hypoxia may cause a radical reduction in work capacity. This notion is supported by MICKERSON (*8*) who found, in all but 12 of a series of 445 patients with hypertension and heart failure, a cause of heart failure in addition to hypertension. Chief among the secondary causes were valvular heart disease, renal disease, alone or combined with cardiac lesions, malignant hypertension, and respiratory infections. Significantly, TAYLOR et al. (*9*) and VARNAUSKAS (*10*) found no relationship between arterial pressure and cardiac reserve.

Thus, the chronic stimulus of hypertension causes concentric hypertrophy with an increase in fibers and muscle mass in the heart. Experimental data suggest that minute work capacity may be greater in the heart with simple hypertrophy, but evidence concerning man in this regard is not clear.

One final point should be made, relative to the supposedly close correlation of hypertrophy of the heart and diastolic pressure in the hypertensive. In a recent analysis of clinical records and x-rays of 535 male hypertensives, RAMIREZ and GARCIA PONT (*11*) demonstrated that correlation between the systolic and diastolic pressures and the transverse diameter of the heart is relatively poor. Indeed, such correlation as existed was better between systolic pressure and heart size than between diastolic pressure and transverse diameter. This is perhaps significant, since SARNOFF et al. (*12*) have shown that external cardiac work is directly proportional to myocardial oxygen consumption only when the increase in work is caused by a rise in mean systolic pressure. When work increase results from an increase in flow, oxygen consumption does not change, and the ratio of extrinsic work to oxygen consumption indicates a high external myocardial efficiency. In contrast, systolic hypertension causes increased oxygen consumption, which leads to relative myocardial hypoxia. The ratio of extrinsic work to oxygen consumption is decreased, indicating a low external myocardial efficiency. SARNOFF's group found, however, that the mean systolic pressure is not the fundamental determinant of myocardial oxygen consumption, which actually correlates best with the tension-time index, a product of the mean systolic pressure and the duration of the tension state.

RAMIREZ and GARCIA PONT (*11*) suggested that the systolic pressure increase, associated with reduced distensibility of large arteries (resulting, for instance, from arteriosclerosis), could account for a major component of the cardiac enlargement in hypertensives. An alternative explanation might be that overfilling of the distended aorta in patients with hypertension leads to a maximal stretching of the aortic wall, which restricts further distension and causes systolic hypertension and hypertrophy. While RAMIREZ and GARCIA PONT's study did not clarify this matter, it did show that the association of systolic pressure with transverse diameter was independent of age. This suggests that a disease process associated with age – such as atherosclerosis – might not be a major factor in the production of the elevated systolic pressure. The matter is not settled, however, for in a very fine epidemiologic study, HUMERFELT (*13*) found that there was almost a linear increase in heart volume with age in women, and a sharp increase in volume in men in the sixth and seventh decades.

There is little question that, in the vast majority of hypertensives, cardiac output measured by any of the conventional methods is usually normal or, in far advanced disease, reduced, whereas peripheral vascular resistance is elevated. Nevertheless, for years it has been known that increased peripheral vascular resistance, induced acutely in experimental animals, is attended initially by an augmented cardiac output (*14*). Interest in the possibility that some forms of essential hypertension in man may also begin with a high cardiac output was kindled by EICH et al. (*15*), who found a distinct elevation of cardiac output in 16 labile hypertensives. They also found that some labile hypertensives, as well as patients with fixed hypertension, had cardiac indices in the normal range. Peripheral vascular resistance was reduced in the high-output group. Other studies have shown that such findings are not isolated (*10*, *16*, *17*). In this regard, it is of interest that the majority of patients with coarctation of the aorta not in congestive heart failure have high cardiac outputs and large stroke volumes (*18*). Similarly, the acute hypertension of glomerulonephritis is caused by an increased cardiac output with elevated right atrial pressure and normal peripheral resistance (*19*).

Four years after the initial report, EICH et al. published the results of follow-up studies from the high-output patients, at which time there was no indication that these individuals were developing into the usual normal-output, high-resistance hypertensives (*20*). However, in a personal communication, EICH recently indicated that re-evaluation now in progress reveals that patients of this group have, in fact, developed into stable hypertensives with high resistance and normal outputs.

These findings certainly suggest that the heart may play a more important role than is normally accorded to it in the pathogenesis of hypertension and, indeed, that cardiac-output elevation precedes increased peripheral vascular resistance in the development of hypertension. Parallel studies by LEDINGHAM (*21*), GUYTON (*22*), FLOYER (*23*), and ULRYCH (*24*) and their co-workers have led to widespread speculation that the heart – by increasing its output in response to, firstly, expansion of the circulating compartment, secondly, alterations in tone of the capacity vessels, or, thirdly, myocardial contractility – may set the stage for hypertension.

BORST and BORST-DE GEUS (*25*) explain the participation of the heart in hypertensive disease on the basis of STARLING's theory of fluid balance and circulatory homeostasis. In this complex scheme, hypertension is part of a reaction to "deficient renal sodium output". When sodium balance is positive, in spite of a normal cardiac performance, the increase in volume of extracellular fluid brings about a rise in cardiac output which results in increased sodium excretion by the kidney. STARLING's theory cannot explain why increased cardiac performance results in a rise in arterial pressure, but not in cardiac output; therefore, BORST and BORST-DE GEUS considered the initial increase in pressure to be maintained, first, by autoregulation with increased resistance in the periphery, and then by a slow resetting of the baroreceptors, leading to less resistance to the rise in arterial pressure. They used the experimental model of hypertension produced in man by liquorice and demonstrated that an increase in central venous pressure preceded the rise in arterial pressure. BORST and BORST-DE GEUS postulated that cardiac performance was enhanced later by cardiac hypertrophy, which occurred without change in central venous pressure, perhaps as a result of the heart's functioning on a higher function curve or because of upward resetting of baroreceptors.

LEDINGHAM and COHEN (*26*), as well as PETERS (*27*), have attacked BORST's hypothesis, their chief objections being to the difficulty in defining some of the terms and to BORST's insistence that there must be "deficient sodium output".

In a series of articles, LEDINGHAM and COHEN (*28*, *29*) reported a transient fall in cardiac output when renal artery constriction and the consequent hypertension were relieved. They also demonstrated that, in the early phase of hypertension associated with experimental renal artery stenosis, there is an increase in extracellular fluid and a transient increase in cardiac output. These studies in rats did not include numerous data on cardiac output. A bradycardia accompanied the increased output, making it unlikely that angiotensin or increased peripheral vascular resistance initiated the changes.

These investigators felt that the rise in cardiac output in renal arterial hypertension could result from increased myocardial contractility or from an increased atrial filling pressure. The latter, in turn, could follow an increase in extracellular fluid and plasma volume compartment or a rise in venous tone. The rise in cardiac output, if unchecked, could lead to a rise in blood pressure, since accommodation of baroreceptor responses occurs. The rise in blood pressure could bring about a myogenic constriction of the arterioles, such as had been observed by Folkow (*30*), which would cause the blood pressure to rise to even greater heights. Ledingham and Cohen believe that behind the stenotic area in the renal circulation there is a negative-feed-back mechanism which initiates mechanisms to restore the blood pressure behind the stenosis to its normal level. They postulate that the initial fall in pressure results in expansion of extracellular fluid and plasma compartment or increased venous tone of capacitance vessels of myocardial contractility. Cardiac output increases and a rise in arterial pressure follows. As has already been mentioned, hypertension produced in this way stimulates autoregulatory responses from the resistance vessels and raises blood pressure further. When the blood pressure behind the renal artery stenosis is restored to normal, the stimulus to increase cardiac output is lost. The increase in peripheral resistance is then maintained by an inherent property of the arterioles, while the cardiac output remains in the normal range.

Such a sequence of circulatory events has not been recorded in patients with *renal artery* hypertension. The difficulty of demonstrating various elements of the renin-angiotensin system in patients with renal artery stenosis suggests that other mechanisms may sustain the hypertension after initial renin-angiotensin stimulation. If the events suggested by Ledingham and Cohen do occur, the peripheral arteriolar effects of angiotensin may be less important in instituting hypertension than its ability to retain salt under certain conditions and the inotropic action of aldosterone. Obviously, the possibility exists that humoral substances other than these, acting on capacitance vessels, are responsible for the cardiac effect and hypertension.

The situation regarding the role of the heart in initiating *essential* hypertension is even less clear. Eich's observations suggest that it might be an important early factor in some instances, but experimental evidence on this point is very sparse. Russian investigators (*31*) suggest that a fruitful area of future investigation would be the study of the influence of central nervous stimuli on the heart, particularly in regard to the development of essential hypertension. In psychogenic hypertension, however, as in most other varieties of known experimental and human hypertension, the heart plays a secondary role.

Summary

Hypertrophy of the heart may represent a useful adaptation to the circulatory stress of hypertension. It is clear, however, that when coronary artery disease and decreased myocardial perfusion occur, dilatation of the heart is seen and cardiac reserve falls sharply. Hypertrophy of the heart is poorly correlated with the height of the diastolic pressure, less poorly with systolic pressure, and probably best with the tension-time index. The influence of age on the development of cardiac hypertrophy in hypertensives is not settled.

The heart plays a secondary role in the genesis of most hypertensive diseases. A major uncertainty is whether the cardiac and circulatory abnormalities observed in renal and essential hypertension arise from changes in resistance or capacitance vessels or from changes in the heart itself produced by neural influences. We badly need a better understanding of the sequence of circulatory events in all forms of hypertension and more precise knowledge about the effect of the central nervous system and humoral substances on the heart and circulation to provide support for current theories regarding the cause of elevated blood pressure.

Zusammenfassung

Hypertrophie des Herzens kann eine zweckmäßige Anpassung an die Belastung des Kreislaufs beim Hochdruck darstellen. Es ist jedoch offensichtlich, daß bei Auftreten einer Erkrankung der Koronararterien und einer verminderten Durchblutung des Myokardes das Herz dilatiert und die Herzreserve stark abnimmt. Die Herzhypertrophie ist kaum mit der Höhe des diastolischen, etwas besser mit derjenigen des systolischen Blutdrucks, und am besten mit dem Spannung-Zeit-Index korreliert. Der Einfluß des Alters auf die Entwicklung einer Herzhypertrophie beim Hochdruck ist noch nicht klargestellt.

Das Herz spielt eine sekundäre Rolle bei der Genese der meisten mit Hochdruck einhergehenden Zustände. Recht unsicher ist, ob die beim renalen und essentiellen Hochdruck beobachteten Herz-Kreislauf-Störungen auf Änderungen der Widerstands- oder Kapazitätsgefäße zurückzuführen sind oder auf Änderungen im Herzen selbst, die durch nervöse Einflüsse hervorgerufen werden. Um die heute üblichen Theorien über die Ursache eines erhöhten Blutdruckes zu stützen, ist ein besseres Verständnis für den zeitlichen Ablauf der Kreislaufveränderungen bei allen Formen des Hochdruckes ebenso notwendig wie eine genauere Kenntnis der Einflüsse des Zentralnervensystems und humoraler Stoffe auf Herz und Kreislauf.

Résumé

Le cœur peut efficacement s'adapter à l'obstacle circulatoire de l'hypertension en s'hypertrophiant. Il est cependant évident que lorsque survient une maladie coronarienne et une diminution de l'irrigation du myocarde, le cœur se dilate et sa réserve énergétique s'effondre. L'hypertrophie du coeur n'est que médiocrement liée au niveau de la pression diastolique, moins médiocrement à celui de la pression systolique; elle est probablement le plus en relation avec un index tension-temps. Le rôle de l'âge dans le développement de l'hypertrophie cardiaque chez les hypertendus n'est pas démontré.

Le cœur joue un rôle secondaire dans la genèse de la plupart des maladies hypertensives. Une incertitude majeure est la question de savoir si les anomalies cardio-circulatoires observées dans l'hypertension rénale et dans l'hypertension essentielle résultent de modifications des vaisseaux conditionnant la résistance périphérique ou le volume vasculaire disponible, ou bien de modifications du cœur lui-même, provoquées par des influences nerveuses. Nous aurions grandement besoin d'une meilleure compréhension de l'enchaînement des phénomènes circulatoires dans toutes les formes d'hypertension et de connaissances plus précises sur les effets du système nerveux central et des substances humorales sur le cœur et la circulation, pour pouvoir étayer les théories actuelles sur la pathogénie de l'hypertension artérielle.

Acknowledgement

This work was supported in part by grants T1 HE 5577 and T1 HE 5367 from the National Institutes of Health.

References

1. Linzbach, A. J.: Amer. J. Cardiol. **5**, 370 (1960). — 2. Sandler, H., and H. T. Dodge: Circulation Res. **13**, 91 (1963). — 3. Badeer, H. S.: Amer. J. Cardiol. **14**, 133 (1964). — 4. Dieckhoff, J.: Arch. exper. Path. Pharmak. **182**, 268 (1936). — 5. Hasenfeld, A., and E. Romberg: Arch. exper. Path. Pharmak. **39**, 333 (1897). — 6. Beznak, M.: Circulation Res. **6**, 207 (1958). — 7. Yurchak, P. M., W. B. Hood, Jr., E. L. Rolett, R. B. Hickler, and R. Gorlin: Amer. J. Med. Sc. **247**, 42 (1964). — 8. Mickerson, J. N.: Amer. Heart J. **65**, 267 (1963). — 9. Taylor, S. H., K. W. Donald, and J. M. Bishop: Clin. Sc. **16**, 351 (1957). — 10. Varnauskas, E.: Scand. J. Clin. Laborat. Invest. **7**, Suppl. **17** (1955). — 11. Ramirez, E. A., and P. H. Garcia Pont: Circulation **31**, 542 (1965). — 12. Sarnoff, S. J., E. Braunwald, G. H. Welch, Jr., R. B. Case, W. N. Stainsby, and R. Macruz: Amer. J. Physiol. **192**, 148 (1958). — 13. Humerfelt, S.: Acta med. Scand. **175**, Suppl. **407** (1963). — 14. Katz, L. N., and C. J. Wiggers: Amer. J. Physiol. **82**, 91 (1927). — 15. Eich, R. H., R. J. Peters, and R. H. Lyons: In: Hypertension. Vol. VII. Ed. by F. R. Skelton. Amer. Heart Assoc., New York, 1958, p. 100. — 16. Finkielman, S., M. Worcel, and A. Agrest: Circulation **31**, 356 (1965). — 17. Werkö, L., and H. Lagerlöf: Acta med. Scand. **133**, 427 (1949). — 18. Culbertson, J. W., J. W. Eckstein, W. M. Kirkendall, and G. N. Bedell: J. Clin. Invest. **36**, 1537 (1957). — 19. deFazio, V., R. C. Christensen, T. J. Regan, L. J. Baer, Y. Morita, and H. K. Hellems: Circulation **20**, 190 (1959). — 20. Eich, R. H., R. J. Peters, R. P. Cuddy, H. Smulyan, and R. H. Lyons: Mod. Med. **30** (10), 81 (1962). — 21. Ledingham, J. M.: In: Hypotensive Drugs. Ed. by M. Harington. Pergamon Press, London, 1956, p. 183. — 22. Guyton, A. C.: Amer. J. Cardiol. **8**, 401 (1961). — 23. Floyer, M. A., and P. C. Richardson: Lancet 1961/I, 253. — 24. Ulrych, M., J. Hofman, and Z. Hejl: Amer. Heart J. **68**, 193 (1964). — 25. Borst, J. G. G., and A. Borst-de Geus: Lancet 1963/I, 677. — 26. Ledingham, J. M., and R. D. Cohen: Lancet 1963/I, 887. — 27. Peters, G.: Lancet 1963/I, 1270. — 28. Ledingham, J. M., and R. D. Cohen: Clin. Sic. **22**, 69 (1962). — 29. Ledingham, J. M., and R. D. Cohen: Lancet 1963/II, 979. — 30. Folkow, B.: Circulation Res. **15**, Suppl. **1**, 19 (1964). — 31. Simonson, E., and J. Brozek: Ann. Int. Med. **50**, 129 (1959).

Introduction to the General Discussion

By

V. Puddu

For the clinician, this afternoon's subject, the behaviour of the cardiovascular system, is probably the key-point in the problem of hypertension.

In the absence of cardiac and vascular involvement, hypertension would not be a clinically manifest disease, but merely a curiosity, detectable only with the aid of the manometer. The problem is to know when and why a person will fall a victim to hypertension, and why his heart or vascular tree will suffer the consequences of the disease.

Our knowledge of the prognosis and natural history of hypertension and hypertensive disease is scant. Often, people with high blood-pressure levels survive for years without developing complications, while in others, complications appear within a short time. Often, we are faced with a combination of hypertension and atherosclerosis, and, here again, we are not sufficiently familiar with the natural history of the disease.

It is my impression that atherosclerosis is not such a chronic disease as it is generally held to be. Not infrequently, we may encounter patients in whom the aorta is enlarged at a relatively early age but thereafter remains the same size for many years. Similarly, it is not uncommon for patients to show signs of angina for some months and then remain asymptomatic for years afterwards. In the course of hypertension, symptoms and complications may develop and persist for a time and then give way to a silent period which may last for years.

In this disease, it seems that the factors of evolution that we can evaluate are in the minority in relation to the multitude about which we know nothing.

I think we must admit that it would be worth while not to restrict measurements of basal blood pressure to specific investigations on hypertension, but to adopt this procedure in all epidemiological studies of cardiovascular disease. The blood-pressure measurements made in the Framingham survey and in similar studies are casual or semi-casual: interesting correlations are evident between these findings and the incidence of cardiovascular disease. It would probably be wise to investigate the possible modifications that might occur in these correlations if basal blood pressures were measured.

A few days ago, I had the pleasure of meeting Dr. M. SOKOLOW of San Francisco, who told me some of the details of his well-known investigations with a machine for the continuous measurement of blood pressure. It seems that in many subjects with elevated blood-pressure levels under conditions of rest there is a fall in blood pressure during work, if the work is pleasant and readily acceptable to the subject. This is just the contrary of what we should expect.

How would the correlations change if in our epidemiological surveys we could observe the behaviour of blood pressure continuously? This is only one of the unknown factors in the development of this disease I had in mind before. But surely there are many others that, if we knew them, could supply answers to many of the unsolved questions relating to the aetiology of the disease.

When we consider the care taken by research groups engaged in epidemiological studies of hypertensive disease to avoid "observer-errors", e.g. the "blind" system of blood-pressure measurement adopted by the London School of Hygiene, and the establishment of central laboratories all over the world for the purpose of blood cholesterol measurement, it is astonishing how rarely spontaneous fluctuations of blood pressure are taken into account in such investigations.

General Discussion

Reubi: I should like to add one remark to Dr. Kirkendall's paper. I think there is little doubt that in established hypertension the cardiac output is normal or perhaps somewhat decreased. Nevertheless, it is quite possible that in the initial stage of hypertensive disease there is some increase. Unfortunately, such an increase is very difficult to prove. Any procedure involved in the measurement of cardiac output is likely to produce an elevation in cardiac output itself. This occurs particularly in patients with the neurogenic type of hypertension, in whom emotional factors may play an important role.

Anyway, the hypothesis presented by Dr. Kirkendall is very interesting and attractive, and I should like to make a comparison with what we find in chronically treated patients. Most of the antihypertensive drugs used today initially produce a drop in the cardiac output, at least in the standing position; but after several months or years, cardiac output tends to rise again, and the peripheral resistance diminishes. I still don't know why after long-term treatment the initial drop in cardiac output is replaced by a decrease in peripheral resistance; but certainly it means a sequence of events which is exactly the reverse of that described by Dr. Kirkendall. In other words, it suggests that the decrease in cardiac output itself makes the blood pressure drop and that the drop in blood pressure makes the peripheral resistance decrease. This may be called homoeostasis.

Page: This sounds plausible.

Taquini: With regard to the cardiac output, it is well established that it is normal in experimental chronic hypertension. Dr. Page will probably discuss his experiments on the development of renal hypertension, the results of which he published recently[1]. In essential hypertension we have found that in one and the same patient cardiac output varies from one moment to the next — even though the patients are previously made familiar with the procedure to be used — without any relation to their oxygen consumption. The variations in cardiac output are accompanied by changes in peripheral resistance in the opposite direction; thus, blood pressure doesn't change, in spite of the changes in cardiac output. It seems that, as in normal subjects, the level of the blood pressure is maintained by baroreceptors. I do not know of any clear-cut evidence to the effect that the increase in the cardiac output *per se* is responsible for the development of hypertension.

Pickering: May I ask how Eich and Borst measured the cardiac output?

Kirkendall: Eich measured cardiac output by the Fick principle. Borst did not report cardiac-output studies in his most recent paper.

Pickering: I am highly sceptical of drawing conclusions about the behaviour of the cardiac output in man under ordinary conditions of life from this elaborate procedure. It seems just like a remark that I heard made

[1] Page, I. H.: Circulation Res. **16**, 134 (1965).

last week, namely that judging the behaviour of rats from what they do in experimental cages is like judging the behaviour of the human race from that of the one-armed bandit in Las Vegas. I think it's not surprising that people whose blood pressures go up and down, whom therefore we call labile, should tend to have rather higher outputs under this circumstance. I think there is one condition which is known to be associated with a high cardiac output, and that is severe anaemia. You can't get away from it. And I should like to ask whether you or anybody else knows what happens to blood pressure in long-continued severe anaemia. Does it go up?

KIRKENDALL: Mean pressure certainly doesn't go up regularly, although pulse pressure does increase.

WERKÖ: During the late forties and early fifties we studied cardiac output in about 100 patients with established arterial hypertension. The results of these studies were published by VARNAUSKAS in 1955[1]. About half of the patients had a slightly elevated cardiac output, and the calculated total peripheral resistance came out within so-called normal limits. The elevated output was most certainly not due to the procedure of study, and the rest of the patients had normal or low outputs with raised peripheral resistance.

About 20 of these cases have been studied again approximately ten years later. At an age of around 40 years, the cardiac index was about 4 l./min.; now, at an age of 50, the output is lower and the cardiac index around 3 l./min., with about the same blood pressure as before. This means that they now have elevated resistance.

I do not think that you can draw very many conclusions from such a highly selected material. There is, however, no doubt that there are patients with high blood pressure who have a hyperkinetic circulation, with fairly normal peripheral resistance, and do not seem to be able to adjust the periphery to the increase in output as normal subjects do. So they have a higher blood pressure, because there is no decrease in peripheral resistance in response to the increased rate of flow.

SMIRK: Some years ago, we made studies of the type Dr. PUDDU was suggesting, measuring the casual and the basal blood pressures of hypertensive patients in relationship to the presence or absence of cardiac hypertrophy at the time. Cardiac hypertrophy was closely related to the basal blood pressure and was entirely unrelated to what we call the supplemental blood pressure (the casual minus the basal). Likewise, the presence of cardiac failure was closely related to the basal pressure and not to the supplemental blood pressure, and at any one level of the basal blood pressure the incidence of heart failure was higher in the male than in the female. The degree of retinopathy was also related to the basal, but not to the supplemental, blood pressure. Dr. HAMILTON is here with us now and will remember that together with DOYLE and MCQUEEN in the early stages of hexamethonium and pentolinium therapy we made an experiment[2] which bears on what Dr. KIRKENDALL has been saying: we treated hypertensive left ventricular failure with ganglion blockers, without digitalis, and without diuretics. In the great majority of cases, left ventricular failure attacks ceased and remained absent on continued treatment by blood-pressure reduction only. In general congestive

[1] VARNAUSKAS, E.: Scand. J. Clin. Laborat. Invest. 7, Suppl. 17 (1955).

[2] SMIRK, F. H., M. HAMILTON, A. E. DOYLE, and E. G. MCQUEEN: Amer. J. Cardiol. 1, 143 (1958).

heart failure due to hypertension we tried the same experiment; about 50% of the patients managed without digitalis or diuretics. In those days, many of the heart-failure patients died later. But they didn't die from heart failure, the majority of them died from stroke.

Page: That's a great therapeutic achievement!

Wilson: Dr. Byrom showed some years ago in rats with chronic hypertension produced by clipping one renal artery after removing the opposite kidney that when the clip is removed, the blood pressure comes down to normal in a few hours[1]. It is difficult to believe that the heart is primarily producing the hypertension, if under those circumstances this restoration of the renal circulation to normal abolishes the hypertension.

Page: The rat is not typical of the response to inducing renal hypertension in some other animals if it raises its arterial pressure by elevating cardiac output when a clip is applied. In the dog, the cardiac output goes down, not up, immediately after hypertension is initiated. If an Olmsted electromagnetic flow-meter is put on the dog's aorta and an arterial cannula implanted to measure cardiac output continuously, along with stroke volume and calculated total peripheral resistance, and then a Goldblatt clamp placed on the renal artery or cellophane used to develop a perinephric hull around the kidney, the accompanying hypertension is associated with an initial drop in cardiac output and an increase in peripheral resistance. Then with the passage of time — within about three to eight days — the cardiac output returns to normal: the peripheral resistance remains elevated, thus accounting for the rise in blood pressure. Our results obtained in the dog by continuous registration of cardiac output are thus different from those of Ledingham[2] on rats.

Wilson: I think that there is a species difference in this response of cardiac output to renal artery constriction. Ledingham has made recent observations which suggest, in fact, that in the rat there may be a short period of reduced cardiac output, followed by a rise before the cardiac output turns to normal.

Hood: This session is on hypertension and vascular disease. Let us go back for a moment to the relationship between atherosclerosis and hypertension. Deming tried to bridge the gap between the people who have been studying one disease or the other separately. He presented work on the rat, but what do we know about conditions in man? We know that if we have got both high lipids and high pressure in long-term prognostic types of study the risk is several times higher as regards coronary disease. What levels of lipids do we have in man in hypertension? I think this is a difficult question to answer now, but we can turn it round the other way and look at patients with hypercholesterolaemia and at their pressures. Out of about 500 patients with hypercholesterolaemia that we studied, half had elevated diastolic levels; 60% or 70% (some difference between the two sexes) had levels in the upper quartile of the normal range for their age. Of these, initially selected owing to their having high cholesterol, 40% have high triglyceride levels. You can study it this way, or you can go in for a closer or more intimate study. If you have high-quality aortograms, you can study the renal arteries and a big part of the abdominal aorta and try to correlate the radiological appearance of the

[1] Byrom, F. B., and L. F. Dodson: Clin. Sc. 8, 1 (1949).

[2] Ledingham, J. M., and R. D. Cohen: Lancet 1963/II, 979.

aorta and renal artery and the lipid parameters. In proximal renal artery stenosis you will naturally find a very extensive abdominal atherosclerosis, and you will find a statistical increase, not in cholesterol levels, but in triglyceride levels. You will also find a different behaviour in fat-tolerance tests, as BERKOWITZ did in unspecified hypertensives in the Second Philadelphia Symposium[1]. We have used another technique and found the same. Is this a result of the elevated fasting triglyceride level ? Because there is a close correlation between the response to a fat-load and the fasting level. Well, it seems so, but there are examples of exaggerated response to a fat-load even in those with a fasting triglyceride level in the low normal range. Thus, in man, you can study this correlation either from the point of view of the lipid elevation or from the point of view of hypertension.

[1] BERKOWITZ, D.: In: Hypertension. Recent Advances. The Second Hahnemann Symposium on Hypertensive Disease. Ed. by A.N. BREST and J. H. MOYER. Lea and Febiger, Philadelphia, 1961, p. 169.

General principles in antihypertensive treatment

Assessment of antihypertensive therapy

By

W. I. Cranston

By far the most important criterion in assessing the efficacy of antihypertensive treatment is the extent to which it improves the prognosis. This aspect will not be considered now, as it will be discussed later on in the symposium. If, as seems probable, the improvement in prognosis is proportionate to the reduction in arterial pressure, it is clearly important to attempt to measure the effects of the drugs used upon the blood-pressure level. Although it is easy, in man and in animals, to determine the acute effects, it is more difficult to measure the long-term effects over a period of weeks or months, and the longer the trial period lasts, the greater this difficulty becomes. Several of the factors responsible for this difficulty are purely technical: for instance, repeated measurement of blood pressure calls for the use of some form of sphygmomanometry; this method is subject to errors, and it is uncertain to what extent these errors are random and to what extent they are predictable over a period of time. Biological factors are probably more important: studies involving continuous blood-pressure recording have shown that blood pressure varies considerably in normal as well as in hypertensive patients at different times throughout the day (*1*), and this must also be taken into account in assessing the efficacy of treatment; repeated measurements also reveal that blood pressure usually falls progressively over several weeks in response to medication, and even placebo therapy may cause an apparent fall in pressure in some patients (Fig. 1).

At present no completely satisfactory drug is available for the treatment of hypertension. Generally speaking, the more potent the remedy or the lower the controlled blood pressure, the greater becomes the problem of side effects. It is pertinent to consider the aims of treatment, so far as we can determine them at present. In patients with benign hypertension, death rate is related to the diastolic blood-pressure level (*2*). The relationship between the degree of blood-pressure control achieved and the prognosis is much less distinct, but there is evidence to suggest that there is a connection.

One interesting point emerged from LEISHMAN's first study of survival in treated hypertensive patients (*2*): male patients with diastolic blood pressures of 130–149 mm. Hg, but without papilloedema, were treated with pentolinium and reserpine, in response to which the standing diastolic blood-pressure level fell to 110 mm. Hg in about two thirds of the patients. The survival rate in these patients was quite similar to that found in untreated men with diastolic blood pressures of 100–119 mm. Hg. If there is any general validity in this observation, a reduction of 10–20 mm. Hg in diastolic blood pressure may confer a considerable benefit in terms of survival.

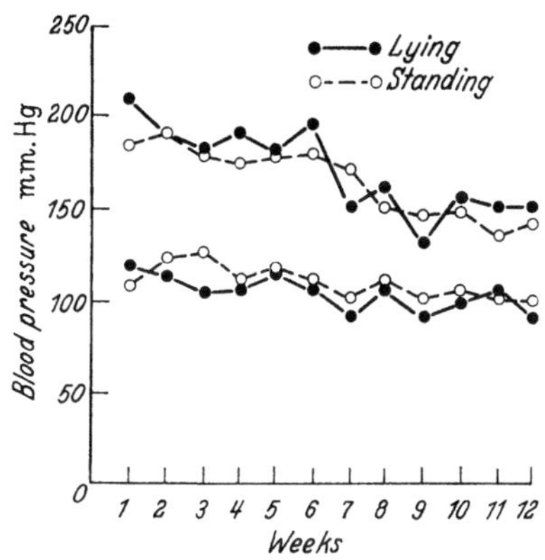

Fig. 1. Blood pressure, measured weekly, in a patient receiving placebo tablets [from PICKERING et al (*8*)].

We have conducted several trials on a double-blind cross-over basis, mainly with the less potent antihypertensive drugs, which can be given in a fixed daily dosage. Placebos and the drugs under comparison were administered in random order. After an initial period of three to six weeks on placebos, each patient was given each drug or placebo, for 12 weeks at a time in trials involving Rauwolfia alkaloids, and for six weeks at a time in trials involving diuretics. Patients were seen every week, and the blood pressure was measured at the same time of day by the same observer; every two weeks, blood samples were taken for determination of urea, creatinine, and electrolytes. The mean blood pressure recorded during the period in which the patient was receiving inert tablets was taken as the control level. In trials involving Rauwolfia alkaloids, only the average blood-pressure levels over the last six weeks of each 12-week period were compared, to allow the effects of the administration or withdrawal of the alkaloids to become stable. The effect on blood pressure of each drug or combination is expressed as the change, in mm. Hg, as compared with the control level (*3*, *4*). Fig. 2

shows the results of two separate trials: in one, the effects of reserpine and phenobarbitone were compared, in the other, the effects of reserpine, deserpidine, and rescinnamine. It is clear that reserpine, administered in a relatively large dose of 0.5 mg. three times daily, causes a significant fall in systolic and diastolic pressures, the average reductions in response to this drug being 19/16 mm. Hg in the

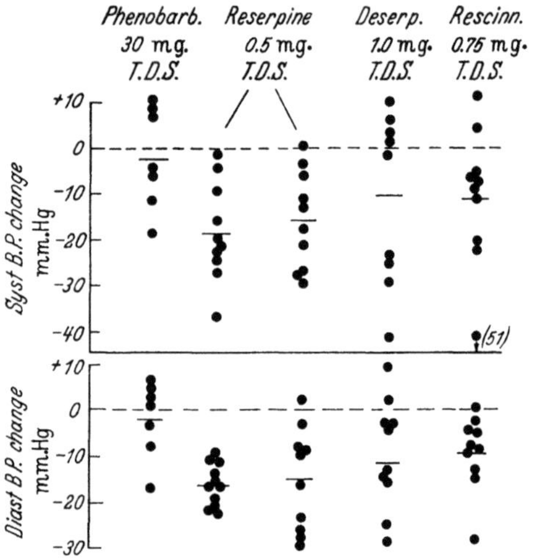

Fig. 2. Blood-pressure change in patients receiving phenobarbitone, reserpine (results from two separate trials), deserpidine, and rescinnamine [from PICKERING et. al (8)].

first trial and 16/15 mm. Hg in the second. Phenobarbitone, on the other hand, had no significant effect upon blood pressure when given in this way. This reflects upon the still common practice of giving small doses of barbiturates to patients with essential hypertension. In the second trial, the effects of reserpine, rescinnamine, and deserpidine were similar. The doses of Rauwolfia alkaloids used in these trials were larger than those commonly employed in the long-term treatment of hypertension; nevertheless, during the trial, side effects were not marked. Tiredness or depression was observed in six patients receiving reserpine, in one receiving rescinnamine, in four receiving deserpidine, and in three receiving placebos. The similarity of the effects of reserpine in two different trials encouraged us to believe that this kind of trial is fairly reliable.

Similar trials have also been carried out with various diuretics, as it would be a great advantage to have an effective diuretic which would lower blood pressure, but would not cause hypokalaemia. The effects of spironolactone in doses of 500 mg. daily and of chlorthalidone in doses of 50 mg. daily were compared in ten patients. Chlorthalidone caused an average fall in blood pressure of 21/10 mm. Hg, spironolactone a fall of 18/7 mm. Hg, and both drugs together a fall of 30/12 mm. Hg. Spironolactone thus appeared to be slightly, though not significantly, less effective than chlorthalidone as regards lowering blood pressure, but it did prevent hypokalaemia (*5*). Triamterene, in a daily dose of 150 mg., has also been compared with chlorthalidone in a daily dose of 50 mg. In this trial, triamterene caused a non-significant reduction of 6/3 mm. Hg in the average blood pressure, compared with a fall of 18/8 mm. Hg in response to chlorthalidone; both drugs in combination lowered the average blood pressure by 24/9 mm. Hg. Thus, triamterene also seems to have little place in the routine treatment of essential hypertension.

In each of these trials, the higher the control blood-pressure level was, the greater was the decrease in pressure in response to medication. In addition to this, however, there was a marked degree of similarity between the effects of the various drugs on the blood pressure. If one diuretic caused an appreciable fall in blood pressure in a particular patient, the other ones tended to do the same. This could imply that the drugs acted in a similar way, or it might merely mean that some patients respond better to any drug than others. An attempt was made to decide this by comparing the effects of two drugs thought to act in different ways. We administered cyclopenthiazide in a single daily dose of 1.5 mg. and methoserpidine in a single daily dose of 40 mg. Rather to our surprise, methoserpidine in this dose had no significant effect on the average blood pressure, though a fairly marked reduction was noted in some patients. Cyclopenthiazide lowered blood pressure by 17/8 mm. Hg on the average; the patients in whom one drug caused a marked fall in blood pressure, also responded in the same way to the other drug. Thus, it is unlikely that similar responses to different drugs imply a common mode of action.

A further trial involving 24 patients was carried out in order to determine how the relationship between control blood pressure and the fall in blood pressure following the administration of a diuretic might be affected by varying the dose; at the same time the effects of three different diuretics were compared (*6*). Each patient received placebos and either bendrofluazide, chlorthalidone, or cyclopenthiazide, which were given in three dosage levels (bendrofluazide: 1.25, 2.5, and 5 mg. three times daily; cyclopenthiazide:

0.25, 0.5, and 1.0 mg. three times daily; chlorthalidone: 50, 100, and 200 mg. once daily). The order of administration of placebos and active drugs in high, intermediate, and low doses was random. These patients, however, unlike those treated in the previous trials, received supplementary potassium (39 mEq./day) throughout the trial.

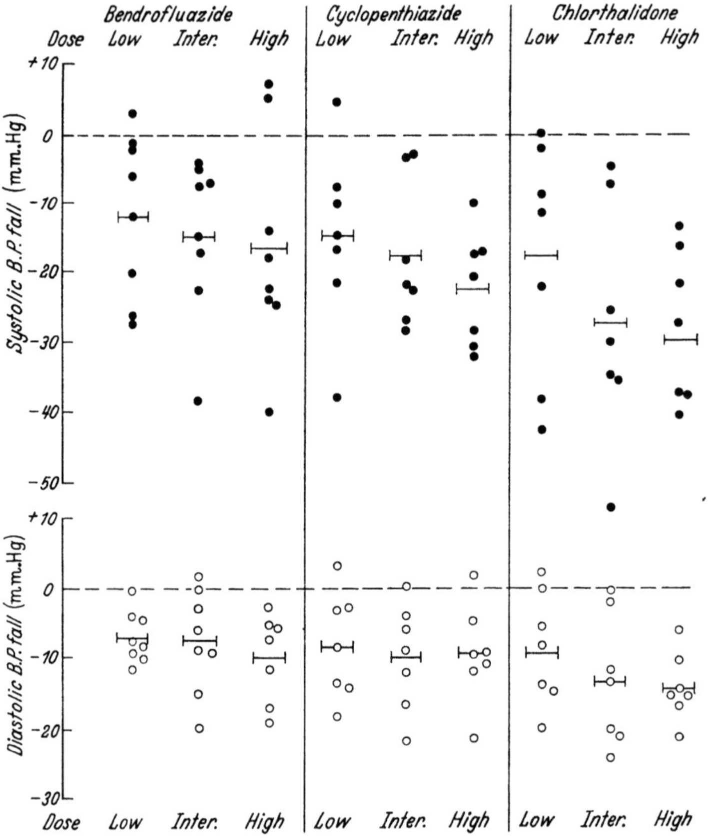

Fig. 3. Blood-pressure change in patients receiving bendrofluazide, cyclopenthiazide, and chlorthalidone in three different dosage levels [from Cranston et al. (6)].

The effects on arterial pressure are shown in Fig. 3. The high dose of each drug was slightly more effective than the low or intermediate dose, but the dose-response curve remained very flat. In these patients, there was a significant relationship between the control blood-pressure level and the blood-pressure fall induced by the drug (Fig. 4). Increasing the dose of the drug did not cause any change in slope in the line relating control blood pressure to blood-pressure fall, but did cause a significant change in intercept (Fig. 5). This implies that in patients with a relatively low control

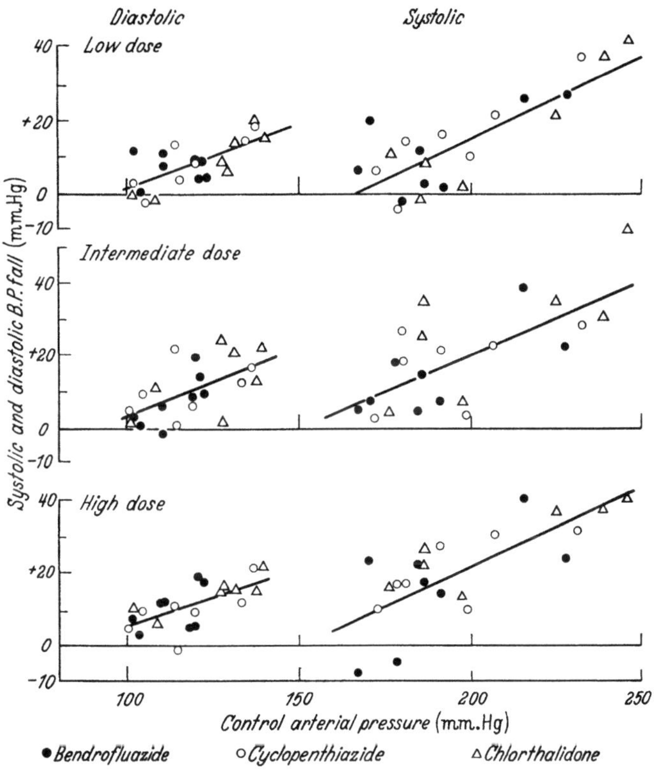

Fig. 4. Relation between control blood pressure and the fall in blood pressure induced by three diuretics administered in three dosage levels [from CRANSTON et al. (6)].

blood pressure larger doses of diuretic will be required in order to induce a given fall in blood pressure than in patients whose control diastolic blood pressure is relatively high.

These trials were all of relatively short duration, and the numbers of patients were limited, mainly owing to the difficulty of ensuring regular attendance. Nevertheless, the results proved to be fairly reproducible when the same drug was evaluated in different trials. This type of trial has the advantage that each patient acts as his own control, and probably provides a fair representation of the long-term effects of the drugs. The results obtained are similar to those observed by Smith and colleagues (7) in more prolonged trials, in which patients made their own blood-pressure measurements.

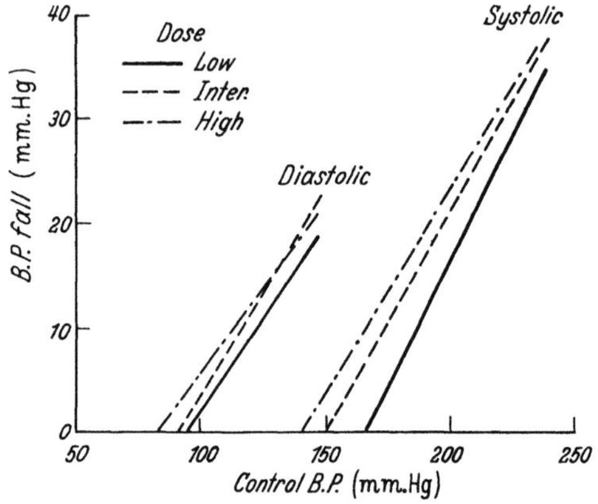

Fig. 5. Regression lines relating control blood-pressure levels to blood-pressure fall, as shown in Fig. 4 [from Cranston et al. (6)].

It is much more difficult to organise satisfactory trials of the more potent antihypertensive drugs, the dosage of which requires titration. In addition, it is not at all easy to assess tolerance of these drugs: in some patients, the dosage has to be increased, because otherwise their blood pressures rise progressively as time goes on; but it is often very hard to decide whether tolerance has developed, and also to compare different agents in this respect. The patterns of response differ considerably from patient to patient; unless placebos are given at intervals, it is impossible to assess the extent to which tolerance is due to a change in the underlying condition rather than to any change in effectiveness of the drugs used.

There is evidence that in some patients who have received prolonged treatment with effective antihypertensive drugs the blood pressure may remain at a relatively low level even after medication has been withdrawn. It may therefore be that the benefit to be gained by treatment is sometimes over-estimated. Probably the only way to assess this is to administer placebos from time to time. There is no doubt that this requires close supervision, and if a patient has been seen at infrequent intervals for some years and is then seen frequently, this change alone may influence the level of his blood pressure. So far no completely adequate solution to this problem has been found.

All hypotensive drugs provoke some side effects; and the exact evaluation of side effects, particularly subjective ones, is a very difficult matter. If the patients are asked leading questions, a number of placebo reactors will be disclosed; on the other hand, if one waits for the patients to complain of side effects, the incidence of such complications will be under-estimated. With a few exceptions, there is no way of predicting which patients will develop side effects. It therefore appears that an approximate estimate of the probability of side effects may provide an adequate basis for the choice of drug in the treatment of hypertension. It seems to me, however, much more important to establish that a drug does have a significant effect upon blood pressure. If it has not, it should not be used.

Summary

This paper is concerned with the assessment of the effects of various agents upon the level of arterial blood pressure. Some of the difficulties of measuring the long-term effects of therapy are discussed, and a number of double-blind, cross-over trials involving diuretic agents and Rauwolfia alkaloids are described. Phenobarbitone had no significant effect upon arterial pressure when given in doses of 30 mg. t.d.s. over periods of 12 weeks. Rauwolfia alkaloids and thiazide diuretics had effects which were consistent from trial to trial. Spironolactone had no clear advantage over thiazide diuretics, and triamterene, in the doses used, was still less effective. The assessment of tolerance and side effects are discussed generally.

Zusammenfassung

Die vorliegende Arbeit befaßt sich mit der Beurteilung der Wirkungen verschiedener Substanzen auf die Höhe des arteriellen Blutdruckes. Einige der Schwierigkeiten, den Einfluß einer Langzeittherapie zu bestimmen, werden besprochen und eine Reihe von doppeltblinden, gekreuzten Versuchen mit Diuretika und Rauwolfiaalkaloiden beschrieben. Phenobarbital in Dosen von dreimal täglich 30 mg, während 12 Wochen gegeben, hatte keinen signifikanten Effekt auf den Blutdruck, Rauwolfiaalkaloide und Thiazid-Diuretika führten zu übereinstimmenden Resultaten von Versuch zu Versuch. Spironolacton ließ keinen eindeutigen Vorzug gegenüber Thiazid-Diuretika erkennen, und Triamteren war in den angewendeten Dosen noch weniger wirksam. Die Beurteilung von Gewöhnung und die Nebenwirkungen werden allgemein besprochen.

Résumé

Cet article a trait à l'évaluation des effets de divers produits sur les chiffres tensionnels. On y discute quelques-unes des difficultés de mesurer les effets à long terme de la thérapeutique et on y décrit un certain nombre d'essais croisés à double insu comportant des diurétiques et des alcaloïdes du

Rauwolfia. Le phénobarbital n'a pas eu d'effet significatif sur la pression artérielle à la dose de 30 mg trois fois par jour pendant des périodes de 12 semaines. L'effet des alcaloïdes du Rauwolfia et des diurétiques thiazidiques a été constant. La spironolactone n'eut pas d'avantage net sur les diurétiques thiazidiques, et le triamtérène, aux doses administrées, fut encore moins efficace. L'évaluation de la tolérance et les effets secondaires sont discutés d'une façon générale.

References

1. Richardson, D. W., A. J. Honour, G. W. Fenton, F. H. Stott, and G. W. Pickering: Clin. Sc. **26**, 445 (1964). — 2. Leishman, A. W. D.: Brit. Med. J. 1959/I, 1361. — 3. Cooper, E. H., and W. I. Cranston: Lancet 1957/I, 396. — 4. Cranston, W. I., B. E. Juel-Jensen, and G. de J. Lee: Brit. Med. J. 1961/I, 950. — 5. Cranston, W. I., and B. E. Juel-Jensen: Lancet 1962/I, 1161. — 6. Cranston, W. I., B. E. Juel-Jensen, A. M. Semmence, R. P. C. Handfield-Jones, J. A. Forbes, and L. M. M. Mutch: Lancet 1963/II, 966. — 7. Smith, W. M., A. N. Damato, N. J. Galluzzi, C. F. Garfield, E. G. Hanowell, W. H. Stimson, R. H. Thurm, J. J. Walsh, and L. Bromer: Ann. Int. Med. **61**, 829 (1964). — 8. Pickering, G. W., W. I. Cranston, and M. A. Pears: In: The Treatment of Hypertension. Ed. by I. N. Kugelmass. Thomas, Springfield, Ill., 1961, p. 124.

Discussion

PAGE: We all recognise that it has been difficult over the past 20 or 30 years to assess the value of definitive treatment. The problem began with the treatment of patients by sympathectomy. Although the situation is now much better, we still do not have a standard method of deciding on the relative merits of different treatments. I think one of the great difficulties is that, inexplicably, some patients respond very satisfactorily, whereas others do not respond at all; yet there seem to be no observable differences in their clinical condition. I am convinced that here lies an important truth waiting to be discovered. We have all seen how, one by one, groups of hypertensives have been separated out; for instance, at one time we called all patients with renovascular hypertension "essential hypertensives", simply because we did not know that the vascular lesion was present.

Study of the haemodynamics of animals with induced renal hypertension with the aid of electromagnetic flow-meters shows that the animal uses different combinations of cardiac output, stroke volume, and total peripheral resistance to maintain the elevated blood pressure as time passes. The combinations at different hours of the day, or even during sleep, have no invariable pattern.

So it is not surprising that when a drug acting on a specific mechanism is used, it may prove ineffective for the particular mechanism which is predominant at the time. This may explain why some patients respond beautifully, and other patients hardly at all, to one and the same drug. It is to be expected, then, that one investigator will claim that a drug shows excellent results and another will find no effects at all. There have been perfectly reliable investigators reporting negative results with α-methyldopa, while others report excellent effects; some think it is very good in malignant hypertension, others that it is useless.

I should like to bring up the question of home blood-pressure measurements. I think Dr. DUSTAN and I agree that, by and large, home blood pressures are much lower than those taken in the clinic. We go to considerable pains to teach our patients how to measure their own blood pressure. We check their measurements, both in their homes and while in the hospital. They send the readings to us by mail every two to four weeks and report by telephone if their pressures are not being properly controlled. In this way the patients themselves take some of the responsibility for, and an interest in, the control of their own blood pressures. I know of no better way of ensuring adherence to our plan of treatment and the constant attention to regulation of the amounts of antihypertensive drugs to be given. I feel convinced that if the patient does not participate actively in long-term treatment, he will eventually default; but when he himself measures the success of his own treatment, he seldom does.

Practising physicians must be persuaded that treatment of hypertension is tedious, exacting, and fairly expensive. It is not worth doing unless it is done with care. Simply to prescribe some pills and occasionally measure the blood pressure is, I think, a waste of time and money. Unfortunately, there are a few people who are not capable of taking their medicine or their blood pressures, but this is a small number. All in all, I submit that drug treatment of hypertension has been successful. And as you know, I think we have reversed the hypertensive process in some patients by rigid insistence on arterial pressure being maintained at or near normal as measured in the supine position.

FREIS: We have recently been impressed by the frequency with which some of the clinic patients failed to take their medicines regularly. This is a matter of concern in improving the techniques for running clinical trials. I imagine that the frequency of non-cooperative patients will vary from one type of patient population to another, that the incidence of such cases in charity clinics might be quite different from that found in populations drawn from private practice. I would urge, as an important technique, the utilisation of tablet-counts as a standard method of procedure in running therapeutic trials on hypertensive patients.

DEMING: I should like to agree with Dr. FREIS on the importance of determining whether the patient is taking the medication and mention, as one possible technique, a method that LUNTZ and AUSTIN[1] developed in outpatient therapy of tuberculosis, namely measurement of the drug in the urine. If a chemical method is available, this can be helpful, although it, too, is fallible, since, with enough imagination and purpose, the patient can restrict his medicine-taking to the day of urine collection.

LEE: I was interested in the linear relationship of the blood-pressure response to chlorthalidone and to spironolactone, because recently in a randomised cross-over study with α-methyldopa, guanethidine, and pargyline, we have found more or less the same thing.

Statistical results or responses to an antihypertensive drug may be disappointing. As a scientist, I can see that a blood-pressure fall of 9 mm. Hg in diastolic pressure may be of great statistical significance, but I can visualise a point in the management of a patient, where it could be of no medical value at all. I think this is very important, because we could conceivably go ahead and attempt to use test drugs of proved statistical ability which would fall flat on their faces when they came out for clinical trials.

It is true that a patient's blood pressure will vary; this has been known since the time of Hippocrates, and we are all finding it out again. Which blood pressure do you treat? Do you treat the lowest or the highest levels that a patient may reach? My feeling is that it is important to know how *high* a patient's pressure may go, and also to use that knowledge from the viewpoint of management.

PEART: I always know when my patients are not taking their drug, because they come and tell me that they feel well. And I think this is a very important point about cross-over trials, anyway, because the patients do know. I am very surprised, Dr. FREIS, that you rely on tablet-counts. That did surprise me a little. — But I disagree with Dr. LEE, because one of the real problems we are up against is that you assess the patient's response to a drug either by its effects or by changes in the pathology of the condition in a comparison trial. I think if you believe that a drug is producing a fall in blood pressure, it is your duty to demonstrate it, which is, in fact, the whole purpose of this sort of trial.

---

[1] LUNTZ, G. R. W. N., and R. AUSTIN: Brit. Med. J. 1960/I, 1679.

GROSS: Dr. CRANSTON, in drawing up your treatment schedule for the comparison of different diuretics, did you consider the fact that these drugs have different half-lives and different durations of action? There are quite substantial variations in this respect between cyclopenthiazide and chlorthalidone, for example, and if you had included the short-acting furosemide in this comparison, you would have had the two extremes. In comparing low, medium, and high doses of drugs, the results may be influenced by differences in the half-life time of the individual compounds.

PETERS: Do you have any data on electrolyte and water balance in your patients? What is the renal response to diuretics in patients who do not react to antihypertensive treatment with these drugs? Is the natriuretic effect of the drugs correlated with antihypertensive efficacy? In experimental animals, the correlation seems to hold well. Thus, the absence of an antihypertensive effect of thiazides in rats with nephrogenic hypertension, mentioned yesterday by Dr. BEIN, may well be related to the depression of the diuretic effect of these drugs in the "unclamped" kidney[1].

CRANSTON: As to home blood pressure, the difficulty about this, Dr. PAGE, is that we have seen patients whose home blood pressures have been running at around 105 to 110 mm. Hg diastolic on treatment, who have developed retinopathy, and who, when they have come to hospital, had very much higher levels. This is why we have been a little bit frightened of this method.

As regards Dr. LEE's point about the measurement of response, I think that when you do double-blind trials, you find that the responses are a good deal smaller than you thought they would be beforehand. Until we know what sort of response is necessary to affect survival, it is very difficult to know what sort of response is significant, or what we are aiming at. And I think that we must obtain information about the effectiveness of the drugs.

The half-lives of various thiazides is a point that I perhaps did not bring out properly. In the trials on three diuretics, we gave chlorthalidone once daily and the other two agents three times daily, but in the other trial, which was later in time, we used cyclopenthiazide in the same dose, 1.5 mg. a day, and on this occasion we gave it only once a day. Relating blood-pressure falls to control-level blood pressure, we could not detect any difference between giving cyclopenthiazide three times or once a day.

We have no data on sodium balance; we tried to collect 24-hour urine specimens in out-patients and found considerable variations in creatinine output; so we do not think they are reliable. The only information that we have was derived from the last trial I mentioned. We did measure extracellular fluid volume with radio-active sulphate, which did not show any significant change. Variations in extracellular fluid volume or weight were not correlated with blood-pressure changes, but I have no evidence about sodium balance.

---

[1] PETERS, G.: Nephron **2**, 95 (1965).

Selection of patients for antihypertensive therapy

By

M. Hamilton

Every patient who knows that his or her blood pressure is elevated requires treatment. In the majority of cases, this will consist only of reassurance, combined with simple measures, such as weight reduction and possibly sedation; in a few cases, however, treatment with hypotensive drugs will be necessary, and the problem of deciding which patients should be treated remains a difficult one. Nevertheless, two points are clear:

1. Once started, treatment with a potent drug will be required for the rest of the patient's life, except in a small proportion of those treated.

2. The more time and care devoted to treatment by the doctor, and the more co-operative the patient, the better will be the results obtained.

Within a very few years of the introduction of hexamethonium, the benefits of hypotensive therapy were clearly established. The side effects produced by ganglion blocking agents were so severe that their administration was virtually restricted to the treatment of the complications associated with hypertension. However, since the introduction of thiazides, adrenergic blocking agents, and α-methyldopa, it has been possible to control hypertension without fear of causing major side effects due to drug administration. Hence, the indications for hypotensive treatment have broadened.

Table 1. *Percentage of total number of hypertensive patients in whom treatment was introduced within three months of referral to the out-patient clinic*

	1957/58	1959/60	1961/62	1963	1964
Total number	123	116	135	110	111
Number treated	55	51	96	68	79
Percentage of total treated	46	44	71	62	71

This is confirmed by Table 1, which shows that there has been an increase in the proportion of patients in whom treatment has been initiated within three months of their being referred to an out-patient clinic. The introduction of thiazides, in particular, has simplified treatment, and the increasing use of drug therapy in recent years is in part attributable to the value of thiazides as hypotensive agents (Table 2).

Table 2. *Percentage of patients starting treatment with thiazides*

	1957/58	1959/60	1961/62	1963	1964
Total number treated	55	51	96	68	79
Number treated with thiazides	14	15	53	36	47
Percentage of total treated with thiazides	25	29	55	53	59

However, the complications of hypertension still demand priority in respect of treatment, which, in some cases, should be initiated as soon as the diagnosis has been established, i.e. in the presence of

a) malignant hypertension,
b) hypertensive encephalopathy,
c) cardiac asthma.

Malignant hypertension should be regarded as a medical emergency calling for the immediate introduction of hypotensive therapy, which in this instance should precede any investigation into the aetiology of the elevated blood pressure unless there is reason to assume that a phaeochromocytoma is responsible. I personally still start with parenteral treatment in such cases, using pentolinium in order to establish control of the blood pressure within 36 hours of diagnosis.

Hypertensive encephalopathy is a diagnosis which is frequently abused. There are physicians who still maintain that a stroke occurring during the course of hypertension constitutes a contraindication to the use of hypotensive drugs and yet employ such treatment, justifying their decision by diagnosing a stroke as an encephalopathic attack. I confine the diagnosis of encephalopathy to attacks of confusion and severe headache — often with minor focal neurological signs — proceeding to epileptiform fits and coma. It may be impossible to distinguish these symptoms from those occurring in cerebral haemorrhage and, in fact, a definite diagnosis of encephalopathy can often only be made in retrospect, following the remarkable improvement shown by such patients in response to blood-pressure reduction.

The relief afforded by parenteral pentolinium or α-methyldopa in *pulmonary oedema* due to hypertensive left ventricular failure can be quite dramatic.

If the finding of *papilloedema* constitutes an indication for immediate blood-pressure reduction, such treatment is no less urgently required in cases with evidence of vascular damage resulting from hypertension, such as the appearance of retinal exudates in a patient previously without retinopathy or the finding of soft exudates in a newly examined hypertensive.

In many publications *heart failure* is reported to be the main single cause of death in untreated hypertensives, accounting for between 40 and 50% of the total mortality; but it should no longer be a cause of death in treated patients (1, 2). Heart failure must therefore be regarded as an absolute indication for hypotensive therapy, the urgency with which treatment is introduced being determined by the severity of the failure.

The association of hypertension and *ischaemic heart disease* perhaps requires special mention. Twelve years ago, DOYLE and KILPATRICK (3) demonstrated that the lowering of blood pressure reduced the frequency of anginal attacks, and this must by now be commonplace experience. I have treated 80 patients in whom angina was the predominant complaint, and 48 of them were able to discontinue trinitrine entirely following blood-pressure reduction. Five died, three as a result of coronary thrombosis and two as a result of stroke. I also recommend blood-pressure reduction in patients with persistent hypertension following cardiac infarction. Although I have no evidence of benefit resulting from this policy, I am convinced that it does not provoke further coronary thrombosis.

Treatment has thus been recommended solely for the complications of hypertension, but obviously evidence of deterioration in the patient's condition should reveal the need of therapy before such complications become established. Hence, the appearance of retinal lesions or of clinical, radiological, or cardiographic changes associated with ventricular hypertrophy, or the onset and progression of dyspnoea, requires that the blood-pressure level be reduced in order to prevent the development of cardiac failure or the malignant phase.

The relief afforded by blood-pressure reduction in cases of headache due to hypertension is dramatic. Admittedly, it has been shown that in the majority of patients such headaches may be relieved by a placebo (4); however, if a patient is suffering, as a result of hypertension, from headaches severe enough to interfere with his normal activities, I do not consider it justifiable to withhold hypotensive therapy, even if no complications are demonstrable. If headaches cannot be relieved rapidly by simple measures, such as sedation, weight reduction, and reassurance, then the blood pressure should be reduced. I see no reason to depart from the accepted principles of therapeutics which recommend that, whenever possible, the underlying disease should be treated rather than the symptoms alone.

The decision to treat asymptomatic, uncomplicated hypertension is one which should not be taken lightly. It is no longer adequate merely to reassure such patients of the absence of complications. Full investigation is obligatory, and the aim should be to exclude any remediable cause of the raised blood pressure. If no such cause is found, then one must decide which patients will require treatment in order to prevent the development of complications and whether the evidence available at present in fact justifies the use of hypotensive therapy for this purpose.

When the blood pressure is raised as a result of renal disease – chronic glomerulonephritis or pyelonephritis – early reduction of blood pressure can retard the development of renal failure, and Moyer et al. (5) have produced evidence to support this view.

The position with regard to the administration of hypotensive drugs to a patient who has had a stroke is still obscure. To my knowledge, there is no evidence to show that blood-pressure reduction, unless excessive, causes cerebral thrombosis. Of 67 patients in whom treatment was begun following a cerebral thrombosis, only 15 died; nine of these deaths were due to stroke, five of these being thrombotic. I consider that cerebral thrombosis is an added indication for blood-pressure reduction, provided that the stroke has left no appreciable physical or mental deterioration. However, the problem is whether blood-pressure control, if it is established early in the course of the disease, will prevent the development of stroke. For many years, the prognosis in hypertension associated with stroke remained uncertain. By comparing consecutive series of patients, Leishman (6, 7) provided convincing proof of improved prognosis in this respect, but the study of consecutive cases is always open to some doubt. In an attempt to resolve this prognostic dilemma, my colleagues and I (8) conducted a therapeutic trial, the object of which was to determine whether blood-pressure reduction influenced the incidence of complications, including strokes, in patients with essential hypertension.

In selecting the subjects for the trial it was essential to include only hypertensive patients in whom atherosclerosis was not a dominant feature – as far as could be judged by the crude methods available to the clinician. It was also imperative that the subjects should show a sustained manometric hypertension. Moreover, it was clearly indefensible to include in such a trial any patient with complications of hypertension or symptoms severe enough to require treatment at the time of the patient's reference to the out-patient clinic.

The subjects were therefore selected from patients referred to the out-patient clinic because of asymptomatic hypertension which was considered in all cases to be essential. None had symptoms of arterial disease, i.e. all denied having angina, claudication, rest-pain in the limbs, or transient symptoms suggestive of cerebro-vascular disease. In all of them the carotid and foot pulses were palpable, and no bruit was audible over the carotid or femoral arteries; none displayed cardiographic changes suggesting the presence of cardiac infarction.

In all of the subjects included, the diastolic blood pressure maintained a level of at least 110 mm. Hg over a period of out-patient observation lasting three months and entailing at least three visits to the clinic. In view of the difficulty of obtaining accurate blood-pressure recordings, all readings were made to the nearest 5 mm. Hg.

The potential subjects were all submitted to clinical examination and investigation to eliminate a) those requiring immediate hypotensive treatment owing to the presence of symptoms or complications, and b) those in whom some other condition known to be associated with hypertension was demonstrable. Known causes of secondary hypertension were excluded by routine investigation, including, if necessary, renal arteriography. Retinal examination revealed no complications of the disease, such as papilloedema, exudate, or haemorrhage, and there were no clinical, radiological, or cardiographic signs of cardiac enlargement. Urinalysis showed no albuminuria or casts; all had normal levels of serum urea.

The trial was continued for six years, and no new cases were included during the last two years, so that all the treated patients received a minimum of two and a maximum of six years' therapy. The subjects — all of whom were under 60 years of age — were allocated alternately to the treatment group and the control group in order to maintain equal numbers in the two groups. At the conclusion of the trial, however, three cases were rejected; one patient was found to have been aged 62 at the time of his admission to the series, and in the other two cases there was some doubt as to the aetiology of the hypertension. Hence, the numbers in the two groups do not balance exactly. The final assessment thus involved 61 patients — 39 females and 22 males (Tables 3 and 4) — with severe, sustained, asymptomatic, uncomplicated, benign essential hypertension, showing no detectable evidence of atherosclerosis. The treated series consisted of 20 females and 10 males, and the control series of 19 females and 12 males. Despite the slight discrepancy in the numbers, there was no significant difference between the two groups in respect of age, weight, and blood-pressure levels.

Table 3. *Comparison of male patients*

	No.	Age	Blood pressure		Weight (lb.)
			systolic	diastolic	
Control	12	47 ± 4	212 ± 28	127 ± 10	162 ± 23
Treated	10	49 ± 5	229 ± 30	135 ± 16	154 ± 14

Table 4. *Comparison of female patients*

	No.	Age	Blood pressure		Weight (lb.)
			systolic	diastolic	
Control	19	49 ± 6	223 ± 18	130 ± 10	150 ± 30
Treated	20	49 ± 7	245 ± 26	136 ± 5	146 ± 29

No indication was made in the patients' clinical notes of their inclusion in the trial, and the list of participants was deliberately kept remote from the clinics and wards in order to avoid possible prejudice against introducing treatment in a patient included in the control series. It was thought that if such information were available when the patients attended the clinic, it might weigh against other considerations favouring the introduction of hypotensive therapy, such as the appearance of symptoms or complications.

In assessing the efficacy of blood-pressure control in the treated series, the following criteria were adopted:

— Good control implies a diastolic pressure consistently below 100 mm. Hg.
— Fair control implies a diastolic pressure maintained between 100 and 110 mm. Hg.
— Poor control implies a diastolic pressure consistently over 110 mm. Hg.

In all the treated males, the degree of blood-pressure control was considered adequate, being good in nine cases and fair in one. None suffered a stroke or developed any other complications of the disease. Of the 12 untreated males, four suffered strokes; in one case this proved fatal and necropsy showed a cerebral haemorrhage.

Three other patients developed hemiplegia; two of them made a complete objective recovery and were ultimately able to resume work, but the third, a schoolmaster, was left with slight dysarthria and weakness of the hand, which unfortunately prevented him from returning to his former occupation. Although the incidence of four strokes among 12 subjects appears high, the numbers are small and the difference between the two groups is not statistically significant. Of the remaining eight untreated patients, one had a coronary arterial thrombosis after which the blood pressure fell to normal levels, another began to suffer from headaches of increasing severity and intensity which required treatment with hypotensive drugs to control them, and in two further cases clinical and cardiographic signs of increasing left ventricular hypertrophy developed, making it necessary to introduce hypotensive therapy in order to prevent hypertensive cardiac failure. Thus, eight of the 12 untreated male patients developed complications of hypertension during the course of the trial (Table 5), as compared with none of the ten treated patients. This difference is highly significant, exceeding the 2.5% level.

Table 5. *Male control: 12 cases, eight complications*

Age (yrs)	Blood pressure (mm. Hg)	Weight (st. and lb.)		Complications
51	240/140	13	11	Cerebral thrombosis
51	180/110	12	7	Coronary thrombosis
52	200/120	10	3	Cerebral thrombosis
44	260/130	9	5	..
41	210/120	14	2	Blood-pressure reduction; increasing left ventricle
45	190/130	11	8	Blood-pressure reduction; symptoms
46	180/120	12	11	Blood-pressure reduction; increasing left ventricle
42	210/125	12	6	..
49	220/120	9	11	Cerebral thrombosis
52	200/130	11	10	..
51	260/150	11	0	Cerebral haemorrhage (died)
44	190/130	9	10	..

Of the 19 females in the control group, three suffered a stroke; two made a full objective recovery following a presumed cerebral thrombosis, but one died from rupture of an intracranial aneurysm 15 months after the commencement of treatment introduced to control headaches of increasing severity. In five others, complications arose; in two cases, coronary thrombosis (with a subsequent fall in blood pressure) occurred, and in three cases, increasing left ventricular hypertrophy necessitated the introduction of treatment. Thus, eight of the 19 patients developed complications (Table 6).

Table 6. *Female control: 19 cases, eight complications*

Age (yrs)	Initial blood pressure (mm. Hg)	Weight (st. and lb.)		Complications
54	250/140	10	5	..
41	210/130	12	11	Blood-pressure reduction after stroke
48	210/110	9	1	..
56	230/130	9	9	..
50	190/110	12	9	..
44	220/130	8	11	Blood pressure fell after coronary artery thrombosis
47	260/140	7	11	..
40	200/130	8	1	..
47	220/125	9	0	Blood-pressure reduction because of increasing left ventricle
56	230/130	13	12	Blood pressure fell after coronary artery thrombosis
53	240/140	11	5	..
48	240/130	17	3	..
58	240/140	11	2	..
42	210/120	9	7	Blood-pressure reduction because of increasing left ventricle
57	220/125	10	6	..
41	210/130	9	4	Blood-pressure reduction because of symptoms
50	210/120	11	5	Cerebral thrombosis
39	220/130	11	3	Blood-pressure reduction because of symptoms with subsequent death from subarachnoid haemorrhage
57	230/150	11	4	..

Of the 20 females in the treated series, five developed complications of the disease, consisting of a stroke in three (two instances of cerebral thrombosis with recovery and one fatal cerebral haemorrhage), coronary thrombosis in one, and increasing heart size in one (Table 7). The difference between the treated group and the control group is clearly not significant.

However, in four members of the treated group, the blood-pressure control was considered poor, i.e. the diastolic pressure was never maintained below 110 mm. Hg. Thus, if we consider the females from the point of view of the adequacy of blood-pressure control, complications arose in only one of a total of 16 patients in whom blood-pressure was adequately controlled (one case of pro-

Table 7. *Female treated: 20 cases, five complications*

Age (yrs)	Initial blood pressure (mm. Hg)	Control of blood pressure	Weight (st. and lb.)		Complications
60	260/125	Fair	14	0	..
49	220/120	Good	11	6	..
41	240/120	Good	11	2	..
46	240/140	Fair	8	9	..
47	240/150	Fair	7	10	..
52	300/135	Poor	9	10	Increasing left ventricle
36	230/140	Good	9	4	..
45	240/130	Good	9	3	..
50	260/140	Good	10	4	Coronary thrombosis
47	180/110	Fair	9	4	..
47	250/150	Poor	12	1	Cerebral thrombosis
32	220/110	Good	7	1	..
54	270/140	Poor	12	5	Cerebral thrombosis
51	230/135	Fair	13	3	..
53	260/170	Fair	9	4	..
34	220/130	Good	10	2	..
50	270/150	Good	13	0	Carcinoma cervix (died)
58	270/150	Poor	7	5	Cerebral haemorrhage (died)
53	260/140	Fair	10	9	..
51	230/135	Good	13	3	..

gressive left ventricular hypertrophy), whereas in 23 patients with inadequately controlled blood pressure (19 in the control series plus four inadequately treated), there were 12 complications, including six strokes (Table 8). The difference, both in respect of the incidence of strokes and the over-all incidence of complications, is highly significant.

Table 8. *Effect of adequate blood-pressure control upon the incidence of strokes and all complications*

Female	Adequate B.P. control	Inadequate B.P. control
No. of cases	16	23
No. of strokes	0	6
No. of complications	1	12

There is therefore no doubt that adequate blood-pressure control, maintaining the diastolic pressure below 110 mm. Hg in younger patients, reduces the over-all incidence of complications, including stroke.

As to whether it is justifiable to treat patients with even less severe grades of hypertension or whether any benefit is likely to follow blood-pressure reduction in a young person between the ages of 20 and 40 years who has a diastolic pressure level of 90–100 mm. Hg, I have as yet no evidence to offer. It has, however, been suggested that such patients should be treated according to the level of diastolic pressure, i.e. if their blood pressure persists at levels associated with a known increased mortality. PICKERING et al. (*9*) quote the following levels of diastolic pressure as justifying hypotensive therapy:

Age	*Male*	*Female*
Under 40 years	106 mm. Hg	115 mm. Hg
Over 40 years	110 mm. Hg	120 mm. Hg

Certainly, in pregnancy, I believe that greater latitude is needed in respect of the introduction of drug therapy. The presence of maternal hypertension greatly increases the risk of foetal death. Prior to the introduction of α-methyldopa, I was unable to maintain an adequate degree of blood-pressure control in any severely hypertensive pregnant woman. Although my facilities in this respect are unfortunately restricted, in the past three years I have been able to treat seven women during pregnancy. All were hypertensive before pregnancy. The raised blood pressure was attributed to renal vascular disease in one case and to pyelonephritis in three others; the remaining three were considered to be suffering from essential hypertension. The diastolic blood pressure in all of these women was maintained throughout pregnancy at a level not exceeding 90 mm. Hg; all the pregnancies were induced

Table 9. *Influence of blood-pressure control upon course of pregnancy in seven hypertensive patients*

Age in years	Aetiology of hypertension	B. P. before pregnancy		Number of pregnancies	Number of miscarriages	Greatest birth weight		Duration of present pregnancy (weeks)	Birth weight of child		Fate of child
		S	D			lb.	oz.		lb.	oz.	
41	Essential	190	120	5	1	7	12	38	6	13	Live
25	Pyelonephritis	180	110	2	2			38	7	1	Live
23	Pyelonephritis	160	120	—	—			36	5	12	Live
42	Essential	220	130	9	3	7	8	36	6	15	Live
21	Essential	220	140	—	—			37	5	15	Live
25	Pyelonephritis	150	115	4	2	7	4	38	5	14	Live
21	Vascular	220	130	—	—			36	6	1	Live

between the 36th and 38th week and all produced a live infant of satisfactory birth weight (Table 9).

It may therefore be concluded that although the main importance of drug therapy still lies in the treatment of complications of hypertension, the recent introduction of new compounds capable of achieving blood-pressure control with few side effects has broadened the indications for such therapy, and its role in preventing the development of complications of the disease is now firmly established.

Summary

The role of antihypertensive therapy in the treatment of established complications of hypertension is discussed. Evidence is presented to justify the treatment of uncomplicated hypertension. A therapeutic trial confirmed the role of adequate blood-pressure control in preventing complications, including stroke.

Blood-pressure reduction also reduces the severity of angina in hypertensive subjects and increases the chances of live birth from hypertensive pregnancies.

Zusammenfassung

Die Bedeutung der antihypertensiven Therapie für die Behandlung von Komplikationen, die im Verlaufe eines Hochdruckes aufgetreten sind, wird besprochen. Die vorliegenden Daten rechtfertigen die Behandlung des unkomplizierten Hochdruckes. Eine kontrollierte therapeutische Untersuchung bestätigte die Bedeutung einer wirksamen Blutdrucksenkung für die Verhinderung von Komplikationen mit Einschluß der Apoplexie.

Senkung des Blutdruckes vermindert auch die Schwere der Angina pectoris bei Patienten mit Hypertonie und verbessert die Aussichten dafür, daß bei Schwangerschaftshochdruck ein lebendes Kind geboren wird.

Résumé

Le rôle de la thérapeutique antihypertensive dans le traitement des complications confirmées de l'hypertension est discuté. Il existe des arguments justifiant la légitimité du traitement de l'hypertension non compliquée. Une expérimentation thérapeutique a confirmé l'importance d'un traitement adéquat de l'hypertension artérielle dans la prévention des complications, y compris l'attaque d'apoplexie.

La réduction de la tension artérielle diminue également la gravité de l'angine de poitrine chez les sujets hypertendus et augmente les chances d'accouchement d'un enfant vivant dans les hypertensions gravidiques.

References

1. Smith, K. S., and P. B. B. Fowler: Lancet 1955/I, 417. — 2. Smirk, F. H.: High Arterial Pressure. Blackwell Scientific Publications, Oxford, 1957, p. 693. — 3. Doyle, A. E., and J. A. Kilpatrick: Lancet 1954/I, 905. — 4. Stewart, I. McD. G.: Lancet 1953/I, 1261. — 5. Moyer, J. H., C. Heider, K. Pevey, and R. V. Ford: Amer. J. Med. **24**, 177 (1958). — 6. Leishman, A. W. D.: Brit. Med. J. 1959/I, 1361. — 7. Leishman, A. W. D.: Lancet 1963/I, 1284. — 8. Hamilton, M., E. N. Thompson, and T. K. M. Wisniewski: Lancet 1964/I, 235. — 9. Pickering, G. W., W. I. Cranston, and M. A. Pears: In: The Treatment of Hypertension. Ed. by. I. N. Kugelmass. Thomas, Springfield, Ill., 1961, p. 124.

Discussion

Bock: With regard to the question of prognosis in treated and untreated hypertensive patients, I should like to add an observation that we made in a series of 92 patients with known pre-existing hypertension and acute myocardial infarction. There is a difference in the mortality rate in the first week between patients who have previously had effective antihypertensive treatment and those who have not (see Table 1).

Table 1. *Mortality rate from acute myocardial infarction in hypertensive patients with and without effective antihypertensive therapy*

	n	Age (mean)	Blood pressure on admission (mm. Hg)	Mortality (%)	Age of patients who died (mean)
Patients with previous effective antihypertensive treatment . . .	28	68.2	175/100	17.8[1]	70.6
Patients without effective treatment	64	65.4	178/103	43.7[1]	66.9

[1] $P < 0.05$

Thus, effective antihypertensive treatment not only reduces the incidence of complications, but also seems to improve the early prognosis in myocardial infarction. Noteworthy are the almost identical blood pressures in both groups on admission to the hospital.

Furthermore, I should like to ask Dr. Hamilton whether he thinks there are any strict contra-indications for antihypertensive therapy.

Mach: Dr. Hamilton, did you restrict the patients' salt intake during treatment?

Brod: I should like to comment upon the treatment of hypertension in cases of primary renal disease. You have mentioned that in the course of chronic renal disease the development of uraemia can be delayed. I think this is true, especially in those cases who do not present manifestations of malignant hypertension. I am not so sure that it is necessary to treat mild hypertension in renal patients, especially if renal function is rather restricted; and we nearly always have to consider the possibility that by lowering the blood pressure we might get into trouble by reducing renal function still further. There is one renal disease in which we have particular experience with antihypertensive agents, and that is polycystic kidney disease. My colleague Dr. Prát[1] has collected a relatively large series of these patients and has found that their prognosis depends on two things: one is control of the infection and the other is control of high blood pressure. In these cases we should probably always use hypotensive agents.

Dustan: We should agree that the treatment of hypertension has been rather effective in controlling complications of hypertension in most patients.

[1] Prát, V.: Čas. lék. česk. **99**, 1332 (1960).

As you know, in treated malignant hypertensives who receive adequate therapy the incidence of atherosclerotic complications is also lower. Now, whether, in the long run, one prevents the development of atherosclerosis or merely slows its progress, only time can tell. To find this out we must examine patients sequentially with arteriographic and other techniques.

As regards the assessment of therapy, I should like to know which diastolic pressure you use in your assessment — the lying or the standing. We have always used the lying diastolic pressure, because we have had some patients in whom we have been able to reduce only the standing pressure, but not the lying pressure, and we feel that the adequacy of blood-pressure control must be judged according to every pressure the patient has, regardless of whether he is in the lying or the standing position.

Lee: Dr. Brod has touched on an extremely important point that is never emphasised in the literature or in discussions of this sort. There must be a great difference between the severe hypertension one finds in chronic nephritis and that associated with renal disease due to vascular impairment resulting from the hypertensive process. In our clinic, if a patient with malignant hypertension arrives with an original blood urea nitrogen of 60, we estimate the average time of survival without therapy at five days. On the other hand, we have many patients with chronic nephritis and hypertension who appear to be otherwise in good health, yet whose blood urea nitrogen is regularly in the nineties. I have one such patient, whose work consists in operating a steam shovel. There is therefore a basic difference here in the mechanism of the hypertensive process and especially in the extent to which these patients can tolerate renal impairment.

Leishman: We have recently taken stock of our patients who had been treated with guanethidine for some five and a half years. These were cases of severe or moderately severe hypertension, and in relation to what Dr. Brod said regarding renal function, a slightly disquieting feature has emerged. Although we have been satisfied with the progress of these patients — in that mortality has been very low, there has been an improvement in angina, and the patients seem comfortable — the position is less satisfactory with regard to renal function. Eighty-two of 142 patients whose initial blood urea levels were normal now have raised blood ureas, and 40 out of 68 patients who started with raised blood ureas now have even higher levels. So it does rather look as if this may be the limiting factor in the continuing survival of these severe cases of hypertension that we are keeping going with guanethidine.

Dollery: How much higher, Dr. Leishman; are you speaking in terms of 5 mg. or of 50 mg.?

Leishman: Commonly, increases of more than 10 mg. each year; in a number of cases the blood urea is now in the neighbourhood of 100 mg. %.

Dollery: Are these people treated only with guanethidine or with diuretics as well, because they always increase the blood urea?

Leishman: Rather less than half the cases have been treated with diuretics as well, and there is no relationship between this rise in blood urea and treatment with diuretics, nor indeed with a primary renal cause of the hypertension. Neither is it related to the height of the blood pressure nor to the dose of guanethidine.

Lee: Is a mild rise in the blood urea important?

Leishman: Well, that is what we are going to see in the next five years.

Hoobler: May I bring the discussion back to the prevention of stroke? I am delighted that Dr. Hamilton's paper suggests that there is in fact a substantial reduction in the subsequent mortality rate due to stroke in patients who have severe hypertension but whose blood pressures are reduced by treatment. I think the stage is now past where there is any question about the value of lowering blood pressure in a person with a high sustained diastolic pressure, such as 120 mm. Hg.

At the moment we are entering another period, in which the tendency will be to try to treat those people in whom diastolic blood pressure is between the near normal and a level of 110 mm. Hg. By treating such persons who have had one small cerebral episode we hope to see whether, at this lower level of blood pressure, protection against the recurrence of stroke can be demonstrated. It is a field of investigation that we have been hesitant to go into, because neurologists have told us that we should not lower the blood pressure in such cases. I personally do not believe that. All I can say at this stage is that for between six and eight months we have had one half of a group of 20 patients on treatment in this relatively low blood-pressure range. None of them has had any recurrences, and none of them has been suffering from any ill effects due to the rather substantial lowering of their blood pressures. So I submit that we should go ahead now and look at the very mild hypertensives and see whether treatment of their blood pressure will reduce the rate of stroke recurrence.

Wilson: We have been particularly concerned with the treatment of severe hypertension in patients with primary renal disease, and out of this emerges the very obvious fact that the effect of lowering the blood pressure on renal function depends largely on the activity of the renal lesion. Patients who have a stationary renal lesion, such as chronic pyelonephritis which has burnt out, or chronic glomerulonephritis which is in a quiescent stage with hypertension as its chief manifestation, do very well, showing very little deterioration of renal function, and may survive for many years, even after the development of malignant hypertension if this is promptly treated. On the other hand, in progressive nephritis, especially membranous glomerulonephritis, blood pressure can be controlled, but the curve of renal function undergoes an inevitable progressive deterioration. Blood-pressure reduction does not alter the natural history of the underlying nephritis. Some patients with malignant hypertension of primary renal origin are extremely resistant to hypotensive drugs, even in large doses. Using intermittent dialysis, the blood pressure can, however, be controlled by sufficient fluid depletion. I think here is a second factor which comes into operation with impaired renal function. There is some disorder of volume control which, if corrected, may allow the blood pressure to be dealt with.

Smirk: Our experience with renal cases corresponds almost exactly to that of Dr. Wilson. We do not get much nephritis, but pyelonephritis is common. Comparatively few of our patients die of uraemia, except those who already have a considerably raised blood urea nitrogen when they first report to us. Our practice in introducing hypotensive drugs has been to lower the blood pressure gradually, ascertaining the lowest satisfactory level of the blood pressure which is unassociated with further increase in the blood urea.

I should like to make a point about the use of the casual blood pressure in deciding whether a person will be treated or not. Although the casual blood pressure may vary considerably, basal pressure is relatively constant, and the five-year mortality is very closely related to the basal blood pressure but much less so to the casual blood pressure. It does not take long to determine the basal blood pressure, and it can be done in the patient's own home. When using powerful drugs, reduction of the casual blood pressure to below the level of the basal blood pressure is an indication that an effective dose has been reached.

In assessing the degree of blood-pressure control in hypertensive patients we use all-day tests conducted by trained technicians who measure the blood pressure at approximately hourly intervals. In particular, we like to know the lowest pressure in the standing posture and the average for the day, together with the corresponding pressures in the lying posture. It is important, as Dr. DUSTAN pointed out, to decide whether you are reducing only the standing pressure. If only the standing pressure can be reduced, then it is most important to use posture therapeutically, i.e. to have the patient propped up in bed at a 45-degree tilt at night and adopt the sitting or standing posture during the daytime in order, deliberately, to make use of postural hypotension as a means of reducing the blood pressure.

HAMILTON: Regarding the contra-indications, these are numerous and include the patient's age, co-operation, mental state, any physical disability, e.g. a substantial legacy from a stroke, or substantial mental impairment following stroke; all these must be considered, and I don't think you can easily define any specific contra-indications if they are all-embracing.

I don't restrict the patients' salt intake, as I think they have a sufficiently difficult life taking tablets and being dependent upon regular visits to the clinic without my imposing the additional burden of salt restriction on them when I don't consider this essential. I feel we should restrict the imposition upon the patient to the minimum.

As regards renal function, I was deliberately evasive and non-committal, and I am glad that I was so; but I agree that there are very many factors which influence the fate of the patient with renal hypertension and that, in particular, infection is a terribly important one in chronic renal disease. I appreciate Dr. WILSON's point about the activity of the renal lesion and, in the light of the little experience I have had, I should certainly agree with that.

In respect of the state of the blood pressure and the position of the patient, many years ago I came under Dr. SMIRK's influence and I tried to measure basal pressures initially, but in the organisation which I have in a peripheral hospital in England, this is not physically possible. When I was dependent on the ganglion blocking agents for the treatment of patients, I did assess the control of blood pressure by day-test as recommended by Dr. SMIRK. I should perhaps point out that many of the patients received different treatments during the course of the trials. The treatment employed was the one which maintained the most satisfactory level of blood pressure; thus, a patient might have started on ganglion blocking agents, in which case the pressure I would regard as significant would be the standing pressure; use was, in fact, made of posture along the lines described by Dr. SMIRK, and the habit of sleeping propped up in bed or having the head of the bed raised was therefore one transferred from New Zealand to mid-Essex among hypertensives in receipt of ganglion blocking agents. However, when they changed from ganglion blocking agents to perhaps α-methyldopa or a thiazide, I found that in the majority there was a much less pronounced postural effect; but I still recorded the lowest pressures in the standing position, even though in later years the postural effect is probably not nearly so significant as in the initial stages of the trial.

Zaimis: What did you mean by using the term chemotherapy?

Hamilton: By chemotherapy I implied treatment by chemical agents. It was simply easier to use this term than to refer continually to "hypotensive therapy" or "blood-pressure reduction", and I consider it infinitely preferable to "antihypertensive therapy".

Methodology of blood-pressure recording

By

S. B. Humerfelt

In recent years, there has been a growing interest in epidemiological studies of blood pressure. One of the reasons is the controversy about the aetiology of essential hypertension. Attempts have been made to elucidate the shape of frequency distribution curves of blood pressure and compare the mean pressures of different population groups.

The continuous distribution of blood pressure in the general population led Pickering (*7*) to conclude that what has been called *essential* hypertension is a purely arbitrary segregation of subjects whose arterial pressure is in the higher ranges, and that the inheritance of blood pressure is probably multifactorial.

The alternative view expressed by Platt (*8*) is that essential hypertension is a specific disorder characterised by its age-incidence and its hereditary nature. This opinion has been supported by the demonstration of bimodality in the distribution of pressure in relatives of hypertensive propositi and in the offspring of parents who died in middle age [Morrison and Morris (*6*)].

Unfortunately, the conventional apparatus used in measuring blood pressure is apt to give rise to systematic and unpredictable errors that may seriously detract from the value of this approach to the problem. The principal sources of blood-pressure variation may be summarised as follows:

According to Rose et al. (*9*), the variations in the arterial pressure may be true variations, some of which are known, others unknown, or they may be due to measurement errors, which in turn are partly *instrumental* and partly attributable to "*observer-errors*". The latter may be the result of:

a) systematic errors, whereby one observer tends habitually to read higher or lower pressures than another. This leads to false estimation of the *mean* pressure. Thus, Lowe and McKeown (*5*) have found that there is a consistent and substantial difference between readings made by different doctors. Mean pressures recorded by four doctors showed a difference of 15 mm. Hg between the lowest and the highest reading.

b) terminal digit preference. In the Bergen survey (*1*) the nurses recorded the blood pressure to the nearest multiple of ten on the scale six to seven times more frequently than to the nearest multiple of five. These errors distort the frequency distribution curves.

c) prejudice in favour of or against certain pressure values, which tends to give a bimodal distribution curve.

It is, therefore, not surprising that the pooling of measurements made by different observers may give irregular distributions.

To eliminate these sources of serious observer-bias, a new instrument has been developed by the epidemiologists at the London School of Hygiene and Tropical Medicine [Rose et al. (*9*)].

The final version of this instrument is shown schematically in Fig. 1.

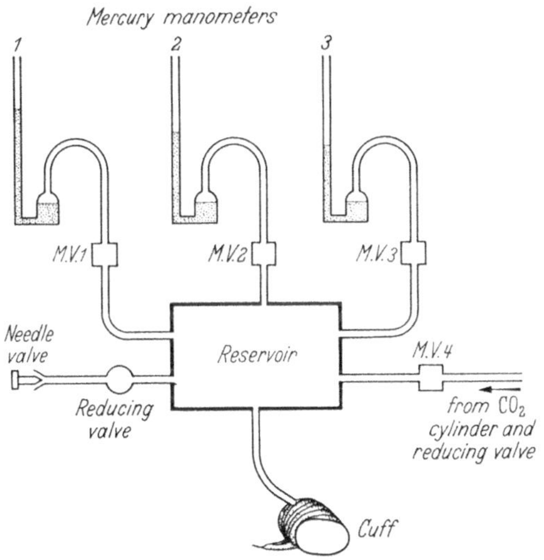

Fig. 1. Diagram of the apparatus.

It consists essentially of three standard mercury manometers connected to a gas reservoir. Each manometer can be isolated from the reservoir by means of a separate valve. The input of the reservoir is connected via a valve to a pressure cylinder fitted with a reducing valve. The output is connected to a standard blood-pressure cuff.

On inflating the cuff, the pressure rises in the reservoir and in all three manometers at a constant speed. When the maximum is reached, deflation starts, and the rate of decline of pressure (2 mm./Hg/sec.) is also constant (Fig. 2). As the pressure in the cuff drops, the Korotkoff sounds appear at the systolic pressure; the observer then closes the valve for the first manometer, and the

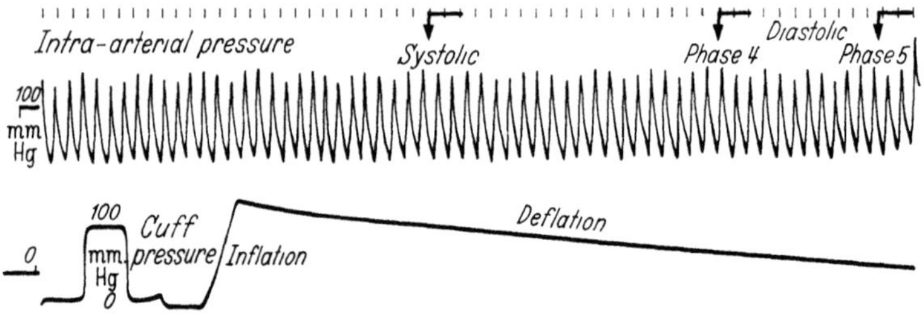

Fig. 2. Intra-arterial pressure (upper curve) and pressure within cuff (lower curve). Note constant speed of inflation and deflation. The arrows mark the signals for systolic and diastolic pressures.

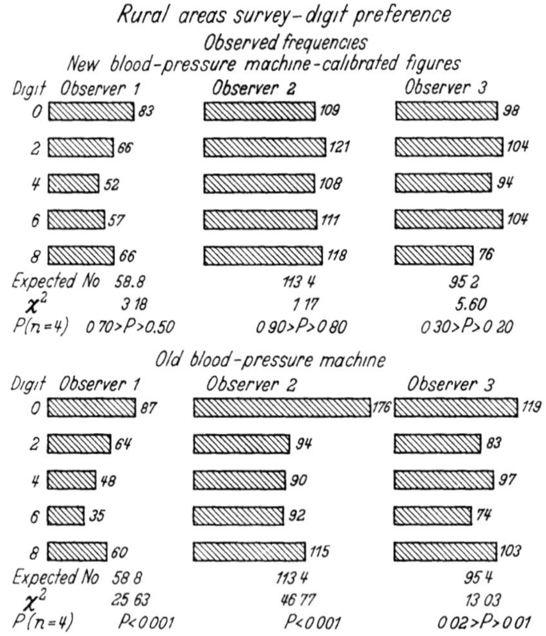

Fig. 3. Frequency of recording even digits using the usual and new methods of measurement.

mercury ceases to fall. The same procedure is adopted when measuring the two diastolic pressures, Phases 4 and 5 (D 4 and D 5).

No readings can be taken with the "door" of the apparatus open, and the observer's decisions are all made "blind", i.e. when recording the systolic and diastolic end-points, he has no means of knowing the cuff pressure.

This new equipment has been compared with the old apparatus in several surveys [HOLLAND (*2*)].

While each of three observers (one British, one Norwegian, and one Egyptian doctor) showed significant digit preference when using the conventional method, this preference was markedly reduced with the new method (Fig. 3).

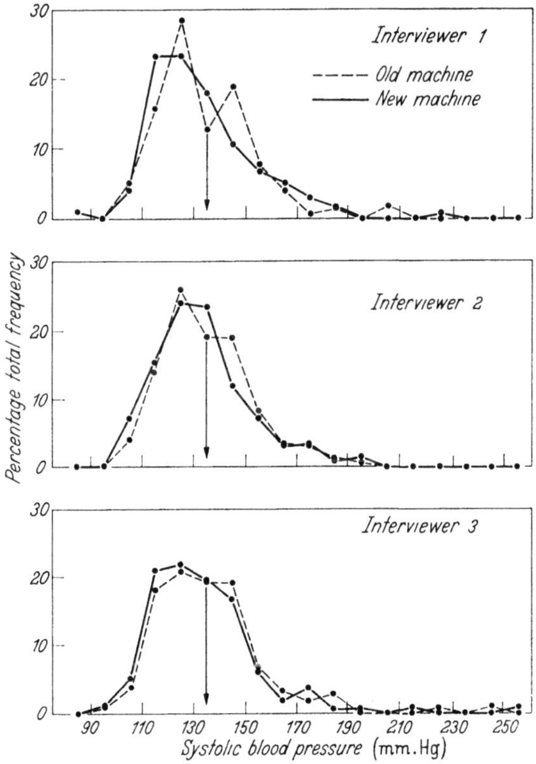

Fig. 4. Frequency of distribution of readings of systolic pressure by different observers.

Furthermore, each of the three doctors obtained a bimodal frequency distribution of the systolic blood pressure when using the conventional apparatus. The dip at 135 mm. Hg occurred at the same point with each observer. Using the new apparatus, there is no bimodality in the frequency distribution (Fig. 4).

The advantages of this new apparatus are that it ensures uniform inflation and deflation of the cuff and eliminates subjective bias. This is of particular importance in *epidemiological* studies, in which population groups may be examined by many observers. It may also be of use in *therapeutic* trials, in which both conscious and unconscious bias may affect the results.

Returning to the errors due to the instrument itself, we all know that the readings given by the ordinary sphygmomanometer are inaccurate in comparison with direct intra-arterial readings. This has been shown by numerous reports. Provided all observers use a standard instrument and cuff in a standard way, all would be liable to make the same errors. A systematic bias can be accepted as long as it is constant.

Recent work [HOLLAND and HUMERFELT (*3*)], involving the use of the new apparatus designed at the London School of Hygiene and Tropical Medicine and a Tybjerg Hansen capacitance manometer for the direct intra-arterial pressure, has verified these discrepancies between direct and indirect readings.

Although there are differences between the arterial and cuff pressures, there is a high correlation between the direct and indirect systolic blood pressure (correlation coefficient 0.95) (Fig. 5).

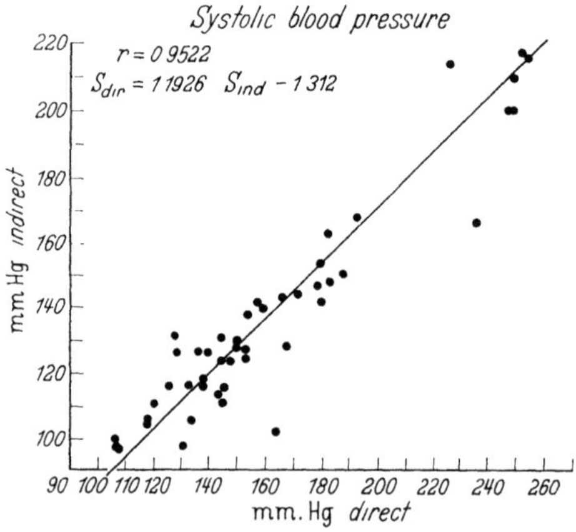

Fig. 5. Relationship and regression line of intra-arterial and cuff systolic pressures.

Good correlations are also found in the diastolic pressures; they are, however, better for Phase 5 (D 5) (0.93) than for Phase 4 (D 4) (0.83), as can be seen in Fig. 6.

The question whether the difference between intra-arterial and cuff pressures could be explained in terms of age, height of blood pressure, arm circumference, and skinfold thickness was investigated by calculating the correlation and regression coefficients between these parameters and the difference in intra-arterial and cuff pressures.

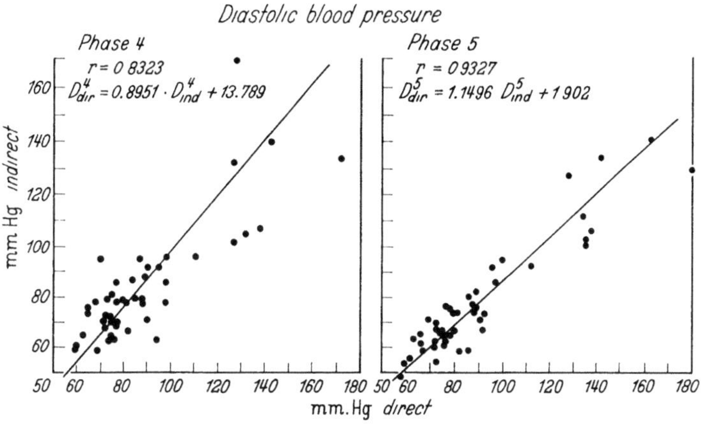

Fig. 6. Relationship and regression lines of intra-arterial and cuff diastolic pressures.

I shall not go into all the details, but the difference between direct and indirect readings could not be accounted for by age, arm circumference, or skinfold thickness. There was a low correlation between the difference in direct and indirect diastolic blood pressure and the height of blood pressure (Table 1).

Table 1. *Correlation of intra-arterial blood pressure and difference between intra-arterial and cuff blood pressures*

Measurement	Correlation coefficient
Systolic intra-arterial pressure and difference between systolic intra-arterial and cuff pressures	+0.22*
Diastolic (Phase 4) intra-arterial pressure and difference between diastolic (Phase 4) intra-arterial and cuff pressures.	+0.39†
Diastolic (Phase 5) intra-arterial pressure and difference between diastolic (Phase 5) intra-arterial and cuff pressures.	+0.64‡

* $P < 0.1$ † $P = 0.01$—0.001 ‡ $P < 0.001$

There was also some relation between the arm circumference and the level of the direct intra-arterial blood pressure. On an average, with each increase of 2.5 cm. in arm circumference, the intra-arterial blood pressure rises by 14 mm. Hg systolic and by

Table 2. *Difference between intra-arterial and auscultatory blood-pressure measurements in 52 subjects, with cuffs of two sizes*

	Systolic			Diastolic					
				Phase 4			Phase 5		
	Small		Large	Small		Large	Small		Large
	Biceps	Triceps		Biceps	Triceps		Biceps	Triceps	
Mean pressure difference between cuff and intra-arterial pressures (mm. Hg)	0.5	5.5	—3.0	17.7	16.6	12.2	7.6	4.6	1.4
Standard deviation	12.3	13.8	8.4	15.1	14.5	10.1	14.4	17.0	9.1
P	0.01	0.001	—	0.01	0.01	—	0.01	0.001	—

P = Probability of no difference from the variation with the large cuff.

8.4 mm. Hg diastolic. However, the rather low correlation coefficient shows that only one fifth of the difference can be ascribed to the increase in arm circumference.

In this study, we used a standard cuff (12 × 24 cm.) connected to the manometer. In a recent study, Karvonen (*4*) pointed out the importance of the *length* of the cuff. He compared the commercially available standard cuff with a bag 40 cm. in length in a series of 52 hospital patients. The main results are shown in Table 2. The difference between direct and indirect measurements of both systolic and diastolic pressures shows the smallest standard deviation when the large cuff is used. The scatter was significantly higher with the small cuff in either position. Table 2 also shows that mean systolic pressure comes closest to the intra-arterial pressure when the short cuff is applied over the biceps, while for the diastolic pressure the large cuff gave the best approximation, when the disappearance of sound is taken as a criterion.

When planning the new blood-pressure survey of the Bergen population in 1963/64, we decided to avoid as far as possible all the mistakes made in our first survey (1950/51). The most important shortcomings were:

a) insufficient representativeness: the blood pressure was measured in 75% of a total of 88,339 persons;

b) technique of measuring the blood pressure.

First of all, we decided to start on a longitudinal survey of a 10% sample of the adult population (both sexes) and not only of that part of the population which attends mass radiography examinations. Although mass radiography is compulsory in Norway, we never get a complete population sample. We therefore wanted to record the blood pressure in those who did not attend the mass radiography units, and this was done by calling on such persons at home or at work.

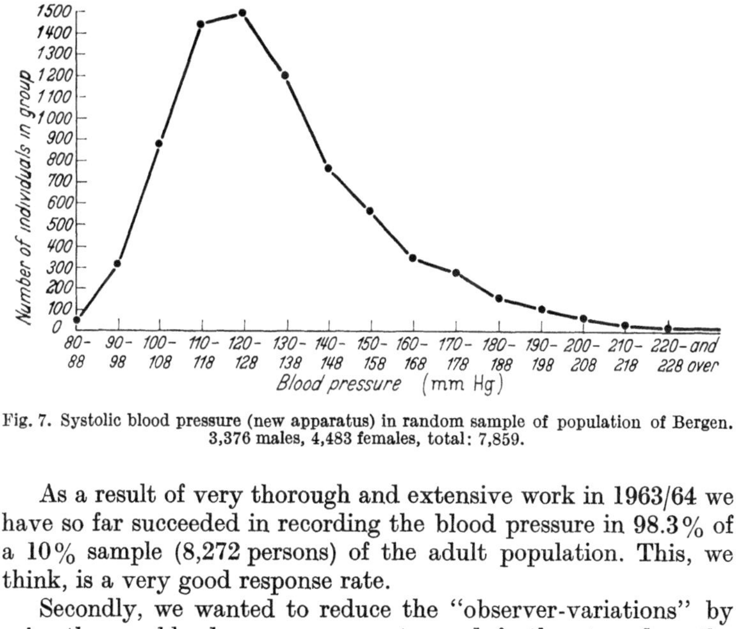

Fig. 7. Systolic blood pressure (new apparatus) in random sample of population of Bergen. 3,376 males, 4,483 females, total: 7,859.

As a result of very thorough and extensive work in 1963/64 we have so far succeeded in recording the blood pressure in 98.3% of a 10% sample (8,272 persons) of the adult population. This, we think, is a very good response rate.

Secondly, we wanted to reduce the "observer-variations" by using the new blood-pressure apparatus and, further, to reduce the "instrumental" errors by employing a cuff sufficiently long (40 cm.) to encircle the arm.

We are now very busily engaged in making all sorts of calculations. It is not possible to present complete data yet, but I should like at least to show one of the distribution curves obtained with the aid of the new apparatus in this population sample (Fig. 7). In this figure there is no tendency at all to bimodality. Neither is there any bimodality when this population is split into different age groups (Fig. 8).

We are therefore convinced that the bimodality of the frequency distribution curves presented in earlier series is an artefact attributable to such factors as small numbers in the series and measurement errors.

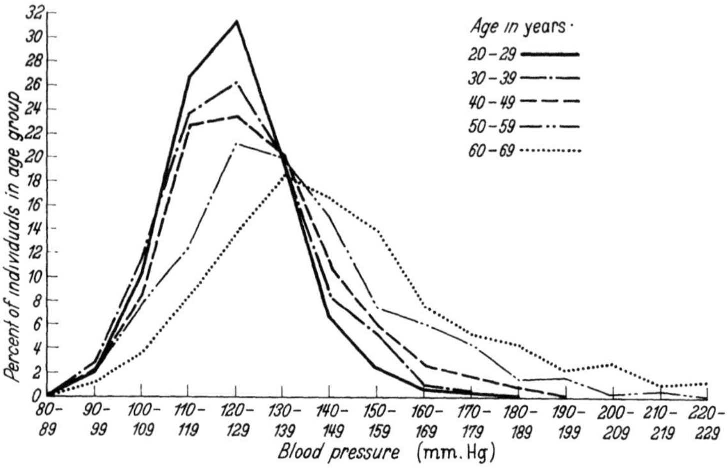

Fig. 8. Systolic blood pressure (new apparatus) in different age groups of males. Random sample.

Summary

The conventional blood-pressure-measuring instrument is subject to systematic and unpredictable errors. These errors lead to false mean pressures, terminal digit preference, and prejudice in favour of or against certain values, distorting the frequency distribution curves.

A new apparatus has been developed at the London School of Hygiene and Tropical Medicine which ensures uniform inflation and deflation and eliminates subjective bias. This instrument, supplied with a cuff 40 cm. in length, has been used in a blood-pressure survey of the Bergen population in 1963/64. The blood pressure has been recorded in 98.3% of the subjects of a 10% sample of the adult population, in all, 8,272 persons.

The results are presented briefly. There is no tendency to bimodality in the distribution curves in the different age groups.

It is concluded that the bimodality of the frequency distribution curves presented in earlier series is an artefact attributable to such influences as small numbers in the studied series and measurement errors.

Zusammenfassung

Das übliche Blutdruckmeßgerät ist mit methodischen und unvorhersehbaren Fehlerquellen behaftet. Diese Fehler führen zu falschen mittleren Druckwerten, einer Bevorzugung bestimmter Endzahlen und einem Vorurteil für oder gegen bestimmte Werte, so daß die Häufigkeitsverteilungskurve verfälscht wird.

An der London School of Hygiene and Tropical Medicine ist ein neues Gerät entwickelt worden, das ein gleichmäßiges Aufblasen und Entleeren der Manschette gewährleistet und subjektive Einflüsse eliminiert. Dieses Instrument, versehen mit einer Manschette von 40 cm Länge, wurde in einer Blutdruckstudie bei der Bevölkerung von Bergen in den Jahren 1963/64 verwendet. Der Blutdruck wurde bei 98,3% aller Individuen eines 10%igen Anteils der gesamten erwachsenen Bevölkerung gemessen, insgesamt 8272 Personen.

Aus den Resultaten geht hervor, daß die Verteilungskurve keinen Hinweis auf eine bimodale Form innerhalb der verschiedenen Altersgruppen erkennen läßt.

Daraus wird geschlossen, daß der in früheren Untersuchungen gefundene bimodale Verlauf der Häufigkeitsverteilungskurve ein Artefakt ist, das auf die kleine Zahl dieser Versuchsreihen und auf Meßfehler zurückzuführen ist.

Résumé

La mesure de la tension artérielle au moyen de l'appareil classique est entachée d'erreurs systématiques et imprévisibles. Ces erreurs conduisent à des moyennes de pression fausses, à des chiffres "arrondis" de façon arbitraire et à des erreurs en plus ou en moins sur certaines valeurs, d'où perturbation des courbes de distribution de fréquence.

Un nouvel appareil a été mis au point à la London School of Hygiene and Tropical Medicine; cet appareil assure un gonflement et un dégonflement uniforme et élimine toute influence subjective. Cet instrument, pourvu d'un brassard de 40 cm de long, a été utilisé à une large échelle au cours d'un examen systématique de la tension artérielle dans la population de Bergen en 1963—64. La pression artérielle a été mesurée chez 98,3% des sujets d'une tranche de 10% de la population adulte, soit en tout 8.272 personnes.

Les résultats sont brièvement rapportés. Il n'y a pas de tendance à la bimodalité dans les courbes de distribution dans des groupes d'âges différents.

On peut conclure que la bimodalité des courbes de distribution de fréquence rapportée dans les séries précédentes est un artéfact attribuable à certaines influences telles que le petit nombre des séries étudiées et les erreurs de mesure.

References

1. Bøe, J., S. B. Humerfelt, and F. Wedervang: Acta med. Scand. **156—159**, Suppl. **321** (1957). — 2. Holland, W. W.: In: Epidemiology. Reports on Research and Teaching. Ed. by J. Pemberton. Oxford Univ. Press, London, 1963, p. 271. — 3. Holland, W. W., and S. B. Humerfelt: Brit. Med. J. 1964/II, 1241. — 4. Karvonen, M. J.: Bull. World Health Org. N. Y. **27**, 805 (1962). — 5. Lowe, C. R., and T. McKeown: In: Epidemiology. Reports on Research and Teaching. Ed. by J. Pemberton. Oxford Univ. Press, London, 1963, p. 131. — 6. Morrison, S. L., and J. N. Morris: Lancet 1959/II, 864. — 7. Pickering, G. W.: The Nature of Essential Hypertension. Churchill Ltd., London, 1961. — 8. Platt, R.: In: Essential Hypertension. An International Symposium. Ed. by K. D. Bock and P. T. Cottier. Springer, Berlin, 1960, p. 39. — 9. Rose, G. A., W. W. Holland, and E. A. Crowley: Lancet 1964/I, 296.

Discussion

Puddu: I should like to stress again the importance of having a complete knowledge of the behaviour of the blood pressure in the individual. Casual pressure is very different from basal pressure in many persons, and, moreover, in some people basal pressure is not the lowest value. The ideal would be to attach to each patient to be studied a small machine which would register the blood pressure continuously throughout the 24 hours. This was done by Kain et al.[1], but their method is neither simple nor cheap enough to be adopted on a large scale. Furthermore, it is not so easy for the busy practitioner to determine the basal pressure.

To get an idea of the spontaneous fluctuations in the blood-pressure values in my patients, I devised a very elementary, but still useful, method: I measure the blood pressure of every patient entering my office, as soon as he lies on the couch, before the registration of the electrocardiogram (which is the first step of my examination). I then take a second blood-pressure reading, with the patient still lying, after noting the history and making the clinical examination, by which time the patient is relaxed and an atmosphere of mutual understanding has been established. The difference between these two readings is often pronounced, and they give me a rough, but still useful, idea of the spontaneous fluctuations in blood-pressure values in the individual patient, and of the character of his disease.

Dollery: I should like to ask two questions, Dr. Humerfelt. The first concerns methodology. Does changing your method of recording the blood pressure mean that you cannot compare the data from your earlier survey with your current data? I hope not. The second question is whether you have any data on the rate of rise of blood pressure in subjects with a raised blood pressure in the first survey who were re-examined in the second.

Smirk: I should like to comment on the relation between blood pressure and age following what Dr. Puddu said about casual and basal pressures. We undertook studies on the first casual blood pressure (taken without rest or explanation) in 370 persons attending clinics for illnesses unlikely to be associated with blood-pressure changes. In the same 370 persons we also studied the near basal pressure[2]. The two graphs, relating age to the first casual and the near basal blood pressures respectively, are widely separated, the former lying well above and the latter well below most published graphs dealing with this relationship. The differences between first casual and near basal pressures at age 25 were 24/19 mm. Hg in males and 25/16 mm. Hg in females; at age 65, 34/18 mm. Hg in males, 45/23 mm. Hg in females. Had basal blood pressures been taken, the differences would have been greater, by about 15/7 mm. Hg at age 25 and probably more at age 65, as the basal blood pressure is lower than the near basal pressure.

---

[1] Kain, H. K., A. T. Hinman, and M. Sokolow: Circulation **30**, 882 (1964).

[2] Veale, A. M. O., M. Hamilton, R. O. H. Irvine, and F. H. Smirk: N. Zealand Med. J. **61**, 65 (1962).

PICKERING: May I just make one comment and ask one question? Many years ago, a paper was published which alleged an association between diabetes and essential hypertension[1]. We went into this in the diabetic clinic of St. Mary's and found that there was about 20 mm. difference between the pressure as recorded by the physician in the clinic and the pressure as we recorded it in the out-patient waiting hall, as we had done in our population survey. This, I think, emphasises what Dr. PUDDU said.

I should like to ask a question. COMSTOCK[2] noted that there was a sex effect, in other words, males taking female pressures got higher readings than females taking female pressures and vice versa. Have you noticed that?

TAQUINI: One difficulty in evaluating the differences between casual and basal pressures is that, in one and the same subject, they may be due to changes either in cardiac output or in peripheral resistance. In fact, the increase in blood pressure may be due to an increase in cardiac output on one occasion, and on another occasion merely to an increase in peripheral resistance or perhaps to a combination of both mechanisms.

HUMERFELT: As to Dr. DOLLERY's remarks, I said that one of the shortcomings of our first survey (1950/51) was that it was not sufficiently representative. This is owing to the fact that the epidemiologists require a better attendance than we had (75—80%). We do not think we could improve on the distribution curves to any great extent by selecting a sample and going to all the trouble — and expense — of getting in touch with all the people involved. As the previous curves have shown, the difference between the blood-pressure distributions in the two surveys is very small; I therefore do not think we can disregard the Bergen survey of 1950/51. Secondly, I can assure you that we are very much interested in the group we studied in 1950/51 and in seeing what has happened to them in the intervening period. This is very important. A lot of studies have been based on this epidemiological survey. Some randomly selected groups have been followed up for many years by one of us. Others have investigated a new sample. We have had some of the cases brought into the department for a very thorough examination, including renal function tests and attempts to find out how many have secondary hypertension.

To reply to Dr. PICKERING's question, yes, I have seen that paper. In the Bergen surveys we have consistently used very well trained nurses but no men.

PICKERING: That was in the first survey. Does the same apply to the second?

HUMERFELT: Yes, it does. There is very little difference in blood pressure between those who attended the mass radiography and the subjects whose pressures were measured in their homes. However, I have no data to show you here, as we are still working out all the figures at present.

---

[1] BALME, H. W., and L. COLE: Quart. J. Med. (New Series) **20**, 335 (1951).

[2] COMSTOCK, G. W.: Amer. J. Hyg. **65**, 271 (1957).

Spontaneous blood-pressure variations in hypertension; the effect of antihypertensive therapy and correlations with the incidence of complications

By

K. D. Bock and W. Kreuzenbeck

Since indirect methods of measuring blood pressure were introduced into clinical practice at the end of the last century, many investigators have studied the variations in blood pressure occurring during the day and over longer periods (cf. summaries of the literature by Menzel, 1961, 1962; and Richardson et al., 1964). The earliest studies, e.g. the findings of Zadek, published in 1881, were of limited value, owing to the technical inadequacy of the apparatus available; in others, the blood pressure was measured only at fairly long intervals, or not consistently over 24 hours. Although the results are divergent in a few cases, most of these investigations reveal that blood pressure may vary considerably, not only from day to day, but also in the course of one and the same day, the lowest values appearing during the night and the highest in the morning or, as is more frequently the case, in the early evening. The following factors, however, which may well exert an influence on the results, were left unconsidered by all but a few of the investigators:

1) the presence of an observer to make the measurements,
2) subjective errors that are inherent in the auscultatory method of blood-pressure determination, and
3) the possibility that sleep might be disturbed by the process of measurement.

The first attempt to eliminate these potential sources of error was made in 1922 by Katsch and Pansdorf, who led long tubes from the stethoscope and the cuff on the patient's arm through a hole in the wall into a neighbouring room, in which the observer made the measurements. This was undoubtedly a simple and effective method; unfortunately, however, the blood pressure was measured during the night only, and at fairly long intervals. In the last few years, several automatic blood-pressure-recording devices have been developed which permit measurements to be made at

Table 1. *Classification of hypertensive patients according to clinical course and cause*

Clinical course	n	Age, Mean (Range)	Blood press. Mean	Cause	n	Age, Mean (Range)	Blood press. Mean
Benign	*57*	40 (17—68)	189/112	*Primary*	*51*	43 (17—67)	190/113
mild	25	35 (17—57)	175/102	*Secondary*	*15*	38 (19—56)	214/131
moderate + severe . . .	32	43 (17—68)	202/127	renal	12	41 (19—56)	207/126
Malignant	*9*	48 (43—67)	232/147	aortic coarctation . . .	2	23 (20—26)	220/125
				porphyrinuria	1	32	220/140
Total	66			Total	66		

any desired intervals without an observer being present. Results obtained with apparatus of this type have recently been published by SHAW et al. (1963), RICHARDSON et al. (1964), and by ourselves (BOCK and KREUZENBECK, 1965).

On the basis of 24-hour blood-pressure measurements in a large number of patients, we shall try to answer the following questions:

1) Are differences in blood-pressure variation over a 24-hour period found in different forms of hypertension?

2) Is the blood-pressure variation over 24 hours influenced by antihypertensive therapy?

3) Is there any correlation between the 24-hour blood pressure and the incidence of complications?

Material and methods

The investigations involved 13 healthy normotensive subjects of an average age of 52 years, 66 untreated hypertensives of an average age of 42 years, and eight patients of an average age of 67 years with evidence of generalised arteriosclerosis. Most patients in the last-mentioned group had a history of apoplexy, myocardial infarction, or peripheral arterial occlusion; their blood pressures were normal or only slightly elevated. The classification of the hypertensive patients is given in Table 1. The group with benign hypertension was subdivided into mild or labile cases, in which normal pressure values were occasionally found prior to therapy, and moderately severe to severe cases, in which the pressure was consistently elevated and organic lesions secondary to hypertension were present. The criteria on which the diagnosis of malignant hypertension was based were evidence of advanced hypertensive disease and the presence of hypertensive retinopathy of Grade III or IV. The group with secondary hypertension includes 12 cases of renal hypertension (three of chronic glomerulonephritis, five of chronic pyelonephritis, three of renal artery stenosis, and one of polycystic kidney disease) as well as two cases of aortic coarctation and one case of acute intermittent porphyrinuria.

The patients were hospitalised in an open ward and kept under bed-rest conditions while the 24-hour measurements were being made, except for occasional visits to the toilet. They were allowed to lie or sit up in bed and could move almost freely. Blood pressure was measured at intervals of 15 minutes.

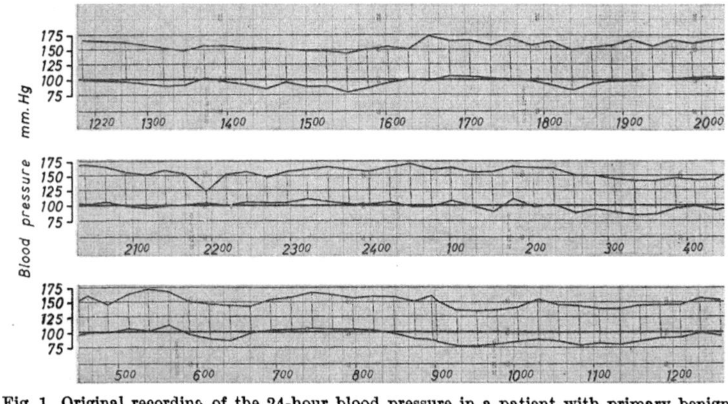

Fig. 1. Original recording of the 24-hour blood pressure in a patient with primary benign hypertension. To facilitate comparison the individual readings of systolic and diastolic pressures have been connected.

The apparatus used was designed by von Uexküll and Killing (1959) and von Uexküll and Wick (1962). At preselected intervals, it automatically inflates a cuff on the patient's upper arm, and, when the cuff pressure falls, records the Korotkoff sounds, which are picked up by means of a microphone. In contrast with other equipment on the market, this device has the advantage that it records all the Korotkoff sounds and not only the first and last, so that artefacts, which are unavoidable with all these devices, can be recognised more easily and eliminated. An original recording is shown in Fig. 1.

The curves showing the mean 24-hour blood-pressure values of the various groups were calculated as follows: in each case, the mean one-hour blood-pressure value was calculated from four 15-minute values, and the results were used to obtain the mean values for the whole group. The use of this method of calculation and the fact that the minimum and maximum blood pressures in the various patients do not coincide exactly result in the flattening of the mean-value curves and conceal the much larger individual variations.

Results and discussion

1. Blood-pressure variations in different forms of hypertension

The mean 24-hour blood-pressure curves for 13 normotensives, eight patients with arteriosclerosis, 57 with benign hypertension, and nine with malignant hypertension are given in Fig. 2. In all groups, the minimum blood pressures were recorded during the night, between 1 a.m. and 5 a.m. The maximum pressures were reached in the morning or in the evening. During the night, the systolic pressure decreased more than the diastolic, resulting in a fall in pulse pressure. The differences between the various groups are quantitative rather than qualitative and apply only to the height of the pressure and the extent of the nocturnal fall in blood pressure.

In Fig. 3, the hypertensive patients are classified according to the *severity* of hypertensive disease, i.e. as a) mild benign, b) moderate and severe benign, and c) malignant cases. Here, too, differences mainly in degree but no fundamental differences in the course of the 24-hour blood-pressure curve are seen. The more advanced the hypertensive disease, the higher are the average pressures on admission and the over-all levels of the blood pressure, and the less pronounced is the nocturnal drop in pressure. Some malignant cases show slight increases, others slight decreases in pressure during the night, with the result that the mean-pressure curve for the whole group is virtually straight. That the relative "fixation" of the pressure, especially of the diastolic values, is mainly functional, or, if organic, at least in part reversible, can be concluded from its reduction following successful therapy.

When the hypertensive patients are classified according to the *suspected origin of the disease* in primary and secondary forms

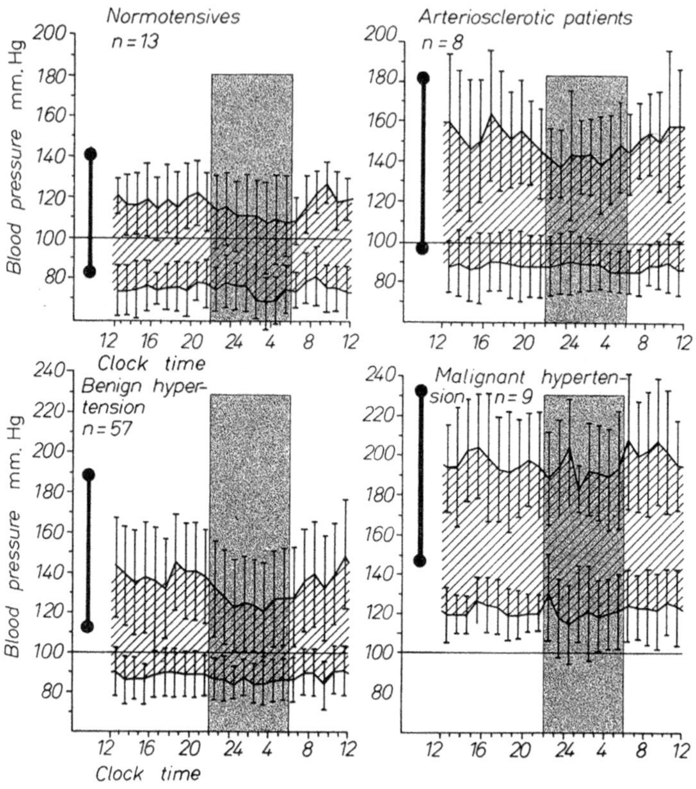

Fig. 2. 24-hour systolic and diastolic blood-pressure curves for 13 normotensives, eight arteriosclerotic patients, 57 patients with benign and nine patients with malignant hypertension. Mean values ± standard deviation. The vertical bar (↕) indicates the average blood pressure on admission to the hospital.

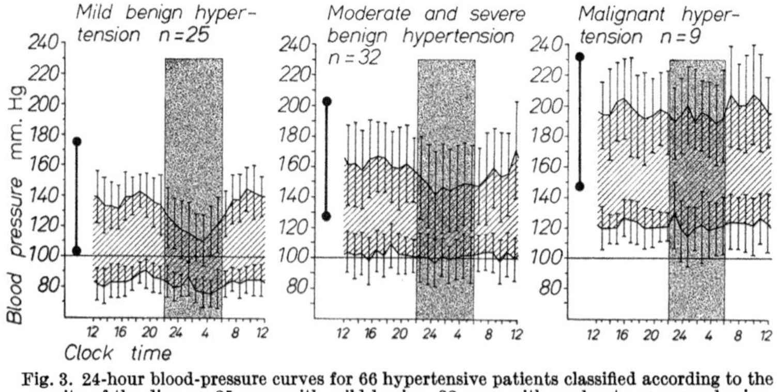

Fig. 3. 24-hour blood-pressure curves for 66 hypertensive patients classified according to the severity of the disease: 25 cases with mild benign, 32 cases with moderate or severe benign, and nine cases with malignant hypertension. Mean values ± standard deviation. The vertical bar (↕) indicates the average blood pressure on admission to the hospital.

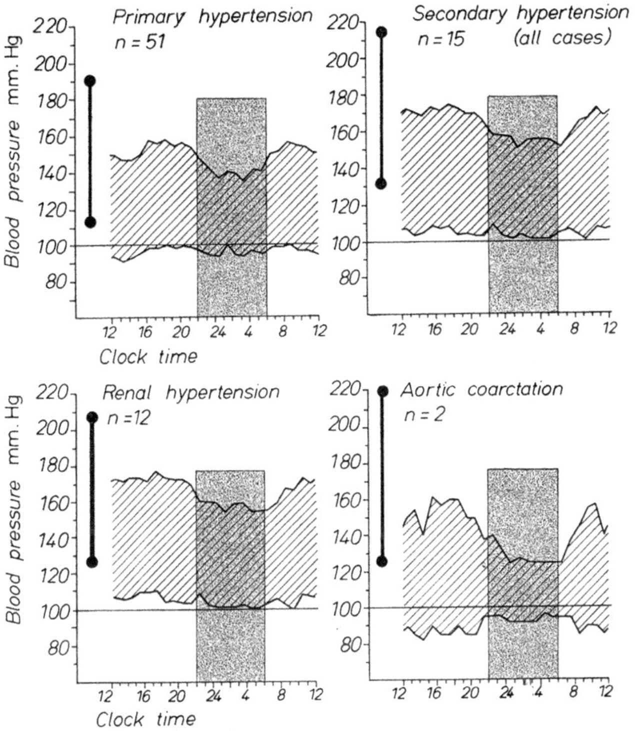

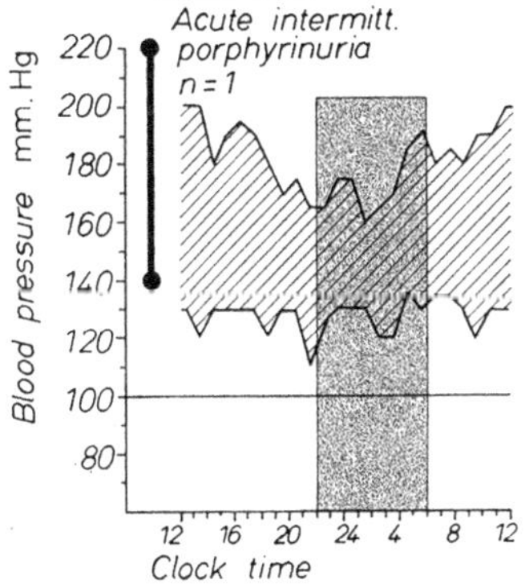

Fig. 1. 24-hour blood-pressure curves for 66 hypertensive patients classified according to the suspected origin: 51 cases with benign and 15 cases with secondary hypertension, the latter including 12 cases of renal hypertension, two cases with aortic coarctation, and one case with acute porphyrinuria. Mean values. The vertical bar (|) indicates the average blood pressure on admission to the hospital.

(Fig. 4), the 24-hour blood-pressure curves are very similar. Even further subdivision of the cases with secondary hypertension (renal hypertension, aortic coarctation, acute intermittent porphyrinuria) reveals no fundamental differences. The same applies

Table 2. *Lowest blood pressures in 24 hours*

	n	Mean (mm. Hg)	Lowest single value (mm. Hg)
Normotensives	13	102/70	80/55
Arteriosclerotics	8	134/86	100/80
Hypertensives	66		
Benign (all cases)	57	124/85	85/70
mild	25	113/75	85/70
moderate + severe	32	138/95	110/80
Malignant	9	178/118	150/100
Primary	51	130/87	85/70
Secondary (all cases)	15	141/101	100/80
renal	12	142/100	100/80
aortic coarctation	2	125/95	125/95
porphyria acuta	1	160/130	160/130

Table 3. *Maximum variations in blood pressure over a period of 24 hours under bed-rest*

	n	Age (Mean)	B.P. Variation mm. Hg Mean (Range)	
			Syst.	Diast.
Normotensives	13	52	24[1] (15—40)	14 (5—20)
Arteriosclerotics	8	67	35 (15—80)	15 (0—30)
Hypertensives	66	41	38[1] (10—90)	15 (0—30)
Benign (all cases)	57	40	39[1] (15—90)	16 (5—30)
mild	25	35	36 (15—55)	16 (5—30)
moderate + severe	32	43	42 (20—90)	16 (5—30)
Malignant	9	48	31 (10—50)	10 (0—20)
Primary	51	43	37 (15—90)	16 (5—30)
Secondary (all cases)	15	38	43 (10—90)	13 (5—30)
renal	12	41	45 (10—90)	15 (0—30)
aortic coarctation	2	23	42 (35—50)	5
porphyria acuta	1	32	30	5

[1] The difference in systolic blood-pressure variation between normotensive and hypertensive subjects (whole group and all cases with benign hypertension) is significant ($p < 0.005$); all others are not.

to the different forms of renal hypertension (glomerulonephritis, pyelonephritis, renal artery stenosis, polycystic kidney disease).

The *lowest systolic and diastolic blood pressures* recorded during 24 hours in the various groups of patients are summarised in Table 2. The more advanced the hypertension is, the higher are both the mean values and the lowest single values; but there are no significant differences between the primary and secondary forms.

In Table 3, the *maximum differences in the 24-hour blood pressure* in the various groups of patients are listed. The variation in systolic pressure is greater in the patients with benign hypertension than in the normotensive group and smaller again in patients with malignant hypertension. The first-mentioned difference is statistically significant ($p < 0.005$); all others are not.

It should be mentioned here that the variations in blood pressure become greater with increasing age (MENZEL, 1961, 1962; RICHARDSON et al., 1964). In contrast, sex seems to have no influence. Some of these results agree with previous findings reported by MÜLLER (1921), KATSCH and PANSDORF (1922), MUELLER and BROWN (1930), HAMMARSTRÖM (1947), KILPATRICK (1948), MENZEL et al. (1949), SHAW et al. (1963), and RICHARDSON et al. (1964) as far as the experimental procedure is comparable. There are other unimportant differences which, however, cannot be discussed here.

2. Influence of antihypertensive treatment on 24-hour blood-pressure variation

In order to find out whether effective antihypertensive treatment influences the 24-hour blood-pressure variation, investigations were carried out in 15 hypertensive patients. The treatment consisted in the administration of α-methyldopa in combination with cyclopenthiazide; two patients received small doses of guanethidine in addition. The 24-hour blood-pressure recordings were made before treatment and after a clear-cut fall in blood pressure had been obtained.

One individual case and the mean values for all patients before and during treatment are shown in Figs 5 and 6. The over-all blood-pressure level is lowered by treatment; the characteristic 24-hour course is, however, still present. As can be seen from Table 4, no significant reduction in the 24-hour pressure variation takes place. It must be stressed, however, that these results are only valid for treatment with α-methyldopa in combination with a saluretic and

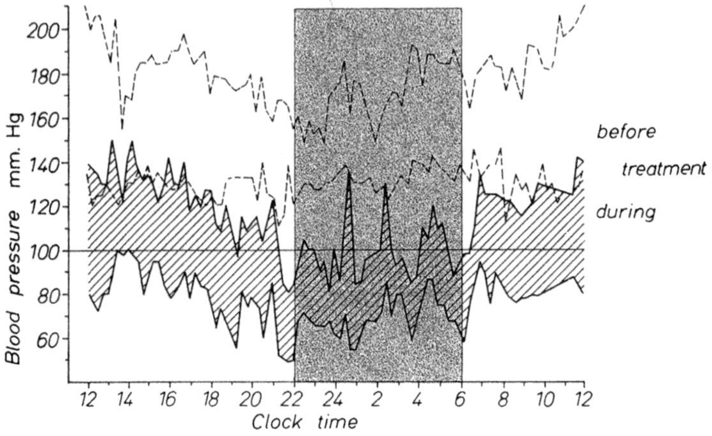

Fig. 5. 24-hour blood pressure of a 34-year-old patient with polycystic kidneys before (dotted lines) and during (solid lines) treatment with α-methyldopa in combination with cyclopenthiazide.

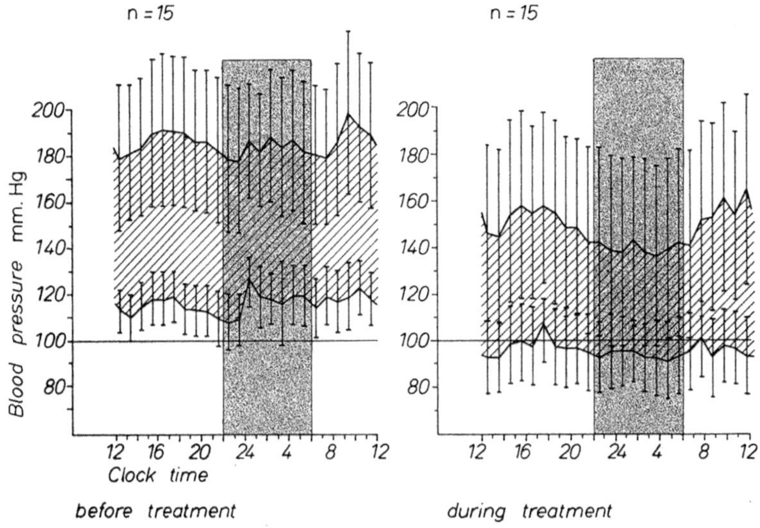

Fig. 6. 24-hour blood-pressure curves of 15 hypertensive patients before and during treatment with α-methyldopa in combination with cyclopenthiazide. Mean values ± standard deviation.

only under conditions of bed-rest. Treatment with a potent sympathetic blocking agent, e.g. guanethidine, and/or normal physical activity would probably result in a much greater variability in blood pressure.

Table 4. *Maximum variations in blood pressure over a period of 24 hours (bed-rest) before and during successful treatment*

n = 15	B.P. Variation mm. Hg Mean (Range)	
	Syst.	Diast.
Before treatment	38 (15—65)	17 (10—40)
During treatment	31 (10—60)	17 (5—30)

3. Correlation between the 24-hour blood-pressure variations and the incidence of myocardial infarction and stroke

The opinion is widely held that a sudden fall in blood pressure is an important factor in the pathogenesis of myocardial infarction and stroke and that these are consequently more apt to occur during the night, when blood pressure decreases. In our clinical experience, however, these complications occur — at least in hypertensive patients — far more frequently when the blood pressure is particularly high. It is difficult to reach an objective conclusion on this question, because only in extremely rare cases is the actual blood pressure at the onset of a stroke or myocardial infarction known. Even pressures measured only a very short time afterwards may be quite different.

Apart from casuistic observations, the only evidence available is indirect. If one assumes that the incidence of myocardial infarction or stroke is equally distributed over the 24 hours of the day, one third of them should happen during the eight hours between 10 p.m. and 6 a.m. This, however, is not the case (Fig. 7). Of 204 myocardial infarctions and 229 strokes in which the time of onset was known, 38% and 51% respectively began between 6 a.m. and 2 p.m.; 31% of the myocardial infarctions and only 20% of the strokes (less than one would expect) took place during the night, between 10 p.m. and 6 a.m., i.e. when the blood pressure was lowest. Similar figures relating to the distribution over 24 hours have been obtained by Pell and d'Alonzo (1963) for myocardial infarctions, and by Scheid and Wolf (1959) and Reuter (1964) for strokes. Differentiation in the strokes, between cerebral haemorrhages and malacias, shows that haemorrhages occur somewhat less frequently during the night, but, since haemorrhages account for only 10–20% of the total number of strokes, no significant difference in the above-mentioned percentage distribution is apparent. Convincing evidence has recently been put forward by Kendell and Marshall (1963) and Fazekas and Alman (1964)

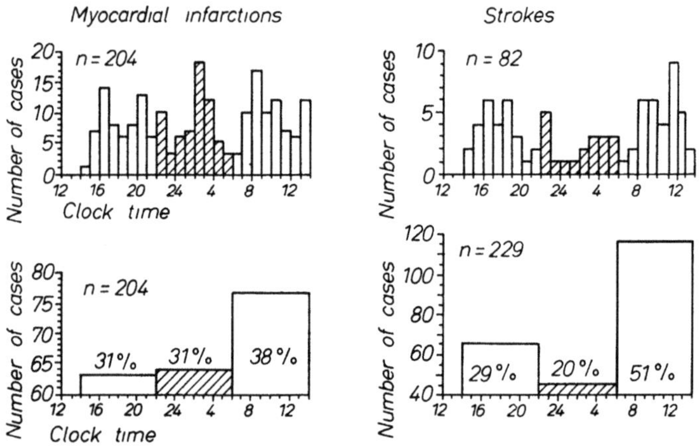

Fig. 7. Distribution of myocardial infarctions (204) and strokes (82 and 229 resp. in two groups) over 24 hours. Above: Classification in one-hour intervals. Below: Classification in eight-hour intervals. The differences in the number of strokes occurring in the morning (51%), in the afternoon (29%), and at night (20%) are statistically significant ($p < 0.01$ and < 0.05 resp.). As regards myocardial infarctions, the differences are not significant.

to show that, even in patients subject to recurrent transitory ischaemic cerebral attacks, relapses occur only in extremely rare cases (one in a total of 46), when an appreciable fall in blood pressure is induced experimentally.

The reason for bringing up this question here is that the fear of inducing myocardial infarction or strokes still sometimes precludes the application of an effective antihypertensive treatment and, moreover, even encourages the administration of pressor substances in normotensive arteriosclerotic patients. Although occasional observations leave no doubt that a sudden drop in blood pressure to subnormal values may induce myocardial infarction or a stroke – most of us know of such cases – the statistical evidence available so far indicates that lowering of the pressure to the normal range and, in particular, the physiological nocturnal fall in blood pressure are of no importance in the majority of cases.

Finally, I should like to comment briefly on the significance of automatic blood-pressure-recording devices with regard to diagnosis and therapy in hypertensive disease. These machines are very expensive, and none of them is free of artefacts, so that the records have to be critically evaluated. Moreover, patients can seldom be expected to submit to recordings over periods of more than 24 hours. Owing to the necessity of maintaining bed-rest, the conditions are somewhat artificial, and the fluctuations in pressure are certainly smaller than in patients who are allowed to move freely within the ward or to live under normal day-to-day conditions. Furthermore, none of the existing publications relating to investigations in which automatic recording devices have been used has brought forth any fundamentally new observations as compared with the results obtained by older methods. The main advantage of the automatic recording devices is that they eliminate subjective errors and the oberserver's influence on blood pressure. In addition, they permit 24-hour records to be made with relatively little work. For the reasons just mentioned, the lowest pressures recorded in this way are more important than the highest ones. They are lower than the so-called "basal" blood pressures determined by the method described by Alam and Smirk (1943) and Smirk (1944) or by methods recommended by some medical societies, or by a combination of both (Smirk, 1957). If we assume that the maximum spontaneous decrease of a patient's arteriolar tone is indicated by the lowest blood pressure recorded under resting conditions, this lowest pressure is at present best determined with the aid of an automatic recording device.

Summary

1. In 13 normotensives, eight arteriosclerotic and 66 hypertensive patients, 24-hour blood-pressure determinations were made at 15-minute intervals with an automatic blood-pressure recorder.

2. The 24-hour blood-pressure curves do not differ qualitatively in various forms of hypertension.

3. The more severe the hypertensive disease, the less pronounced is the nocturnal fall in blood pressure, the latter often being completely absent in malignant hypertension.

4. Under conditions of bed-rest, the maximum variation in the 24-hour blood pressure is, on the average, greater in arteriosclerotic patients and patients with benign hypertension than in normotensives. Cases of benign hypertension show a greater diurnal variation than cases of malignant hypertension, whereas no difference is apparent between primary and secondary hypertension in this respect.

5. Successful antihypertensive treatment with α-methyldopa in combination with a saluretic lowers the over-all 24-hour blood-pressure level, but does not reduce the maximum daily variation (under bed-rest).

6. The statistical distribution over 24 hours for 204 cases of myocardial infarction and 229 cases of stroke shows a lower incidence of these complications during the night than one might expect. This is taken as indirect evidence that the nocturnal fall in blood pressure is of no pathogenic importance in the majority of these cases.

Zusammenfassung

1. Mit Hilfe eines automatischen Meßgerätes wurde der Blutdruck während 24 Std. in 15minutigen Zeitabständen bestimmt, und zwar bei 13 Normotonikern, acht Patienten mit Arteriosklerose und 66 Patienten mit Hochdruck.

2. Bei den verschiedenen Formen von Hochdruck zeigen die während 24 Std. aufgenommenen Blutdruckkurven keine qualitativen Abweichungen.

3. Je schwerer der Hochdruck, um so weniger deutlich ist der nächtliche Blutdruckabfall, der bei maligner Hypertension vollständig fehlen kann.

4. Während Bettruhe ist die maximale Variation des 24-Std.-Blutdrucks bei arteriosklerotischen Patienten und bei Kranken mit benignem Hochdruck im Durchschnitt größer als bei Normotonen. Fälle von benignem Hochdruck weisen größere Tagesschwankungen auf als solche von malignem Hochdruck, während zwischen primärem und sekundärem Hochdruck in dieser Hinsicht kein Unterschied nachweisbar ist.

5. Die Behandlung des Hochdruckes mit α-Methyldopa zusammen mit einem Saluretikum senkt zwar die während der gesamten 24-Std.-Periode gemessenen Blutdruckwerte, ändert jedoch nicht die maximalen Tagesschwankungen (bei Bettruhe).

6. Bei 204 Patienten mit Herzinfarkt und bei 229 Patienten mit Apoplexie ergab die statistische Verteilung über 24 Std. eine geringere Häufigkeit dieser Komplikationen in den Nachtstunden als zu erwarten wäre. Dies ist ein indirekter Hinweis dafür, daß der nächtliche Blutdruckabfall keine pathogenetische Bedeutung für die Mehrzahl dieser Komplikationen besitzt.

Résumé

1. Chez 13 normotendus, huit artérioscléreux et 66 hypertendus ont été effectuées des mesures de la pression artérielle sur une période de 24 heures, à intervalles d'un quart d'heure, avec un sphygmomanomètre automatique.

2. Les courbes des 24 heures ainsi obtenues ne présentent aucune différence qualitative dans les diverses formes d'hypertension.

3. Plus la maladie hypertensive est grave, moins la chute nocturne est prononcée, manquant souvent complètement dans l'hypertension maligne.

4. Dans les conditions de repos au lit, la variation maximum de la pression artérielle dans les 24 heures est, en moyenne, plus importante chez les artérioscléreux et les hypertendus "bénins" que chez les normotendus. Dans les cas d'hypertension bénigne la variation dans la journée est plus grande que dans les cas d'hypertension maligne, alors qu'il n'apparaît pas de différence à cet égard entre l'hypertension primaire et l'hypertension secondaire.

5. Un traitement antihypertenseur efficace à l'α-méthyldopa associée à un salidiurétique abaisse le niveau général de la tension artérielle des 24 heures, mais ne diminue pas la variation journalière maximum (au repos au lit).

6. La distribution statistique, dans les 24 heures, des heures de début de 204 cas d'infarctus du myocarde et de 229 cas d'ictus apoplectique montre une

fréquence de survenue nocturne de ces complications plus faible que celle à laquelle on devrait s'attendre, ce qui est considéré comme une preuve indirecte que la chute nocturne de la pression artérielle n'a pas d'importance pathogénique dans la plupart de ces cas.

Acknowledgement

We are indebted to Mr. H. VENNEWALD for his valuable technical aid.

References

ALAM, M., and F. H. SMIRK: Brit. Heart J. **5**, 156 (1943). — BOCK, K. D., and W. KREUZENBECK: In: Hochdruckforschung, II. Symposion in Freiburg, Juli 1964. Ed. by L. HEILMEYER and H. I. HOLTMEIER. Thieme, Stuttgart, 1965, p. 72. — FAZEKAS, J. F., and R. W. ALMAN: Amer. J. Med. Sc. **248**, 567 (1964). — HAMMARSTRÖM, S.: Acta med. Scand. **128**, Suppl. **192** (1947). — KATSCH, G., and H. PANSDORF: Münch. med. Wschr. **69**, 1715 (1922). — KENDELL, R. E., and J. MARSHALL: Brit. Med. J. 1963/II, 344. — KILPATRICK, J. A.: Brit. Heart J. **10**, 48 (1948). — MENZEL, W., R. TIMM, and G. HERRNRING: Verh. Dtsch. Ges. Kreisl.forsch. **15**, 256 (1949). — MENZEL, W.: Med. Welt **12**, 560 (1961). — MENZEL, W.: Menschliche Tag-Nacht-Rhythmik und Schichtarbeit. Benno Schwabe, Basel-Stuttgart, 1962. — MUELLER, S. C., and G. E. BROWN: Ann. Int. Med. **3**, 1190 (1930). — MÜLLER, C.: Acta med. Scand. **55**, 381 (1921). — PELL, S., and C. A. D'ALONZO: J. Amer. Med. Ass. **185**, 831 (1963). — REUTER, J. P.: Dtsch. med. J. **15**, 77 (1964). — RICHARDSON, D. W., A. J. HONOUR, G. W. FENTON, F. H. STOTT, and G. W. PICKERING: Clin. Sc. **26**, 445 (1964). — SCHEID, W., and G. WOLF: Med. Klin. **54**, 2243 (1959). — SHAW, D. B., M. S. KNAPP, and D. H. DAVIES: Lancet 1963/I, 797. — SMIRK, F. H.: Brit. Heart J. **6**, 176 (1944). — SMIRK, F. H.: High Arterial Pressure. Blackwell Scientific Publications, Oxford, 1957. — VON UEXKÜLL, T., and F. KILLING: Münch. med. Wschr. **101**, 380 (1959). — VON UEXKÜLL, T., and E. WICK: Zschr. Kreisl.forsch. **51**, 184 (1962). — ZADEK, I.: Zschr. klin. Med. **2**, 509 (1881).

Discussion

Werkö: One important question is how much of the daily variation in blood pressure is due to changes in blood flow — cardiac output — and how much to changes in peripheral resistance. The influence of psychic stress

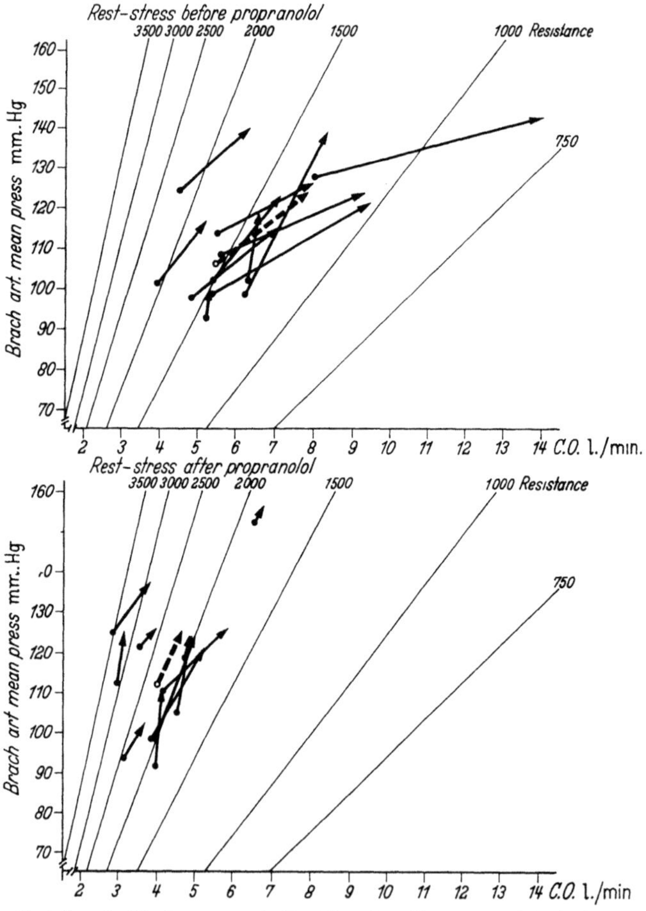

Fig. 1. Variations in blood pressure (ordinate) and cardiac output (abscissa) under the influence of a defined stress (flight simulation in a link trainer). Upper part before, lower part after the injection of the β-adrenergic receptor blocker, propranolol. The increase in cardiac output under the influence of stress is almost completely inhibited.

on flow and resistance has been studied by ELIASCH, ROSÉN, and SCOTT[1], using a standardised form of such stress as occurs in everyday life, and they have granted me permission to show some of their so far unpublished results (Fig. 1). The persons studied were pilots in the Swedish Air Force who volunteered to take part in this experiment, and the stress consisted of a difficult, simulated flight in a link trainer. Blood pressure was measured intra-arterially, and blood flow using a dye-dilution technique. Several observations were made before, during, and after the stress period. In all subjects, the cardiac output during the stress period rose, concomitantly with an increase in heart rate and blood pressure. Usually, the increase in blood flow was more marked than the rise in pressure.

In some cases the observations were repeated after the injection of a β-adrenergic blocking agent, propranolol: here, the same stress gave rise to much the same increase in blood pressure, but this time without — or with very little — change in blood flow or heart rate.

Under ordinary conditions the increase in pressure can thus be explained in terms of an increase in flow, but if the increase in flow is prevented by β-adrenergic blockade, the blood pressure still rises, presumably owing to an increase in resistance. This is different from what is seen during exercise, where β-adrenergic blocking does not interfere with the augmentation of flow.

ZANCHETTI: I have studied spontaneous blood-pressure variations in animals, and I should like to emphasise how valuable it is that similar studies are being done in healthy human subjects and in hypertensive patients as well. I must congratulate Dr. BOCK upon his interesting data, which usefully complement the information recently provided by Dr. PICKERING and his co-workers[2]. I am fully aware of the difficulties involved in carrying out these studies in man, but it would be exciting if somebody tried in the future to record blood pressure continuously in man by direct catheterisation of an artery. Indeed, during sleep associated with rapid eye movements there are considerable and sudden variations in arterial pressure and heart rate — a phenomenon which is common to experimental animals and man. I am afraid that most of these swift changes may not be recorded when blood pressure is monitored at five-minute or half-hourly intervals.

At any rate, it is evident from Dr. BOCK's figures that larger variations in blood pressure occur in hypertensive subjects, with the exception of malignant hypertensive patients, than in normotensive ones. This is consistent with our experience in comparing normotensive animals with animals subjected to carotid sinus and aortic deafferentation. May I suggest that the greater variability in arterial pressure shown by hypertensive patients might result from a resetting of baroceptive reflexes, i.e. from a decreased activity of these reflexes in hypertension, as has been suggested by several authors?

If an attempt were made to combine the information on blood pressure during sleep that we have gathered in animal experiments with the data provided by Dr. BOCK and Dr. PICKERING as a result of their research on human subjects, I think it would not be impossible to assess the importance of neural control of circulation in normotensive and hypertensive human subjects. It would be enough to study blood-pressure changes during sleep,

---

[1] ELIASCH, H., A. ROSÉN, and H. SCOTT: Circulation **32**, Suppl. **2**, 81 (1965).

[2] RICHARDSON, D. W., A. J. HONOUR, G. W. FENTON, F. H. STOTT, and G. W. PICKERING: Clin. Sc. **26**, 445 (1964).

before and after bilateral cocainisation of the carotid sinuses — a procedure which a lot of authors have used for other purposes in man without any danger to the patient.

Finally, Dr. BOCK has emphasised that a small number of myocardial infarctions or strokes occurs during sleep hours, and his figures are very clear on this point. However, it seems to me that, even in the group he studied, the incidence of these accidents is not reduced as much as blood pressure is. May I suggest as a tentative hypothesis that a good proportion of the vascular accidents during sleep might be concentrated in the recurrent episodes of rapid-eye-movement sleep, the extreme variability of blood pressure during these periods being the precipitating cause of the vascular accidents.

TAQUINI: Going back to Dr. WERKÖ's comments about cardiac output, I should like to say that in the data presented by Dr. BOCK, there is some evidence that there might be changes in the cardiac stroke volume. In fact, the changes in systolic pressure are higher than those in diastolic pressure; moreover, in the cases of coarctation of the aorta, it was only the systolic pressure that was lowered.

HOOBLER: I have two questions for Dr. BOCK. Looking at the curves, I was struck by the fact that only in the normotensives was there a substantial diastolic reduction during the night: systolic pressure fell, but diastolic did not, in cases mostly of mild benign or moderately severe essential hypertension. I should like to know whether there is a qualitative difference here between the normal and the hypertensive.

The other question has to do with the incidence of strokes at different times of the year. Dr. SCHUMAN[1] of the School of Public Health at the University of Michigan has collected statistics for several major cities of the United States indicating that the incidence of strokes is greatly increased during the summer months, in hot weather. I wonder whether Dr. BOCK has analysed his data with respect to seasonal variations, as he has so many cases so well documented. It would be easy to confirm or refute this interesting and hitherto unexpected relationship between temperature and stroke.

DONTAS: I should also like to ask two questions, Dr. BOCK. Firstly, have you observed any longer-lasting blood-pressure waves, either systolic or diastolic, of the type described by SCHMID et al.[2], that is to say, lasting several days rather than several hours; are such waves more obvious in the systolic or in the diastolic phase? Secondly, are these waves present in essential hypertensives or arteriosclerotic hypertensives, as opposed to normotensives?

BROD: May I take up the point made by Dr. TAQUINI and Dr. WERKÖ about the relative contributions of cardiac output and peripheral vascular resistance? Peripheral vascular resistance is not a single parameter; it consists of very many parallel resistances, and in the conditions under which blood pressure rises, mainly during emotion and during exercise, these regional resistances change in opposite ways; there is always vasoconstriction in the viscera, kidneys, and partly also in the skin, and there is always vasodilatation in the muscles. What happens to the total peripheral vascular resistance depends on the balance of these vasodilating and vaso-

[1] SCHUMAN, S. H., C. P. ANDERSON, and J. T. OLIVER: J. Amer. Med. Ass. **189**, 733 (1964).

[2] SCHMID, A., R. SAUTER, and F. REUBI: Schweiz. med. Wschr. **84**, 760 (1954).

constricting components. In some instances, especially during emotion, the total peripheral vascular resistance might rise, and in these instances the cardiac output usually tends to drop. However, there are emotional states where the degree of muscular vasodilatation is such that the total resistance decreases, and then the cardiac output increases. So I should think that all this is one pattern influenced only by the relative magnitude of the individual haemodynamic components.

PICKERING: I should like to ask Dr. BOCK whether the differences which he has found between waking and sleep are similar to those which we found. It seemed to me, looking at his figures, as though they were smaller. I wondered whether he had any electro-encephalographic record of the depth of sleep, because this is, as Dr. ZANCHETTI showed yesterday, extremely important with regard to the level of arterial pressure. I also wondered about the circumstances in which he measured these changes. Does the patient go to the machine or does the machine come to the patient?

BOCK: The maximal diurnal variations we have found are, in fact, somewhat smaller than those you have observed, Dr. PICKERING; the reason for this I do not know. Certainly the patients slept during the night, although this was not controlled by E.E.G. recordings. — The machine came to the patient in his room.

I agree with Dr. ZANCHETTI that it would be ideal to have some method for making long-term, continuous, direct blood-pressure recordings in man, but unfortunately there is none. Direct determinations would probably reveal a greater blood-pressure variation over short periods of time, but I doubt whether the 24-hour variation would increase very much. The main advantage would be the elimination of the errors inherent in the indirect methods. — The greater diurnal variation in blood pressure in hypertensives as compared with normotensives is not necessarily due to an alteration in neurogenic control, as you have suggested. An alternative explanation could be that in arterioles with a reduced lumen (as is the case in hypertension), even very small additional changes in diameter will result in considerable changes in peripheral resistance and blood pressure.

As to Dr. HOOBLER's questions, the extent of the nocturnal fall in blood pressure does not allow us to distinguish clearly between normotensives and hypertensives, because patients with mild, or even occasionally those with moderately severe, hypertension may show nocturnal blood-pressure levels similar to those of normotensives. On the other hand, the failure to lower the blood pressure during the night seems to indicate a severe form of hypertension. — With regard to seasonal variations in the occurrence of strokes it can be stated that the 323 cases we have investigated showed a uniform distribution over the 12 months of the year, except for a (statistically insignificant) lower incidence in October. This material may, however, be a non-representative selection, because it includes hospitalised patients only and none who died immediately or was treated at home.

In reply to Dr. DONTAS' questions, the phasic blood-pressure fluctuations formerly described by SCHMID extend over a longer period than 24 hours. We are not convinced of the existence of these waves; in any case they are different from the 24-hour blood-pressure rhythm we have investigated.

Effect of a simple therapeutic regimen on blood pressure and its variability in mild hypertension

By

H. Schwartz, G. A. Eadie, R. D. Remington, and S. W. Hoobler

The effects of prolonged outpatient treatment in persons with quite mild and variable forms of hypertension have not, to our knowledge, been carefully studied by double-blind techniques. The problem nevertheless presents itself, because some patients, in an intermittently hypertensive episode, may exhibit neurological features suggestive of cerebrovascular insufficiency. Following such an event, the blood pressure may fall to normal under conditions of bed-rest, yet remain on the border line between normal and hypertensive levels on successive visits to the clinic. Since recurrence of such very high blood pressures might represent a renewed threat to the patient, it is important to know whether treatment would reduce the peak level of blood pressure or its spontaneous variability. The therapeutic regimen which we have found to cause the fewest side effects and which has the maximum antihypertensive action consists of a combination of thiazide and deserpidine (*1*). A slight modification of this regimen was therefore used in the treatment of patients with mild to moderate elevations of blood pressure.

Methods

Twenty-two patients, aged between 32 and 54 years and having some recent elevation in blood pressure, were selected from persons attending the clinics at Wayne County General Hospital. The first blood-pressure readings varied between 140/92 and 200/100 mm. Hg (average 161/102 mm. Hg). Six of the patients exhibited minimal electrocardiographic abnormalities, but none showed albuminuria or major retinopathy, and none had a history of important vascular complications. In the two groups described below, there was approximately an equal number of males and females, and of Negroes and whites.

After the initial selection was made, the patients were asked to return at monthly intervals to an examining clinic established for this purpose at the Wayne County Health Department, Eloise, Michigan. They were given placebo tablets and instructed to take one a day for the first four months. At each visit to the clinic, a series of tests was performed to determine the level of blood pressure and its variability. The measurements noted included the difference between the casual recumbent and the 20-minute resting levels, and the difference between recumbent and standing readings, before and after three minutes of graded exercise, and before and after a stressful mirror-drawing test.

The first four-month period was followed by a period of six months, during which either placebo or active drug was administered according to a random allocation made by R. D. REMINGTON. Details of this schedule were unknown to the investigator (H. SCHWARTZ). The active drug consisted of a tablet containing 100 mg. chlorthalidone[1] and 1.0 mg. deserpidine[2]; the placebo tablet was identical in appearance and in taste[3]. At the end of this period, the placebo group was switched to the active drug, and *vice versa*.

Observations

Changes in the casual recumbent blood pressures recorded in Groups 1 (those who received the drug first) and 2 (those who received the placebo first) are shown in graphic form in Figs 1 and 2 respectively; the same information is given in tabular form in Tables 1 and 2. In Group 2, the mean blood pressure fell slightly (average 10/7 mm. Hg) during the last three months of the placebo period, but declined by a further 25/13 mm. Hg when the chlorthalidone-deserpidine combination was given. In Group 1, treatment with the active drug (4th to 10th months) produced a marked blood-pressure reduction (average 33/17 mm. Hg). Perhaps this represented a summation of the effects of placebo, increasing familiarity with the clinic, and the drug, for when the active drug was replaced by placebo, blood pressure failed to return to the previous levels. The final readings during the 14th to 16th months of observation were, on the average, 12/8 mm. Hg less than the levels recorded during the initial observation period. This decline is approximately equal to the fall of 10/7 mm. Hg, noted in Group 2

[1] Kindly supplied as Hygroton, brand of chlorthalidone, by Geigy Pharmaceuticals, Division of Geigy Chemical Corporation, Ardsley, N. Y.

[2] Kindly supplied as Harmonyl, brand of deserpidine, by Abbott Laboratories, North Chicago, Ill.

[3] The compounding of the placebo and of the active tablet was performed through the courtesy of Dr. THOMAS ROWE, Dean, School of Pharmacy, University of Michigan, and his colleagues.

between the end of the initial observation period and the end of the placebo period.

The graphic data represent the month-to-month variation in blood pressure. The intra-individual variation for the groups as a

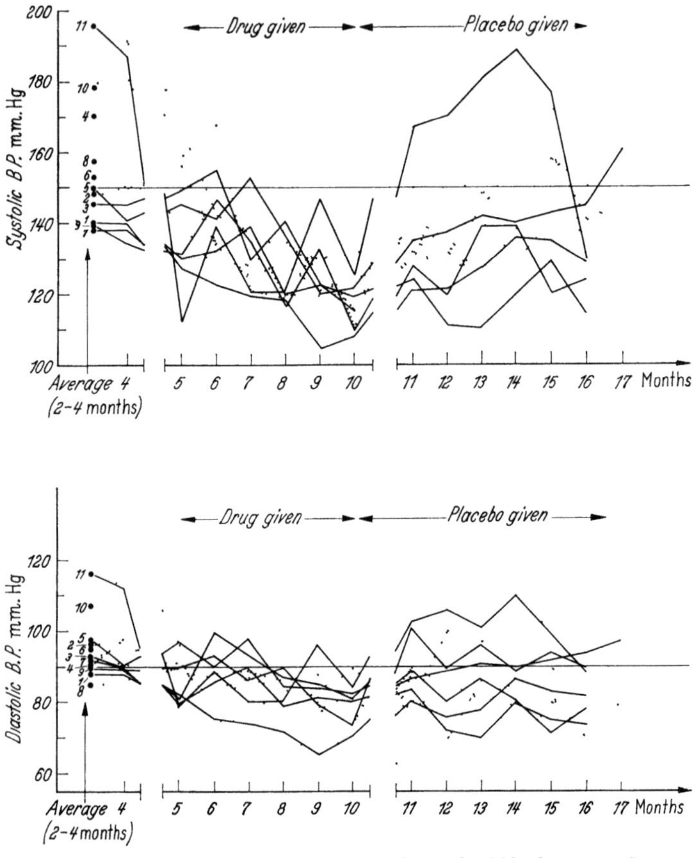

Fig. 1. Month-by-month effect of treatment on casual recumbent blood pressure. Group 1 — drug first.

whole declined, particularly in Group 1, with the result that those patients with the highest blood pressures showed the best response. In Table 1, the cases are arranged in descending order of initial systolic blood pressure; the column headed "change 1—2" shows a similar trend towards a decreasing drug effect. The same trend is apparent, though to a lesser extent, in Table 2 (the column headed "change 1—3"). In both instances, the ultimate effect of the treatment was to restore blood pressure to below the upper "normal" limit of 140/90 mm. Hg in all but one subject.

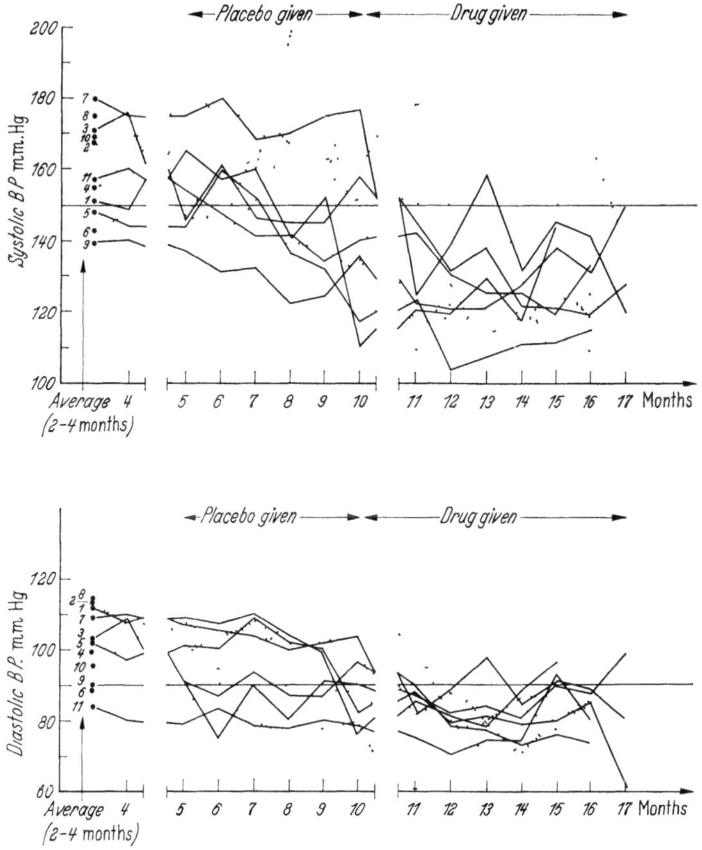

Fig. 2. Month-by-month effect of treatment on casual recumbent blood pressure. Group 2 — drug second.

Maximum blood-pressure reduction in response to the active drug was apparently not reached until the fourth month of treatment in the "drug first" group (Fig. 1). However, when the placebo was given first (Fig. 2), a slow decline over the first five months was also seen; further blood-pressure reduction, probably due

Table 1. *Effect of active drug and placebo on the blood-pressure level and its variability. Group 1 (drug first)*

Patient No.	Initial casual recumbent B.P. and changes in periods 2 and 3					Av. change in B.P.: casual recumbent to 20-min. rest			Av. change in B.P.: 3-min. standing to exercise		
	B.P.$_1$[1]	B.P.$_2$ (drug)	Change 1—2 (drug)	B.P.$_3$ (placebo)	Change 1—3	Period 1 mm. Hg	Period 2 mm. Hg (drug)	Period 3 mm. Hg (placebo)	Period 1 mm. Hg	Period 2 mm. Hg (drug)	Period 3 mm. Hg (placebo)
1	196/116	131/86	—65/—30	165/100	—31/—16	— 3/—1	—12/—4	—12/—5	+31/—29	+20/—17	+26/—20
2	178/107	120/78	—58/—29	177/103	— 1/— 4	— 2/+4	— 3/+1	—13/ 0	+68/—12	+33/—12	+59/—17
3	170/ 91	121/68	—49/—23	149/ 77	—21/—14	—11/—1	— 6/—1	— 8/—1	+70/—16	+44/— 8	+47/— 8
4	157/ 85	125/66	—32/—19	143/ 80	—14/— 5	— 6/+3	—10/+2	— 4/+1	+36/—26	+39/—11	+21/—28
5	151/ 92	132/83	—19/— 9	143/ 87	— 8/— 5	— 4/ 0	—11/—7	—11/—1	+66/—35	+38/—25	+55/—26
6	149/ 97	125/84	—24/—13	150/ 95	+ 1/— 2	— 3/ 0	— 4/+3	— 6/—2	+40/—11	+21/— 5	+21/—12
7	149/ 96	125/83	—24/—13	121/ 82	—28/—14	+ 1/+4	— 2/—1	0/+2	+33/— 3	+17/—13	+14/— 7
8	145/ 93	126/81	—19/—12	151/ 91	+ 6/— 2	0/—3	0/+4	— 7/+1	+54/— 3	+40/—10	+31/— 6
9	140/ 90	120/84	—20/— 6	127/ 77	—13/—13	—15/—5	— 1/—4	—11/+2	+41/—20	+29/—12	+40/—16
10	140/ 88	110/69	—30/—21	133/ 84	— 7/— 4	— 5/—2	— 4/—2	— 4/—2	+37/—19	+41/— 1	+51/—13
11	138/ 92	120/80	—18/—12	121/ 76	—17/—16	— 6/—7	—15/—9	— 9/—2	+42/—14	+19/—16	+21/—14
Mean	156/ 95	123/78	—33/—17	144/ 87	—12/—8	— 5/—1	— 6/—2	— 8/—1	+47/—17	+31/—12	+35/—15

[1] B.P.$_1$ = Average B.P. for each patient during 2nd to 4th months of observation.
B.P.$_2$ = Average B.P. during 8th to 10th months of observation.
B.P.$_3$ = Average B.P. during 14th to 16th months of observation.

Table 2. *Effect of active drug and placebo on the blood-pressure level and its variability. Group 2 (drug second)*

Patient No.	Initial casual recumbent B.P. and changes in periods 2 and 3					Av. change in B.P.: casual recumbent to 20-min. rest			Av. change in B.P.: 3-min. standing to exercise		
	B.P.₁[1]	B.P.₂ (placebo)	Change 1—2	B.P.₃ (drug)	Change 1—3 (drug)	Period 1 mm. Hg	Period 2 mm. Hg (placebo)	Period 3 mm. Hg (drug)	Period 1 mm. Hg	Period 2 mm. Hg (placebo)	Period 3 mm. Hg (drug)
12	180/109	159/ 95	—21/—14	135/87	—45/—22	—17/—1	—11/ 0	—13/— 1	+44/—10	+30/— 9	+40/—16
13	175/114	155/103	—20/—11	114/75	—61/—39	— 6/+1	— 4/—6	— 7/— 9	+40/— 4	+40/—13	+20/—20
14	171/104	149/ 91	—22/—13	122/78	—49/—26	— 7/—1	—10/—2	—13/— 2	+58/—11	+53/—20	+31/—11
15	170/ 93	168/ 92	— 2/— 1	152/82	—18/—11	— 8/—2	—12/—6	—12/— 4	+75/—26	+82/—30	+54/—26
16	168/113	155/102	—13/—11	114/86	—54/—27	— 1/ 0	— 3/ 0	— 1/— 2	+33/— 7	+40/— 4	+19/—10
17	157/ 84	138/ 79	—19/— 5	125/82	—32/— 2	—18/—4	— 6/—4	— 8/—13	+61/—26	+48/—18	+33/—22
18	156/112	151/104	— 5/— 8	130/87	—26/—25	— 1/—2	— 4/—1	—12/— 2	+66/—28	+53/—30	+ 8/—26
19	155/ 99	171/100	+16/+ 1	119/78	—36/—21	— 9/—2	—11/—3	— 5/— 5	+37/—14	+32/—15	+31/—26
20	148/101	128/ 95	—20/— 6	112/74	—36/—27	— 7/—1	— 4/+2	— 4/+ 1	+31/— 7	+29/— 2	+17/—20
21	143/ 88	149/ 78	+ 6/—10	130/71	—13/—17	— 6/—2	—23/ 0	—16/— 1	+52/—13	+39/—28	+42/—17
22	139/ 90	123/ 96	—16/+ 6	123/88	—16/— 2	— 3/+3	— 5/—8	+ 5/— 3	+23/—12	+25/—16	+19/—27
Mean	160/101	150/ 94	—10/— 7	125/81	—35/—20	— 8/—1	— 8/—3	— 8/— 3	+47/—14	+43/—17	+29/—20

[1] B.P.₁ = Average B.P. for each patient during 2nd to 4th months of observation.
B.P.₂ = Average B.P. during 8th to 10th months of observation.
B.P.₃ = Average B.P. during 14th to 16th months of observation.

solely to the active drug, was, on the other hand, completed within two months. The delayed response seen in Group 1 is therefore probably a result of the summation of a placebo effect, acting during the 4th to 10th months of treatment, and an additional component, due to the active drug and working chiefly in the first two months after the beginning of active-drug treatment.

Some further useful generalizations may be made. There were only four "non-responders" to drug treatment, i.e. patients who showed an average decline of less than 10 mm. Hg in diastolic blood pressure; most hypertensive patients, including five out of eight patients with an average pretreatment blood pressure below 150/100 mm. Hg, exhibited a greater decline in blood pressure in response to the drug than in response to placebo. Inter-individual variability of blood pressure from month to month was not altered by treatment, even if the usual level was reduced. Furthermore, we were able to detect a change in blood-pressure responsiveness during treatment in only one of the variability tests discussed below. One test, the decline in blood pressure from the casual recumbent to the 20-minute resting state, is illustrated in Tables 1 and 2. Perhaps we failed to demonstrate a difference because the variations in blood pressure were minimal.

In another test of variability, the post-exercise rise in systolic blood pressure, significantly reduced levels were recorded (Tables 1 and 2), whereas the diastolic change was unaffected. Despite these results, the apparent capacity for work performance (the task set was to step up 20 cm. every two seconds for three minutes) was not influenced.

With the exception of two patients who had transient symptoms suggestive of hypokalemia but were later able to tolerate a full dosage, none of the subjects felt poorly during the period of active-drug treatment. Casual questioning by the nurse and the examining physician did not reveal any of the characteristic side effects of thiazide or Rauwolfia. Electrocardiograms were recorded, and serum uric acid and electrolytes were determined in most subjects. Except for unimpressive changes in the expected direction, nothing unusual appeared. It must be remembered, however, that the patients were relatively young and in good health.

To detect possible effects of deserpidine on mood, the Clyde mood-scale was utilized. In this test, the patient selects cards which he believes reflect his current mood. The period during which deserpidine was taken was not apparent by any evidence of mental depression[1].

[1] We are indebted to Dr. DEAN CLYDE, University of Miami, for assistance in making this analysis.

Discussion

The observations reported above indicate that a simple combination of chlorthalidone and deserpidine effectively lowered the blood pressure in nearly all of a group of 22 patients with mild hypertension, often barely in excess of the critical level of 160/95 mm. Hg specified by the World Health Organization as the threshold for essential hypertension (*2*). A further, mild, placebo effect, which continued beyond the fourth month of placebo administration until the tenth month was also evident. Although the reduction was minimal (average 11/8 mm. Hg), this phenomenon obviously cannot be ignored in studies of the effects of chronic antihypertensive treatment. However, in addition to this response, the patients showed a further, clear-cut and sustained reduction in blood pressure of 23/11 mm. Hg, when the active drug was superimposed. In this type of patient, no side effects of consequence occurred. If these conclusions are supported in later studies, a treatment program of one tablet per day could be employed with relative impunity in large numbers of patients with early, mild hypertension.

Although blood-pressure levels are reduced, individual blood-pressure variability is not influenced. In this respect, our findings confirm those of Shapiro (*3*), who showed that neither reserpine nor thiazides materially affected the responsiveness to various pressor stimuli. We also agree with Shapiro's conclusion that prophylactic therapy of this kind would greatly reduce the likelihood that the blood pressure under stress would exceed a particular level. If, as is possible, the elevation of blood pressure above a critical point is sufficient to trigger a serious cerebrovascular disturbance, such prophylaxis would be useful. Clinical experience, particularly in a Negro community (*4*), suggests that an acute rise in pressure may create a focal or diffuse cerebral lesion, and this hypothesis is supported by experimental studies in animals (*5*). Therefore, in the treatment of young persons with mild hypertension who have had cerebral attacks in the past or have a marked familial susceptibility to cerebrovascular disease, a preventive-treatment program, such as the one outlined, may well prove helpful, even when the usual elevation of blood pressure is not impressive.

The only instance of alteration in cardiovascular responsiveness which could be demonstrated was a reduction in the peak systolic blood pressure immediately after exercise. The study carried out by Varnauskas et al. (*6*) has already demonstrated the influence of thiazides in diminishing the blood-pressure rise which follows exercise. Moreover, this study showed that, after graded physical exertion, the increase in cardiac output is less and the reduction in total peripheral resistance greater when the patient is receiving diuretic drugs. The net result is that when a subject under treatment is called upon to do heavy exercise, the increase in cardiac work is substantially reduced. Under these circumstances it is not surprising that our patients did not complain of inability to perform the exercise as effectively as before. This relative reduction in cardiac work has been postulated to play a role in the reduction in exercise angina observed when thiazides are administered (*1*). A similar reduction in cardiac work during exercise has been reported after the administration of guanethidine in the treatment of angina pectoris (*7*).

The response of the casual blood pressure to thiazides has been described by others and will not be reviewed here (*8*). We wish only to repeat the major observations: nearly every patient with mild hypertension treated with chlorthalidone and deserpidine exhibited some blood-pressure reduction, the extent being commensurate with the height of the initial pressure; the maximum response was observed by the second to third month; no resurgence of blood pressure was evident during the six-month period of drug treatment; a rise in blood pressure towards the previous level can generally be expected to take place within two months of the withdrawal of therapy; a slight placebo effect on blood pressure can be demonstrated between the fourth and tenth month of observation; no orthostatic gradient is created by the administration of either deserpidine or chlorthalidone.

The almost complete absence of side effects was unexpected. This probably would not have been the case in patients with more severe disease. Biochemical observations showed only minor deviations from the normal. We made no effort to limit the salt intake, and this may have prevented development of the more severe hypokalemia with its attendant weakness reported by others.

A simplified treatment can therefore be highly effective in persons with mild hypertension. Moreover, such a program can be applied in the treatment of people still at work and apparently otherwise in good health, without fear of causing drug-induced disability. Neither mental acuity nor the capacity to perform the usual physical tasks was impaired. Furthermore, if there is a direct correlation between the mean level of blood pressure and subsequent cardiovascular morbidity and mortality (*9*), and if this correlation is linear from 140/90 mm. Hg to much higher levels of blood pressure, then the value of treatment initiated at such a relatively low blood-pressure level in preventing the development of the late complications of hypertension may be just as great as that of treatment confined to patients with severe, established hypertension. A long period of observation will, of course, be required in order to establish a significant difference in morbidity and mortality rates. Nevertheless, SMIRK's recent observations (*10*) suggest that the survival rate over a five-year period in subjects with Grade I or Grade II hypertension is improved by treatment. The data provided by the double-blind studies conducted at the Veterans Administration Hospitals (*11*) likewise indicate that a substantial lowering of blood pressure leads to a decrease in mortality rate when a thiazide is used to treat hypertensive patients with a good prognosis. We therefore suggest, in view of the overall effectiveness of the regimen prescribed, that treatment of hypertension be extended, on an experimental basis only, to younger members of the population with less severe forms of the disease.

Summary

1. Twenty-two patients with very mild, uncomplicated hypertension (average blood pressure 161/102 mm. Hg) were observed at monthly intervals for 16 months. The casual blood pressure and its variability under different tests were determined regularly during a four-month initial placebo period, and a subsequent six-month trial of active drug (chlorthalidone 100 mg. and deserpidine 1.0 mg.), which was given first to half of the subjects, the other 11 patients receiving placebo during this period. The treatment programs were reversed after six months. Neither the patients nor the investigator were informed of the medication schedule, and there were no symptoms or side effects sufficient to indicate that active drug was being given.

2. After two months' treatment with active drug, the blood pressure had fallen in all cases (mean reduction 33/17 mm. Hg). Those treated with placebo showed a reduction of 10/7 mm. Hg during the same period. When the placebo group received active drug during the second six-month period, a further drop of 25/13 mm. Hg was observed. We therefore conclude that in the prolonged follow-up of hypertensive patients, a small placebo effect may be evident between the 4th and 10th month of observation, but that a uniform and substantial blood-pressure reduction, averaging approximately 20/10 mm. Hg, occurs in nearly all subjects receiving a Rauwolfia-thiazide combination.

3. Changes in blood-pressure variability were not generally observed. However, because of the lower starting point, peak blood pressures after pressor tests were considerably reduced. Furthermore, a substantial reduction of about 17 mm. Hg in the rise in systolic pressure brought on by exercise was observed. Consequently, it may be presumed that the peak blood-pressure levels reached in mildly hypertensive patients, particularly after exercise and to a lesser extent after the usual stresses, can be lowered by treatment. The relationship between such prophylactic therapy and subsequent cardiovascular and cerebrovascular morbidity is discussed.

Zusammenfassung

1. Zweiundzwanzig Patienten mit leichter, unkomplizierter Hypertonie (mittlerer Blutdruck 161/102 mm Hg) wurden in monatlichen Zeitabständen während 16 Monaten untersucht. Der unter üblichen Bedingungen gemessene Blutdruck sowie seine Veränderungen unter verschiedenen Testanordnungen wurden regelmäßig während einer anfänglichen viermonatigen Placeboperiode und anschließend während einer sechs Monate langen Periode aktiver Behandlung (100 mg Chlorthalidon und 1 mg Deserpidin täglich) verfolgt. Die Medikamente wurden zuerst der Hälfte der Patienten gegeben; die anderen 11 erhielten während dieser Zeit Placebos. Die Behandlungsprogramme wurden nach sechs Monaten ausgetauscht. Weder die Patienten noch der Untersucher waren über das Behandlungsschema informiert, und es traten weder Symptome noch Nebenwirkungen auf, die Hinweise für die Verabreichung der aktiven Substanzen gegeben hätten.

2. Nach einer zweimonatigen Behandlung mit den aktiven Substanzen war der Blutdruck in allen Fällen abgesunken (mittlere Senkung 33/17 mm Hg). Die mit Placebos behandelten Patienten zeigten während derselben Zeitspanne eine Reduktion um 10/7 mm Hg. Erhielt die Placebogruppe während der zweiten Sechsmonatsperiode die beiden Medikamente, so ergab sich ein weiterer Druckabfall um 25/13 mm Hg. Wir schließen daraus, daß bei der langzeitigen Verfolgung von Hochdruckpatienten zwar ein geringer Placebo-Effekt zwischen dem vierten und zehnten Beobachtungsmonat nachweisbar sein kann, daß aber eine einheitliche und deutliche Blutdrucksenkung von durchschnittlich 20/10 mm Hg bei nahezu allen Patienten auftritt, die eine Rauwolfia-Thiazid Kombination erhalten.

3. Änderungen in den Blutdruckschwankungen wurden im allgemeinen nicht beobachtet. Auf Grund des niedrigeren Ausgangswertes war jedoch der maximale Blutdruckanstieg nach den Pressortests beträchtlich vermindert. Weiterhin fand sich eine deutliche Reduktion von etwa 17 mm Hg des systolischen Druckanstieges infolge körperlicher Belastung. Es kann somit angenommen werden, daß die Blutdruckspitzen, die leicht hypertone Patienten, besonders nach körperlicher Tätigkeit und in einem geringeren Maße nach den üblichen Belastungen, erreichen, durch die Behandlung vermindert werden. Die Beziehungen zwischen einer derartigen prophylaktischen Behandlung und der späteren cardiovaskulären und cerebrovaskulären Morbidität werden besprochen.

Résumé

1. Vingt-deux malades présentant une hypertension très modérée et sans complication (tension artérielle moyenne à 161/102 mm Hg) ont été suivis pendant 16 mois à intervalles d'un mois. Les variations spontanées de la pression artérielle et les variations provoquées par différents tests ont été déterminées régulièrement tout d'abord pendant une période initiale de quatre mois de prescription d'un placébo, puis pendant une période consécutive de six mois de prescription d'un produit actif (100 mg chlorthalidone et 1 mg déserpidine), cette médication active ayant d'abord été administrée à la moitié des sujets, l'autre moitié recevant le placébo, et ces traitements ayant ensuite été croisés au bout de six mois. Ni les malades ni l'expérimentateur n'étaient au courant du schéma de traitement, et aucun symptôme ni effet secondaire n'a été suffisant pour permettre l'identification du produit actif.

2. Après deux mois de traitement avec le produit actif, la pression artérielle avait diminué dans tous les cas (diminution moyenne de 33/17 mm

Hg). Les malades traités par le placébo ont montré une réduction de 10/7 mm Hg au cours de la même période. Lorsque le groupe soumis au placébo a reçu le produit actif pendant la deuxième période de six mois, une baisse supplémentaire de 25/13 mm Hg a été observée. Nous pouvons donc conclure que dans le traitement au long cours de l'hypertension un léger effet placébo peut se manifester entre le quatrième et le dixième mois, mais qu'une baisse de pression artérielle appréciable, d'environ 20/10 mm Hg en moyenne, survient dans la presque totalité des cas soumis à l'association Rauwolfia-thiazide.

3. Des modifications dans la variabilité de la tension artérielle n'ont généralement pas été observées. Cependant, en raison des valeurs de départ plus basses, les élévations de pression artérielle au cours de tests vasopresseurs ont été considérablement atténuées. De plus, on a observé une réduction notable, d'environ 17 mm Hg, de l'élévation de la pression systolique à l'effort. En conséquence, on peut admettre que les bouffées hypertensives se produisant chez les malades porteurs d'une hypertension légère, en particulier après effort et, à un moindre degré, après les "stresses", peuvent être diminuées par le traitement. On discute enfin l'incidence d'un tel traitement prophylactique sur la morbidité vasculaire cardiaque et cérébrale.

Acknowledgements

We wish to acknowledge the services of Mrs. Freda Fick, without whose assistance this study could not have been completed. For the statistical analysis, we express our indebtedness to Miss Martha Sommerfeld and Miss Judy Bean. We are grateful for the assistance of the Wayne County Hospital and Health Department, where the observations were made, for the statistical service provided by the Department of Biostatistics, University of Michigan School of Public Health, and for the consultant services of the Department of Internal Medicine, University of Michigan, Ann Arbor, Mich.

References

1. Hoobler, S. W., and L. Ruiz: Amer. Practitioner **13**, 373 (1962). — 2. Hypertension and Coronary Heart Disease: Classification and Criteria for Epidemiological Studies. First Report of the Expert Committee on Cardiovascular Disease and Hypertension. World Health Org. Techn. Rep. Ser., No. 168, Geneva (1959). — 3. Shapiro, A. P.: Circulation **26**, 242 (1962). — 4. Moser, M., R. Morgan, M. Hale, S. W. Hoobler, R. D. Remington, H. Dodge, and A. Macaulay: Amer. J. Cardiol. **4**, 727 (1959). — 5. Byrom, F. B.: Lancet 1954/II, 201. — 6. Varnauskas, E., G. Cramer, R. Malmcrona, and L. Werkö: Clin. Sc. **20**, 407 (1961). — 7. Georgopoulus, A. J., F. M. Sones, Jr., and I. H. Page: Circulation **23**, 892 (1961). — 8. Rosenbloom, S. E., R. P. Shapera, R. S. Goldbloom, J. Pincus, and A. P. Shapiro: N. England. J. Med. **264**, 164 (1961). — 9. Society of Actuaries: Build and Blood Pressure Study. Peter F. Mallon, Inc., Long Island City, N. Y., 1959, Vol. 1, p. 122. — 10. Smirk, F. H.: N. Zealand Med. J. **63**, 413 (1964).— 11. Veterans Administration Cooperative Study on Antihypertensive Agents: Arch. Int. Med. **110**, 222 (1962).

Discussion

Dengler: With regard to these blood-pressure variations, I should like to mention some biochemical findings that we made in a particular group of hypertensive patients. Most of them were admitted to the hospital for exclusion of phaeochromocytoma, since they had had hypertensive attacks superimposed on their elevated basal blood pressure. The urinary noradrenaline excretion was determined daily. During the first few days after admission to the hospital the noradrenaline values were increased up to 100 to 120 μg. per day, so that the possibility of a phaeochromocytoma could not be excluded. Later on, they gradually dropped and finally approached so-called normal values. At the same time, the hypertensive attacks became less frequent, and the casual blood pressures became lower but not normal. During this period, the patients were confined to bed for part of the time; no drugs were administered. Perhaps I should add that this particular group of hypertensive patients consisted mainly of women in or shortly after the menopause.

As regards the study of urinary catecholamine excretion in primary hypertension, there are two different types of approach. We can compare the urinary output of noradrenaline in a population of hypertensive patients with that in normotensives. As you all know, this statistical approach yields no clear-cut differences, since only about 15% of hypertensive subjects have an elevated urinary noradrenaline excretion. But if, on the other hand, we do a sort of follow-up study on individual hypertensive patients, we can observe — at least in the cases I was referring to — a correlation between blood-pressure variations and noradrenaline excretion. It would be most interesting to learn more about other characteristics of this group of patients.

Cottier: Dr. Hoobler, did you give potassium to your patients; if not, did you observe any hypokalaemia in this group of very mild hypertensives? It is important to know this when submitting mild hypertensives to such prolonged hypotensive therapy with saluretics.

Brod: Dr. Hoobler, do you still give a sphygmomanometer to your patients to take their blood pressures at home? If I remember correctly, you and Dr. Freis were trying this about five years ago and were talking about the advantages of this procedure at the Symposium in Berne[1].

Peart: I am very interested in the statement that there is a considerable variation in the noradrenaline output in the urine of people with hypertension. I was wondering whether we could know the method you adopted for measuring the noradrenaline. Using biological assay I investigated people with hypertension for years, and, as in the normal, the range is very wide if you measure the pressor amine in the urine. I think one has to be very careful as to what one is measuring in the urine. I therefore wonder whether you are using a biochemical method or biological method. Those employing methods involving measurement of metabolic products of both noradrenaline

[1] Essential Hypertension. An International Symposium. Ed. by K. D. Bock and P. T. Cottier. Springer, Berlin, 1960, p. 300.

and adrenaline do not report an increase in people with hypertension of any sort.

Dengler: We used a trihydroxyindole method after absorbing the catecholamines on alumina.

Taquini: As I reported yesterday, we have found that 25% of the hypertensive patients show an increase in urinary excretion of catecholamines — mean value 159 μg. per 24 hours; the other 75% have a normal range of excretion.

Cranston: A small practical point: I should like to ask Dr. Hoobler whether he has any evidence about the reliability with which people take tablets twice a week as opposed to once a day. We often find that people forget more frequently. Do you find this?

Page: I wonder whether it is true that the fall in blood pressure with antihypertensive drugs in all patients is directly proportional to the height of the arterial pressure. It might even be the percentage fall rather than the absolute fall. At the back of this lies a concept — I do not know whether it is true or not — implying that the mechanisms maintaining hypertension are always the same. I suggest that this is a soluble problem, but let's first get more factual data on a variety of patients.

It has been said that the arterial pressure of patients with malignant hypertension is more difficult to lower than that of patients with essential hypertension. Again I know of no quantitative studies to prove this. This is all in line with my trying to persuade you to discuss and define new mechanisms among the great miscellaneous group we call essential hypertensives.

I am personally convinced that the response of patients to such treatments as strict low-salt diets varies so much as almost to suggest different diseases. Many of us are still aware that hypertension from renal stenotic lesions was not recognised by bedside methods, even when the latter were most carefully applied. Remember that the mosaic characterising the many possible mechanisms of hypertensive disease may find many applications in human beings suffering from hypertension.

Hoobler: In reply to Dr. Cottier's question, we did measure the potassium levels. The reductions were relatively small, 0.2—0.4 mEq./l. We did not give potassium supplements. The point of the whole regimen was to make it as simple as possible for the patient. We did not restrict salt either, during this programme of treatment. This may be the reason that potassium did not fall as much.

I agree with the comment that it's a lot easier to remember to take a tablet once a day than twice a week. I don't know how to get around that difficulty, but if there is any potential toxicity — I don't think anybody has discovered it yet — then naturally it would be better for a mild hypertensive to take less of the drug.

In response to Dr. Brod's question, we are still very much interested in home blood-pressure readings. We did, in fact, try the method in this population, but I wasn't the one that talked to the patients, and the nurse wasn't familiar with the technique, so it did not work out well. But a great many of our current studies are being conducted employing the home blood-pressure measurement technique, which has the enormous advantage that many readings may be made each week, so that an occasional error gets lost among something like 28 weekly blood-pressure readings. You can very quickly arrive at statistically significant information, if you believe that the blood-pressure readings made by the patients are correct, which I personally do.

I should like to comment on Dr. PAGE's point. I think some of these patients were so near normotensive that on the basis of a single casual reading one might almost say they were normotensive. Yet in most instances, in fact in all instances, they showed a substantial blood-pressure reduction, although this was not so great when the pressures were in the lower range. There was no clear-cut relationship, just a general tendency for the fall to be greater when the initial pressure was high. The point I am making is that I have often thought we should review the concept that a normotensive's pressure doesn't drop at all in response to thiazides, as I think Dr. FREIS claimed originally, and I'm not sure whether his study has ever been repeated. I suspect that you would find that in people with pressures of 130/80 mm. Hg the level would drop by a little bit less, but would nonetheless drop, and percentagewise the reduction would perhaps be the same. My conclusion is the opposite of Dr. PAGE's; I believe that everybody shows some blood-pressure reduction in response to a diuretic programme. I am opposed to the view that one type of hypertensive will respond to thiazides and another will not.

FREIS: I agree with Dr. HOOBLER. We also found reductions in blood pressure after chlorothiazide in patients who were only slightly hypertensive. Lack of reduction in mean arterial pressure was found in completely normotensive young or early-middle-aged adults who were free from any evident cardiovascular disease.

In regard to Dr. PAGE's question, co-operative study results did show that the reduction was approximately percentagewise when we took the means of large numbers of patients, but there were tremendous individual variations. These are due to a number of causes. In our clinic group we find that some pressures do not fall, because the patients are not taking their tablets. When we put them into hospital and give them the same dose, they respond. Then we find that other patients who are put into hospital and given their usual dosage don't show a fall, although they are taking their tablets properly. Among these patients, however, I cannot detect any characteristics which differentiate them from others.

Introduction to the General Discussion

By

J. Brod

In introducing the discussion on general principles in antihypertensive treatment, I should like to touch upon two points. The first concerns the need for an exact diagnosis of the pathological basis of hypertension. It is obvious that coarctation of the aorta and the various well-defined endocrinological disorders call for the use of a specific therapeutic approach which is beyond the scope of the present discussion. These are rarities compared with hypertension of renal origin, including renovascular hypertension, and with essential hypertension. In the great majority of cases, it is possible to differentiate these by relatively simple laboratory means which were discussed at a W.H.O. meeting of experts in 1961 and published in a W.H.O. pamphlet (*1*).

There is no doubt that even hypertension of renal origin can be brought under control with the aid of modern antihypertensive therapy (Fig. 1). There are, however, important differences between renal and essential hypertension which have to be kept in mind. In essential hypertension the kidneys are, at least at the beginning, morphologically intact, and the changes in renal blood flow and other parameters have a functional basis. This can be normalised by a well-chosen therapy, so that the fall in blood pressure does not induce a reduction but may even increase the renal blood flow. The situation is slightly more complicated in the late phases of the disease, in which there is a marked organic reduction of the renal vascular bed by nephrosclerosis, especially in cases of malignant hypertension. Here, lowering of the high blood pressure may further diminish the low renal blood flow and glomerular filtration rate and may precipitate the development of uraemia. Although in cases of malignant hypertension this might be unavoidable for the sake of arresting the malignant course of the disease and might even necessitate temporary peritoneal dialysis, it is certainly an undesirable complication of the treatment of hypertension in patients suffering from primary renal disease with a partial obliteration of the renal vascular tree. The slight decrease in renal function due to hypotensive agents in patients whose glomerular filtration rate has been restricted to levels above 40—50 ml./min. is of no practical significance, but might constitute a serious danger in patients who are on the verge of chronic renal failure (filtration rates below 30 ml./min.).

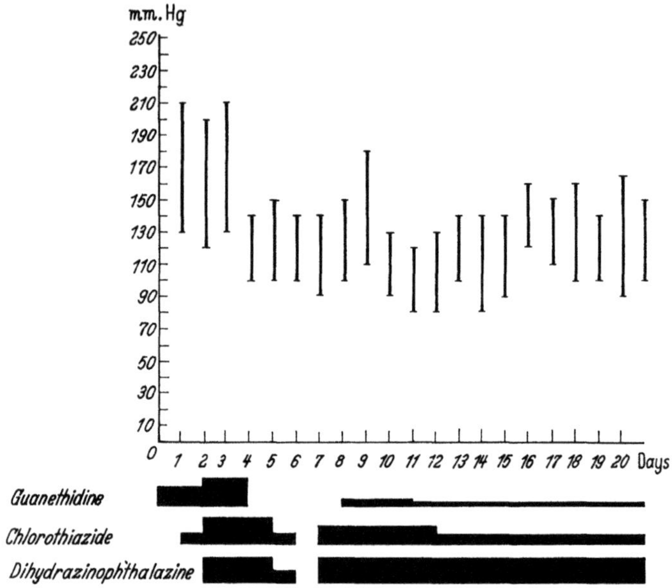

Fig. 1. Therapeutic effect of antihypertensive drugs in a case of renovascular hypertension.

It seems that this danger is greatest (even if transient) with the sympathetic blockers, whereas it is probably absent with Rauwolfia extracts (reserpine), and hydrazinophthalazines are even said to have a vasodilator effect in the kidneys (*2*). These are, therefore, the agents of choice in patients with severe degrees of hypertension of renal origin. Moderate hypertension of renal disease we prefer to leave untreated, and even in severe hypertension our therapy does not aim at a full normalisation of blood pressure, for the reasons stated above. It is obvious that frequent tests of renal function (endogenous creatinine clearance) are necessary in the course of the treatment before blood pressure is properly controlled.

My second point concerns the general management of patients with essential hypertension. Even if its aetiology and pathogenesis remain — in spite of extensive experimental work in numerous laboratories — an unsolved problem, and even if it is true that the ultimate prognosis depends much more on the basal than on the casual pressure levels (influenced, no doubt, by environmental factors), extensive clinical experience amplifies the fact that adverse environmental factors affecting the individual through the central nervous system — i.e. factors causing dissatisfaction, tension, anxiety, fear, anger or uncertainty, difficult situations, emotional conflicts, etc. — may be connected with the appearance or accentuation of symptoms known to accompany hypertension and may even lead to acute catastrophes. The reverse is equally true. Numerous examples of normalisation of blood pressure and disappearance of symptoms after the solution of individual problems are known from the literature (*3*) and have probably been encountered by each of us in his clinical practice. Moreover, the well-known spontaneous lowering and even normalisation of the blood pressure in many hypertensive subjects during the first days of hospitalisation, without any particular treatment or enforced bed-rest, is probably due to the removal of the subject from a stressful domestic or occupational atmosphere (Fig. 2).

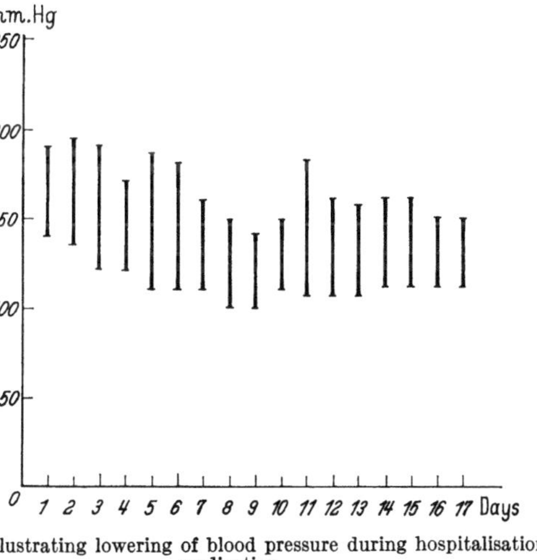

Fig. 2. Example illustrating lowering of blood pressure during hospitalisation without any medication.

All this emphasises the necessity of the regularisation of life in all subjects with essential hypertension — a point which occasionally tends to be forgotten now that potent hypotensive drugs are available. Probably the unquestionably beneficial effect of treatment in the various spas is also based on the influence of a favourable change of the patient's environment much more than on the vasodilating effect of the carbon dioxide bath, which acts only very transiently. Proper controls are missing in practically all studies dealing with this form of balneotherapy and attributing the effect to carbon dioxide. Attempts to replace the visit to a spa by a carbon dioxide bath twice or three times a week in the evening, after the patient has finished his regular day's work, are therefore valueless.

Claims that treatment involving protracted sleep, for a period of two to three weeks, could cure the basic disorder in essential hypertension and permanently normalise blood pressure could not be substantiated by a well-controlled investigation in our institute (*4*), and this form of therapy has now been almost generally abandoned.

There is no evidence that physical work is harmful, unless symptoms and signs of a severely damaged cardiovascular system are present; and regular, mild physical exercise or sport has been reported to have beneficial effects with regard to blood pressure and symptoms (*5*). This is also important as a means of preventing obesity, which was asserted by several participants at the Chicago Symposium on the Epidemiology of Hypertension in 1964 to be somehow connected with hypertension. Even if this point is still unsettled, and there are voices to the contrary, it seems certain that for a heart already overburdened by hypertension any additional overload due to excess weight is undesirable. Moderation in dietary habits is, therefore, equally important.

Experimental reasons for salt restriction, a procedure favoured by many clinicians since the beginning of the century (*6*), have been provided in recent years by PERERA and BLOOD (*7*), DAHL (*8*, *9*), MENEELY (*10*), and others, and this line of therapy has reached its extreme in KEMPNER's (*11*) rice-diet. We have never been much in favour of this therapeutic approach, which presupposes some masochistic traits on the part of the patient, and there is no doubt that we can obtain today at least the same benefit from modern oral saluretic agents without spoiling the patient's life by prescribing an unpalatable diet.

There seems to be no reason to forbid the patient small quantities of beer or wine, and there are also no grounds why he should not be allowed an occasional cup of black coffee (which is even recommended by ZÁRDAY (*12*) on the strength of its assumed coronary vasodilating effect). Although smoking has not been found to aggravate the degree of hypertension, its unquestionable connection with vascular disease makes great moderation or complete abstinence recommendable in hypertension, which in itself enhances the development of atherosclerosis.

Two final remarks: except in cases in which severe vascular changes interfere with the blood supply to organs, we are always aiming at a normalisation of blood pressure. With patience, careful and slow increase in the dosage of the individual drugs, and frequent medical check-up, this is possible in the majority of patients without causing undue side effects. In most cases, the routine prescription of one tablet of reserpine t.d.s. is valueless and a sheer waste of money. The second mistake, which is equally frequent, is to discontinue therapy the moment blood pressure has been brought under control by a carefully built up therapeutic combination of various agents. Generally, the blood pressure very soon returns to its original level, and the patient is back where he started several weeks previously.

References

1. Arterial hypertension and ischaemic heart disease. World Health Org. Techn. Rep. Ser., No. 231, Geneva (1962). — 2. Reubi, F. C.: Proc. Soc. Exper. Biol. Med. **73**, 102 (1950). — 3. Wolf, S., P. V. Cardona, Jr., E. M. Shepard, and H. G. Wolff: Life stress and essential hypertension. A study of circulatory adjustments in man. Williams and Wilkins, Baltimore, 1955. — 4. Ehrlich, V., and Z. Harantová: Čas. lék. česk. **94**, 247 (1955). — 5. Adamírová, J., I. Kopšík, and A. J. Chrástek: Tělových. sbor. **4**, 309 (1959). — 6. Ambard, L., and E. Beaujard: Arch. gén. méd. **1**, 520 (1904). — 7. Perera, G. A., and D. W. Blood: J. Clin. Invest. **26**, 1109 (1947). — 8. Dahl, L. K.: In: Essential Hypertension. An International Symposium. Ed. by K. D. Bock and P. T. Cottier. Springer, Berlin, 1960, p. 53. — 9. Dahl, L. K.: Presented at the Symposium on Epidemiology in Cardiovascular Disease. Chicago, 1964. — 10. Meneely, G.: Presented at the Symposium on Epidemiology in Cardiovascular Disease. Chicago, 1964. — 11. Kempner, W.: Amer. J. Med. **4**, 545 (1948). — 12. Zárday, I.: Praktische Kardiologie. Steinkopff. Dresden, 1964.

General Discussion

Kincaid-Smith: I should like to enlarge on the question of the investigation and treatment of patients with renal hypertension in whom the blood urea is raised. The diagnosis of the underlying disease is of great importance, and something which hasn't been mentioned this morning is the question of underlying renal vascular disease. We feel that, in this group, uraemia may sometimes be an even better indication for renovascular surgery than hypertension. We have seen definite improvement in renal function resulting from renovascular surgery.

In other hypertensive patients with high blood ureas, we found renal biopsy of great value. One may detect, for example, a curable form of renal hypertension, such as nephrocalcinosis, in a few patients. On the other hand, one may detect severe vascular changes, due to malignant hypertension, of such a degree that one can predict that even with treatment the patient will become uraemic and die. In addition, one may find a whole variety of other underlying renal lesions which require different methods of treatment and in which the prognosis differs.

Lee: The comments made by Dr. Page during this morning's discussion seem to "mosaic" with some made by others. You referred to the basal blood pressure, Dr. Brod, and we certainly have to have some base-line as a reference for judgement of therapy. But the thought has occurred to some that there may be hypertensive patients in whom the peak blood pressure is more important than the basal blood pressure. Hypertension is marked by lability, and more than half of the cerebrovascular accidents we have observed have occurred in patients with labile hypertension at peak blood pressures and, moreover, at blood-pressure elevations that others tolerate as a steady level with ease. For example, in one person with a blood pressure of 170/110 mm. Hg, a sudden rise in pressure to 200/120 mm. Hg may cause a stroke, yet there are thousands with the latter blood pressure who have no real problems. It may therefore be crucial to evaluate spontaneous variations in hypertension — especially the highest peak levels attained — in determining which patients should be treated. Few people spend their waking hours at the "basal pressure" already described in the literature.

Page: There is one other aspect of treatment which ought to be seriously considered, and that is the problem of renal transplantation. The transplant of a kidney into a patient with malignant hypertension of renal origin has been followed by severe damage to the normal, transplanted kidney, suggesting that there is something about malignant hypertension itself which is damaging to the kidney. Everybody should be alert to the problem of whether, if we make a transplant in a patient with chronic nephritis and/or malignant hypertension, the kidney will be damaged by the original disease process.

Hood: I should like to ask Dr. Page about this implanted kidney. Were the damaged kidneys left in the patient after transplantation, and what was the pressure?

PAGE: The subjects I referred to were JOHN MERRILL's patients, with whom you are familiar.

WILSON: I think MERRILL showed quite clearly that the development of a malignant change was associated with a state of overhydration in the patient; when he was able to reduce this, the patient no longer had hypertensive encephalopathy, and heart failure also was relieved.

PAGE: Yes, but we are concerned with the vascular lesions themselves. Dr. DUSTAN and I recently published a paper[1] describing the effects of changing blood volume on blood pressure in patients without kidneys. When renal transplants were made, the close relationship immediately disappeared. In short, good kidneys make people relatively independent of blood volume, as this is related to blood pressure. If the height of the blood pressure is related to the vascular lesions, then reducing it could reduce vascular damage.

PICKERING: May I return to this morning's subject? And may I make general comments and ask two questions? — I should like to congratulate the people who have done the work presented this morning. This is an extremely difficult and extremely complicated field, and I think the amount of thought that they have given to the design of their experiments and to the accuracy and reliability of their measurements is wholly admirable. We shall soon, I'm sure, have facts on which we can base our opinion, rather than hunches or clinical impressions; and that, I think, is a good thing.

My first question will make me the most unpopular man at this conference, if I am not that already. It is this: can anybody tell me whether there is a good reason why we should go on calling the complications that happen in the vessels with elevated arterial pressure either arteriosclerotic or atherosclerotic? The function of a technical term is to convey an idea precisely. I am not sure what idea these convey. The common use, for example, of atherosclerosis is to describe a common disease of the intima of large arteries, associated with plaque formation and thrombi, and that is a quite specific disease. But there are two other common diseases of arteries in hypertension which are totally different. One is the cerebral micro-aneurysms which affect a different order of size of vessel and a different coat and produce an aneurysm rather than a stenosis; clearly a totally different disease. The other comprises the variety of vascular lesions occurring in the kidney, of which fibrinoid necrosis is, of course, by far the most important. I think that if we are going to talk about these in one breath, we ought to call them vascular or arterial, but not arteriosclerotic or atherosclerotic, because there is no unity in these three diseases. My second question is: can anybody here distinguish between a cerebral thrombosis and a cerebral haemorrhage? I used to think I could, but now I am absolutely certain that I cannot without angiography.

DEMING: I agree that the terms atherosclerosis and arteriosclerosis lack the precision they pretend to have, for me and for most clinicians, although some pathologists think that they know what the terms mean. What I should like to raise a question about is Dr. PICKERING's assertion that because the lesion looks different, and particularly because it occurs in a vessel of a different size, we should necessarily assume that it is a different lesion. I am interested, as I think he is, in how the lesion begins. That it will look different is, I think, inevitable. If we look at a lesion in the arch of the aorta and at

[1] DUSTAN, H. P., and I. H. PAGE: J. Laborat. Clin. Med. **64**, 948 (1964).

one in an arteriole, they must be different. The vessels themselves are different, but I don't feel confident in the statement that, because an aneurysm occurs in a small vessel, it must have a different aetiology from a stenosis occurring in a large vessel. We see aneurysms with atheroma, we see stenoses with atheroma. The question is: what started the lesion in the intima of the vessel? I am not insisting that it is the same, I am simply raising this point because I don't feel quite sure that it's different because the vessels are of a different size. I am not certain that large-vessel atheroma, arteriolosclerosis, or aneurysms in small cerebral vessels necessarily have a different pathogenesis.

Hood: To elaborate on the point raised by Dr. Deming, we could, for instance, say this: in vascular disease in diabetic patients we have been accustomed to looking at the small vessels, whether in the peripheral nerves, in the stomach, in the joints, in the eyes, or in the kidney. But if we care to look for the deposits in the aorta we shall find them, in some individuals at least. The biochemical change is more or less the same, but the anatomical change may differ according to the part of the vessel wall in which the deposits occur; and the symptoms provoked vary greatly. Dr. Pickering, the other day, actually drew our attention to the vast difference in the results of an anatomical alteration in provoking symptoms in the brain as compared with less sensitive and thus more silent areas.

Smirk: I agree entirely, from a functional standpoint, with Dr. Pickering in regard to his criticism of the term atherosclerosis. Admittedly, I use it myself. Functionally, there seems to be a remarkable difference between the coronary arteries and the cerebral vessels. If we compare the experience in the United States with that in Japan and, I understand, China also, we find that the incidence of cerebral vascular accidents and the incidence of coronary disease vary remarkably. Furthermore, in hypertensives, treatment affects the incidence of these two conditions in a very different way. So it is perhaps better not to rely entirely upon the difference in structure between the responsible lesions in cerebral or coronary vessels. It may be pointed out that there is also a difference in behaviour, and this is supported by the difference in function.

With regard to the remarks that Dr. Page made about malignant hypertension, I am sure he has encountered many more patients than I have who are irresponsive even to very large doses of drugs such as hexamethonium. And perhaps I might refer him to his own work with nitroprusside and also to some work which was done by Black et al.[1] on the use of sodium azide. Now, we have encountered a number of patients with malignant hypertension and severe hypertensive crises of various types whose blood pressures resist very large, indeed frightening, doses of hexamethonium. But blood pressure in those patients comes down perfectly well with sublingual sodium azide and also, as I am sure Dr. Page knows from his wide personal experience, with nitroprusside given intravenously or even by mouth.

Peart: I should like to come back to the remarks that Dr. Page made about the possibility that a transplanted kidney may somehow be destroyed in patients with malignant hypertension. Considering Scribner's original work on chronic haemodialysis and recent experience in transplanting normal kidneys from cadavers and other sources, I should regard the presence of

---

[1] Black, M. M., B. W. Zweifach, and F. D. Speer: Proc. Soc. Exper. Biol. Med. **85**, 11 (1954).

malignant hypertension in the prospective transplantee as an indication for removing the kidneys if I could not control the blood pressure with drugs or by dialysis so as to reduce the circulating blood volume. In some of the patients in whom we have reduced the blood volume we failed to control the blood pressure. It is most people's experience that with nephrectomy in patients with malignant hypertension the blood pressure will come down. It does not necessarily come down from one day to the next, but it will come down within a week. And I think one must not forget that in transplanting a kidney from any source that kidney itself is liable to vascular disease by an immunological process. Therefore one cannot simply say that damage to the kidney following transplantation is somehow related to hypertension; I feel fairly certain that it is much more closely related to an immunological process.

KINCAID-SMITH: I should like both to agree and disagree with what Dr. PEART said about the malignant hypertension and renal transplantation. We have not found that bilateral nephrectomy invariably reduces the blood pressure in patients with malignant hypertension. However, it does seem to make them more sensitive to reduction of the blood pressure by manipulation of the salt and water intake, although they do not appear to be more sensitive to hypotensive drugs. As far as the vascular lesions which develop in transplants are concerned, having studied repeated biopsies from renal transplants, I am quite sure that the vascular lesions represent immunological damage, as Dr. PEART has said, and not hypertensive damage. They may appear when the blood pressure is low and occur in relation to rejection phenomena rather than to episodes of hypertension. They also occur in patients who have not had malignant hypertension previously. Histologically, however, the vessel changes may be quite indistinguishable from those of malignant hypertension.

CRANSTON: May I go back to another point that Dr. PAGE made? This concerns the relationship between the control blood pressure and the fall of blood pressure, and the question whether there is a percentage change or not. With the methods we have used I have no doubt that it is not a percentage change, because if this were so, you would expect to find a relationship between the control blood pressure and the fall of blood pressure, to be expressed by a regression line going through zero. Now this is not so. The regression line crosses the abscissa at a diastolic pressure somewhere between 80 and 100 mm. Hg.

PETERS: A relationship between blood urea concentrations and prognosis has been mentioned several times this morning. Nobody would think that urea concentration in body fluids had any direct influence on the fate of the patients: measuring blood urea is simply a short and admittedly imperfect way of estimating the glomerular filtration rate. Thiazide diuretics *reversibly* depress glomerular filtration rate and, to an even greater extent, the clearance of urea in normal animals as well as in those with reduced glomerular filtration. If the same applies to patients with renal disease, the blood urea concentrations in patients treated with these drugs will tend to exaggerate the degree of renal failure present. The functional state of the kidneys should, therefore, be assessed by repeated measurement of glomerular filtration rate after diuretic therapy has been interrupted for a few days. Alternatively, one may try to find another simple test that is not influenced by the thiazides. Furosemide and ethacrynic acid may not depress glomerular filtration rate or urea excretion.

Taquini: Patients with essential hypertension in whom renal failure occurs are different from those with pyelonephritis. Renal failure in association with essential hypertension is characterised by generalised disease of the kidney: all the units are involved. In pyelonephritis, many units maintain normal function, even in the presence of severe renal failure. This explains, in part at least, the difference in the evolution between the two groups.

Brod: As to the comment by Dr. Taquini, in the last few months we have studied the problem of very low glomerular filtration rates in patients with pyelonephritis. Histologically, these cases differ very markedly from glomerulonephritis or severe vascular nephrosclerosis. In the last two categories the glomeruli are destroyed at this stage of functional reduction. The pyelonephritic patient with a filtration rate of 2 or 3 ml. and severe uraemia still has very many glomeruli which look perfectly normal. It seems that the drop in filtration rate in these patients has a vascular basis and that it is due to compression of vessels bringing blood to the glomeruli, and probably also partly to the obstruction of some of the nephrons.

Hoobler: Dr. Peters, would you consider the procedure I use in distinguishing renal deterioration under conditions of thiazide therapy valid? This is a simple 15-minute phenolsulphonephthalein (P.S.P.) excretion test which does not even require overnight urine collection. Frequently, we see patients in the hospital with some azotaemia, but with a normal P.S.P. excretion test. Now, do you know whether the P.S.P. test is altered by thiazide therapy?

Peters: P.S.P. excretion would probably be a bad test of renal function in individuals receiving thiazide diuretics. P.S.P. is secreted by the same mechanism as P.A.H. and competes with P.A.H. for tubular secretion. Chlorothiazide, on the other hand, is secreted by the same mechanism as P.A.H. and is known to inhibit P.A.H. secretion competitively. Other thiazide diuretics have also been shown to depress tubular P.A.H. secretion. They must, therefore, be expected to interfere also with P.S.P. secretion.

Taquini: Dr. Peters, do you think that urea clearance or inulin clearance can reveal any difference between a kidney with normal and abnormal units and other kidneys with a generalised disease?

Peters: Certainly not.

Taquini: Then, in certain cases, other tests, such as overload of the kidney, are needed.

Peters: Yes.

Hood: If we are looking for a simple test which would give an approximate measurement of the filtration rate, this could be done with a single injection of inulin or vitamin B_{12}. Urine collection is not necessary. We have tried the inulin slope as compared with conventional inulin and P.A.H. clearance tests performed within a few days of each other. Although the inulin slope is a simple thing, we can simplify it a little further: basing the results on the calculated surface area of the individual, we find the best point occurs 180 minutes after injection. This involves one injection of inulin followed by removal of a blood sample 180 minutes afterwards. What will this give us? It will decrease the error we made in appraising glomerular filtration rate to one half or one third of the error which results even with a combination of such tests as repeated serum creatinine measurements or Pitressin tannate concentration tests. We shall thus reduce the number of serious mistakes resulting from the impression that the filtration rate is higher than it actually is, especially in the region between 40—90 ml./min. The reproducibility looks fairly good if the repeated tests are done in a steady state. It may be that this would provide a fairly simple test which could be applied in large-scale clinical work.

Reubi: I must say that I have become a little bit confused about this discussion. I don't quite understand why it is such an important problem or why speakers think it is one. If you want to know the glomerular filtration rate, you have to use the conventional inulin method. But if you are interested in the renal function from a clinical point of view, you have to remember that a moderate azotaemia corresponds to a range of filtration rate between 10 and 25 ml./min. In these cases you need only determine blood urea nitrogen, N.P.N., or creatinine. It doesn't matter which. Of course, that is semi-quantitative, but I think that is quite sufficient for clinical purposes. If you apply antihypertensive treatment to a patient with a low filtration rate, of course blood urea will rise. If you are not sure about the technique, you can determine simultaneously blood creatinine. If, after several weeks of antihypertensive treatment, blood urea goes down again, as we see it do many times, you need not worry about the fate of the patient, at least for the immediate future. And that is the most important point.

Dustan: I should like to suggest that, if one tries, one can find out something about the various controlling mechanisms in hypertension, and in this regard I should like to describe some studies that we have done in a hypertensive patient with terminal renal failure who subsequently received a successful renal homograft[1]. This man had chronic glomerulonephritis; we had followed him for a period of two years, during which time his kidney function had progressively decreased. His hypertension had originally been easily controlled with reserpine, but as renal failure became more severe his arterial pressure rose. His brother wished to donate a kidney, and therefore the patient was started on intermittent haemodialysis to prepare him for the transplantation. After the first six weeks, both kidneys were removed, and he was maintained in a renoprival state for four subsequent weeks before the homotransplantation was carried out. During the ten weeks of the dialysis prior to transplantation, we measured blood volumes in response to haemodialysis and, of course, arterial pressure, plasma renin levels, and responses to trimethaphan, the short-acting ganglion blocker. During this time we were able to show that, whether he had kidneys or whether his kidneys were absent (that is, whether he had renal or renoprival hypertension), his blood pressure was a direct function of the intravascular volume. However, during the phase of renal hypertension, at any given blood volume, arterial pressure was higher than it was during the renoprival phase.

During the phase of renal hypertension we were able to demonstrate renin in his plasma and we, therefore, suggest that hypertension accompanying chronic renal diseases is a combination of renal and renoprival mechanisms. What nephrectomy does is to remove the supply of renin, but it does not in any way modify that strange problem of inability to regulate blood pressure in response to changes in intravascular volume.

---

[1] Dustan, H. P., and I. H. Page: J. Laborat. Clin. Med. **64**, 948 (1964).

Clinical pharmacology and short-term treatment

Haemodynamic analysis of some principles applied in the treatment of arterial hypertension

By

R. Sannerstedt, G. Schröder, and L. Werkö

The human pharmacology of hypotensive drugs is as complex as the experimental pharmacology (*21, 28*). Many drugs act by interfering with physiological mechanisms necessary for the maintenance of the arterial blood pressure, others by mechanisms that are unknown and can only be speculated about. The only way to test the usefulness of a drug in the treatment of high blood pressure is to try it in patients with hypertensive cardiovascular disease, because the complex clinical situation characteristic of such patients cannot be simulated in the laboratory.

As many of the drugs used interfere with physiological mechanisms necessary to maintain the ability to stand, walk, and work, we have designed a standardised exercise test in order to study the influence of hypotensive drugs in hypertensive patients. The purpose of this test is primarily to allow haemodynamic analysis of the systemic circulation and its reaction to moderate exercise.

I would rather describe our experiences with this test in a few words and present some of our results than try to give a more comprehensive discussion on the human pharmacology of all different hypotensive drugs. For comparison, I shall show the results obtained in control patients not treated with hypotensive agents and in patients treated with saluretic agents, α methyldopa, a monamine-oxidase inhibitor, and a sympatholytic drug, as well as the effects of β-adrenergic blocking agents. The treatment period in this study has been about one week; consequently, only the more immediate effects of the drugs in question have been analysed.

Each group of patients treated consists of seven to ten patients, with the exception of the control group, in which we have so far only four patients with hypertension. The reproducibility of the results of the haemodynamic study has, however, been established in a larger series of subjects who displayed almost exactly the same values for heart rate, cardiac output, and blood pressures at rest and during exercise, when studied repeatedly at intervals of about one week (*23*).

Methods and procedure

The studies were carried out in the morning, with the patients in a postprandial state. A polyethylene catheter was inserted into a brachial artery. If possible, a radio-opaque catheter was placed in the right atrium through an antecubital vein under fluoroscopy, according to the Seldinger technique; otherwise, a polyethylene catheter was placed in the axillary vein.

Intravascular blood pressures were recorded on a multichannel oscillograph with a variable-inductance transducer (Elema), and the systolic, diastolic, and mean pressures were calculated from the tracings obtained. Reference pressure was placed at the level of the third intercostal space when the subjects were sitting. The electrocardiogram was recorded simultaneously.

Cardiac output was determined in the sitting position after half an hour of rest by a dye-dilution technique with sulphobromophthalein or cardiogreen. The dye concentrations in the fractioned plasma samples were read on a Beckman B densitometer. The expired air, collected in a Douglas bag during the dye-dilution procedure, was analysed in a Scholander apparatus to determine oxygen consumption and carbon-dioxide elimination.

After another half-hour of rest, exercise was performed in the sitting position for ten minutes on an electrically braked bicycle ergometer. Towards the end of this period, cardiac output and oxygen consumption were measured. Blood pressure was recorded every two minutes throughout the exercise period. In some patients, a second period of exercise was performed after at least half an hour of rest, and the same observations were made.

After this preliminary study, the test drug was given by mouth in adequate doses for about one week. The haemodynamic study was then repeated one to two hours after the morning dose.

Results

The patients with arterial hypertension and the normal subjects reacted to exercise with an increase in cardiac output of about similar magnitude. During exercise, this increase was accompanied by an increase in arterial blood pressure roughly proportional to the amount of exercise performed or to the increase in cardiac output.

The main difference between patients with hypertension and normal subjects seems to be that the blood-pressure rise for a given increase in flow is greater in the former than in the latter (*21*). This might be regarded as being indicative of the higher peripheral resistance in arterial hypertension, and of the reduced ability to decrease vascular resistance under conditions of physical exercise.

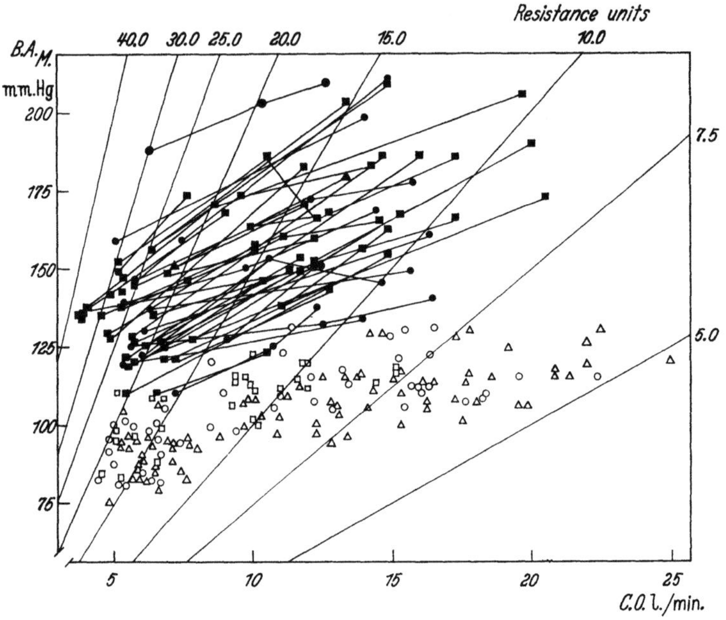

Fig. 1. Pressure-flow relationship at rest and during exercise in the sitting position. Results in 45 male patients with stabilised arterial hypertension (black symbols) and 59 normotensive male controls (white symbols), divided into three different age groups. △ = 16—30 years; ○ = 31—45 years; □ = 46—60 years; B.A.$_{M.}$ = mean brachial artery pressure in mm. Hg; C.O. = cardiac output in litres per min.

To a certain extent, the ratio of flow to pressure is related to the age of the population studied. A comparison of the exercise reaction in normotensive males and male patients with hypertension between the ages of 16 and 60 is given in Fig. 1.

Diuretic drugs cause a rapid decrease in blood volume, cardiac output, and arterial blood pressure (*1, 5, 8, 17, 32*). During standard exercise, both blood pressure and cardiac output were lower than in the control study, concomitant with a decreased blood volume (Fig. 2.) The restitution of plasma volume to the control value by plasma infusion gave an increase in cardiac output, both at rest and during exercise, without any augmentation of the lowered blood pressure (*30*). This was interpreted as indicating a peripheral action of thiazide diuretics, though the calculated value for peripheral resistance was unaltered after treatment.

In order to provide some new data for discussion, I should like to describe the results obtained by the administration of some

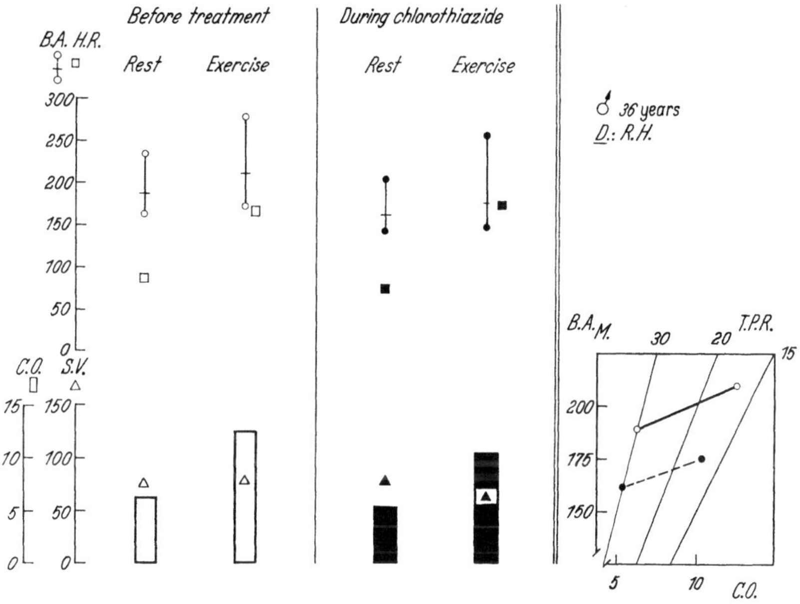

Fig. 2. Systemic haemodynamic profile at rest and during standard exercise test in the sitting position before and during treatment with *chlorothiazide*. Results obtained in a male patient with renal hypertension, treated orally with 0.5 g. twice daily for five days. B.A. = brachial artery pressure in mm. Hg; H.R. = heart rate in beats per min.; C.O. = cardiac output in litres per min.; S.V. = stroke volume in ml. per beat; $B.A._M$ = mean brachial artery pressure in mm. Hg; T.P.R. = total peripheral resistance in arbitrary units.

drugs that are of theoretical rather than practical interest. It is improbable that either β-adrenergic blocking agents or monamine-oxidase inhibitors will come to play any greater role than they do at present in the routine treatment of hypertension. It is quite clear that the sympatholytic drug, acetabutone, will not be used in treatment because of the side effects it provokes and the fact that resistance to this drug develops rapidly. The results of treatment with these drugs are demonstrated more as examples of what different types of hypotensive agent accomplish when studied in this manner.

β-Adrenergic blocking agents have been produced in increasing numbers during the last few years, but only a few have gained general acceptance. They have been recommended in special types of arrhythmia and in anginal pain, and also as a means of treating arterial hypertension, though experience with this type of drug has only been gathered in small clinical series (*3*, *14*, *15*, *16*, *25*). Nethalide, also called pronethalol or Alderlin, has already been followed by other similar drugs. The results are shown as representing this group of substances rather than nethalide itself.

The patients with arterial hypertension showed a decrease in blood pressure, both at rest and during exercise, a decrease in cardiac output at rest, and in peripheral resistance during exercise.

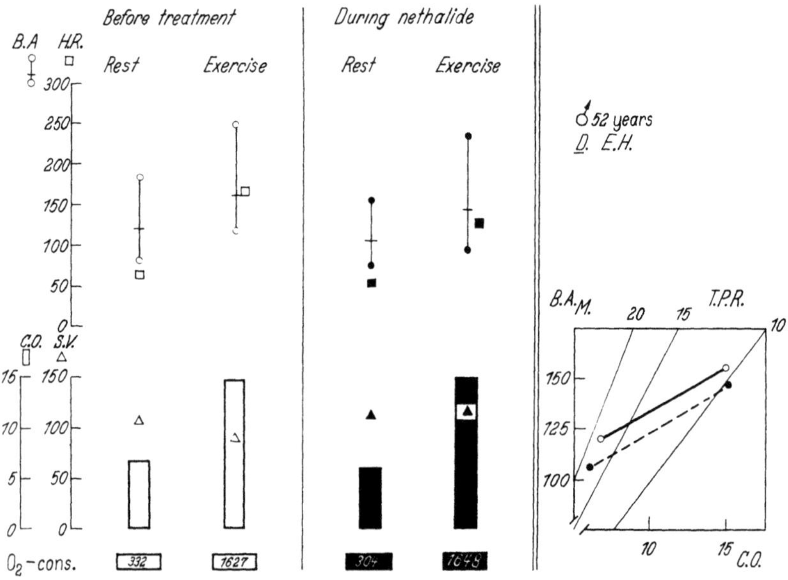

Fig. 3. Systemic haemodynamic profile at rest and during standard exercise test in the sitting position before and during treatment with *nethalide*. Results obtained in a male patient with essential hypertension, treated orally with 0.2 g. t.i.d. for five days. Abbreviations as in Fig. 2. O_2-cons. = oxygen consumption in ml. per min.

Left ventricular work was considerably less, both at rest and during exercise, after one week of nethalide treatment (mean dose: 0.6 g. daily). The blood pressure decreased from 189/103 mm. Hg, mean pressure 134 mm. Hg, to 171/96 mm. Hg, mean pressure 122 mm. Hg (*24*). The data obtained in a male patient with hypertension before and after one week of nethalide treatment are shown in Fig. 3.

When given intravenously in experimental studies, sympathetic blocking agents, such as guanethidine, have a biphasic effect. After a short period of tachycardia and blood-pressure increase, the hypotensive action begins. Heart rate decreases, cardiac output diminishes, and blood pressure is lowered. The haemodynamic changes are thus similar to those found during acute ganglionic blockade, with orthostatic potentiation due to peripheral pooling of blood and decreased venous return (*4*, *6*, *9*, *29*). Under treatment with guanethidine, the normal rise in blood pressure during exercise in the erect position may be abolished.

As a *sympatholytic agent*, dibenamine has been widely studied. Similar new drugs have been synthesised. Acetabutone is one of

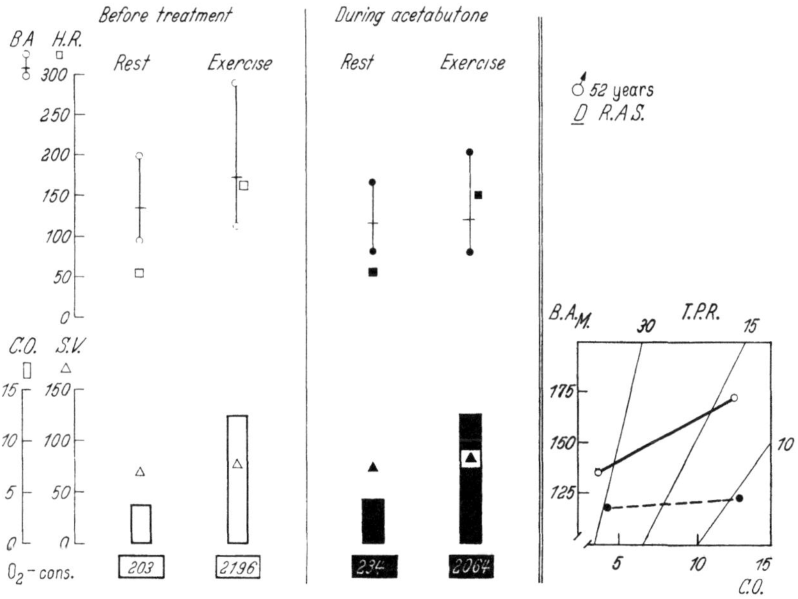

Fig. 4. Systemic haemodynamic profile at rest and during standard exercise test in the sitting position before and during treatment with *acetabutone*. Results obtained in a male patient with renal artery stenosis, treated orally with 5 mg. q.i.d. for eight days. Abbreviations as in Figs 2 and 3.

these, and its action in animal experiments resembles that of dibenamine.

In experiments in the dog, acetabutone has given rise to tachycardia and an elevated cardiac output together with a marked hypotensive action, and thus differs from guanethidine, for example (*22*).

Resistance to treatment has, however, been reported to occur in clinical trials (*18*). The findings in a typical case after one week of oral treatment with this sympatholytic agent are shown in Fig. 4.

Pargyline was chosen to represent the *monamine-oxidase inhibitors*. Pargyline hydrochloride lowers arterial blood pressure by uncertain mechanisms (*10*, *13*, *27*). It has been suggested that a

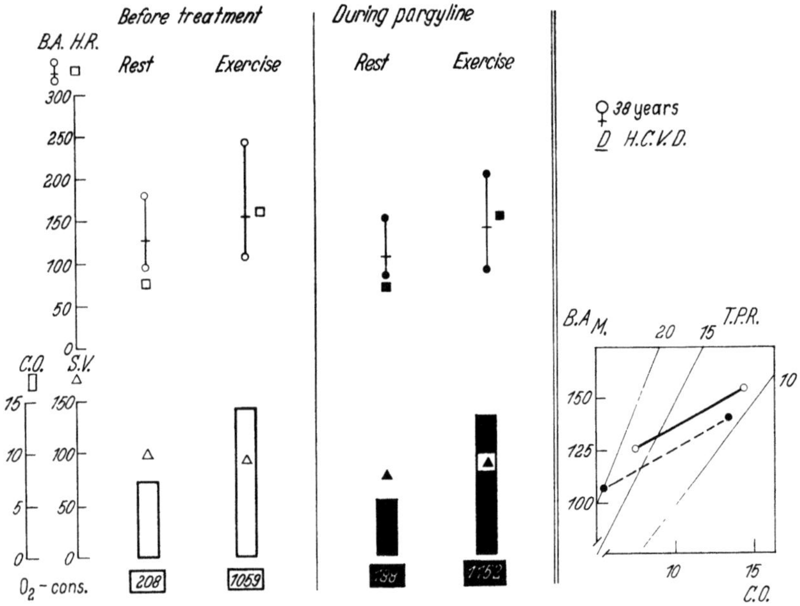

Fig. 5. Systemic haemodynamic profile at rest and during standard exercise test in the sitting position before and during treatment with *pargyline*. Results obtained in a female patient with hypertensive cardiovascular disease, treated orally with 15 mg. q.i.d. for ten days. Abbreviations as in Figs 2 and 3.

sympathetic ganglionic block may account for the hypotensive effect of the drug. The pronounced orthostatic effect is similar to that found with ganglionic blocking agents.

During exercise, the ability to increase cardiac output is impaired and the ratio of flow to pressure follows roughly the same line as in the control state. The blood-pressure increase is thus less than before treatment, but the smaller increase in pressure is due to a smaller augmentation of blood flow (Fig. 5).

α-Methyldopa lowers the blood pressure by an unknown mechanism (*2*, *7*, *26*). Probably it interferes with the catecholamine metabolism in some way. Its haemodynamic action is similar to that of ganglionic and sympathetic blocking agents, though the orthostatic influence is less pronounced and its effect on heart rate perhaps slightly more marked (*4*, *9*, *11*, *12*, *19*, *20*, *31*, *33*). The study during exercise showed a normal rise in cardiac output with less increase in heart rate and blood pressure as compared with control data (Fig. 6).

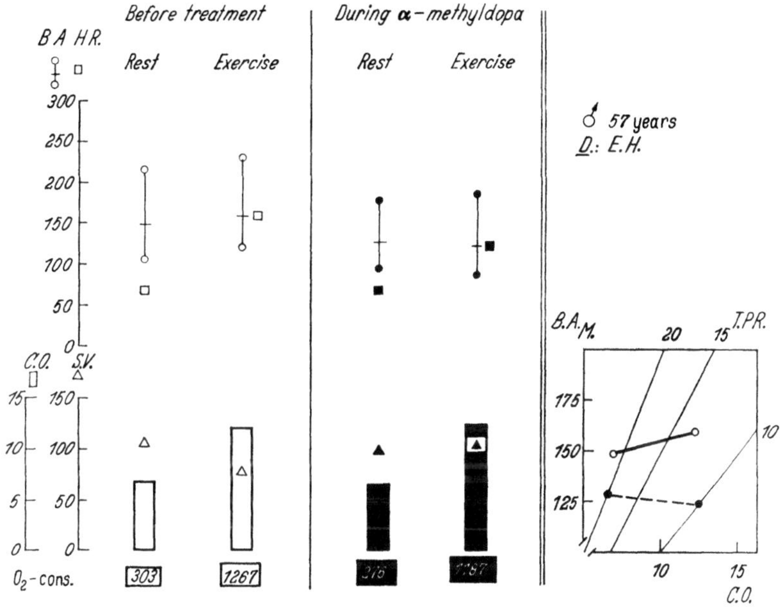

Fig. 6. Systemic haemodynamic profile at rest and during standard exercise test in the sitting position before and during treatment with *α-methyldopa*. Results obtained in a male patient with essential hypertension, treated orally with 0.5 g. t.i.d. for 13 days. Abbreviations as in Figs 2 and 3.

Comparison of the haemodynamic effects of different blood-pressure-lowering drugs

The following figures illustrate the mean values and differences of significance of heart rate (Fig. 7), stroke volume (Fig. 8), and peripheral resistance (Fig. 9) at rest and during exercise in the control state and after treatment with the different drugs mentioned. The blood-pressure decrease obtained with α-methyldopa and acetabutone is usually caused by a reduction in peripheral resistance, especially during exercise. With saluretic agents and pargyline, however, the decrease in cardiac output at rest or reduced ability

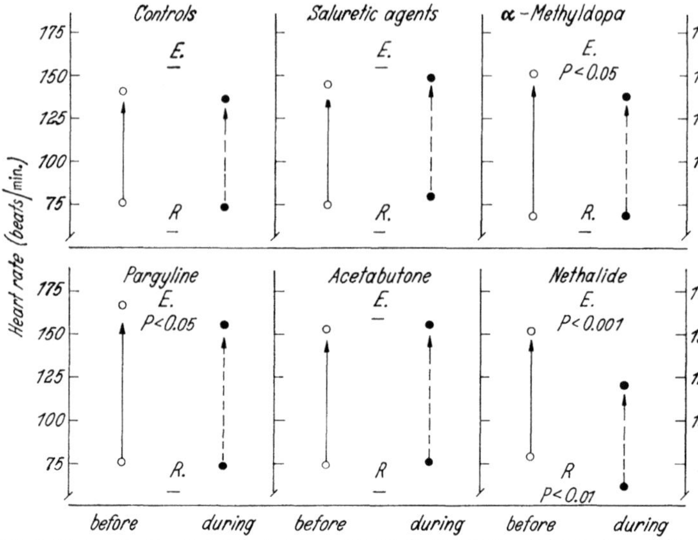

Fig. 7. Heart rate at rest and during standard exercise test in the sitting position before and during treatment with different hypotensive drugs as compared with that found in a control group of untreated hypertensive patients. Mean values are given, together with P-values for significant differences. R. = rest; E. = exercise.

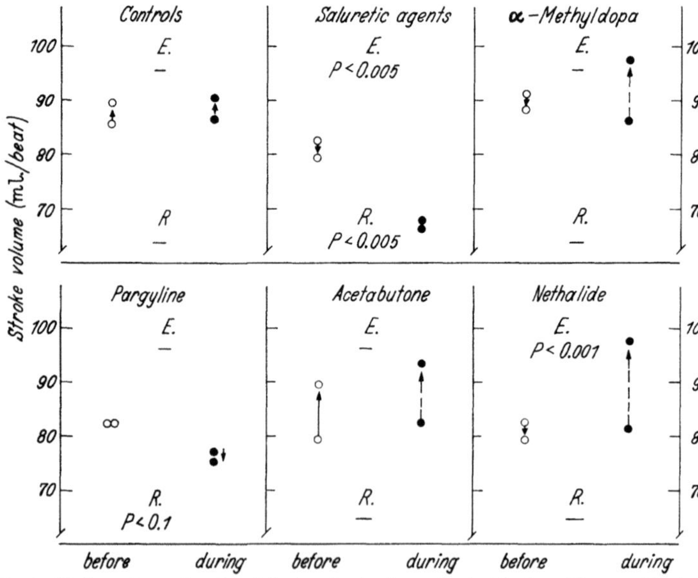

Fig. 8. Stroke volume at rest and during standard exercise test in the sitting position before and during treatment with different hypotensive drugs as compared with that found in a control group of untreated hypertensive patients. Mean values are given, together with P-values for significant differences. R. = rest; E. = exercise.

to increase it during exercise makes the blood-pressure fall observed dependent on a decrease in both flow and resistance. It should be noted that diuretic agents lower the cardiac output without much interference with heart rate or peripheral resistance. On the contrary, β-adrenergic blocking agents or α-methyldopa

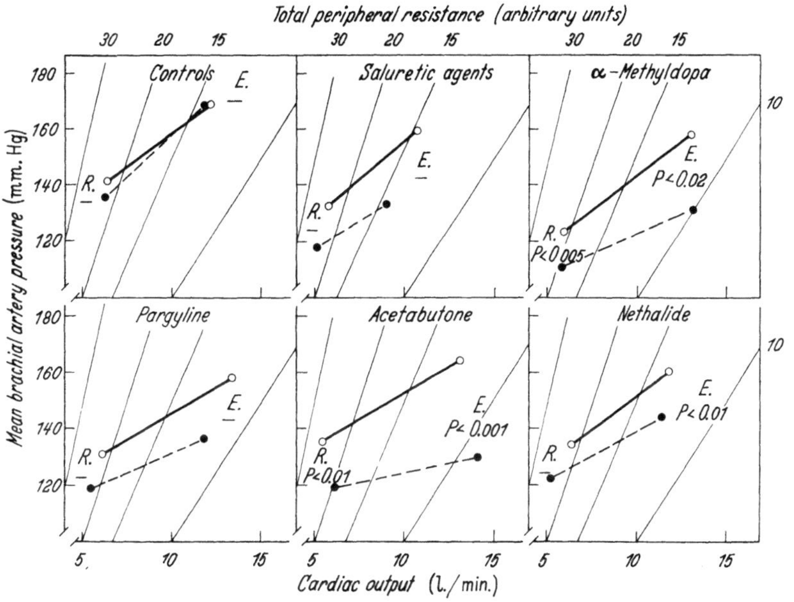

Fig. 9. Pressure-flow relationship at rest and during standard exercise test in the sitting position before and during treatment with different hypotensive drugs as compared with a control group of untreated hypertensive patients. Mean values for mean brachial artery pressure and cardiac output are given, together with P-values for significant differences in calculated total peripheral resistance. R. = rest; E. = exercise.

lower heart rate, and α-methyldopa the peripheral resistance, without causing much change in blood flow. This was most noticeable during exercise.

The drugs used interfere with blood-pressure regulation in different manners. As long as the cause of high blood pressure is unknown, non-specific forms of treatment have to be resorted to. These substances have one thing in common: interference with physiological mechanisms must be so slight that the regulation of flow and pressure can still operate under the daily stresses of standing and performing mild physical exercise. This is essential if these drugs are to be used to any effect in the treatment of such a chronic disorder as hypertensive cardiovascular disease.

The haemodynamic analysis performed in the manner described here is of necessity crude and does not yield any data about the distribution of peripheral blood flow and its possible alteration during treatment. It does, however, give some useful information by demonstrating the maintenance of an adequate cardiac output during exercise in the erect position. In this way the analysis also indicates which agent may involve the least risk of impaired peripheral circulation in treatment of arterial hypertension.

Summary

Haemodynamic recordings have been performed in patients with raised arterial blood pressure and in normal individuals, at rest and during standardised exercise on an electrically braked bicycle ergometer. Blood pressure in the brachial artery (and sometimes in the right atrium) was recorded by means of a variable-inductance transducer, together with the electrocardiogram. Cardiac output was determined by dye-dilution technique, and oxygen consumption and pulmonary ventilation by collection of expired air in a Douglas bag.

The same measurements were repeated in several of the patients after they had been treated with a blood-pressure-lowering drug, given orally for five to 13 days.

A common finding in the patients with raised arterial pressure was a marked further increase in blood pressure during exercise; this was more pronounced than in those with normal pressure, especially in relation to the increase in blood flow (cardiac output).

Diuretic agents lowered the arterial blood pressure and the cardiac output, both at rest and during exercise. When the decrease in plasma volume caused by these agents was compensated by infusion of plasma, the cardiac output reverted to its earlier value, whereas blood pressure remained lower.

Nethalide, a β-adrenergic blocking agent, decreased arterial blood pressure moderately, both at rest and during exercise, but cardiac output only at rest. Heart rate was lowered, especially during exercise.

Acetabutone, a sympatholytic agent, decreased blood pressure without interfering with cardiac-output regulation, either at rest or during exercise.

Pargyline, a monamine-oxidase inhibitor, reduced arterial blood pressure, both at rest and during exercise, and gave rise to a decrease in cardiac output, especially during exercise.

α-Methyldopa, a decarboxylase inhibitor, reduced arterial blood pressure, both at rest and during exercise, without inducing any change in cardiac output. Heart rate was lowered, especially during exercise, in some patients receiving α-methyldopa.

While, in short-term administration, some of the studied drugs exerted a very satisfactory blood-pressure-lowering effect from the haemodynamic point of view, none was found to be free of side effects or to exclude the development of tolerance. This necessitates the use of combined treatment and further investigation of possible antihypertensive agents.

Zusammenfassung

Bei Patienten mit erhöhtem Blutdruck und bei normalen Versuchspersonen wurden verschiedene hämodynamische Größen in der Ruhe und während standardisierter Arbeit am elektrisch abgebremsten Fahrradergometer registriert. Der Blutdruck in der Arteria brachialis (gelegentlich auch im rechten Vorhof) wurde mit Hilfe eines Induktionsmanometers, zusammen mit dem Elektrokardiogramm, aufgezeichnet. Das Minutenvolumen wurde mit Hilfe der Farbverdünnungsmethode bestimmt, der Sauerstoffverbrauch und die Ventilationsgröße durch Sammlung der Ausatmungsluft im Douglas Sack.

Die gleichen Messungen wurden bei einigen der Patienten wiederholt, nachdem sie peroral während fünf bis 13 Tagen mit blutdrucksenkenden Mitteln behandelt worden waren.

Ein gemeinsamer Befund bei den Patienten mit erhöhtem Blutdruck war ein beträchtlicher zusätzlicher Blutdruckanstieg während der Arbeit; dieser Anstieg war deutlicher als bei den Personen mit normalem Blutdruck, besonders im Verhältnis zur Zunahme des Minutenvolumens.

Diuretika senkten den Blutdruck und das Minutenvolumen sowohl in Ruhe als während Arbeit. Wenn die durch Diuretika hervorgerufene Abnahme des Plasmavolumens durch Infusion von Plasma aufgehoben wurde, kehrte das Minutenvolumen auf die Ausgangswerte zurück, während der Blutdruck erniedrigt blieb.

Nethalid, ein adrenergischer β-Blocker, senkte sowohl in Ruhe als während Arbeit den Arteriendruck mäßig, das Minutenvolumen dagegen nur in Ruhe. Die Herzfrequenz war erniedrigt, besonders während Arbeit.

Acetabuton, ein Sympathikolytikum, verminderte den Blutdruck sowohl während Ruhe als auch während Arbeit, ohne die Regulation des Herzminutenvolumens zu beeinträchtigen.

Pargylin, ein Monaminooxydasehemmer, senkte den Blutdruck während Ruhe und während Arbeit und verminderte das Minutenvolumen besonders während Arbeit.

α-Methyldopa, als Decarboxylasehemmer, senkte den Blutdruck sowohl in Ruhe als auch während der Arbeit, ohne daß gleichzeitig Änderungen im Minutenvolumen auftraten. Bei einigen Patienten war unter α-Methyldopa die Herzfrequenz herabgesetzt, besonders während der Arbeit.

Während bei kurzdauernder Gabe einige der untersuchten Stoffe in hämodynamischer Hinsicht eine nahezu ideale blutdrucksenkende Wirkung zeigten, war keiner von ihnen frei von Nebenwirkungen, noch ließ sich die Entwicklung einer Gewöhnung ausschließen. Daraus ergibt sich die Notwendigkeit zu einer kombinierten Behandlung und zur weiteren Untersuchung von blutdrucksenkenden Substanzen.

Résumé

Des enregistrements hémodynamiques ont été effectués chez des malades hypertendus et chez des sujets normaux, au repos et au cours d'un effort physique standardisé sur une bicyclette ergométrique freinée électriquement. La pression artérielle au niveau de l'artère humérale (et parfois dans l'oreillette droite) a été enregistrée au moyen d'un manomètre à induction variable, conjointement à l'électrocardiogramme. Le débit cardiaque a été calculé par une technique de dilution de colorant, et la consommation d'oxygène ainsi que la ventilation pulmonaire par collection de l'air expiré dans un sac de Douglas.

Les mêmes enregistrements ont été répétés chez plusieurs malades après traitement par un agent hypotenseur, administré oralement pendant cinq à 13 jours.

On a observé de façon constante chez les hypertendus une hypertension supplémentaire marquée lors de l'effort musculaire; cette élévation a été plus importante que chez les sujets normotendus, surtout en comparaison avec l'accroissement de flux sanguin (débit cardiaque).

Des agents diurétiques ont diminué la pression artérielle et le débit cardiaque, à la fois au repos et à l'effort. Quand la réduction de volume plasmatique provoquée par ces agents a été compensée par une perfusion de plasma, le débit cardiaque est revenu aux valeurs antérieures, alors que la pression artérielle restait abaissée.

La néthalide, un inhibiteur des récepteurs adrénergiques β, a modérément abaissé la tension artérielle, aussi bien au repos qu'à l'effort, mais n'a diminué le débit cardiaque qu'au repos. La fréquence cardiaque a été diminuée, principalement à l'effort.

L'acétabutone, un agent sympatholytique, a diminué la pression artérielle sans modifier la régulation du débit cardiaque, aussi bien au repos qu'à l'effort.

La pargyline, un inhibiteur de la monoamino-oxydase, a diminué la pression artérielle au repos et à l'effort et a provoqué une diminution du débit cardiaque surtout à l'effort.

L'α-méthyldopa, un inhibiteur de la décarboxylase, a diminué la pression artérielle au repos et à l'effort sans modifier le débit cardiaque. La fréquence cardiaque s'est abaissée, principalement à l'effort, chez quelques malades recevant de l'α-méthyldopa.

Alors que dans des traitements à court terme quelques-uns des produits utilisés se sont montrés d'excellents hypotenseurs du point de vue hémodynamique, aucun ne s'est montré dénué d'effets secondaires ou du risque d'accoutumance. Ce fait commande l'utilisation de traitements associés et la poursuite de l'expérimentation d'agents antihypertenseurs.

References

1. ALEKSANDROW, D., W. WYSZNACKA, and J. GAJEWSKI: N. England J. Med. **260**, 51 (1959). — 2. BUHS, R. P., J. L. BECK, O. C. SPETH, J. L. SMITH, N. R. TRENNER, P. J. CANNON, and J. H. LARAGH: J. Pharmacol. Exper. Therap. **143**, 205 (1964). — 3. CHAMBERLAIN, D. A., and J. HOWARD: Brit. Heart J. **26**, 213 (1964). — 4. CHAMBERLAIN, D. A., and J. HOWARD: Brit. Heart J. **26**, 528 (1964). — 5. CONWAY, J., and P. LAUWERS: Circulation **21**, 21 (1960). — 6. DOLLERY, C. T., D. EMSLIE-SMITH, and M. D. MILNE: Lancet 1960/II, 381. — 7. DOLLERY, C. T., and M. HARINGTON: Lancet 1962/I, 759. — 8. FROHLICH, E. D., H. W. SCHNAPER, I. M. WILSON, and E. D. FREIS: N. England J. Med. **262**, 1261 (1960). — 9. KIRKENDALL, W. M., and W. R. WILSON: Amer. J. Cardiol. **9**, 107 (1962). — 10. MOSER, M., W. PLAINS, B. BRODOFF, N. ROCHELLE, A. MILLER, and A. G. GOLDMAN: J. Amer. Med. Ass. **187**, 192 (1964). — 11. ONESTI, G., A. N. BREST, P. NOVACK, H. KASPARIAN, and J. H. MOYER: Amer. Heart J. **67**, 32 (1964). — 12. ONESTI, G., A. N. BREST, P. NOVACK, and J. H. MOYER: Amer. J. Cardiol. **9**, 863 (1962). — 13. ONESTI, G., P. NOVACK, O. RAMIREZ, A. N. BREST, and J. H. MOYER: Circulation **30**, 830 (1964). — 14. PRICHARD, B. N. C.: Brit. Med. J. 1964/I, 1227. — 15. PRICHARD, B. N. C.: Amer. Heart J. **69**, 716 (1965). — 16. PRICHARD, B. N. C., and P. M. S. GILLAM: Brit. Med. J. 1964/II, 725. — 17. ROWE, G. G., C. A. CASTILLO, A. P. CROSLEY, Jr., G. M. MAXWELL, and C. W. CRUMPTON: Amer. J. Cardiol. **10**, 183 (1962). — 18. SANNERSTEDT, R.: To be published. — 19. SANNERSTEDT, R., G. BOJS, E. VARNAUSKAS, and L. WERKÖ: Acta med. Scand. **174**, 53 (1963). —

20. SANNERSTEDT, R., E. VARNAUSKAS, and L. WERKÖ: Acta med. Scand. **171**, 75 (1962). — 21. SANNERSTEDT, R., and L. WERKÖ: Med. Clin. North America **46**, 1639 (1962). — 22. SCHAPER, W. K. A., A. H. M. JAGENEAU, and R. XHONNEUX: Arzneimittel-Forsch. **12**, 1015 (1962). — 23. SCHRÖDER, G.: Scand. J. Clin. Laborat. Invest. **16**, 559 (1964). — 24. SCHRÖDER, G., and L. WERKÖ: Clin. Pharmacol. Therap. **5**, 159 (1964). — 25. SCHRÖDER, G., and L. WERKÖ: Amer. J. Cardiol. **15**, 58 (1965). — 26. SJOERDSMA, A., A. VENDSALU, and K. ENGELMAN: Circulation **28**, 492 (1963). — 27. SUTNICK, A. I., J. W. FEWELL, J. H. ESBENSHADE, and L. A. SOLOFF: Clin. Pharmacol. Therap. **5**, 167 (1964). — 28. TAYLOR, S. H., and K. W. DONALD: Quart. J. Med. **29**, 631 (1960). — 29. TAYLOR, S. H., G. R. SUTHERLAND, D. C. S. HUTCHINSON, B. S. L. KIDD, P. C. ROBERTSON, B. M. KENNELLY, and K. W. DONALD: Amer. Heart J. **63**, 239 (1962). — 30. VARNAUSKAS, E., G. CRAMÉR, R. MALMCRONA, and L. WERKÖ: Clin. Sc. **20**, 407 (1961). — 31. WEIL, M. H., B. H. BARBOUR, and R. B. CHESNE: Circulation **28**, 165 (1963). — 32. VILLARREAL, H., J. E. EXAIRE, A. REVOLLO, and J. SONI: Circulation **26**, 405 (1962). — 33. VINCENT, W. A., U. KASHEMSANT, R. P. CUDDY, H. SMULYAN, and R. H. EICH: Amer. J. Med. Sc. **246**, 558 (1963).

Discussion

Hoobler: Have you studied guanethidine in the same context?

Werkö: We have, but only in a few patients. We don't have enough material to make any statistical comparison. A decrease both in flow and in resistance has been found in those patients.

Hoobler: At rest?

Werkö: And during exercise, yes; more pronounced during exercise.

Humerfelt: Do the subjects react differently to different grades of exercise?

Werkö: Some of these patients have performed two or three bouts of exercise involving different degrees of effort, but they have usually not done what might be called very light exercise; 300 kpm. is quite a lot for a patient with cardiovascular disease. The most taxing exercise has amounted to 600 or 800 kpm./min. This increases the total oxygen consumption to between 1.5 and 2.5 l./min. The reaction to heavy exercise does not seem to differ from the reaction to light exercise.

Gross: What was the average duration of treatment, for example of the diuretic treatment as compared with nethalide or α-methyldopa?

Werkö: In all cases, the interval between the two studies was around eight days, between seven and 12 days. We have repeated some studies after a longer time, with much the same effect. However, only a few cases were involved.

Cottier: Dr. Werkö, did the severity of hypertension, i.e. the grade of hypertension, have any influence on the haemodynamic response?

Werkö: I really cannot answer this question, because we don't have enough data to draw valid comparisons between different degrees of hypertension.

Page: It is often said that you shouldn't use an antihypertensive drug that lowers cardiac output. Most of them do lower cardiac output, and I have never been sure that I understood why this was an undesirable thing. Would you say that it is just as satisfactory to lower arterial pressure by lowering cardiac output as by lowering the total peripheral resistance? This is a mean question, I know. It's one that many people in our labour union have asked me.

Werkö: Here I can only make a guess. I think some people subscribe to the opinion that it is undesirable to decrease the cardiac output. This view may be based on the fact that congestive failure, or shock, is characterised by a lowered cardiac output. I don't believe that you disturb the circulation too much if you lower the cardiac output a little; but the important thing is that the patient should be able to regulate his peripheral blood flow, even when he is under the influence of an antihypertensive drug. If he does that on a slightly lower cardiac output level, I don't think it will hurt him. We have seen patients with mitral stenosis who have had a low cardiac output for a long time without its developing into congestive failure, and they can regulate their peripheral circulation. It is thus not necessarily injurious to the patient if the output decreases somewhat. On the other hand, it might be important that he does not have any large overshoot of cardiac output, because that would create increases in both the volume load and the pressure load on his left ventricle.

TAQUINI: Cardiac output is related to oxygen consumption under physiological conditions. If you treat the patient with drugs that lower the cardiac output, you are disturbing physiological conditions. If you treat the patient by lowering the peripheral resistance, a lower blood pressure can maintain a normal flow, and thus you maintain physiological conditions. The patient must be treated with drugs that lower the peripheral resistance and not with those that decrease cardiac output.

I should like to ask Dr. WERKÖ whether patients under long-term treatment with chlorothiazide have a low or a normal cardiac output, because I understand that the cardiac output becomes normal after prolonged treatment.

WERKÖ: The first point you raised about the oxygen consumption and the cardiac output may seem self-evident, but it isn't; because if there is a change in the peripheral distribution of blood flow from some areas to others, there may be a change in total blood flow without any alteration in total oxygen consumption. The important question is how much of such a change in the distribution of blood flow the patient can stand without further impairment.

We don't have enough data to say whether there is a continued decrease in cardiac output in response to diuretic agents, when they are studied in this manner, but there is some indication that the standing or sitting cardiac output may be lower even during a fairly long term of treatment.

TAQUINI: I know that arteriovenous difference varies in different parts of the body. In some of them, such as the heart, very wide differences have been found; on the other hand, in the skin and the kidney the arteriovenous difference is very small. But God knows better than we how the arteriovenous differences in the various parts of the body have to be.

REUBI: I think Dr. TAQUINI has made a very important point by stressing that the long-term effect may be very different from the short-term effect. We have some data on this subject. Unfortunately, they are too few to allow us to make statistical comparisons, but we have the definite impression that the haemodynamic pattern observed eight days from the start of therapy is different from what we see after one year of treatment. This has been admirably demonstrated by Dr. HOOBLER and his associates in connection with chlorothiazide[1]. But I think it is a general phenomenon, also occurring with guanethidine and most of the modern drugs, with the possible exception of ganglionic blocking agents. Not only the cardiac output behaves in this way; if you measure the renal blood flow and follow the electrocardiographic changes, you find a similar trend. The blood flow first goes down during the initial weeks of treatment and then goes up again.

WERKÖ: I shan't argue about that; there is no doubt that you get different responses in very acute treatment, when you inject the drug intra-

[1] CONWAY, J., and P. LAUWERS: Circulation **21**, 21 (1960).

venously, and after eight days of treatment, and then you may get another response after one year of treatment. The difficulty is that if you re-examine a patient after one year, you don't know whether the influence of the drug is the only factor at work. It requires quite a large control material to ensure that the conditions are comparable when the time interval between studies is long.

Hartmann: We have some information on juvenile hypertension, and we were very much impressed by the individual variability of the haemodynamics. Fig. 1 shows the variability of the cardiac output; the stroke volume especially varies in the 23 cases. Fig. 2 shows the same for peripheral

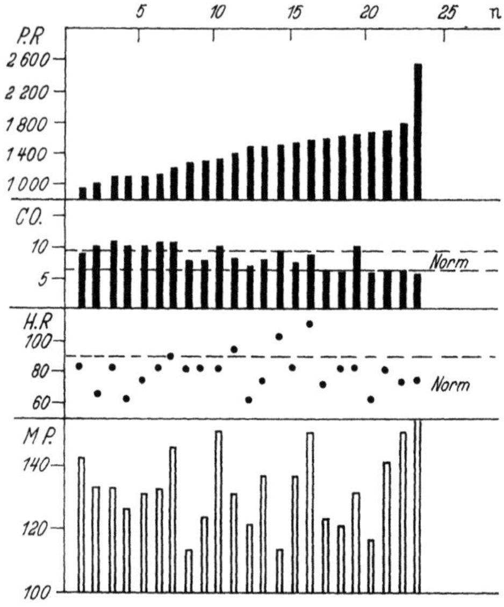

Fig. 1. Variation of peripheral resistance (P.R.), cardiac output (C.O.), heart rate (H.R.), and mean pressure (M.P.) in 23 patients with juvenile hypertension.

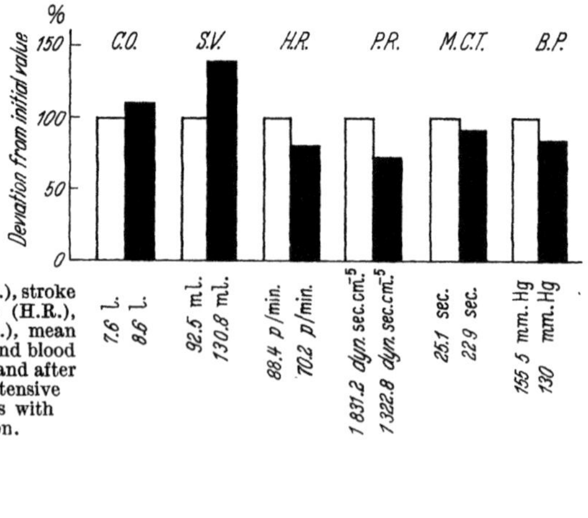

Fig. 2. Cardiac output (C.O.), stroke volume (S.V.), heart rate (H.R.), peripheral resistance (P.R.), mean circulation time (M.C.T.), and blood pressure (B.P.) before (□) and after (■) prolonged antihypertensive treatment in 42 patients with essential hypertension.

resistance. We gave a combination of Rauwolfia and saluretics to 42 patients, most of whom had juvenile hypertension, for periods of four or six months. The diminution in the mean systolic blood pressure and in the peripheral resistance before and after this treatment are indicated. The stroke volume goes up, and the cardiac output remains the same within statistical limits. The data were obtained by means of the I^{131}-albumin method.

Hoobler: Since the work at Michigan has been discussed, I should like to point out that it was Dr. Conway and Dr. Lauwers whose studies on thiazides were referred to. As regards the question on the effects of long-term treatment, I should like to mention some early work that I was involved in directly, in which we measured the output and resistance changes after long-term administration of pentolinium[1]. In this situation, where the patient's blood pressure is constantly fluctuating as he moves from the recumbent to the upright posture over a period of at least a year, we found no adjustment of the peripheral resistance. Cardiac output was reduced, and it remained reduced, and peripheral resistance apparently was constant or slightly increased, at least during a year of chronic pentolinium treatment. The changes were reversed whenever the drug was discontinued. A differentiation, I submit, might be that during pentolinium treatment there was a constant flux in cardiac output, when the patient was recumbent or upright, whereas with chlorothiazide, where there is a constant reduction in pressure, a possibly homoeostatic and autoregulatory mechanism might come into play. This autoregulation may only occur when a continuous steady state of reduced blood pressure is maintained for many weeks, the kind of thing that doesn't happen with a drug that is reducing or altering resistance and output sharply as position is changed.

Peart: I wonder whether Dr. Werkö has seen the sort of patient who has very marked hypotension during relatively mild exercise — the sort of thing you see particularly with guanethidine. Superficially it has always been said that this happens because the patients are unable to compensate for the muscular vasodilatation that occurs. I wonder whether you have any actual observations on that sort of patient which would tell us about the circulation.

Werkö: We have seen some patients behave like that, especially on guanethidine, but it is very difficult to determine the cardiac output at the time when they collapse or seem to collapse. So we don't have any data we could submit to explain what is really going on.

Brod: I should just like to comment on your finding that after muscular exercise there was a smaller decrease in peripheral vascular resistance in hypertensives than in normotensives. Many years ago, we did some studies with Dr. Fencl and Dr. Fejfar[2], with dibenamine in normotensives and hypertensives, and found that we couldn't reduce total peripheral vascular resistance in hypertensive subjects to the same extent as in normotensive controls, and I wonder whether you have any explanation for this finding.

Werkö: I don't have any explanation, but this might be a question of changes in the vascular wall that may be more or less permanent.

---

[1] Smith, J. R., and S. W. Hoobler: Circulation **14**, 1061 (1956).
[2] Fencl, V., J. Brod, and Z. Fejfar: Čas. lék. česk. **93**, 729 (1954).

Some biochemical aspects of treatment and diagnosis of hypertension

By

A. Sjoerdsma

The catecholamine hormone norepinephrine (N.E.) lies at the center of most recent developments in the chemotherapy of hypertension. Drugs such as reserpine, guanethidine, α-methyldopa, and the monamine-oxidase (M.A.O.) inhibitors, by varying mechanisms, interfere with processes which govern the availability of this sympathetic nerve transmitter to receptor sites (e.g. blood vessels) and thereby lower the blood pressure. Although it has not been shown that N.E. plays a primary role in the pathogenesis of essential hypertension, this hormone and its N-methylated derivative, epinephrine, are responsible for the occurrence of the hypertensive syndrome in patients with pheochromocytoma. Chemical assay of these catecholamines and their major metabolites in urine provides the most definitive means of diagnosing this condition.

No attempt will be made here to review the many extensive studies on catecholamine biochemistry in relation to treatment and diagnosis. It is felt, however, that a meaningful cross-section of the available information and the newer developments can be brought forth by dealing with two major topics. The first of these concerns attempts to block the endogenous synthesis of N.E. in animals and man, culminating in recent success via the inhibition of tyrosine hydroxylase. The second major topic will concern another amine, tyramine, which has been shown to interact with N.E. under a variety of experimental and clinical circumstances.

Inhibition of catecholamine synthesis

The sequence of reactions involved in the biosynthesis of N.E. is now well established and all the catalysts concerned have been isolated and their properties studied (Fig. 1). Sympathetically innervated organs, such as the heart, have been shown to contain the three catalysts required to form N.E. from tyrosine (Spector et al., 1963), and the step from tyrosine to dopa has been shown to be the rate-limiting one (Levitt et al., 1965). Coincidently with the elucidation of the nature of the biosynthetic reactions, inhibitors of each of the enzymes have been found.

Several potent inhibitors of the decarboxylase enzyme have been studied, but only two, α-methyldopa and α-methyl-meta-tyrosine, have been found to lower N.E. levels markedly *in vivo* (HESS et al., 1963). However, their depleting actions appear to be unrelated to enzyme inhibition. Available inhibitors of dopamine β-oxidase have also been relatively ineffective in inhibiting normal N.E. synthesis in the intact animal (NICODIJEVIC et al., 1963). We have studied the biochemical effects in man of several agents which inhibit dopa decarboxylase or dopamine β-oxidase or both, but in no instance could marked inhibition of catecholamine biosynthesis be shown (SJOERDSMA et al., 1963; ENGELMAN and SJOERDSMA, 1964a). Nonetheless, one of these compounds, α-methyldopa, proved to be an extremely useful antihypertensive drug. Its mechanism of action will be discussed briefly under the section on tyramine.

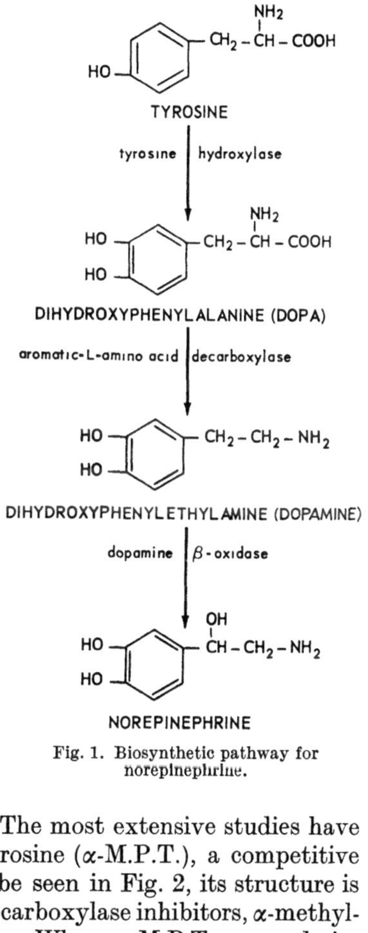

Fig. 1. Biosynthetic pathway for norepinephrine.

Recently, successful inhibition of catecholamine biosynthesis has been achieved in experimental animals (SPECTOR et al., 1965) and in man with inhibitors of tyrosine hydroxylase. The most extensive studies have been done with α-methyl-para-tyrosine (α-M.P.T.), a competitive inhibitor of the enzyme. As may be seen in Fig. 2, its structure is strikingly similar to those of the decarboxylase inhibitors, α-methyldopa and α-methyl-meta-tyrosine. When α-M.P.T. was administered repeatedly to animals in order to maintain enzyme inhibition throughout several $T^1/_2$'s of tissue N.E., owing to blockade of N.E. synthesis, levels of the amine close to zero resulted. The effects of single doses of α-M.P.T. on N.E. levels in the brain and

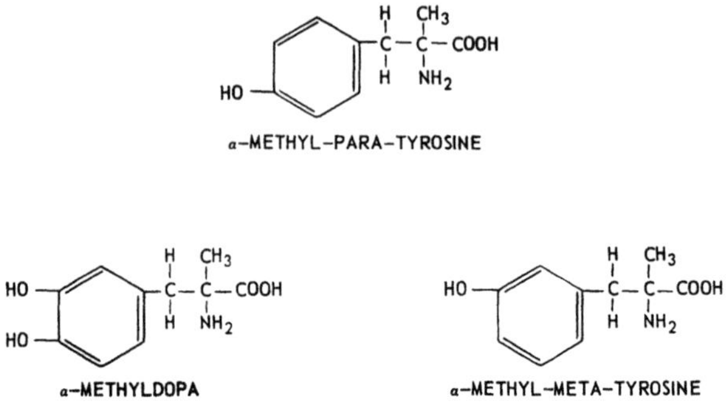

Fig. 2. Structures of three α-methylated aromatic amino acids.

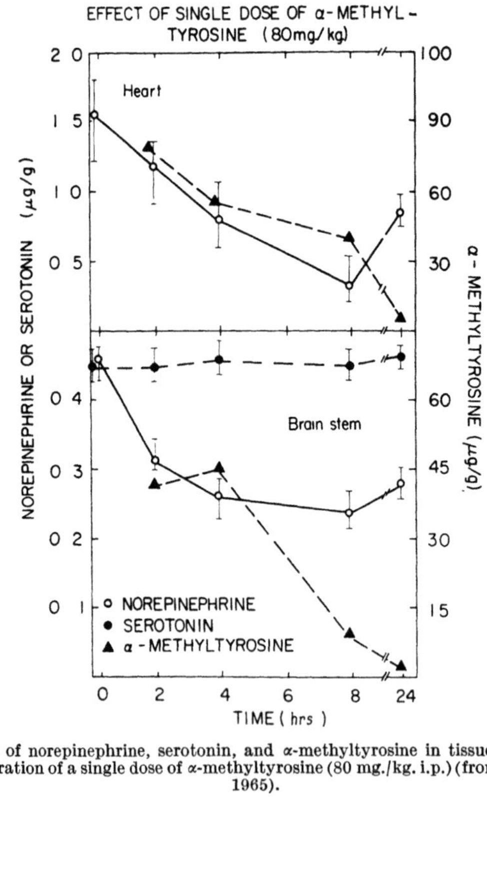

Fig. 3. Levels of norepinephrine, serotonin, and α-methyltyrosine in tissues of guinea-pigs after administration of a single dose of α-methyltyrosine (80 mg./kg. i.p.) (from Spector et al., 1965).

heart of guinea-pigs are shown in Fig. 3. Concurrently with the appearance of α-M.P.T., tissue levels of N.E. fell and reached minimum values about eight hours after administration of the inhibitor. Repletion was appreciable within 24 hours. Serotonin levels in the brain and other tissues were unaffected. Pharmacological effects which have been observed in animals include impairment of motor activity, mild sedation, and a reduction in tyramine pressor responses (SPECTOR et al., 1965). To date it has not been possible to lower blood pressure with this agent in laboratory animals.

We have now administered α-M.P.T. orally in a maximum dose of 400–1,200 mg./24 hours for periods up to three weeks to 11 hospitalized patients with hypertension; three had pheochromocytoma and eight had essential hypertension. Generally, catecholamine biosynthesis was inhibited by at least 50%, as was indicated by decreases in the urinary excretion of vanilmandelic acid (V.M.A.). Results obtained in the first patient with pheochromocytoma to

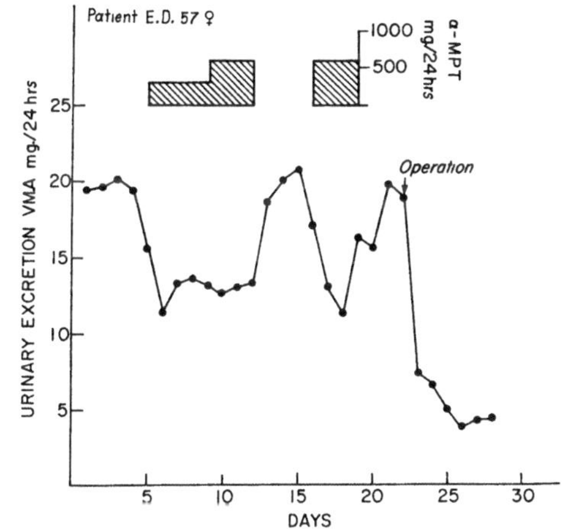

Fig. 4. Effect of α-methyl-p-tyrosine (α-M.P.T.) on urinary vanilmandelic acid (V.M.A.) excretion in a patient with pheochromocytoma.

receive the drug are shown in Fig. 4. Note that V.M.A. fell markedly during initial treatment with 300 and then 600 mg./24 hours. Treatment was then interrupted owing to a respiratory infection, and V.M.A. rose. The effect of drug was then shown again. Finally, V.M.A. declined to normal levels following operative removal of the tumor. The maximum tolerated dosage has not yet been achieved. At the doses employed, sedative effects were detected in most of the patients, but little effect on blood pressure was observed except in the cases of pheochromocytoma. In the latter, concomitantly with the fall in V.M.A. excretion, there was a decrease in blood pressure; both V.M.A. excretion and blood pressure rose when the drug was withdrawn. It would be premature to ascribe the sedative effects observed to central inhibition of N.E. synthesis, since preliminary studies indicate that about 1% of the α-methyltyrosine administered is excreted in the urine as a catechol acid, presumably α-methyldopa. In the light of current studies, the main therapeutic application appears to reside in the treatment of pheochromocytoma; rendering the tumor less functional or even non-functional would be of value in the chronic management of cases of metastatic disease and should make the preoperative and surgical management of benign cases less hazardous.

The many facets of tyramine

1. Naturally occurring intermediate. Tyramine is a sympathomimetic amine which is produced normally in body tissues by the decarboxylation of tyrosine. The enzyme responsible for this reaction is aromatic-L-amino-acid decarboxylase (LOVENBERG et al., 1962); this enzyme also forms several other amines from their amino-acid precursors, e.g. dopamine from dopa (Fig. 1). Bacterial decarboxylases also form tyramine from tyrosine (GALE, 1940), which accounts for the presence of the amine in certain foods and its production in the intestinal lumen. Tyramine was the first compound shown to be metabolized by monamine oxidase (M.A.O.), of which it is an excellent substrate. The action of M.A.O., coupled with that of aldehyde dehydrogenase, yields a final inactive urinary end-product, parahydroxyphenylacetic acid.

2. Clinical research tool in studying antihypertensive drug mechanisms. CARLSSON and his associates demonstrated several years ago (1957) that animals whose tissues had been depleted of N.E. by treatment with reserpine were no longer sensitive to the action of tyramine. Subsequently, the thesis was elaborated by BURN and RAND (1958), and it was amply confirmed that tyramine owes its sympathomimetic effects to the release of N.E. from sympathetic nerve-endings (cf. POTTER and AXELROD, 1963; STJÄRNE, 1964). Tyramine has proved to be a useful tool in evaluating the status of peripheral stores of N.E. in patients receiving various antihypertensive drugs. Reserpine, guanethidine, and α-methyldopa will be considered here; because of other interesting relationships of tyramine to the action of M.A.O. inhibitors, these drugs will be dealt with in a later section. It should be emphasized that pressor responses to N.E. are unchanged or enhanced during treatment with the various drugs to be discussed.

a) Reserpine. Reserpine appears to act by inhibiting transport and binding of N.E. at an intraneuronal level (Potter and Axelrod, 1963; Stjärne, 1964), the resultant depletion of N.E. stores leading to failure of impulse transmission at the sympathetic neuro-effector junctions. Confirmation of the N.E.-depleting effects of reserpine in the human myocardium has been obtained by Chidsey et al. (1963). Utilizing tyramine pressor response as an index of peripheral N.E. stores, it can easily be shown that treatment with reserpine results in suppression of response in patients (Abboud and Eckstein, 1964; Pettinger et al., 1963; McCurdy et al., 1964; also Fig. 8 below).

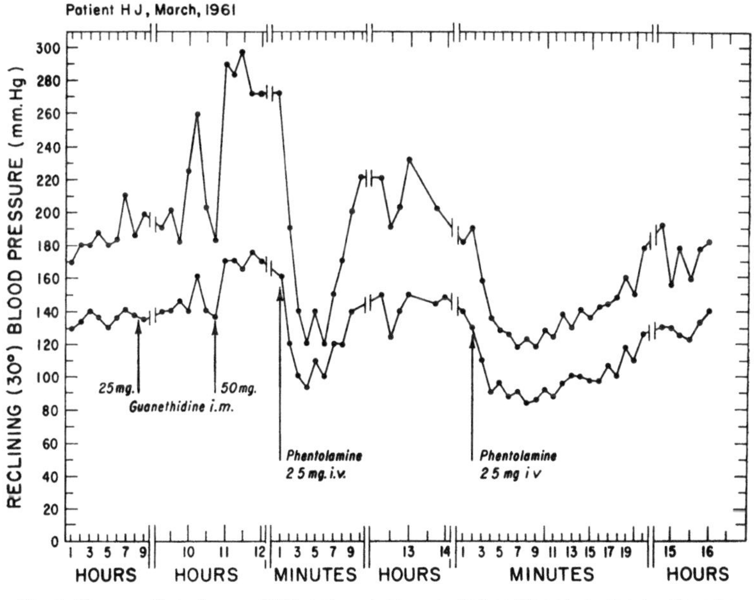

Fig. 5. Pressor effect of guanethidine given intramuscularly with antagonism by the adrenergic blocking agent, phentolamine.

b) Guanethidine. Large doses of this powerful sympathetic inhibitor may, like tyramine, cause an initial rapid release of N.E. and a marked sympathomimetic effect. This N.E.-releasing action is observed in man following parenteral administration of the drug (Cohn et al., 1963); an example is given in Fig. 5. Prolonged tissue

N.E. depletion has been observed in animals, but of lesser degree than with reserpine, and, in addition, the drug has been found to block the release of N.E. from sympathetic nerve-terminals (BRODIE, 1963). Direct measurements of tissue N.E. levels in man during chronic treatment with guanethidine apparently have not been made. At least two reports have appeared (COHN et al., 1963; HORWITZ, 1965), however, showing that therapeutic doses of guanethidine do not alter pressor responses to tyramine, and thus suggesting that N.E. depletion is not an important factor in the mechanism of the antihypertensive effect in man. Evidence has accumulated recently that adrenergic blockade with guanethidine is related primarily to the accumulation of the drug in sympathetic neurons, the loss of N.E. being secondary and insufficient to account for the sympatholytic effect (CHANG et al., 1965).

c) α-Methyldopa. In 1958, a number of compounds were known to have the property of inhibiting the decarboxylation of aromatic

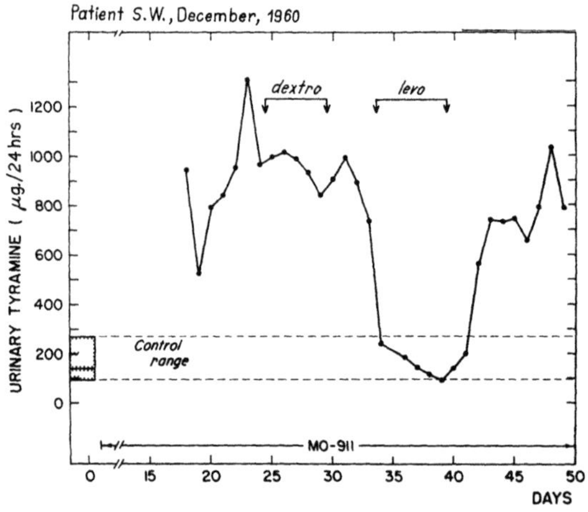

Fig. 6. Urinary excretion of tyramine during administration of 75 mg./day of an M.A.O. inhibitor (pargyline, MO-911) alone and in combination with dextro- (3.0 g./day) and levo- (0.75—1.25 g./day) isomers of α-methyldopa (from GILLESPIE et al., 1962).

amino acids to their corresponding amines in animals (Symposium, 1959); of these, α-methyl-DL-dopa was selected for clinical studies. In addition to decarboxylase-inhibiting properties, unexpected sedative and blood-pressure-lowering properties were demonstrated; these were first reported from this department by OATES et al. (1960). Decreases in the urinary excretion of tyramine represented one of the indices of enzyme inhibition in patients. In early studies, using urinary tyramine as an index, it was possible to show that the decarboxylase-inhibiting as well as the pharmacological effects of α-methyl-DL-dopa resided in the L-isomer (methyldopa, Aldomet) (SJOERDSMA, 1961; GILLESPIE et al., 1962); the differential effects on tyramine excretion are shown in Fig. 6. It is known now that the decarboxylase-inhibiting activity of α-methyldopa is not responsible for either the long-lasting depletion of tissue N.E. observed in

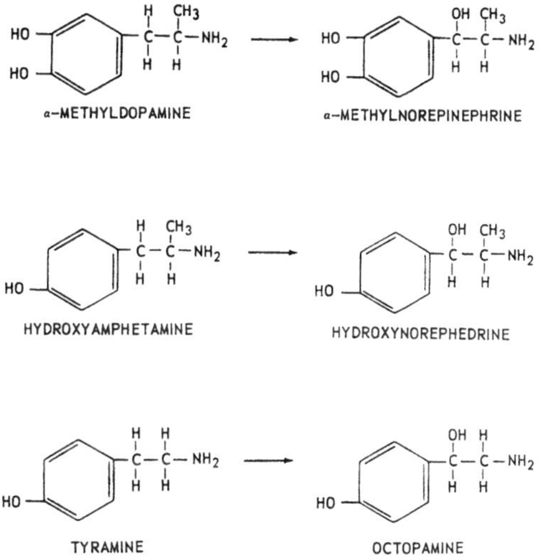

Fig. 7. Three aromatic amines and their β-hydroxylated derivatives.

animals or the blood-pressure effects observed in man (SJOERDSMA et al., 1963). Rather it is because α-methyldopa is itself decarboxylated to α-methyldopamine, which is in turn β-hydroxylated to α-methylnorepinephrine (Fig. 7), that the drug is pharmacologically and biochemically active on sympathetic mechanisms.

Amine metabolites of α-methyldopa seem to account for the fact that tyramine pressor responses are enhanced rather than depressed in patients receiving this drug (PETTINGER et al., 1963; DOLLERY et al., 1963). Furthermore, the formation of amines from α-methyldopa accounts for the finding that the drug can restore the pressor response to tyramine in animals or patients (Fig. 8) previously treated with reserpine (PETTINGER et al., 1963; 1965). Probably the blood-pressure-lowering effect is due to replacement of a potent transmitter (norepinephrine) by a somewhat weaker one (α-methylnorepinephrine), as was first suggested by DAY and RAND (1964), though this explanation still requires some qualification (PETTINGER et al., 1965).

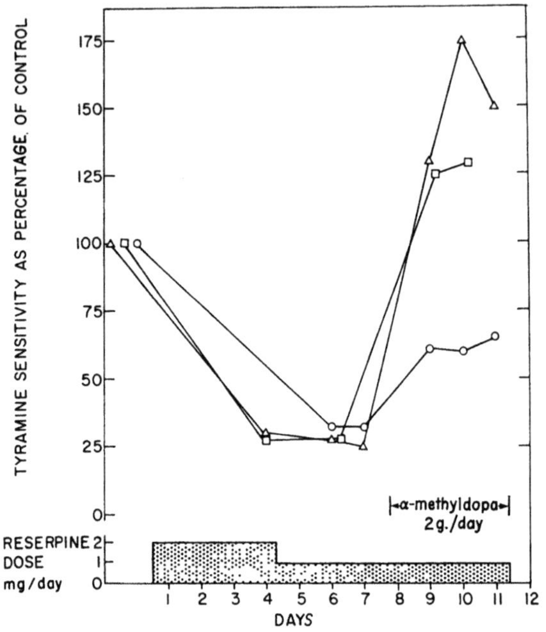

Fig. 8. Depression of tyramine pressor responses in three patients by reserpine and restoration by α-methyldopa (from PETTINGER et al., 1963).

3. Indicator, dietary "toxin", and mediator during treatment with M.A.O. inhibitors. A large number of inhibitors of M.A.O. have been found to produce marked orthostatic lowering of blood pressure. Currently, the M.A.O. inhibitor used mainly as an antihypertensive drug is pargyline hydrochloride (Eutonyl). When M.A.O. is effectively inhibited in man, there is an accumulation of many amines which lack efficient alternative pathways of metabolism. This is reflected by increased levels of their excretion in the urine. Two such amines are tryptamine and tyramine. Elevation of urinary tyramine produced by M.A.O. inhibition is shown in the study with α-methyldopa depicted previously in Fig. 6. In addition, owing to delayed metabolism, the pharmacological effects of such amines are greatly potentiated.

Marked enhancement of the pharmacological effects of tyramine by M.A.O. inhibitors is dramatically illustrated by pheochromocytoma-like pressor crises which may occur following the ingestion of tyramine-containing foods by patients receiving these drugs (Leading Article, 1965). Cheddar cheeses have been the main offenders. Amounts of tyramine sufficient to produce such pressor reactions on ingestion have also been found in certain wines and, most recently, in pickled herring (NEUSSLE et al., 1965). Tyramine in these and probably other food-stuffs is presumably formed by bacterial decarboxylation of tyrosine.

The paradox of blood-pressure lowering by M.A.O. inhibitors in the presence of accumulation of pressor amines has also been related by KOPIN et al. (1965) to alterations in the metabolism of tyramine. These workers obtained evidence that a relatively weak pressor amine, norsynephrine (octopamine), the formation of which by β-hydroxylation of tyramine (Fig. 7) is enhanced during inhibition of M.A.O., accumulates in sympathetic nerve-endings, where it presumably displaces norepinephrine and acts as a weak "false neurotransmitter".

4. Test for pheochromocytoma. In the course of some studies a few years ago on dopamine β-oxidase, we administered a foreign substrate, *p*-hydroxyamphetamine (Paredrine), to a patient with pheochromocytoma in anticipation of an enhanced β-hydroxylation (Fig. 7) of the drug (SJOERDSMA and VON STUDNITZ, 1963). As was indicated by the excretion of the β-hydroxylated metabolite in the urine, this did not occur, but the pressor response was augmented. Paredrine, like tyramine, is an indirectly acting pressor amine. We reasoned that in such a patient the exaggerated response might be due to an increase in the tissue stores of N.E. at sympathetic nerve-endings, resulting from uptake from the blood. If this were so, an enhanced pressor effect might also be expected to follow injection of a sympathomimetic compound such as tyramine. Accordingly, the pressor response to tyramine was also tested in this patient and found to be enhanced. Subsequent studies in four additional patients with pheochromocytoma and in a large number of control subjects (some normal and some with essential hypertension) led us to conclude that pressor responsiveness to tyramine might afford a useful diagnostic test for pheochromocytoma, provided the patients were not receiving some of the aforementioned drugs (ENGELMAN and SJOERDSMA, 1964b). Easier control over the magnitude of pressor response and the absence of untoward effects seemed to afford clear advantages over the histamine provocative test.

Additional observations tend to support the early impression that the tyramine test may be a useful adjunct in diagnosis. Our total experience in pheochromocytoma and in a large number of control cases is summarized in Fig. 9. Responses to two levels of dosage are shown. Generally, our previous suggestion that a systolic pressor response of greater than 20 mm. Hg systolic to an intravenous dose of 1,000 μg. tyramine (or less) warranted further

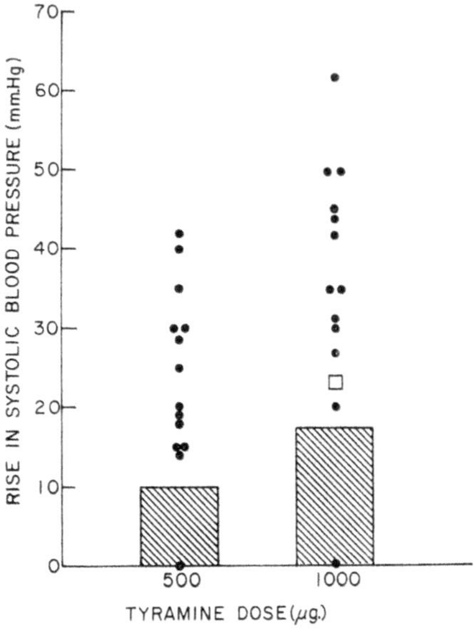

Fig. 9. Individual pressor responses to 500 and 1,000 μg. tyramine i.v. in 14 patients with pheochromocytoma (●), compared to responses for normal and hypertensive control cases. ▨ = Range: Normal and hypertensive patients (> 50); □ = False positive test in a hypertensive patient.

study for pheochromocytoma is supported. As may be seen, only one of 14 patients with pheochromocytoma was negative by this criterion. However, this patient also responded negatively to histamine (50 μg. gave a blood-pressure rise of 8/6 mm. Hg) and phentolamine (Regitine) tests (5 mg. Regitine decreased blood pressure by 16/10 mm. Hg) at a time when the base-line blood pressure was 150/110 mm. Hg. One false positive test has been encountered in a hypertensive patient (Fig. 9) with a blood-pressure rise of 22 mm. Hg following a dose of 1,000 μg.

Summary

Selected aspects of the biochemistry of norepinephrine (N.E.) are dealt with in relation to antihypertensive drug therapy and diagnosis of pheochromocytoma. It is shown that the goal of blockading the synthesis of N.E. in man has finally been achieved with the tyrosine-hydroxylase inhibitor, α-methyltyrosine. Its application in the medical management of pheochromocytoma is suggested. Alterations in pressor responses to tyramine produced by various drugs are cited to illustrate their mechanisms of action on N.E.; the increased responsiveness to tyramine in patients with pheochromocytoma may have diagnostic use.

Zusammenfassung

Einige ausgewählte Gesichtspunkte der Biochemie von Noradrenalin werden in Verbindung mit der therapeutischen Anwendung blutdrucksenkender Substanzen und der Diagnose des Phäochromozytoms behandelt. Es wird gezeigt, daß sich das seit langem verfolgte Ziel, die Noradrenalinsynthese beim Menschen zu blockieren, mit dem Tyrosin-hydroxylasehemmer, α-Methyltyrosin, erreichen läßt. Dessen Anwendung bei der medikamentösen Behandlung des Phäochromozytoms wird vorgeschlagen. Durch verschiedene Pharmaka hervorgerufene Änderungen der Blutdruckreaktion auf Tyramin werden zur Erklärung ihres Wirkungsmechanismus auf Noradrenalin herangezogen; die verstärkte Ansprechbarkeit von Patienten mit Phäochromozytom gegenüber Tyramin eignet sich für diagnostische Zwecke.

Résumé

Certains aspects de la biochimie de la noradrénaline sont envisagés dans leur relation avec la thérapeutique antihypertensive et le diagnostic du phéochromocytome. Il est montré que l'idée de bloquer la synthèse de la noradrénaline chez l'homme a finalement été réalisée par l'inhibiteur de la tyrosine-hydroxylase, l'α-méthyltyrosine. On suggère son application dans le traitement médical du phéochromocytome. On mentionne les modifications de la réponse vasopressive à la tyramine provoquées par diverses substances afin d'illustrer leur mécanisme d'action sur la noradrénaline; la sensibilité accrue à la tyramine chez les malades présentant un phéochromocytome peut avoir son application diagnostique.

References

ABBOUD, F. M., and J. W. ECKSTEIN: Circulation **29**, 219 (1964). — BURN, J. H., and M. J. RAND: J. Physiol. **144**, 314 (1958). — BRODIE, B. B.: Circulation **28**, 970 (1963). — CARLSSON, A., E. ROSENGREN, A. BERTLER, and J. NILSSON: In: Psychotropic Drugs. Ed. by S. GARATTINI and V. GHETTI. Elsevier Publishing Co., Amsterdam, 1957, p. 363. — CHANG, C. C., E. COSTA, and B. B. BRODIE: J. Pharmacol. Exper. Therap. **147**, 303 (1965). — CHIDSEY, C. A., E. BRAUNWALD, A. G. MORROW, and D. T. MASON: N. England J. Med. **269**, 653 (1963). — COHN, J. N., T. E. LIPTAK, and E. D. FREIS: Circulation Res. **12**, 298 (1963). — DAY, M. D., and M. J. RAND: Brit. J. Pharmacol. **22**, 72 (1964). — DOLLERY, C. T., M. HARINGTON, and J. V. HODGE: Brit. Heart J. **25**, 670 (1963). — ENGELMAN, K., and A. SJOERDSMA: Ann. Int. Med. **61**, 229 (1964a). — ENGELMAN, K., and A. SJOERDSMA: J. Amer. Med. Ass. **189**, 81 (1964b). — GALE, E. F.: Biochem. J. **34**, 846 (1940). — GILLESPIE, L., J. A. OATES, J. R. CROUT, and A. SJOERDSMA: Circulation **25**, 281 (1962). — HESS, S. M., R. H. CONNAMACHER, M. OZAKI, and S. UDENFRIEND: J. Pharmacol. Exper. Therap. **134**, 129 (1963). —

HORWITZ, D.: In: Cardiovascular Drug Therapy. Ed. by A. N. BREST and J. H. MOYER. Grune and Stratton, New York, 1965, p. 29. — KOPIN, I. J., J. E. FISCHER, J. M. MUSACCHIO, W. D. HORST, and V. WEISE: J. Pharmacol. Exper. Therap. **147**, 186 (1965). — Leading Article: Lancet 1965/I, 945. — LEVITT, M., S. SPECTOR, A. SJOERDSMA, and S. UDENFRIEND: J. Pharmacol. Exper. Therap. **148**, 1 (1965). — LOVENBERG, W., H. WEISSBACH, and S. UDENFRIEND: J. Biol. Chem. **237**, 89 (1962). — MCCURDY, R. L., A. J. PRANGE, M. A. LIPTON, and C. M. COCHRANE: Proc. Soc. Exper. Biol. Med. **116**, 1159 (1964). — NEUSSLE, W. F., F. C. NORMAN, and H. E. MILLER: J. Amer. Med. Ass. **192**, 726 (1965). — NICODIJEVIC, B., C. R. CREVELING, and S. UDENFRIEND: J. Pharmacol. Exper. Therap. **140**, 224 (1963). — OATES, J. A., L. GILLESPIE, S. UDENFRIEND, and A. SJOERDSMA: Science **131**, 1890 (1960).— PETTINGER, W. A., D. HORWITZ, S. SPECTOR, and A. SJOERDSMA: Nature **200**, 1107 (1963). — PETTINGER, W. A., S. SPECTOR, D. HORWITZ, and A. SJOERDSMA: Proc. Soc. Exper. Biol. Med. **118**, 988 (1965). — POTTER, L., and J. AXELROD: J. Pharmacol. Exper. Therap. **140**, 199 (1963). — SJOERDSMA, A.: Circulation Res. **9**, 734 (1961). — SJOERDSMA, A., A. VENDSALU, and K. ENGELMAN: Circulation **28**, 492 (1963). — SJOERDSMA, A., and W. VON STUDNITZ: Brit. J. Pharmacol. **20**, 278 (1963). — SPECTOR, S., A. SJOERDSMA, and S. UDENFRIEND: J. Pharmacol. Exper. Therap. **147**, 86 (1965). — SPECTOR, S., A. SJOERDSMA, P. ZALTZMAN-NIRENBERG, M. LEVITT, and S. UDENFRIEND: Science **139**, 1299 (1963). — STJÄRNE, L.: Acta physiol. Scand. **62**, Suppl. **228** (1964). — Symposium on Catecholamines: Pharmacol. Rev. **11**, 317 (1959).

Discussion

DOLLERY: I should like to ask Dr. SJOERDSMA a question. It concerns the false-transmitter hypothesis of the action of α-methyldopa and particularly the increased response to tyramine. Patients treated with α-methyldopa are about twice as sensitive to noradrenaline after treatment as they are before. There is also an increase of approximately 50% in their sensitivity to tyramine. If tyramine acts by release of transmitter, it might be expected that release of the false transmitter would produce a smaller effect and not a larger one.

One other point about the action of tyramine in man is that its effects do not resemble those of exogenous noradrenaline. Tyramine causes a tachycardia with an increase in pulse pressure but very little change in diastolic pressure, whereas noradrenaline causes bradycardia and an increase in both systolic and diastolic pressures.

SJOERDSMA: I also have difficulty in explaining some of these phenomena. I should say, however, that in a reserpine-treated animal, where one has eliminated norepinephrine, one can restore the response to tyramine with α-methyldopa or with its amine products. Now it's interesting that α-methylnorepinephrine is more effective in restoring a tyramine response in a reserpine-treated animal, for example in the dog, than norepinephrine itself. I think there is always a temptation to give simple explanations. I don't have one in the case of α-methyldopa. I feel that the evidence indicating that its actions are related to formation of amines is good. The possibility that there may be a central action cannot be entirely ruled out; we certainly observe sedative effects. In man, for whatever the gross effects of α-methylnorepinephrine on blood pressure are worth (admittedly there are both cardiac and peripheral effects), it is interesting that the compound is considerably less active than norepinephrine (about $^1/_5$), whereas these amines are almost equally potent in laboratory animals, such as the dog. Thus, a false-transmitter mechanism may explain the relative sensitivity of the human to the blood-pressure-lowering effects of α-methyldopa. I think Dr. CARLSSON is really in a better position to enlarge on some of the changes which may occur at nerve-endings. Do you have anything to add to this, Dr. CARLSSON?

CARLSSON: I think that many of these apparently confusing things that have been raised now can be explained on the basis of the model I showed you in Fig. 1 of my paper. For example, it is not very difficult to explain why you can restore the tyramine response of reserpine-treated animals by means of α-methylnoradrenaline much more easily than by means of noradrenaline. Within the nerve-endings you have monamine oxidase. Your experiment is as follows: you first give reserpine and get rid of endogenous noradrenaline. Then, when you administer tyramine, there is no response. But when you give noradrenaline, followed by a second dose of tyramine, you find that the response is restored, although it is not so strong as before. After that, you give α-methylnoradrenaline, and then you administer your test-dose of tyramine again; and this time, you get a much better response. The explanation of this is that noradrenaline is pumped into the nerve-ending all right, but owing to the presence of monamine oxidase it is destroyed more or less at the same time as it is pumped in. Thus, when you have finished the noradrenaline infusion and then give the test-dose of tyramine, there is very little noradrenaline left. If you give α-methylnoradrenaline, it is again pumped very efficiently into the nerve-ending; but α-methylnoradrenaline is resistant to monamine oxidase and accumulates there. This can be very convincingly demonstrated histochemically[1]. And now, of course, tyramine has a wonderful opportunity to act, because there is a tremendous accumulation of α-methylnoradrenaline. I think I could go on exemplifying, but, in general, I believe that many of these confusing things — admittedly not all of them — can be explained fairly easily by means of the model we have now.

Sjoerdsma: I agree that they can be, and the explanations you offer may be correct. However, I think that for a group such as we are talking to today, it's very useful to realise that the "models" are changing from year to year. I am sure that in a year or so even your model may be somewhat modified.

Carlsson: Mine has been standing for a couple of years now.

Sjoerdsma: How do you explain, on the basis of your model, haemodynamic differences between the responses to tyramine and norepinephrine in man?

Carlsson: Well, this kind of thing is an everyday nuisance to the pharmacologist. This is much easier to explain than those other things, because, you see, in one case you give noradrenaline, which goes directly to the receptors; in the other case you give a compound which releases noradrenaline and may do so with varying degrees of efficiency in different nerve-endings; these adrenergic nerve-endings are not all alike. It can be shown histochemically that some of them are much more easily affected by certain drugs than others.

Hoobler: I was interested to see that Dr. Sjoerdsma had added one false negative tyramine test in phaeochromocytoma. We have been using the tyramine test in a few cases, finding negative results in essential hypertension. But in one case of phaeochromocytoma, where histamine was positive, the test was negative twice, and yet a tumour was found on exploration.

Sjoerdsma: Do you remember the catecholamine excretion in this case? One accepts, of course, that there would be a certain level below which the peripheral store wouldn't really be sufficiently elevated to enhance a tyramine response; I don't know what this level will prove to be.

Hoobler: Was the catecholamine secretion low in your negative case?

Sjoerdsma: In this case the daily excretion of free catecholamines averaged 300—400 μg.

Dengler: We know that in a number of animal species α-methylnoradrenaline was identified in different tissues when the animals were pretreated with α-methyldopa. But to my knowledge there are no reports on the identification of α-methylnoradrenaline, the "false transmitter", in tissues or body fluids of human beings treated with therapeutic doses of α-methyldopa.

[1] Malmfors, T.: Acta physiol. Scand. **64**, Suppl. **248** (1965).

SJOERDSMA: I don't think anyone has made a really intensive search for small amounts of α-methylnorepinephrine in human urine. We thought we saw a spot corresponding to this substance on a paper chromatogram a few years ago. The decarboxylation percentage of α-methyldopa in man is much lower than in animal species (e.g. rat and mouse); however, since man possesses the enzyme machinery to form α-methylnorepinephrine, I am willing to assume that small amounts are present.

KIRKENDALL: When using the histamine test for the diagnosis of phaeochromocytoma it is very helpful to compare the response of the cardiovascular system to a noxious stimulus, such as the cold pressor test, as well. On occasion, one may find individuals who react to the histamine test with a pronounced response and severe hypertension, but when a non-specific stimulus is used the patient also displays a sharp increase in blood pressure. My question is: would it possibly enhance the usefulness of the tyramine test if one compared the response to that following some non-specific stimulus, such as the cold pressor test? I think if such a comparison did help to exclude hyper-reactors, it might strengthen the test.

SJOERDSMA: I think it will evolve in some direction, as any new test does. We see no need for any such additional tests at the moment, because our control responses in patients with essential hypertension have been rather good, with only one false positive in about 200 patients. This is not true of the histamine test, in which many false positives are observed, even when a cold pressor response is used for comparison. I should simply like to see people evaluate the test and, whenever possible, compare it with other tests, both chemical and pharmacological.

Advantages and disadvantages of combined drug treatment

By

A. N. Brest

Although mild hypertension can usually be controlled by single antihypertensive drug therapy, most cases of moderate or severe blood-pressure elevation require double or triple drug regimens. The successful application of combined drug regimens demands a complete understanding of the clinical pharmacology of the drugs involved. Inherent in this understanding is full recognition of the rationale, as well as of the advantages and disadvantages of combined antihypertensive drug therapy.

Rationale

It is rational to combine antihypertensive drugs, if their anatomic sites of action or their pharmacodynamic activities differ. Accordingly, it is rational to combine a postganglionic blocking drug with a diuretic or with hydralazine, since each of these drug groups interferes with the mechanisms governing hypertension at different sites and by different pharmacological means. On the other hand, the combination of two drugs such as guanethidine and reserpine would probably not have additive or potentiating effects, since they act similarly at the same anatomic site (i.e. both drugs exert their antihypertensive effects by causing an exaggerated release of norepinephrine from the postganglionic nerve fibers, thereby depleting these fibers of their catecholamine stores).

Clinical experiences

Of the several antihypertensive drug groups currently available, the diuretics satisfy the definition of the "ideal antihypertensive drug" most closely. Their attributes may be classified as follows: 1) they lower both the supine and erect blood pressures, 2) the incidence of accompanying side reactions is relatively low, and 3) their antihypertensive activity is sustained despite prolonged drug administration. The potent oral diuretic (thiazide, phthalimidine, and quinazoline) drugs lower blood pressure significantly in 40–50% of randomly selected hypertensive patients (Table 1).

By adding other antihypertensive compounds to diuretic drug therapy, the blood-pressure response can be improved further.

Table 1. *Blood-pressure response to various diuretic drugs*

Drug regimen	No. of patients	Supine				Erect			
		Normotensive[1]		Responsive[2]		Normotensive[1]		Responsive[2]	
		No.	%	No.	%	No.	%	No.	%
Chlorothiazide	50	9	18	18	36	12	24	23	46
Hydrochlorothiazide .	54	11	20	21	39	12	22	21	39
Flumethiazide	17	2	12	7	41	8	47	9	53
Chlorthalidone	30	5	17	12	40	8	27	15	50
Quinethazone	29	5	17	12	41	7	24	12	41

[1] Blood pressure reduced $>$150/90 mm. Hg.
[2] Mean blood pressure reduced $>$20 mm. Hg or normotensive.

Although some investigations have suggested that Rauwolfia compounds, administered orally, lack significant antihypertensive activity (*1*), other studies state that Rauwolfia lowers blood pressure in 25–30% of the hypertensive population (*2*). Our experience with several potent oral diuretic-Rauwolfia combinations has indicated a significant antihypertensive response in approximately 65% of randomly selected hypertensive patients (Table 2). This combined response is what would be anticipated on

Table 2. *Blood-pressure response to various combined diuretic-Rauwolfia regimens*

Drug regimen	No. of patients	Supine				Erect			
		Normotensive[1]		Responsive[2]		Normotensive[1]		Responsive[2]	
		No.	%	No.	%	No.	%	No.	%
Chlorothiazide + Raudixin	18	5	28	10	56	6	33	10	56
Flumethiazide + Raudixin	22	8	36	11	50	13	59	15	68
Hydrochlorothiazide + syrosingopine . . .	27	6	22	16	59	7	26	19	70
Chlorthalidone + reserpine	21	10	48	13	62	11	52	13	62
Quinethazone + reserpine	13	3	23	8	61	4	30	8	61

[1] Blood pressure reduced $>$150/90 mm. Hg.
[2] Mean blood pressure reduced $>$20 mm. Hg or normotensive.

an additive basis and therefore would seem to provide confirmation of the mild, but definite, antihypertensive effectiveness of the Rauwolfia compounds.

The antihypertensive action of hydralazine is generally acknowledged. Its major drawbacks include: 1) the occasional development of a mesenchymal reaction, which simulates idiopathic lupus erythematosus, and 2) the possible development of drug tolerance when used alone. The occurrence of iatrogenic lupus reactions can usually be obviated by using dosages of less than 500 mg. daily, and the likelihood of tolerance can be avoided or reduced by the concomitant use of other drugs (*3*). The combination of hydralazine with thiazides and Rauwolfia drugs is particularly effective, yielding significant blood-pressure reduction in approximately 80% of hypertensive patients (Table 3).

Table 3. *Blood-pressure response to hydralazine administered alone and in combination with chlorothiazide and Rauwolfia*

Therapeutic regimen	No. of patients	Normotensive[1]		Responsive[2]	
		No.	%	No.	%
Hydralazine alone	54	6	11	19	35
Chlorothiazide + hydralazine	38	18	47	25	66
Chlorothiazide + alseroxylon + hydralazine	48	30	63	39	80

[1] Blood pressure reduced $>150/90$ mm. Hg.
[2] Mean blood pressure reduced >20 mm. Hg or normotensive.

Prior to the introduction of guanethidine, the ganglion blocking compounds were the most potent antihypertensive drugs available. Guanethidine and pargyline have tended to displace the ganglioplegic drugs in the current drug armamentarium, since 1) the antihypertensive potency of the newer drugs is similar to that of the ganglionic blocking drugs, whereas 2) the incidence of accompanying side reactions is less, and 3) their more prolonged duration of action makes drug dosage titration somewhat easier (*4*, *5*). On the other hand, both guanethidine and pargyline – like the ganglioplegic drugs – exert a predominantly orthostatic antihypertensive action with only a modest effect on the supine blood pressure. However, the concomitant administration of an oral diuretic lessens the dosage requirement of the more potent drug (thereby decreasing the incidence of side reactions encountered with the latter) and increases the supine antihypertensive response (without compromising the orthostatic antihypertensive effect) (Table 4).

Although α-methyldopa is less potent than guanethidine or pargyline, the drug has a similar, predominantly orthostatic, antihypertensive activity (*6*). As with the other potent drugs, the concomitant use of an oral diuretic lessens the dosage requirement of α-methyldopa and increases the supine antihypertensive response (Table 4).

Table 4. *Blood-pressure response to guanethidine, pargyline, and α-methyldopa, alone and in combination with hydrochlorothiazide*

Therapeutic regimen	No. of patients	Supine				Erect			
		Normotensive[1]		Responsive[2]		Normotensive[1]		Responsive[2]	
		No.	%	No.	%	No.	%	No.	%
Guanethidine	30	5	17	12	40	13	43	27	90
Guanethidine + hydrochlorothiazide	25	6	24	13	52	14	56	22	88
Pargyline	33	5	15	7	21	19	57	27	82
Pargyline + hydrochlorothiazide	11	1	9	4	36	5	45	9	82
α-Methyldopa	38	6	16	13	34	9	24	16	42
α-Methyldopa + hydrochlorothiazide	19	8	42	12	63	10	53	17	89

[1] Blood pressure reduced $>$150/90 mm. Hg.
[2] Mean blood pressure reduced $>$20 mm. Hg or normotensive.

In addition to their effects on blood pressure, the antihypertensive drugs also exert important hemodynamic actions. Thus, whereas certain drugs, such as guanethidine and pargyline, tend to depress renal hemodynamic functions, others, such as α-methyldopa, may improve renal blood flow despite blood-pressure reduction (*4*, *5*, *6*). It is important, therefore, to appreciate these hemodynamic effects, and especially so when antihypertensive drugs are used in combination.

The ultimate aim of antihypertensive therapy is to lower both supine and erect blood pressures to normotensive levels. Triple drug regimens, employing thiazide, guanethidine, and hydralazine, or thiazide, α-methyldopa, and hydralazine, have proved quite useful in instances where thiazide-guanethidine or thiazide-α-methyldopa combinations failed to control both supine and erect blood pressures. The success of these triple regimens serves further to confirm the rationale of combined antihypertensive drug therapy.

Advantages and disadvantages

The clinical experiences described above indicate the following advantages of combined antihypertensive drug therapy: 1) by combining drugs with different antihypertensive actions, additive effects can be obtained, thereby resulting in increasingly effective blood-pressure control; 2) judicious combination of drugs with varying antihypertensive potencies often makes it possible to decrease the total incidence of side reactions by reducing the necessary dosage of the individual drugs (Table 5). In addition, knowledgeable use of drug combinations may reduce side reactions by pharmacological means, e. g. the tachycardiac effect of hydralazine can be reduced by the concomitant use of Rauwolfia or guanethidine, both of which tend to cause bradycardia. Similarly, the combination of a potent, gravity-dependent compound with drugs which possess mild or moderate potency (but have different antihypertensive actions) may achieve improved supine antihypertensive control while permitting the dosage requirement of the more potent drug to be decreased without loss of orthostatic efficacy.

Table 5. *Incidence of side effects with hydralazine alone and in combination with chlorothiazide and Rauwolfia* (percent of patients treated)

Side effect	Hydralazine alone (54 patients)	Thiazide + hydralazine (38 patients)	Thiazide + Rauwolfia + hydralazine (48 patients)
Palpitations	52%	34%	19%
Headache	37%	26%	12%
Angina pectoris	7%	5%	2%
Nausea, vomiting	37%	13%	6%
Anxiety	15%	11%	6%
Weakness	22%	42%	29%

In contrast, the inappropriate selection of drug combinations, such as reserpine plus guanethidine, serves only to expose the patient to the combined side reactions of each drug without the likelihood of increased antihypertensive efficacy, since both drugs possess similar pharmacological actions. In fact, the inappropriate combination of antihypertensive drugs may result in a paradoxical hypertensive response. Thus, the combination of a drug which releases adrenergic stores of norepinephrine (e.g. guanethidine) with a monamine-oxidase inhibitor (e.g. pargyline) may be responsible for sudden blood-pressure elevation (7).

The individual hemodynamic attributes of the antihypertensive drugs may also effect an adverse or beneficial response to combination drug therapy. Reduction in glomerular filtration rate and renal blood flow may accompany the use of potent oral diuretics, guanethidine, pargyline, and/or the ganglion blocking drugs. Combinations of these drugs may therefore aggravate renal functional impairment; consequently these drugs should be used with caution in patients with borderline or lesser renal function. On the other hand, the beneficial renal hemodynamic effects of α-methyldopa and hydralazine commend their combined use in patients with renal hypertension or in hypertensive individuals with renal functional impairment.

Comprehensive regimen for ambulatory patients with diastolic hypertension

Utilizing the clinical experiences herein described, the following regimen has been employed successfully in the management of most patients with diastolic hypertension (Table 6).

Table 6. *Comprehensive therapeutic regimen*

Diastolic blood pressure	Initial therapy	If necessary, add
> 90 mm. Hg but < 110 mm. Hg	Chlorothiazide[1]	Rauwolfia
> 110 mm. Hg but < 130 mm. Hg	Chlorothiazide[1] + Rauwolfia or α-methyldopa	Hydralazine or Veratrum
> 130 mm. Hg	Chlorothiazide[1] + guanethidine or pargyline	Hydralazine or α-methyldopa

[1] Other thiazide, phthalimidine, or quinazoline diuretics produce equally good results.

One of the potent oral diuretics is invariably employed, unless some specific contraindication to their use exists. If the oral diuretic fails to achieve the desired response, a Rauwolfia compound or α-methyldopa should be added to the therapeutic regimen after two weeks. Thereafter, if the blood pressure remains elevated, hydralazine or a Veratrum compound should be given in addition. In instances of severe or rapidly progressive hypertension, it is recommended that guanethidine or pargyline be added to the therapeutic regimen without delay. Most patients with moderate or severe diastolic hypertension require a double or triple drug regimen in order to achieve significant blood-pressure reduction.

Summary

The appropriate (or inappropriate) combination of antihypertensive drugs may result in beneficial (or adverse) effects on 1) blood pressure, 2) side reactions, and 3) hemodynamic actions. The potential advantages generally exceed the disadvantages of combined antihypertensive drug therapy. It is incumbent on the physician, therefore, to understand the rationale of such regimens and the clinical pharmacology of the individual drugs, so that they can be used in combination to fullest clinical advantage.

Zusammenfassung

Die zweckmäßige (oder unzweckmäßige) Kombination blutdrucksenkender Substanzen kann zu günstigen (oder ungünstigen) Wirkungen auf 1) Blutdruck, 2) Nebenerscheinungen und 3) hämodynamische Effekte führen. Die möglichen Vorteile übertreffen im allgemeinen die Nachteile einer kombinierten blutdrucksenkenden Therapie. Der Arzt soll die Grundlagen derartiger Behandlungsschemata verstehen und die klinische Pharmakologie der einzelnen Stoffe beherrschen, damit er sie in Kombination mit größtmöglichem klinischem Vorteil anwenden kann.

Résumé

L'association judicieuse de substances antihypertensives peut donner d'heureux résultats 1° sur la tension artérielle, 2° quant à la moindre fréquence des effets secondaires, 3° dans les actions hémodynamiques; des associations inadéquates, à l'inverse, conduisent à des effets néfastes. Les avantages potentiels des associations dans la thérapeutique antihypertensive sont généralement supérieurs à leurs inconvénients. C'est au médecin qu'il incombe par conséquent de comprendre les principes de tels schémas thérapeutiques et de connaître la pharmacologie clinique de chaque produit, de façon à ce qu'il puisse tirer le maximum de profit de leur association.

References

1. GROLLMAN, A.: Pharmacology and Therapeutics. Lea and Febiger, Philadelphia, 1962, p. 499. — 2. MOYER, J. H., E. DENNIS, and R. V. FORD: Arch. Int. Med. **96**, 530 (1955). — 3. MOYER, J. H., and A. N. BREST: Med. Clin. North America **45**, 375 (1961). — 4. BREST, A. N., P. NOVACK, H. KASPARIAN, and J. H. MOYER: Dis. Chest **42**, 359 (1962). — 5. BREST, A. N., G. ONESTI, C. HEIDER, R. H. SELLER, and J. H. MOYER: Amer. Heart J. **68**, 621 (1964). — 6. ONESTI, G., A. N. BREST, P. NOVACK, and J. H. MOYER: Amer. J. Cardiol. **9**, 863 (1962). — 7. GOLDBERG, L. I.: J. Amer. Med. Ass. **190**, 456 (1964).

Discussion

SMIRK: I think one must agree that using a diuretic with one of the more potent drugs will sometimes lessen the amount of postural hypotension, but I wonder whether you would agree with the observations of my colleague SIMPSON[1] to the effect that there is usually a larger fall in blood pressure in the standing than in the lying posture with most of the diuretics, even when they are the only hypotensive agents given.

BREST: This is true, although the disparity between the supine and the orthostatic response is much less marked than that observed with guanethidine or pargyline or ganglioplegic drugs.

BOCK: I do not agree with the statement Dr. BREST made at the beginning of his paper, saying that it is not rational to combine drugs which are thought to have the same site of action. My main reason for disagreeing is that the mode and the site of action of most antihypertensive agents are in fact by far not so clearly defined as they appear to be in the usual schemes. For instance, the two drugs which were placed in the same category as regards their site of action, α-methyldopa and guanethidine, have an additive effect in hypertensive patients, and this combination — together with a saluretic — has proved to be very useful in severe cases.

BREST: I believe the statement holds good, but I think this is a matter of semantics. If two drugs with precisely the same pharmacodynamic activities are administered, one would not expect an additive effect. On the other hand, many of the available drugs have discrete, albeit small, pharmacodynamic differences, even though they presumably belong to the same or similar drug groups.

CARLSSON: I think Dr. BREST's statement is a very good one in principle, but when we come to the actual drugs, our knowledge of their site of action is often incomplete. For example, we still don't know anything about the antihypertensive site of action of α-methyldopa, nor do we know whether reserpine acts only peripherally or whether there is also a central component in its hypotensive action, as we discussed on the first day.

PETERS: I object to the statement that the action of the maximal effective dose of a drug cannot be intensified by adding another drug, if it has the same site or the same mechanism of action. The "maximal" effect of a drug may or may not be increased by another drug acting at the same site, depending on the binding of the two drugs to the supposedly common receptor and their persistence there, as well as their "intrinsic" activities. There is no definitive relationship between site of action and "intrinsic" activity. A "second" drug acting at the same site may even be given in a dose which does not influence the parameter measured, but may still enhance the maximal effect of the "first" drug.

PAGE: It is fair to say that now that we have had about 15 years' experience in the use of all this variety of drugs we are getting into another

[1] SIMPSON, F. O.: Curr. Ther. Res. **6**, 21 (1964).

era. We have to think not only of the immediate effects of drugs, but of the very long-term effects as well. Drugs we use in medicine as therapeutic agents differ from drugs which might almost be called "public health measures". Very large quantities of the latter are going to be used by millions of people. I remember that when Rauwolfia came in, it was suggested by one very distinguished person in the United States that our Government should buy Rauwolfia and provide it free to the public. This would have been a catastrophe. It is important to begin to weed out the drugs that may have dangerous long-term effects. We are going to treat people for possibly 40 years with a drug. This is another aspect of treatment which has got to be given serious attention. So I would remind you that when dealing with what I call "public health" drugs, the limit of tolerance as regards side effects is very small indeed. This contrasts sharply with the situation in relation to "therapeutic drugs". Ultimately we must prevent as well as treat hypertension.

SMIRK: I should like to ask one more question. With the majority of the diuretics in use at the present time, my colleague SIMPSON[1] finds, as others have done, a rise in the blood urea and a rise in the blood uric acid, sometimes with precipitation of gout and occasionally accompanied by interference with glucose tolerance. Now, our experience has been that these have rarely led to anything of a serious or irreversible nature, so far as the patient was concerned. But have you any views on the question of prolonged use? For example, if the patient is going to have a high blood uric acid for many years, is renal damage likely to occur? I'd like Dr. PAGE to speak about that, too.

BREST: Some of these untoward metabolic effects may occur early and some may occur late; for instance, in our experience with hyperuricaemia following thiazide therapy, we have seen gout develop in as little as three to 21 days, whereas in other cases gout has not appeared for seven to ten months. In this connection, there has been a great deal of interesting speculation which one could discuss here. For example, it is well known that there is an association between hyperuricaemia and the development of atherosclerosis. If one produces hyperuricaemia, and if this is present over a long period of time, and if hyperuricaemia is associated with atherogenesis, then perhaps you are facilitating the development of atherosclerosis. This is the type of speculation I think one could muse upon for quite a long time.

SMIRK: I can add to that some experience from our clinic. We had a look at the question as to whether the occurrence of coronary disease was related to which of the patients were receiving diuretics and which were not, and so far — I emphasise that this is a very preliminary study — we have found no difference in the incidence of coronary disease. I wonder whether Dr. PAGE or Dr. DUSTAN could say anything from their clinic about this.

DUSTAN: I am increasingly impressed with the problems created by the use of oral diuretics, because during the past year we have seen a number of cases of acute gout that have posed very difficult therapeutic problems. Because of these difficulties I seriously raise the question whether the oral diuretics, as we know them now, are not going to be old memories in about ten years. At the present time, we are going back to the use of low-sodium diets, because they afford the same advantages as do the diuretics in terms of enhanced effectiveness of drugs, without, as far as I know, causing hyperuricaemia or diminishing carbohydrate tolerance. So the pendulum swings

[1] SIMPSON, F. O., and H. J. WAAL: N. Zealand Med. J. **63**, 199 (1964).

back again. I realise that low-sodium diets are difficult to take and that patients don't like them, but I do suggest that we perhaps are heading for more difficulty with the oral diuretics than we imagined during those early halcyon days of their use.

PAGE: May I add one more thing? If you reduce the patient's blood pressure to essentially normal levels and keep it there, even though you have to use large doses of drugs, will this result in a state in which ultimately you may be able to withdraw drug therapy entirely? I think that in some of Dr. DUSTAN's and my patients the hypertension has been reversed. We have acted on the principle that if we pushed these people very hard and insisted, not just on orthostatic reduction of blood pressure, but on reduction of blood pressure in the prone position, the regulatory mechanisms might reset themselves and the resetting might be successfully maintained. I think this concept should be very seriously considered by the experts here. We believe that some primary hypertension is reversible if treatment is truly adequate.

SMIRK: I should like to ask Dr. BREST also to comment on that. As far as our experience is concerned, it has been the same. We have always pressed therapy. We have found malignant hypertensive patients over the years (some of them have lasted as long as ten years) who, with continued treatment, can eventually be managed with much less medication — sometimes only a diuretic, sometimes a diuretic and reserpine — and remain very well controlled.

We have had instances of patients with severe hypertension, sometimes malignant, sometimes severe in other ways, who for one reason or another had stopped taking their antihypertensive drugs. We have taken the opportunity to repeat the basal blood-pressure measurements while these patients were off drugs. They may have been off for only two or three weeks, but long enough to have escaped from the normal pharmacological action of the drugs. We found that in many instances such patients do not show the expected rise with age in the level of the basal blood pressure, and that their basal pressure may even fail to rise to the original level, whereas basal blood-pressure recordings repeated in untreated patients from five to 14 years after the original measurement are almost always found to have increased. Basal pressures don't swing about like the casual blood pressures.

I think I have seen in the audience a number of people who have had experience in this field, but I should like to ask Dr. BREST first whether he would care to comment.

BREST: Our own experience suggests that once a hypertensive, always a hypertensive. When we have taken hypertensive patients off drug therapy, we have generally found that their blood-pressure elevation has recurred, although it has taken sometimes days, weeks, months, or years. I think that this is probably similar to the situation with diabetes mellitus; although there may be a remission with drug therapy, the patient remains an inherent diabetic.

KINCAID-SMITH: I should like to question Dr. BREST's statement that certain drugs should be combined and that others should not be used in combination because of their supposed sites of action. As we have heard at this meeting, the site of action of many drugs is not yet clearly understood, which does not support such a line of reasoning. We use virtually any combination of hypotensive drugs in certain patients, and we have found a combination of α-methyldopa and guanethidine, together with a diuretic, particularly valuable in severely hypertensive patients. I should also like to question the use of pargyline. Our own view has been that the necessity to avoid red wine and cheese, together with the unpredictable hypertensive crises which occur in patients taking pargyline, are sufficient reason to use this drug only when all else fails.

SMIRK: It should perhaps be added that dangerous reactions are also liable to occur after ingestion of several other types of food-stuff. For example, HODGE et al.[1], in our clinic, showed that considerable rises in blood pressure may follow the consumption of broad-bean pods in patients on a monamine-oxidase inhibitor.

FREIS: Since the question of hyperuricaemia has been raised, I might mention that we surveyed our clinic patients, and in 66 non-azotaemic hypertensives, one third had hyperuricaemia. By that I mean uric acid elevations of 6.5 mg.% or above. We have treated them with probenecid for four months now. At the end of two months, the average uric acid concentration was reduced from 8.1 mg.% to 5.6 mg.%. Whereas 17 of 20 patients had levels above 7 mg.% before treatment, none had elevations above 7 mg.% at two months, although at four months three patients had such elevations. Though one dislikes adding more drugs to an already complicated regimen, it is possible with probenecid to control the thiazide-induced uric acid elevation in most patients.

HOOBLER: I should like to second Dr. PAGE's comments. I believe we are entering an era in which we shall have to consider the problems inherent in very long-term treatment and the risks that may be associated with such treatment. This is why I think we all have to study the possible toxicity of thiazides, which will be the ultimate drugs in most of these patients under prolonged treatment. Those of us who have long-term experience with thiazide treatment should study these patients extremely carefully to detect any early serious abnormalities. Secondly, we should move toward milder effective regimens, as Dr. DUSTAN mentioned, such as salt restriction or the infrequent administration of thiazides. Also I think our classic problem is that we must treat earlier and earlier if we are to use prophylaxis against atherosclerosis. In our series that I reported, there was no hyperuricaemia, and I think this was partly because we chose patients with excellent renal function. This underlines again the importance of early treatment before the disease becomes established, and early control of blood pressure, if we are to give our patients protection against vascular disease.

[1] HODGE, J. V., E. R. NYE, and G. W. EMERSON: Lancet 1964/I, 1108.

Management of hypertensive crisis

By

R. E. Lee

Hypertensive crisis may result from a variety of causes. These include eclampsia, acute nephritis, misuse of anesthetic equipment in the operating theater, administration of vasopressor drugs, and malignant hypertension.

There is general agreement that in each of these instances, very prompt control of the blood pressure is needed. The delay between the onset of treatment with oral medications and the achievement of blood-pressure control may range from several days to several weeks. For this reason, more rapidly acting intravenous or intramuscular preparations are preferred. The agents available at present may produce troublesome side effects. There are different opinions as to which are the best substances to use, and as to whether intravenous or intramuscular administration is the more worthwhile. The purpose of this paper is to review some of the present-day techniques of managing hypertensive crisis and malignant hypertension and to present new data on the treatment of the latter condition with intramuscular guanethidine.

Review of present techniques

Reserpine, in intramuscular doses of 1–5 mg., will often bring about a prompt blood-pressure reduction within a few hours (*1*). It has been used in the treatment of many types of acute hypertension, including eclampsia and cerebral vascular accidents. Repeated injections may be given at intervals of two to eight hours, if necessary, and oral medication may be employed at the same time. Unfortunately, intramuscular doses of reserpine may produce symptoms ranging from deep stupor to near coma. If stupor is already present owing to an intracerebral hemorrhage, the subsequent course of the patient will be obscured. Nevertheless, this is a popular method of treating acute hypertension and will probably continue to be so in the future.

Hydralazine, given intramuscularly in doses of 5–25 mg., will also bring the blood pressure down appreciably within a few hours

(*2*). Since this product, in contrast to other antihypertensive products available, may increase renal plasma flow, it is often the parenteral drug of choice in the management of hypertension associated with acute nephritis. Some specialists feel that it is not a particularly potent agent and prefer to use other compounds. Hydralazine may cause a rapid heart rate with insufficient cardiac filling and a near cardiac-failure syndrome in some persons. Occasionally, angina pectoris may be aggravated.

Veratrum products are used intravenously in doses of 2–4 mg./l. (*2*). These agents act primarily via nerve reflexes in the mediastinum; they control blood pressure promptly and produce a reflex slowing of the heart as well. The therapeutic index in the case of Veratrum products, however, is quite narrow, and vomiting is frequently encountered. Because of the danger of aspiration pneumonia, these preparations are no longer as popular as they were formerly.

Autonomic blocking agents, such as pentolinium tartrate, have proved useful when given slowly in intravenous doses of 2–200 mg./l. (*3*). These products, however, are known to reduce renal plasma flow and act on the blood pressure primarily via orthostatic mechanisms. Because of interference with the autonomic regulatory function of the bowel, severe ileus is frequently encountered. The intravenous administration of ganglionic blockers is still popular today.

Trimethaphan, when given slowly intravenously in doses of 5–100 mg./l., brings about a very prompt reduction of the blood pressure (*4*). This product is quite safe and has no known serious side effects. Its action is so swift, however, that when the drip is slowed or discontinued, the hypotensive effect disappears very rapidly. For that reason, the use of this product requires the continuous attendance of a nurse or physician during the treatment period in order to prevent overzealous reduction of the blood pressure or escape from therapeutic control.

α-Methyldopa, given intravenously in saline solution by the drip method at various dose levels, brings about a prompt control of the blood pressure in most instances. Although it acts primarily via orthostatic means, reduction of the supine blood pressure also occurs. This product is popular, but the publication of several reports to the effect that it may cause liver damage has detracted from its usefulness (*5*). We have encountered at least three such instances in our clinic.

Guanethidine has recently been introduced as an oral product for the control of severe blood-pressure elevation (*6*). The injectable preparation has been tested in our clinic in a series of 14 patients with malignant hypertension. It was found that intramuscular injections of this material (in some instances a single injection) brought about a prompt reduction of the blood pressure in each case and required a minimum of attendance by medical personnel. Side effects were uncommon and not troublesome. In only one instance were they sufficiently severe to necessitate discontinuation of the preparation.

Methods

The drug was used on patients admitted to The New York Hospital with malignant hypertension. They were relatively young, the average age being 41 years. The group comprised nine males and five females; seven were whites, six were Negroes, and one was an oriental (Table 1). The duration of hypertension was relatively brief, the average being only 5.6 years. The average blood pressure on admission was 220/144 mm. Hg. Obviously, many had blood pressures that were appreciably higher than these levels.

Table 1. *Age, sex, and race distribution in 14 patients with malignant hypertension treated with intramuscular guanethidine*

Age	Sex		Race		Duration of hypertension
	m.	f.	white	non-white	
av. 41 yrs	9 av. 42 yrs	5 av. 41 yrs	7 av. 41 yrs	7 av. 42 yrs	av. 5.6 yrs no "days" included

Results

Nine of the 14 cases responded well to doses of 10–15 mg. (Table 2). In a total of seven instances, however, including two patients who were treated twice and two of those mentioned, 20 mg. were used, either occasionally or routinely. Response to

Table 2. *Effective dose and time lapse until blood-pressure control was achieved*

Effective single dose in mg. 10 15 20	Time required to achieve significant B.P. fall after first (single) i.m. dose	Time required to achieve sustained and significant B.P. fall	Intervals between doses	Duration of i.m. therapy before oral therapy used alone
No. of patients 5 4 7	59 min.	75 min.	13.5 hrs	3.9 days

the intramuscular guanethidine was spectacularly rapid in most instances. Within 59 minutes, all patients given the medication had shown a blood-pressure reduction (supine in all cases) of significant value. The speed of response ranges from ten minutes (three patients) to 180 minutes (one patient). In four of the 14 patients, a *single injection* proved adequate to bring the blood pressure down and hold it there until satisfactory blood-pressure control could be established by oral medication. The remaining ten patients required multiple doses. In these subjects, the interval between the first injection and the achievement of a sustained, significant, blood-pressure reduction considered to be of therapeutic value (one sixth of the mean arterial pressure or more) was 75 minutes. The interval between injections varied from three to 24 hours, the average being 13.5 hours. In the ten patients given more than a single intramuscular injection of guanethidine, the average total duration of intramuscular therapy was 3.9 days. Thereafter, oral medication, usually with guanethidine, controlled the blood pressure satisfactorily.

Side effects were infrequent (Table 3). The immediate unwanted responses were restricted to one case in which diarrhea developed within two to three hours of the injection. The somewhat more

Table 3. *Side effects in 14 patients with malignant hypertension treated with guanethidine*

a. Immediate:	diarrhea (1 case). No other immediate side effects.
b. Delayed: (i.e. occurring 24—48 hrs later)	diarrhea (2 cases) lethargy (1 case) blurring vision (1 case) excessive orthostatic blood-pressure fall and weakness (2 cases)

delayed side effects (appearing 24—48 hours after the injection) included diarrhea in two cases, lethargy in one, and blurred vision in another. Two of the patients displayed an orthostatic blood-pressure fall to very low levels accompanied by weakness in the erect position. In neither case was this sufficiently severe to make discontinuation of the medication necessary. In only one subject was the intramuscular medication discontinued because of severe diarrhea.

Levels of blood pressure attained

The average blood pressure immediately before guanethidine was given was 220/141 mm. Hg. After a single intramuscular dose of guanethidine, it was 172/106 mm. Hg. The sustained blood pressure attained with this medication was 166/106 mm. Hg (Table 4).

Table 4. *Average blood pressure on admission, after a single intramuscular dose, and during continued intramuscular injection of guanethidine*

Average blood-pressure level on admission	Average blood pressure after i.m. guanethidine (Single dose)	Average blood-pressure levels attained on continued i.m. guanethidine
220/141 mm. Hg	172/106 mm. Hg	166/106 mm. Hg

In two instances in which parenteral medication of another type had failed to produce completely satisfactory results, intramuscular guanethidine provided adequate blood-pressure control. In one of these cases, intravenous administration of α-methyldopa produced no blood-pressure fall, whereas intramuscular injection of guanethidine brought about a prompt control of the pressure at satisfactory levels. In the second case, intravenous trimethaphan had lowered the blood pressure from 275/150 to 160/100 mm. Hg. Because of the difficulty of maintaining a stable blood-pressure level, trimethaphan was discontinued, and the patient was treated instead with intramuscular guanethidine. The blood pressure fell from 230/130 to 130/90 mm. Hg and was maintained at this level in a very satisfactory manner.

Discussion

The usefulness of an antihypertensive product at the present time depends on its relative freedom from side effects as well as on its therapeutic efficacy. For these reasons, intramuscular guanethidine seems to be preferable to most of the products that are currently in use. We detected no serious gastrointestinal reactions, apart from one case of diarrhea, no troublesome orthostatic hypotension, nor other events that could be attributed to the medication. As with many antihypertensive products, the administration of guanethidine may, in certain instances, be followed by a rise in blood urea nitrogen concentration. This should be followed carefully in patients treated with this and other agents.

Another, almost equally important aspect of intramuscular guanethidine therapy is its relative ease of use. It may be given by a nurse, and its action, though rapid, is neither so precipitous nor so abruptly terminated that the use of the drug calls for the constant attention of trained medical staff. Shortages of personnel make this an important therapeutic consideration.

Many further data are needed before this product can be used with complete acceptance in such circumstances as acute hypertension with nephritis and toxemia of pregnancy.

Summary

In comparison with current methods for the management of acute hypertensive crises in malignant hypertension, intramuscular guanethidine has, in our experience, proved to be the drug of choice. It is the simplest and at the same time probably the most effective means of achieving prompt blood-pressure control in acute and fulminating hypertension. Side reactions have been minimal, and the interval between the onset of parenteral treatment and the subsequent establishment of blood-pressure control by oral therapy is a matter of one to three days in most cases. The efficiency and the efficacy of intramuscular guanethidine, and its relative freedom from unwanted actions, warrant its trial in other types of hypertensive crisis.

Zusammenfassung

Unter den heute verfügbaren Methoden für die Behandlung der akuten Blutdruckkrise bei malignem Hochdruck ist für uns die intramuskuläre Anwendung von Guanethidin das Mittel der Wahl. Es ist die einfachste und gleichzeitig wohl auch die wirksamste Art, eine rasche Blutdrucksenkung bei akuter und fudroyant verlaufender Hypertension zu erzielen. Die Nebenwirkungen sind gering, und der Abstand zwischen dem Einsetzen der parenteralen Behandlung und der nachfolgenden Einstellung des Blutdruckes durch eine orale Behandlung beträgt in den meisten Fällen ein bis drei Tage. Die Leistungsfähigkeit und die Wirksamkeit von intramuskulär injiziertem Guanethidin sowie die Tatsache, daß es verhältnismäßig frei ist von unerwünschten Wirkungen rechtfertigen auch bei anderen Arten von Hochdruckkrisen einen Versuch damit.

Résumé

En comparaison avec les méthodes actuelles du traitement des poussées hypertensives aiguës dans l'hypertension maligne, la guanéthidine par voie intramusculaire s'est montrée dans notre expérience être le médicament de choix. C'est le moyen le plus simple et probablement le plus efficace de réduire les poussées tensionnelles aiguës. Les effets secondaires se sont montrés minimes, et le passage à la voie orale est possible dans la plupart des cas après un à trois jours de traitement parentéral. L'efficacité de la guanéthidine intramusculaire et l'absence relative d'effets secondaires justifient son essai dans d'autres sortes de crises hypertensives.

References

1. Leonberg, S. C., Jr., J. B. Green, and F. A. Elliot: Ann. Int. Med. **60**, 866 (1964). — 2. Moyer, J. H., and A. N. Brest: In: Hypertension. Recent Advances. The Second Hahnemann Symposium on Hypertensive Disease. Ed. by A. N. Brest and J. H. Moyer. Lea and Febiger, Philadelphia, 1961, p. 516. — 3. Gifford, R. W.: Amer. J. Cardiol. **9**, 880 (1962). — 4. Gifford, R. W.: Med. Clin. North America **45**, 441 (1961). — 5. Sheps, S. G., A. Schirger, P. J. Osmundson, and J. F. Fairbairn: J. Amer. Med. Ass. **184**, 616 (1963). — 6. Page, I. H., R. E. Hurley, and H. P. Dustan: J. Amer. Med. Ass. **175**, 543 (1961).

Discussion

Reubi: Dr. Lee, why do you give reserpine intramuscularly? We have been using this drug in the management of hypertensive crises for more than ten years now, and we have always given it intravenously. In this way time can be saved in emergencies.

Lee: We like to use reserpine intramuscularly if we can, because then the nursing staff can give the product. However, we refrain from using it, if possible, because of the stupor.

Hood: Dr. Lee, couldn't you avoid some of your side reactions due to hydralazine by adopting the technique we have been using in such situations for almost 15 years? We use a slow, continuous, intravenous infusion of hydralazine and then gradually increasing, subcutaneous injections of pentolinium to get a certain pulse pressure. If you want a certain pulse pressure, you can get it with combination in the majority of cases. As far as I could make out, you are discussing every agent singly here. Don't you use a combined treatment right away in the first phase?

Lee: No, we haven't, for several reasons. We do not like to use two (or more) potent agents together. If you saw, for example, some reaction by the patient that you did not wish, you would not know which product was causing it, and you would have to stop therapy completely. Moreover, with only one agent, such as guanethidine, there is the simplicity of management. I certainly have nothing against using three or four drugs, if they work, as we do with chronic oral therapy in forms of hypertension milder than a "crisis".

Dustan: I should like to add to Dr. Lee's experience with parenterally administered guanethidine by saying that we have had some six years' experience with its use and also find it extremely effective in the management of hypertensive crises and, particularly, of malignant hypertension. In a case of hypertensive encephalopathy, when one must lower blood pressure rapidly, we should use intravenous sodium nitroprusside; but in a situation in which one wishes to reduce blood pressure over a few hours, parenterally administered guanethidine is a safe way to produce blood-pressure reduction. You might, Dr. Lee, find that subcutaneous administration is a bit better than intramuscular, because we've had no trouble at all with abrupt rises in pressure, giving the material subcutaneously, whereas certainly we did when we gave it intravenously. In this regard, we have used a standard dose of 0.25 mg./kg. as the first dose and have found this very effective. In the work we did with Dr. Imhof[1], with intravenously administered guanethidine, we used 0.5 mg./kg., but we have found that this dose sometimes reduces blood pressure so low that it has to be maintained for the next 24-48 hours with intravenously administered norepinephrine. Therefore it seems that smaller doses, which can readily be repeated, are helpful.

---

[1] Imhof, P. R., R. C. Lewis, I. H. Page, and H. P. Dustan: In: Symposium on Guanethidine. Memphis, Tennessee. April 1960. CIBA, Summit, N. J., 1960, p. 24.

I should like to make a comment in defence of clinical judgement, because I do not think that it should be deprecated.

LEE: It wasn't deprecated, Dr. DUSTAN, believe me.

DUSTAN: After all, this is what we have to go on, you know, and I think the more experience one has, the better one's clinical judgement is and the more closely it approaches scientific judgement. This can be used at the bedside just as "scientific judgement" is used in the laboratory, if one takes the time to look and be thoughtful.

And, finally, I should like to ask you, Dr. LEE, about the magnitude of blood-pressure fall that you have obtained with parenterally administered hydralazine. When we were giving this compound intravenously, we found the blood-pressure reduction very modest. Do you think that if you administered a β-blocker, such as propranolol or nethalide, you would achieve a better blood-pressure reduction with hydralazine, because you would not have a tachycardia?

LEE: First to answer the question. We have had no experience whatever with propranolol, and very likely this would be a useful drug, given as an adjunct to intramuscular hydralazine.

I didn't know about your use of guanethidine subcutaneously. This is one of the values of conferences like this, because there is very little in the literature, even on intramuscular guanethidine. We should be happy to try it that way.

With regard to swift blood-pressure control, as Dr. SMIRK mentioned yesterday, sodium azide is the most rapidly acting antihypertensive we've ever seen. Fourteen or 15 years ago, we used to give it by spraying it into the nose in a stuporous or comatose hypertensive with hypertensive encephalopathy, and the blood pressure would begin to fall within ten to 12 seconds. But where do you stop, and what is sodium azide? I think that Dr. SMIRK's experience with it, as well as ours, and Dr. PAGE's initially with nitroprusside, has served in a way as a background against which new research today with enzyme poisons or inhibitors is progressing further. I should like to hear more about the use of iodo-acetate: what does iodo-acetate do to the blood pressure in hypertensives? We may now be getting at hypertension by basic mechanisms of therapy that we know nothing about.

LEISHMAN: I wonder whether Dr. LEE would agree that there are certain circumstances in which intramuscular guanethidine may not be the drug of choice. The action of guanethidine is largely dependent on postural hypotension, and I have in mind patients with hypertensive encephalopathy who are in a comatose state in which postural hypotension cannot really be achieved, and likewise cases of acute left ventricular failure. In these conditions we have preferred intravenous α-methyldopa, which has proved very satisfactory. We have given this at intervals of six hours and have usually been able to maintain very satisfactory reduction of blood pressure in the horizontal posture, which, I have no doubt, is desirable.

LEE: That is an excellent point, and I completely forgot to mention it. All the blood pressures that I have recorded are supine. This product works particularly in the supine position, when given intramuscularly, and mean arterial pressures were reduced by one sixth or more with these doses. Again, I have nothing against intravenous α-methyldopa other than the hepatotoxicity.

HAMILTON: Might I defend the apparently poor response of my patients compared with those of Dr. LEE? I hope I said yesterday that in cases of malignant hypertension, using parenteral pentolinium for the initiation of treatment, I could obtain control over the blood pressure within 36 hours and usually within 12 hours. By this I meant that the blood-pressure level was uniformly controlled and not subject to wide variations. I always use pentolinium subcutaneously and always start with a very small dose and increase the dose fairly rapidly during the initial few hours until I can achieve and maintain an adequate reduction of blood pressure. Although I intended to imply this, I clearly did not do so.

FREIS: I'd like to ask Dr. LEE about this matter of hepatitis with α-methyldopa. Did you have any cases in which there were residual signs of liver damage after withdrawing the drug? Our impression is that the hepatitis is very mild and clears completely without damage after the drug is stopped.

LEE: No, we have seen no residual liver damage. But I do not agree that the hepatitis is mild. When a patient spikes a fever to 41° C, when his liver descends down to the iliac crest and he turns a brilliant yellow, and when — on top of this — he has malignant encephalopathy, then even my own blood pressure is less than good!

KIRKENDALL: Dr. LEE mentioned that hydralazine was the only drug he knew which might increase renal blood flow in acute hypertensive emergencies. I should like to mention diazoxide, which will increase cardiac output and, I believe, renal blood flow significantly under acute circumstances. Actually, it is not a bad hypotensive drug when used for hypertensive crises. When given in a dose of 5 mg./kg. of body weight, it will regularly reduce blood pressure within an hour and will keep it down for four to six hours. Patients tolerate it rather well as far as side effects are concerned, except for the devilish one of hyperglycaemia. I do not think anyone knows precisely what the hyperglycaemia means in patients who develop it. The vast majority of them get over the hyperglycaemia after diazoxide is discontinued, but certainly such a complication makes one hesitant to use the drug as the primary agent in the treatment of hypertensive encephalopathy. Nevertheless, it is a drug which, from haemodynamic and practical standpoints, has interesting effects, and it may very well be a precursor of others which we can use with safety.

LEE: We have had no experience with diazoxide, so I did not add that to my list. But in thinking about the use of the extremely potent preparations in the treatment of people, I am reminded of S. C. WANG, who said, "Medical research is like going hunting: you think you have a pussy-cat and you end up with a tiger". You don't know what you are going to find or what you will do to the patient, because you don't know what you know, and you don't know what you don't know.

SJOERDSMA: I was just going to comment briefly on the toxicity of α-methyldopa. I think one of the reasons why we really didn't promote α-methyldopa vigorously as a potential therapeutic agent in hypertension is that in the first ten subjects we treated we observed two untoward reactions, both febrile, one of which was associated with alterations in liver function. And even to this day, in the total of some 200 hypertensives that we have treated for rather prolonged periods of time, we have an over-all incidence of toxicity of about 5%, which is, I think, considerably higher than in the experience of many others in this room. None of these side effects has even approached the point of lethal reactions, and most of them have occurred early, being febrile reactions with or without alterations in liver function. We have had two "liver" reactions that came on very gradually, within a period of two or three months, with progressive rises in transaminases and changes in other hepatic indicators, all of which were completely reversible. It is obvious that with α-methyldopa one is dealing with a very different situation from the one we had in the case of iproniazid some years ago: there were dreadful liver problems then, and patients died. This appears not to occur with α-methyldopa, judging from the amount of this drug being used by practitioners without causing serious problems. But in spite of this very early concern about toxicity, as time has gone by the situation has, if anything, improved, as far as I can see.

WILSON: As it hasn't been mentioned, may I just say a word about venesection? This used to be the classic treatment in the hypertensive encephalopathy of acute nephritis. I really feel that there is a problem of volume here as well as of reduction of blood pressure. I should suggest that if in fact there is hypervolaemia — as in acute nephritis and possibly also in malignant hypertension — which is contributing to the encephalopathy, it would seem rational to correct it.

LEE: In Japan, where malignant hypertension is common, venesection is popular today as a means of managing the acute stage; of course this is pushing us back 200 years, but I am in favour of learning more about it, because it indicates that in malignant hypertension there may perhaps be a change in the partition of blood. We need a product or a technique today that will tell us how much blood is in the arterial tree and how much blood is in the venous tree, and what the role of this possible shift of blood may be in the onset of, let us say, malignant hypertension. Perhaps I appeared oversensitive on the subject of side effects in my previous remarks, but I come from a part of the world where the second favourite indoor sport is suing a physician.

SMIRK: There is one thing that doesn't seem to me to have been referred to, and I think I should mention it, and that is the use of posture. We treat our acute hypertensive crises with the patient in a cardiac bed in the sitting posture, with the back-rest straight up, the feet right down, and the arms resting on a bed-table in front. Now, by using posture in this way, you may reduce the necessary dose of a posturally acting drug by a half or a third. The blood pressure can be brought down very promptly with pentolinium or hexamethonium intravenously in a dose which, under those conditions, carries practically no risk of causing paralytic ileus, especially so as nowadays you can transfer promptly to a drug which does not block the parasympathetic system. Now, if the dose administered brings the blood pressure down excessively, for example in a person with some renal failure, to, say, 120 mm. Hg systolic, you can immediately adjust the blood-pressure level merely by altering the posture of the patient; indeed, you can put it where you want it within 10 mm. Hg systolic or adjust it to some selected diastolic level. Certainly, close control by frequent blood-pressure measurement is necessary. After this, we feel that bethanidine[1], which takes effect, when given orally, in about two hours and attains its maximum effect in about four and a half hours, is a very useful substance. It doesn't produce diarrhoea.

[1] SMIRK, F. H.: Lancet 1963/I, 743.

An ordinary initial dose is about 10 mg., but in a hypertensive crisis we might give 30 mg. orally straight off, because if we got an excessive blood-pressure fall with the patient propped up, we should merely decrease the degree of tilt of the patient, thus raising the blood pressure to the desired level. Later, it is quite easy to change over by degrees to guanethidine, if this is preferred.

I was very glad to hear Dr. LEE stress the importance of the absence of side effects in the treatment of patients, because not only is it important to relieve discomfort, but the absence of side effects is one of the most pertinent of all factors in persuading patients to continue treatment.

Hypertension in pregnancy and its treatment

By

N. F. Morris

Hypertension is often a sign of singular importance, since it is one of the few measurable factors that alert us to the possible presence of serious underlying pathology. In particular, of course, it is the baby that is at risk in association with hypertension.

Most obstetricians are aware that there are many possible causes for a raised blood pressure in pregnancy. I only have time to deal quite briefly with the two most common types of hypertension that confront us, namely essential, or persistent, hypertension which predates the pregnancy, and toxaemia (pre-eclampsia) of pregnancy. I am very conscious of the reservations that many of you have about labelling a blood pressure of 140/90 mm. Hg as essential hypertension, as if it were certain evidence of a pathological state; however, I hope to convince you that it is important for obstetricians to respect such minor increases in blood pressure.

I must also admit that occasionally we may fail to identify the cause of hypertension in pregnancy for the simple reason that it is not always possible to carry out complete investigations on a woman who is found to have high blood pressure for the first time during pregnancy. Therefore, every case of moderate or severe hypertension in pregnancy should be investigated thoroughly once the pregnancy is over.

During 1958, we carried out in Britain a national survey of all births that took place between the 3rd and 9th March. In all, about 17,000 births were analysed (Table 1), together with all stillbirths and neonatal deaths during March, April, and May (7,117). 64.7% remained completely normotensive, and the mortality ratio was 76. Of these women, 2.6% had a diastolic pressure of 90 mm. Hg or more before the 20th week of gestation; the foetal mortality ratio in this group was 134. Pure toxaemia, i.e. those cases in which blood pressure was below 90 mm. Hg before the 20th week, but subsequently rose above 90 mm. Hg, accounted for 12.9%; the mortality ratio here was 108. Finally, 11.9% of the cases were diagnosed as unclassified toxaemia. These were women who were not seen until after the 20th week of gestation, but later showed a rise in pressure to above 90 mm. Hg; the mortality ratio in this group was 135. These figures show quite conclusively that

Table 1. *Blood pressure, incidence of toxaemia, and mortality ratio (see text) in 17,000 births in Britain, 1958* (by courtesy of Livingstone Ltd., Edinburgh, from Perinatal Mortality, 1963)

	Incidence (percentage)	Mortality ratio (M)
Normotensive	64.7	76
Essential hypertension	2.6	134
Corrected	4.6	—
Pure toxaemia	12.9	108
Unclassified toxaemia	11.9	135

hypertension is associated with a greatly increased foetal mortality rate. In order to calculate the absolute number of women who have a raised pressure in early pregnancy, I have applied a correction factor, and this gives an incidence of approximately 4.6%.

The mortality ratio was calculated as follows:

$$\text{Mortality ratio (M)} = \frac{\text{deaths}}{\text{population}} \times \frac{\text{Population (16,944)}}{\text{Deaths (7,117)}} \times 100$$

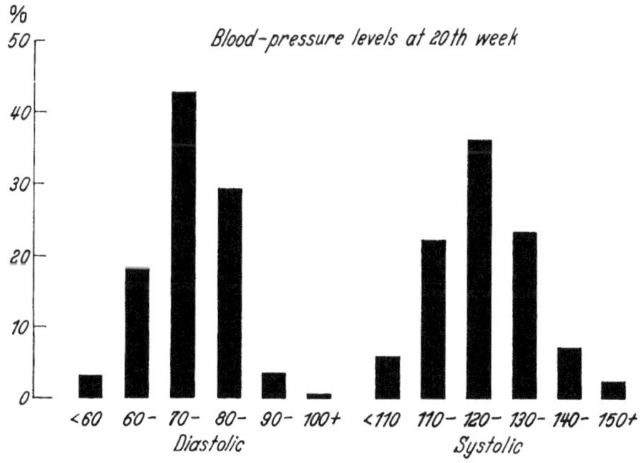

Fig. 1. Analysis of blood pressure in 4,215 primigravidae in Aberdeen (by courtesy of J. Obstetr. Gynaec. Brit. Empire, from MacGillivray, 1961).

Not long ago, MacGillivray (1961) analysed the blood pressure in 4,215 primigravidae in Aberdeen (Fig. 1). The largest group had a blood pressure of 120/70—129/79 mm. Hg. In his series, a pressure of 140/90 mm. Hg occurred in about 4.5%. MacGillivray also analysed the effect of age on blood pressure (Table 2). He showed that the average diastolic pressure does not start to rise until after the age of 30. The systolic pressure, on the other hand, starts rising from the age of 20 onwards.

Table 2. *Average blood pressures at 20th week in 4,215 primigravidae by age* (by courtesy of J. Obstetr. Gynaec. Brit. Empire, from MacGillivray, 1961)

Age	Diastolic mm. Hg	Systolic mm. Hg
Under 20	75	122
20—24	75	124
25—29	75	125
30—34	77	125
35+	78	128

My namesake, W.I.C. Morris (1958), analysed the behaviour of the blood pressure in a series of 480 women with a raised diastolic pressure at the beginning of pregnancy (essential hypertensives) (Fig. 2). He assessed the behaviour in each trimester and obtained four basic patterns. In the majority of his subjects (53.5%), the blood pressure remained stationary. In 18.8%, the blood pressure fell in the second trimester and remained down in the third (usually in these cases it appears to rise quickly in the puerperium). In 11.1%, the pressure fell in the middle, but rose again at the end to its previous or a higher level. In 8.8%, the pressure remained stationary until the end, when it went up. In other words, in 19.9%, the pressure rose at the end of pregnancy.

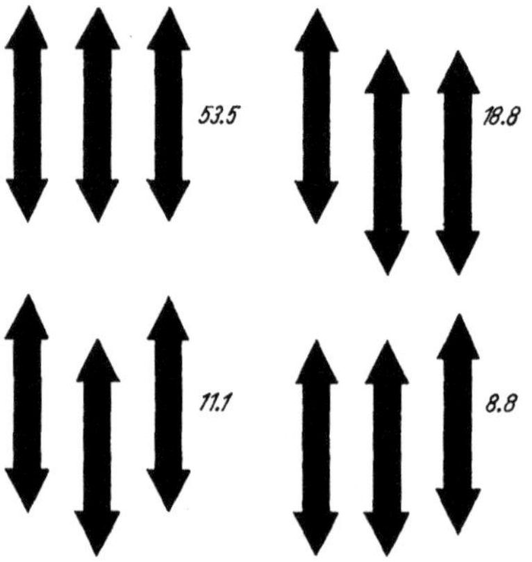

Fig. 2. Response of blood pressure in 480 "hypertensive" pregnancies. Each arrow represents one trimester (by courtesy of Churchill, London, from Morris, 1958).

Coming back to the British Perinatal Survey, an analysis of the cases of so-called essential hypertension is given in Table 3. These results indicate that cases of early essential hypertension are clearly prone to further increases in pressure and the development of proteinuria. It is the associated pathology related to this increase in pressure that is responsible for the high perinatal death rate.

Table 3. *Essential hypertension during pregnancy* (by courtesy of Livingstone Ltd., Edinburgh, from Perinatal Mortality, 1963)

Rise in diastolic pressure	percentage
None	64.5
10—19 mm.	15.1
20 mm.	8.4
Proteinuria ± Rise in pressure	
Confirmed in M.S.U. or C.S.U.	8.8
Unconfirmed	3.2

There has been some argument concerning the nature of the increase in pressure. Is it merely the result of an exacerbation of the basic pressor mechanism already operative in these cases? Or is it, on the other hand, another process, superimposed on the essential hypertension, in other words, *superimposed toxaemia*?

If we examine some of the pathological changes that occur in these two conditions, then I think we can find evidence that the changes associated with uncomplicated essential hypertension in pregnancy are quite different from those occurring in toxaemia, and that in cases of essential hypertension developing a rise in pressure or proteinuria, both types of change may be present together.

For example, biopsy of the *kidney* in an uncomplicated essential hypertensive (POLLAK and NETTLES, 1960) shows sclerosis of the small arteries and arterioles. The glomerulus is normal (Fig. 3). In toxaemia, on the other hand, there are wide-spread changes. The glomeruli are obviously swollen — with a swelling of the endothelial cytoplasm and an amorphous deposit underneath the basement membrane and in the cytoplasm of the endothelial cell. There is also an apparent increase in the number of intercapillary cells. The capillaries are ischaemic. The tubules also show some degeneration, whilst the vessels are sclerotic and swollen (Fig. 4). These findings are summarised in Table 4.

Uterus. It seems fairly clear that it is a disturbance of placental function in association with hypertension in pregnancy that causes the death of the child. Radio-active clearance studies made by MCCLURE BROWNE (1953) and myself (1955) have suggested that there is a reduction in myometrial and placental blood flow in these cases. The higher the blood pressure on the whole, the more the blood flow tends to be reduced. Using a similar technique, I have

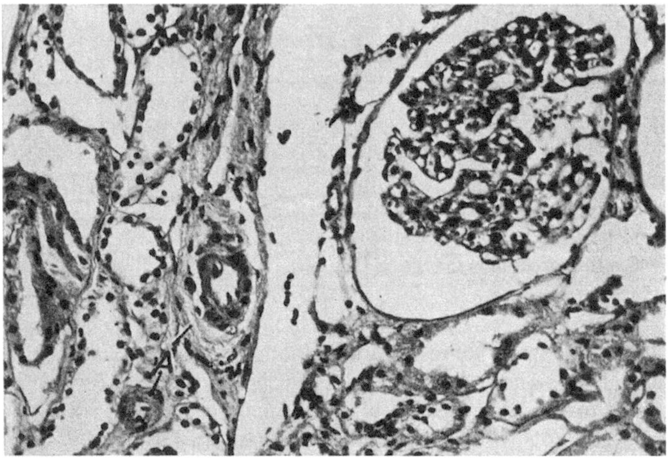

Fig. 3. Renal biopsy in uncomplicated essential hypertension showing sclerosis of small arteries and arterioles. A: Arterioles (by courtesy of Medicine, from POLLAK and NETTLES, 1960).

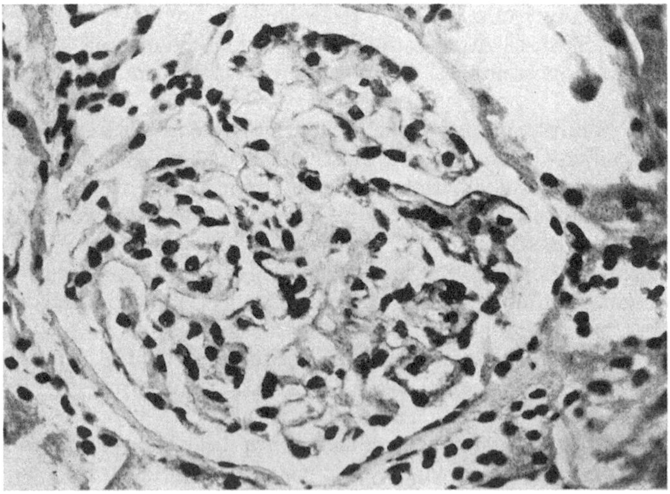

Fig. 4. Renal biopsy in toxaemia of pregnancy with wide-spread changes in glomerulus (by courtesy of Medicine, from POLLAK and NETTLES, 1960).

shown that *during exercise* the blood flow to the uterus appears to be reduced.

Table 4. *Renal lesions found in biopsies in patients with essential hypertension and in toxaemia of pregnancy*

	Essential hypertension	Toxaemia
Glomeruli	Unaffected	Abnormal
Tubules	Unaffected	Abnormal
Vessels	Sclerotic	Sclerotic and swollen

It has been asserted repeatedly that the placenta is severely infarcted in association with hypertension and toxaemia. As LITTLE (1960) and others have shown, however, in a series of 1,000 cases, the placenta is often infarcted in normotensive pregnancies. Nevertheless, there is an increase in the rate of infarction with toxaemia (Table 5).

Table 5. *Placental infarcts in normotensives, essential hypertension, and toxaemia of pregnancy* (LITTLE, 1960)

			percentage
Normotensives			33
Essential hypertension			30
Toxaemia	Mild	64.6	63.2
	Severe	60	

Some of the most interesting changes occur in the placental bed. In this connection, unique studies have been carried out by BROSENS et al. (1965) and DIXON and ROBERTSON (1958). First of all, they have described a physiological change in the spiral arteries that occurs in all pregnancies as term is approached. This involves loss of the muscular and elastic coat and its replacement by fibrinoid material. Giant cells often appear also. In essential hypertension, these changes are seen together with cellular hyperplasia (Fig. 5). In pre-eclampsia, internal hyalinisation occurs, with lipid infiltration of the wall and plaques of foam cells – the so-called acute atherosis. In the basal arteries in essential hypertension there is purely intimal and medial hyperplasia, common to many other vessels elsewhere (Fig. 6). These changes probably explain the reduced blood flow and account for death of the foetus in severe cases.

Finally, I want to consider briefly the *treatment* of hypertension in pregnancy (Table 6). Our main therapeutic weapon in cases of essential hypertension and toxaemia is *rest*. We do not believe that antihypertensive drugs are of much use in essential hypertension, except if the blood pressure is persistently raised above about

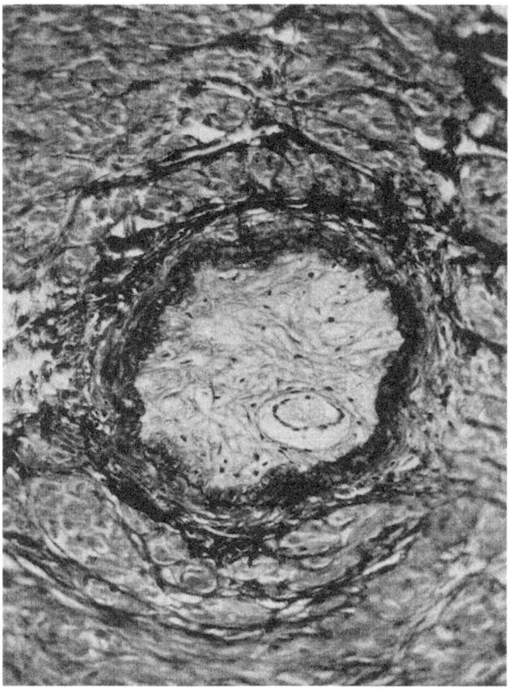

Fig. 5. Artery in placental bed with loose cellular intimal proliferation in essential hypertension (BROSENS et al., 1965).

160/110 mm. Hg. In my experience, they are of no use at all in toxaemia, except to tide over an acute crisis immediately before or after delivery.

Table 6. *Treatment of essential hypertension and toxaemia of pregnancy*

Essential hypertension	Toxaemia
1) Rest	Rest
2) Antihypertensive drugs a) Malignant hypertension b) B.P. 160/110 +	Antihypertensive drugs in crisis only
3) —	Terminate pregnancy

To illustrate my views I should like to recount the story of Mrs. J. W. (Fig. 7). She had two failed pregnancies ending in very severe toxaemia warranting hysterotomy at 26 and 28 weeks.

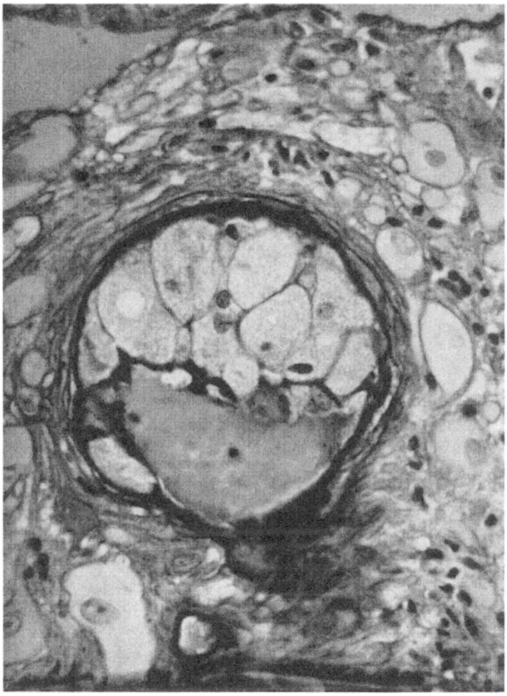

Fig. 6. Arteriole in placental bed with fibrinoid necrosis and lipophage infiltration in pre-eclampsia (BROSENS et al., 1965).

Her obstetrician wanted to sterilise her. Her subsequent diastolic pressure was always above 100 mm. Hg. Investigations, including renal function tests and renal biopsy, showed normal results. Treatment with α-methyldopa was started before she became pregnant for the third time.

During her third pregnancy, she received α-methyldopa until the 31st week. In the 23rd week, she was admitted to hospital and kept there until her baby was delivered. The blood pressure showed a tendency to rise slowly as she approached term. Her placental function was monitored by means of regular pregnanediol estimation of the urine. Suddenly, in the 37th week, the pregnanediol level dropped acutely. I did an immediate caesarean section and delivered a live baby of 7 lbs 3 ozs. The uterus was just about to rupture at the site of the previous hysterotomies. It was an expensive baby, but who is to say our efforts have not been worth while ?

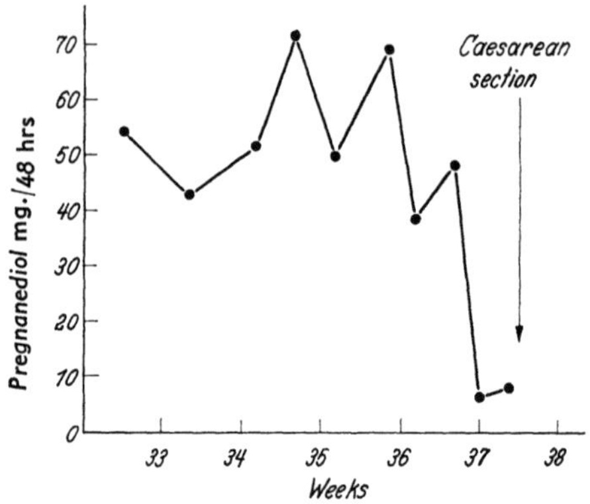

Fig. 7. Mrs. J. W. Pregnanediol excretion during the last weeks of pregnancy. Caesarean section was made after the sharp fall of pregnanediol secretion.

We have had three other cases during the past three years with equally satisfactory results. We tend to wean these patients off α-methyldopa for two reasons. Firstly, we are conscious that hexamethonium accumulates in the liquor, and perhaps α-methyldopa behaves similarly (although there is no special reason why it should). Secondly, we are worried about giving a general anaesthetic to any woman under the influence of powerful antihypertensive agents. Perhaps we are too timid; but these are tricky situations, and we feel that one false step may result in foetal death.

It is possible that antihypertensive therapy is just as effective as rest in these cases, but since our results are so good with rest, we are reluctant to chance our arm by using antihypertensive drugs alone. Although I was one of the first obstetricians to use antihypertensive drugs in the treatment of toxaemia of pregnancy, over the years I have become less and less convinced of the value of these drugs. Perhaps the newer agents at our disposal are more effective than the old ones.

In particular, I have used antihypertensive drugs to lower the blood pressure in acute severe early toxaemia of pregnancy developing in the 28th–32nd week. I have been able to control the blood pressure and produce a clinical improvement, but the foetus has died in nearly every instance three to four weeks after the start of treatment. One of the few survivors is a spastic and is mentally subnormal.

If I could convince myself that antihypertensive drugs can reverse or even halt the pathological changes I have just described, then I should use them with more enthusiasm. As it is, I use them purely to tide the mother over acute crises.

Finally, a word about the ultimate prognosis of women with toxaemia. EPSTEIN (1964) has published his 15-year follow-up studies of 48 women delivered between 1945 and 1948 who had severe toxaemia. He has compared them with 114 controls, whose family history of hypertension was the same. 37% of the toxaemic cases showed a pressure of 150/90 mm. Hg or more, whilst only 7% demonstrated this pressure in the control group. This seems good evidence that severe toxaemia is associated with the ultimate development of hypertension in a significant percentage of women.

Summary

Essential hypertension is a relatively common and serious complication of pregnancy. Careful observation is therefore indicated, particularly in the last trimester, when the blood pressure may rise further and proteinuria may also occur (superimposed toxaemia). When superimposed toxaemia occurs, there are specific changes in both the kidney and the placenta. The interference with placental function is the reason why the foetus is more likely to die when superimposed toxaemia develops. These changes in the placental bed histologically appear relatively irreversible, therefore it seems unlikely that mere reduction of the blood pressure by antihypertensive drugs or thiazide therapy will improve placental function or the outlook for the foetus.

Rest in bed at present seems the most effective method there is of improving the maternal/placental blood flow and therefore placental function.

Antihypertensive drugs are, however, very useful in the treatment of severe hypertension, where the foetal loss is high. Treatment is best started before the pregnancy begins or as soon as the patient is first seen in early pregnancy.

Zusammenfassung

Essentieller Hochdruck ist eine relativ häufige und schwerwiegende Komplikation der Schwangerschaft. Sorgfältige Beobachtung ist daher angezeigt, besonders während des letzten Trimesters, in dem der Blutdruck weiter ansteigen und gleichzeitig eine Proteinurie auftreten kann (aufgepfropfte Toxikose). Wenn eine aufgepfropfte Toxikose vorliegt, bestehen sowohl in der Niere als auch in der Plazenta spezifische Veränderungen. Eine Beeinträchtigung der plazentaren Funktion ist der Grund, warum die Frucht mit größerer Wahrscheinlichkeit abstirbt, wenn sich eine aufgepropfte Toxikose entwickelt. Die Veränderungen im Plazentarbett scheinen histologisch kaum rückbildungsfähig zu sein; deswegen ist es wenig wahrscheinlich, daß lediglich eine Verminderung des Blutdruckes durch antihypertensive

Mittel oder Thiazide die Plazentafunktion und damit die Lebensaussichten für den Fötus verbessert.

Zur Zeit dürfte Bettruhe die wirksamste Behandlungsmethode sein, um die Durchblutung der mütterlichen Seite der Plazenta und damit auch die plazentare Funktion zu verbessern.

Blutdrucksenkende Substanzen sind jedoch zweifellos nützlich bei der Behandlung eines schweren Hochdruckes, bei dem die fötale Sterblichkeit hoch ist. Die Behandlung wird am besten begonnen, ehe die Schwangerschaft eingetreten oder sobald sie festgestellt ist.

Résumé

L'hypertension essentielle est une complication sérieuse et relativement fréquente de la grossesse. Une surveillance attentive est donc indiquée, en particulier au cours du dernier trimestre, où la tension artérielle peut s'élever encore davantage et où peut s'installer une protéinurie (toxémie surajoutée). Dans ce cas surviennent des altérations spécifiques à la fois dans le rein et dans le placenta. L'influence de la toxémie sur la fonction placentaire est la raison du risque de mortalité foetale. Les altérations du réseau vasculaire placentaire semblent à l'histologie être relativement irréversibles, et par conséquent il est peu probable qu'une simple réduction de la pression artérielle par des substances antihypertensives ou des thiazides améliorera la fonction placentaire ou le pronostic foetal.

Le repos au lit semble être actuellement la mesure la plus efficace pour améliorer le flux sanguin maternel placentaire et par conséquent la fonction du placenta.

Les agents antihypertenseurs, cependant, sont très utiles dans le traitement des hypertensions graves, où la mortalité foetale est élevée. On commencera le traitement au mieux avant le début de la grossesse ou dès le diagnostic de celle-ci.

References

Brosens, I. A., W. B. Robertson, and H. G. Dixon: Personal communication (1965). — Dixon, H. G., and W. B. Robertson: J. Obstetr. Gynaec. Brit. Empire **65**, 803 (1958). — Epstein, F. H.: N. England J. Med. **271**, 391 (1964). — Little, W. A.: Obstetr. Gynec. **15**, 109 (1960). — MacGillivray, I.: J. Obstetr. Gynaec. Brit. Empire **68**, 557 (1961). — McClure Browne, J. C., and N. Veall: J. Obstetr. Gynaec. Brit. Empire **60**, 141 (1953). — Morris, N. F., S. B. Osborn, and H. P. Wright: Lancet 1955/I, 323. — Morris, W. I. C.: In: Symposium on Non-Toxaemic Hypertension in Pregnancy. Ed. by N. F. Morris and I. C. McClure Browne. Churchill Ltd., London, 1958, p. 44. — Perinatal Mortality (The First Report of the 1958 British Perinatal Survey). E. and S. Livingstone Ltd., Edinburgh and London, 1963. — Pollak, V. E., and J. B. Nettles: Medicine **36**, 469 (1960).

Discussion

SMIRK: I should like to ask Dr. MORRIS to amplify one matter. He didn't refer to the question of salt depletion.

MORRIS: If you mean whether we use chlorothiazide, then the answer is no.

SMIRK: I meant by the use of a low-salt diet.

MORRIS: Yes, we do use a low-salt diet in cases where there is obvious water retention with gross oedema. By this I mean a proper low-salt diet under the control of the diet kitchen.

KINCAID-SMITH: I have been interested in the subject of hypertension in pregnancy for some years, and even patients with malignant hypertension may now have a successful pregnancy on hypotensive treatment. My reaction has been to treat patients with hypotensive drugs, particularly those women with severe degrees of hypertension during pregnancy. I should like to make one point about the group of patients with so-called essential hypertension in pregnancy. We have followed up a number of women who presented as apparent essential hypertension in pregnancy before the 20th week, and in fact a very high proportion of these have shown underlying renal disease. We have found focal glomerulonephritis on renal biopsies in these patients, and also a fairly high incidence of pyelonephritis. In fact, nearly 50% of those women who have persistent hypertension after pregnancy have shown some underlying renal disease. We have now treated about 60 patients with α-methyldopa during pregnancy; about half these patients have had severe hypertension with diastolic pressures up to 160 mm. Hg, most of them over 110 mm. Hg. We used the drug throughout pregnancy in a number of patients and for shorter periods in others. We haven't had any evidence of foetal malformations or α-methyldopa toxicity in this study. We have treated the patients quite differently from Dr. MORRIS in that we kept them out of hospital. We reduced their blood pressures to near normal levels and treated them as out-patients, partly because of the increased effect of hypotensive agents when they are up and about, and partly because of the difficulty of keeping young mothers in bed for long periods. Superimposed toxaemia was treated by bed-rest.

We think that our results have been fairly good. Three of these patients lost their babies; two of them had severe toxaemia coming on before the 30th week — which, I think every one will agree, is a pretty difficult state of affairs to deal with — and one patient had recurrent habitual abortion. The other patients had live babies; almost all were induced early, between about 36 and 38 weeks. We are at present very interested in finding out whether treatment with hypotensive drugs can reduce the vascular lesions in the placental bed. We feel that it is probably important to treat patients early, and we are now conducting a controlled trial of α-methyldopa in hypertension in pregnancy. We start patients on treatment as soon as they present, and include patients in the trial if they have two blood-pressure readings above 135/85 mm. Hg.

BROD: My first comment concerns Veratrum. This is, of course, a drug which we don't use any more in hypertension, but we still keep it on our list, and perhaps it is our drug of choice in a woman who has toxaemia of pregnancy and comes to us with a severely raised blood pressure and symptoms of an impending cerebral episode. In such cases we resort to an intravenous drip with Veratrum, and so far we have always been able to reduce blood pressure very effectively and very quickly in this way, without any side effects. We don't usually carry on this treatment for more than one or two days, and by that time we have managed to get the blood pressure under control with the other drugs which were mentioned here.

Dr. VEDRA from the Institute for Mother and Child in Prague has been studying the 24-hour renal function rhythm in women with toxaemia of pregnancy, and he has found that very many of them showed a nocturnal increase in urine flow. He thought that this might be due to some inadequacy of the circulation during the day. If this is true, then it might be another reason why these women should be confined to bed. I wonder whether Dr. MORRIS has any further ideas on this point.

My final comment concerns the differential diagnosis. There is no single sign or symptom which would differentiate the various causes of hypertension which we have found in pregnancy. But if we take into account the various renal functions, past history, degree of proteinuria, the excretion of erythrocytes, leucocytes, and casts in the urine, and the relationship between glomerular filtration rate and concentrating power, then we can make a diagnosis in the majority of cases of hypertension occurring during pregnancy, even without biopsy.

MORRIS: May I first answer Dr. KINCAID-SMITH. I should be very worried if I had to rely entirely on antihypertensive drugs without using rest in bed, even if the drugs lowered the blood pressure successfully. Lowering the blood pressure by drugs may produce an entirely false sense of security, since it may lead us to assume that the patient has improved. I am not satisfied that lowering the blood pressure with drugs alters the natural history of this hypertensive condition. I am also not satisfied that the function of the placenta is improved by merely lowering the blood pressure. Perhaps I am wrong about this, but until there is more positive proof of improved placental function I intend to remain sceptical.

Equally, even if we do obtain a living baby in a case where antihypertensive drugs have been used, this is only proof that the drugs have done no apparent harm. It is not proof that they saved the baby, since, occasionally, women with severe hypertension produce quite large, healthy babies after a pregnancy in which no specific treatment — not even prolonged bed-rest — has been given. For these reasons we have to be very critical in the assessment of our results.

In regard to Dr. BROD's questions, I think Veratrum and its extracts are now of historical interest only. I have used preparations of Veratrum alkaloids, and they will lower the blood pressure, but the results are often unpredictable; they also often induce nausea. I believe much better drugs are now available.

One drug in particular that has stood the test of time is the hypnotic Avertin (bromethol) given rectally. This very powerful drug, which is highly effective in severe, fulminating pre-eclampsia and eclampsia, brings the blood pressure crashing down — often to even sub-normal levels — and soon controls the fits if they are present. It is very effective in these cases for dealing with the acute crises.

Regarding the question of 24-hour rhythm, I suspect that this sometimes changes even in some apparently normal pregnancies.

FREIS: Dr. FINNERTY[1] at D. C. General Hospital in Washington has reported a very dramatic decrease in foetal and maternal mortality in patients who were treated with saluretic agents at the first sign of toxaemia. I wondered whether anyone else has done a similar series.

SMIRK: Just to clarify: you mean right from the beginning with the first sign of toxaemia?

FREIS: Yes.

SMIRK: Does that mean blood-pressure increase, oedema, or proteinuria?

FREIS: I believe it was either proteinuria, oedema, or hypertension, and also prophylactically in teen-age pregnant females who usually exhibit a high incidence of toxaemia.

DEMING: I believe he started therapy on the basis of blood pressure. Everybody who had an elevation of blood pressure was treated.

MORRIS: The point I want to emphasise is that although hypertension does increase the number of babies who die just before and just after birth, yet, even so, only relatively small numbers of babies are killed by the hypertensive process. I think the figures I presented from the National Perinatal Mortality Survey give a rather false picture. The use of the mortality ratio tends to over-emphasise the number of babies that are lost. In my view it is a most unfortunate way of presenting these figures. With efficient treatment it is now relatively uncommon to lose a baby, either as a result of persistent hypertension in pregnancy or of toxaemia.

ZANCHETTI: We have seen two hypertensive women in whom renal artery stenosis was subsequently discovered. They had normal blood pressures before pregnancy and became hypertensive during their first pregnancy. We know so little of the natural history of renal artery stenosis, and particularly of fibromuscular hyperplasia, that we cannot say whether there may be some significant relationship between renovascular hypertension and pregnancy. However, we know from recent work by Dr. GROSS[2] and other authors that renin occurs in significant amounts in the placenta. Therefore it would not be impossible to conceive that pregnancy might precipitate hypertension in women with pre-existing renal artery stenosis. I should like to know whether Dr. MORRIS or other people have any experience of cases of renal artery stenosis discovered during pregnancy.

MORRIS: I have so far no personal experience of this. However, it is now our custom to send all patients with severe toxaemia of pregnancy for a complete check-up by my colleague H. DE WARDENER, who, as many of you know, has a special interest in the kidney. As yet we have no detailed figures, but we are already surprised by the number of renal anomalies that we have discovered. It is rather more than we had expected; we hope to publish full details later on.

SMIRK: I am sorry I have to bring this discussion to an end. This paper from Dr. MORRIS has been most helpful. We congratulated ourselves on improving things a bit, but when I hear what he has to say about his results in the absence of specific treatment, I have grave doubts as to whether we have done any good at all in the pregnancy toxaemias. At any rate, we don't seem to have lost any mothers.

---

[1] FINNERTY, F. A., Jr., and F. J. BEBKO, Jr.: J. Amer. Med. Ass. in press.

[2] GROSS, F., G. SCHAECHTELIN, M. ZIEGLER, and M. BERGER: Lancet 1964/I, 914.

Introduction to the General Discussion

By

H. LAGERLÖF

During maximal physical work, about 90% of the cardiac output goes through the working muscles. This means that the blood pressure is governed almost exclusively by the cardiac output and the resistance of the muscle vessels.

The increase in the cardiac output is not sufficient to give an optimal perfusion of the kidneys and the muscles, since renal flow decreases and the arteriovenous oxygen difference in the muscles increases. This indicates that the heart works at maximal capacity and cannot be used as a regulator of the systemic blood pressure. Hence, changes in the resistance of the vessels of the working muscles should be the most important factor in the pressure regulation during work.

At the same time as the resistance of the working muscles decreases about 15 times, the resistance of the kidney vessels increases about three times, as evidenced by the decreased flow. If baroreceptor mechanisms act uniformly on the kidney vessels and the muscle vessels and evoke the same release of noradrenaline from the nerve-endings, and if the resistance is directly proportional to the baroreceptor stimulation, this would mean a decrease in the sensitivity to noradrenaline in the vessels of the working muscle to about 1/45 of that of the kidneys.

This indicates what some speakers have already hinted at – that the sensitivity of the vessel wall in the whole body or in certain areas plays an essential part in the response of the vessels to hitherto known factors which directly influence the vessel tonus, such as vasopressor amines, angiotensin, and vasopressin.

The blood pressure during heavy work in normal individuals is interesting also, because the decrease in renal flow is accompanied by the release of renin. In our clinical physiological laboratory, CASTENFORS and BOŽOVIC (1965) have shown that the arterial renin concentration is almost doubled during short periods of heavy work and is elevated up to four times during prolonged, heavy work, such as long-distance cross-country skiing. This actualises the question of interaction between the low molecular neurohormone, noradrenaline, and the polypeptide, angiotensin.

In the gastro-intestinal tract, similar dual stimulating mechanisms are known to be involved in several different processes.

The vagus stimulates the secretion of pancreatic enzymes, and so does the polypeptide, pancreozymin. The vagus stimulates evacuation of the gall bladder, as does the polypeptide, cholecystokinin. Adrenaline liberates glucose from the liver, and glucagon acts similarly.

Of special interest is the nowadays well-studied relation between vagal and gastrin stimulation of gastric secretion. UVNÄS (1942) has shown that vagal stimulation not only acts directly, but also liberates gastrin. GREGORY and TRACY (1960) have found that combined neural and humoral stimulation gives a much higher response than the sum of the secretions evoked by each of the stimulants separately. In other words, the polypeptide, gastrin, potentiates the effect of the neurohormone, acetylcholine.

I know that Dr. WOLFF has comments to make on the interaction between noradrenaline and angiotensin and I understand that this also applies to Dr. PAGE.

Another factor which may be of major importance and has not yet been discussed is the role of magnesium and calcium. It is also particularly interesting, as regards hypertension, to note that cardiac necrosis, fibrosis and calcification, vascular dilatation and nephrocalcinosis have been found in magnesium-deficient rats. The administration of magnesium to rats on an atherogenic diet decreases the atheromatosis. When myocardial infarct-like lesions were produced by SHIMAMOTO et al. (1959) by giving high molecular polysaccharides together with adrenaline, these lesions were prevented by magnesium.

To this it may be added that decreased serum levels of magnesium have been reported in hypertension and cardiac infarction and, furthermore, that serum magnesium decreases but red-cell magnesium increases during thiazide treatment. HUGHES and TONKS (1965) have also shown that magnesium decreases the aggregation of thrombocytes and increases the coagulation time.

If there is time, I should appreciate some discussion on the role of magnesium (for references see MARTIN, 1965; SELLER et al., 1965; and HUGHES and TONKS, 1965).

References

CASTENFORS, J., and L. BOŽOVIC: personal communication (1965). — GREGORY, R. A., and H. J. TRACY: Amer. J. Digest. Dis. **5**, 308 (1960). — HUGHES, A., and R. S. TONKS: Lancet 1965/I, 1044. — MARTIN, H.: Amer. Heart J. **59**, 932 (1965). — SELLER, R. H., O. RAMIRES-MAXO, A. N. BREST, and J. H. MOYER: J. Amer. Med. Ass. **191**, 654 (1965). — SHIMAMOTO, T., T. FUJITA, H. SHIMURA, H. YAMAZAKI, S. IWAHARA, and G. YAJIMA: Amer. Heart J. **57**, 273 (1959). — UVNÄS, B.: Acta physiol. Scand. **4**, Suppl. **13** (1942).

General Discussion

Wolff: I should like to make a short comment on the functional relationship between angiotensin and catecholamines as suggested by recent observations made by several groups. Distler, Liebau, and I[1] have studied the mode of vasoconstrictor action of angiotensin, using aortic strip preparations from adult rats. The spirally-cut muscle strip was mounted in a perfusion chamber with a total volume of 0.3 ml. and rinsed continuously with Tyrode's solution at 37° C. The upper part of Fig. 1 shows the isometric contraction of the strip while exposed to tyramine, which is known to act by releasing noradrenaline from the adrenergic terminals. Repeated exposures to angiotensin resulted in a stepwise loss of constrictor activity until no response

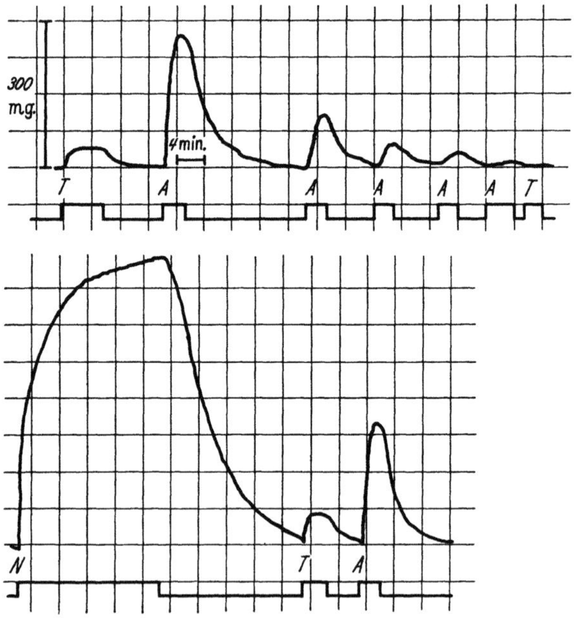

Fig. 1. Strip of rat's aorta, isometric contraction. T: tyramine · HCl 10^{-6} g./ml. A: angiotensin 10^{-6} g./ml. N: noradrenaline 10^{-6} g./ml. Reduced response after repeated exposure to angiotensin and restoration of effect after exposure to noradrenaline.

occurred. At the same time, tyramine also proved ineffective; in other words, a crossed tachyphylaxis between angiotensin and tyramine appeared. If at the same time the strip was rinsed with noradrenaline for 10—15 minutes and

[1] Distler, A., H. Liebau, and H. P. Wolff: Nature **207**, 764 (1965).

thereafter washed with Tyrode's solution, the constrictor action of tyramine as well as that of angiotensin was fully restored (see lower part of Fig. 1). Cocaine, which is known to prevent the action of several sympathomimetic agents, also abolished the action of angiotensin.

These observations suggest that the vasoconstrictor action of angiotensin is mediated, at least partly, by a release of noradrenaline from the post-ganglionic sympathetic nerve-endings in the vascular wall. Consequently, angiotensin must prove ineffective if these stores are depleted to such a degree that noradrenaline cannot be released in amounts sufficient to induce a contraction. After partial repletion of the stores by exogenous noradrenaline, angiotensin regains its activity.

Direct evidence of the noradrenaline-releasing effect of angiotensin was furnished by quantitative fluorimetric estimation of the catecholamine content of the vascular wall before and after exposure to angiotensin. No separate measurement of noradrenaline and adrenaline was attempted, since, according to SCHMITTERLÖW[1], no adrenaline is demonstrable in extracts of most mammalian arteries. For this series of experiments, aortae from rats were cut lengthwise. One part was rinsed with angiotensin, the other with Tyrode's solution, to serve as a control.

Angiotensin caused a decrease in the noradrenaline content of approximately 50% (Table 1). Comparable studies on arteries of cows and pigs indicated that this effect depends on the species, on the type of vessel, and on the concentration of angiotensin.

Table 1. *Effect of angiotensin (10^{-7} g./ml.) on noradrenaline content of rat aortae*

Experiment	Noradrenaline content (μg./g.)		Difference
	Control	After rinsing with angiotensin	
1	0.88	0.30	0.58
2	0.29	0.05	0.24
3	0.37	0.15	0.22
4	0.68	0.47	0.21
5	0.77	0.58	0.19
6	0.82	0.49	0.33
Mean (± S.E.)	0.64 ± 0.09	0.34 ± 0.09	0.30 ± 0.06 $p < 0.01$

Mean of decrease in noradrenaline content 46.7%

The data indicate an indirect vasoconstrictor action of angiotensin by the liberation of noradrenaline from the adrenergic terminals of the vascular wall. The possibility, however, of an adrenergic releasing effect from chromaffin cells, recently found in vascular walls, has to be considered. Besides these indirect effects, the possibility that angiotensin exerts an additional, direct action on vascular smooth muscle cannot be excluded.

PAGE: MCCUBBIN and I[2] found that responsiveness of blood pressure to tyramine is greatly augmented after infusion of angiotensin. We postulated

[1] SCHMITTERLÖW, C. G.: Acta physiol. Scand. **16**, Suppl. **56** (1948).

[2] MCCUBBIN, J. W., and I. H. PAGE: Circulation Res. **12**, 553 (1963).

that angiotensin increased the effectiveness of the transmitter, norepinephrine, because the response to exogenous norepinephrine was not increased. In other words, infused angiotensin does not increase the pressor response of norepinephrine when the latter is injected intravenously, but does increase the effectiveness of the response to injected tyramine. And if it is true that the response to tyramine is wholly due to endogenous norepinephrine, then it follows that angiotensin increases the efficacy of endogenous norepinephrine. We think that this effect of angiotensin represents a bridge between the neural component of hypertension and the humoral renal component.

This became important when we were able to show, along with DE MOURA and OLMSTED[1], that sub-pressor doses of angiotensin, given over a period of eight to ten days, may lead to severe hypertension. This hypertension can be relieved by guanethidine, which suggests it is a neural type of hypertension. We think of this as being a relationship between the renal vasopressor system and the neural control, the two working in concert to regulate tissue perfusion. Herein, of course, can be seen my long-standing bias for the "mosaic" theory of hypertension.

Parenthetically, I think we are using the terms "crisis", "vascular crisis", and "encephalopathy" in a slightly confusing fashion. I usually think of hypertensive encephalopathy as a crisis, and that is why we use sodium nitroprusside in its treatment. This to me is a true emergency. I do not believe malignant hypertension is a crisis, though I strongly believe it should be treated effectively within hours by bringing the arterial pressure down to near normal. The reason that we have little enthusiasm for the usual antihypertensive drugs in the treatment of encephalopathy is that their action is uncertain during a crisis. There is a danger of giving either too much or too little of the drug as well as of finding some of the drugs are ineffective. Sodium nitroprusside has the great advantage of effectively lowering blood pressure to the desired level without fail. Then, too, it is very cheap, which seems to be its chief disadvantage.

SMIRK: Dr. PAGE, I think your first remark was so interesting that I really doubt whether you can withdraw from the discussion; in fact, I should like to direct a question to you. One of my colleagues, LAVERTY[2], published a paper indicating that there was an increase in the sympathetic nervous discharge to hind-limb blood vessels of the rat when angiotensin II was administered. He was working with a preparation[3] in which a hind limb is separately perfused and is only connected with the rest of the rat by nerves. He was able to produce vasoconstriction in that separately perfused hind limb by administering angiotensin to the upper part of the animal, whereas with most pressor drugs the expected result was obtained, namely a homoeostatic vasodilatation in the separately perfused hind limb. I should be glad if you have any additional comment to make.

PAGE: I think it is correct that there is a neural component stimulated by angiotensin. We know from the work of KHAIRALLAH and myself[4] that there is a neural component involved in the intestinal stimulation by angiotensin. This has been quite clearly demonstrated.

---

[1] MCCUBBIN, J. W., R. S. DEMOURA, I. H. PAGE, and F. OLMSTED: Science **149**, 1394 (1965).

[2] LAVERTY, R.: J. Pharmacy Pharmacol. **15**, 63 (1963).

[3] FIELD, L. W., W. DEGRAAF, and A. T. WALLIS: J. Appl. Physiol. **12**, 142 (1958).

[4] KHAIRALLAH, P. A., and I. H. PAGE: Amer. J. Physiol. **200**, 51 (1961).

TAQUINI: If I understood correctly, you said that hypertension appears if angiotensin is infused over a long period of time in small doses, which have no pressor effect. Then it is possible that the increase in pressure is due to the action of angiotensin on the adrenal glands with subsequent aldosterone liberation, ionic changes in the vessels, and secondary hyper-reactivity of them, and not to its direct pressor effect.

PAGE: I recall that you first showed that angiotensin caused release of epinephrine from the adrenal glands. KANEKO, MCCUBBIN, and I[1] found this much enhanced when a ganglion-stimulating agent was given first. Possibly this release of catecholamines aids in the rise in pressure that we found when sub-pressor amounts of angiotensin were infused.

TAQUINI: I consider that the effect you have seen after the infusion of angiotensin is due to some physiological property rather than to a pressor side effect, as you have suggested, since you have used non-pressor doses of the drug.

PAGE: That may well be, yes.

PEART: I think that the question of angiotensin and its relation to noradrenaline was brought out by what Dr. WOLFF said. The work of FELDBERG and LEWIS[2] on the adrenal medulla, showing the effect of close intra-arterial injections of quite small doses not only of angiotensin, but also of bradykinin, with their ability to liberate adrenaline, is highly relevant. This is in the intact animal, which I think is very important. If one looks at the effect on the whole animal of blockers to noradrenaline, it is quite striking how ineffective they are in blocking the pressor actions and, as far as I know, the vasoconstrictor actions of angiotensin. In relation to what Dr. PAGE has been saying, this may only mean sympathetic stimulation would have to act in quite a different way than by liberating noradrenaline — from wherever it is stored — freely and directly in the arterial smooth muscles.

I have my reservations about the action of angiotensin in the whole animal in relation to noradrenaline. I think that what happens to the aortic wall in an electrolyte medium may differ very greatly with a lot of these small peptides. In fact, it is very difficult to find any small peptide which doesn't seem to liberate an amine and *vice versa*. So I'm a bit dubious about this explanation of increasing sympathetic action, and I'm not even convinced that the experiments which PAGE and MCCUBBIN have described on the effects of sympathetic stimulation in renal hypertension mean that angiotensin is really acting through the sympathetic nervous system. It may be a question of the arterial calibre at a particular time and a summation effect of two substances acting at different sites on the smooth muscle.

BEIN: I have the same reservations about explaining the action of angiotensin in terms of the liberation of noradrenaline. On the other hand, one shouldn't forget that a histamine liberator, or the action of histamine in response to a histamine liberator, virtually cannot be inhibited by a histamine antagonist. It seems that endogenous liberation — or liberation of an endogenous substance in the periphery — cannot be as easily antagonised by an otherwise well-known blocker of such an endogenous substance.

---

[1] KANEKO, Y., J. W. MCCUBBIN, and I. H. PAGE: Circulation Res. **9**, 1247 (1961).

[2] FELDBERG, W., and G. P. LEWIS: J. Physiol. **171**, 98 (1964).

Peart: Yes, I agree with that. But here we are getting into the work Dr. Wolff was describing, namely liberation of noradrenaline out of the tissue, just as you get a liberation of adrenaline into the blood stream from the adrenal gland by close intra-arterial injection of angiotensin; so on the one hand there is a liberation and on the other hand you are having to provide another explanation for how angiotensin works in increasing or facilitating, if that is correct, a sympathetic action. As a matter of interest we have infused angiotensin in pressor doses into man and followed the vanilmandelic-acid output. This study is going on at the moment, arising out of the work of Feldberg and Lewis on the adrenal, and so far we haven't found any increase over 12-hour periods.

Long-term treatment

Organization of a long-term multiclinic therapeutic trial in hypertension

By

E. D. FREIS*

The primary purpose of holding conferences such as this is to foster the exchange of ideas and, it is hoped, provide a platform for constructive criticism. It is with this thought that I am presenting our current work, which is still very much in progress. It must be emphasized that I am serving merely as the spokesman for the other cooperating physicians in 14 Veterans Administration Hospitals who, together with our biostatisticians in the V.A. Central Office, are actively engaged in this study.

Objectives

A little over one year ago, the Veterans Administration began a multiclinic trial designed specifically to test the effectiveness of antihypertensive drug treatment on morbidity in so-called mild and moderate hypertension. Although the efficacy of drug treatment in accelerated and other forms of severe hypertension can be regarded as established, its value in the milder forms of the disease is considered by many to remain unproven.

The question we are attempting to answer is admittedly difficult to assess. We believe that the proper approach must make use of the accepted techniques of controlled clinical trials. This means a truly randomized, double-blind experiment, in which a number of clinics with different observers participate.

Some of you may feel that this attempt is unnecessary, because the value of treatment, even in benign hypertension, has already

* Participants in the present study are: Drs L. ARIAS, M. L. ARMSTRONG, A. W. BLOUNT, M. CALABRESI, C. H. CASTLE, L. ELSON, R. E. FREMONT, M. A. HARRIS, D. LITTMAN, A. F. LYONS, H. W. OVERBECK, E. C. PEREZ-STABLE, E. A. RAMIREZ, W. J. TOLLESON, and J. R. THOMAS; biostatisticians: L. W. SHAW and R. B. TEWKSBURY, Ph.D.

been demonstrated. However, many others are unconvinced and will remain so until acceptably designed trials have been carried out. The follow-up studies of HODGE et al. (*1*), LEISHMAN (*2*) and others, while providing valuable evidence that treatment favorably affects prognosis, were not controlled trials in the modern sense of the term. HAMILTON's study (*3*) was better designed but involved small numbers of patients. Doubters can still say, with some justification, that adequate proof has not yet been provided. This lack of conviction is apparent in my section of the world, for example, where many physicians in practice still treat benign essential hypertension casually and sporadically. We believe, therefore, that a carefully designed prospective study is necessary even at this late date and should, if properly carried out, provide much-needed information.

The project was undertaken in full realization of the difficulties involved. The period of follow-up in benign hypertension must necessarily be long. The prognosis varies greatly from patient to patient. The disease often is asymptomatic, and the patients, therefore, may be poorly motivated to continue treatment.

The Veterans Administration has been involved in previous multiclinic trials on antihypertensive agents [ARMSTRONG et al. (*4*, *5*, *6*)]. However, these former studies were designed primarily to evaluate the blood-pressure-reducing ability and side effects of various antihypertensive drugs, both alone and in combination. The trials were relatively short, usually of one year's duration, and no special precautions were taken against drop-outs and uncooperative patients. These studies were of value in providing evidence of the comparative antihypertensive effectiveness of various drug regimens in the control of mild and moderate hypertension. To evaluate the long-term effects on prognosis, however, a different protocol had to be drawn up.

The end-point for assessing the success or failure of treatment can be either morbidity or mortality, or both. We chose morbidity rather than mortality, for the following reasons: 1) The incidence of morbid events should provide an answer more quickly than mortality, which is often preceded by one or more clinically apparent complications. If treatment appears to be beneficial, the trial may be stopped at an earlier date than if mortality were taken as the end-point. 2) Certain complications, such as those associated with accelerated hypertension, are undoubtedly indications for treatment. Patients, therefore, cannot ethically be kept any longer in the randomized trial following such developments. 3) The purpose of treatment should not only be to prevent death but also to permit the patient to live a full, active life. If the treated patients are kept alive but the number of those who become crippled, invalided, or institutionalized is not reduced, then treatment is not very satisfactory.

Classification of patients

Patients who exhibit hypertension on admission to the various hospitals and are not under the care of an outside physician are the source from which the study patients are recruited. Existing drug treatment is withdrawn preceding pretreatment evaluation, the waiting-period depending on the types of drug the patient was taking. The blood pressure is recorded four times daily, and the readings taken between the fourth and the sixth day in hospital after the end of the waiting-period are averaged to give the mean basal blood pressure. Patients who exhibit an average basal diastolic pressure of 90 to 129 mm. Hg are considered for inclusion in the study; all others are excluded. Severity is also graded, according to the degree of detectable involvement in four target organs: the optic fundi, the heart, the brain, and the kidneys. The criteria for grading from I to IV within each panel have been published previously (*4*). After doubling the scores for the basal diastolic pressure and the optic fundi, the scores within each panel are summed to obtain a total severity index. Patients with total scores between 2 and 7 are classified as mild cases, those with scores of 8 to 15 as moderate, and those with scores of 16 or above are regarded as severe cases and are excluded.

Also excluded from the trial are: patients exhibiting eyeground hemorrhages, cotton-wool exudates, or papilledema; those with clinical diagnoses of cerebral or subarachnoid hemorrhage and dissecting aortic aneurysm; those with congestive heart failure which does not clear following digitalis and mercurials and remain clear during the trial-period; and those with blood urea nitrogen levels above 60 mg.% and the clinical diagnosis of acute hypertensive encephalopathy. The criteria adopted in eliminating unreliable patients will be discussed later. Patients with other organic hypertensive complications are not excluded.

Of the first 200 patients who have been admitted to the randomized trial, 36% were classified as having Group II changes in the optic fundi; the remainder showed Group I changes or none at all. Upon assessment according to UNGERLEIDER's criteria, 29% exhibited cardiomegaly and 25% showed electrocardiographic voltage and T-wave modifications indicative of left ventricular hypertrophy; 6% exhibited cerebrovascular complications as manifested by paralysis, paresis, tremor, or unsteady gait. Serum creatinine levels were elevated above 1.7 mg.% in 7% of the patients, and B.U.N. elevations of 30 mg.% or higher were found in 3%.

The excretion of phenolsulfonphthalein is also determined in hydrated patients. Excretion of 45% or less of the dye within two hours is an indication of reduced renal function. Such a reduction was found in 22% of the patients; the majority excreted 40–80% of the dye during this period.

The ages of the patients show a somewhat bimodal distribution with peaks about 25 years apart. The major peak occurs in the 45–54 year range and the minor peak in the 65–75 range. This distribution is characteristic of the veteran population and is due to the two world wars. The inclusion of some younger patients is attributable to the Korean War.

The possibility of limiting the trial to patients without organic complications was considered, but this was not done for the following reasons: 1) The value of antihypertensive treatment in preventing morbidity has not been studied in multiclinic randomized trials in either the complicated or the uncomplicated group. 2) Because of many unknown or undetected variables which might influence prognosis; the less preselection allowed, the more generally applicable will be the results. 3) The elimination of all patients with detectable complications would seriously reduce the size of the trial samples.

A considerable number of patients diagnosed as having essential hypertension on admission are excluded for various reasons. Many exhibit falls in blood pressure to averages below 90 mm. diastolic after the fourth day in hospital. These labile patients have been shown by SMIRK (7) to have a better prognosis than those with elevated basal pressures. Our sample, therefore, is restricted in this respect and also in regard to sex, since the veteran group is limited to males, who have a poorer prognosis in general than females.

Record keeping

The records are designed to make the collection of data as uniform as possible in the various hospitals collaborating in the multiclinic trial. Check-lists are used in place of narrative descriptions to ensure completeness and uniformity and also to facilitate data handling. Spaces are provided for checking or entering numerical data, and each item is numbered. These numbers are code designations, so that the data may be transcribed directly to punch cards by coding clerks. Data analysis, including cross-correlations, can thus be made at any time in the study.

All reports are sent to the chairman who, aided by his staff, reviews them for completeness and consistency. If there are missing or inconsistent data, the forms are returned to the respective clinic. The clinic secretaries in the various hospitals are instructed to submit their completed reports each week, so that no backlog is allowed to accumulate. This permits errors and omissions to be corrected promptly. When records are retained at the participating hospital for long periods, it often becomes impossible to trace missing data. When records are complete and in keeping with the protocol, they are forwarded to the statistician, where they are again reviewed and the data then transferred to punch cards. This procedure, although it makes more work for the chairman, has resulted in great improvement in adherence to the protocol and in the quality and completeness of the reports.

Screening for reliability

After discharge from the hospital, the patient enters on a pre-randomization trial-period of two to four months' duration. During this period he visits the clinic at monthly intervals. The pre-randomization trial-period was instituted for several reasons:

Firstly, in the previous studies (*5*, *6*), the highest percentage of drop-outs occurred during the first two months of follow-up. Since an appreciable number of drop-outs would jeopardize the study, we wished to minimize their occurrence as much as possible. "Skid-row" alcoholics, vagrants, psychopaths, antagonistic personalities, mentally incompetent persons who are not properly cared for at home, and all those who for one reason or another could not return to clinic regularly are therefore excluded from the trial. In addition, the pre-randomization trial-period serves to eliminate other potential drop-outs that are missed during the initial evaluation. While this selectivity narrows the scope of the trial, it should be emphasized that the exclusions are made prior to randomization in order to reduce potential bias. It is considered to be far less serious to lose these cases before randomization than to leave them in and incur a high drop-out rate following randomization.

Secondly, the trial period also provides additional protection for the patients. If, during this interval, the readings made in the clinic show the average diastolic pressure to be above 129 mm. Hg, the patient is referred elsewhere for treatment. The inclusion in the randomized trial of any patient whose diastolic pressures remain at 130 mm. Hg or higher on repeated visits to the clinic would be difficult to justify on ethical grounds.

Thirdly, in this study the cooperativeness and reliability of the patients are assessed by tablet counts. The patients are instructed to bring their medicine bottles with them on each visit to the clinic. The number of tablets remaining in the bottle is counted in private by the clinic secretary. If the patient returns 10% more tablets than he should have, had he taken the prescribed amount, or five tablets less (to allow for breakage or loss), he is considered unreliable. In addition to pill counts, a urine-fluorescence test is made. Riboflavine, which produces a bright yellow fluorescence of the urine, is incorporated in the tablets. A urine sample is examined under ultraviolet light at the time of the visit to the clinic; if fluorescence is found, the physician knows at least that the patient took his medication on that day.

The two indices of pill counts and urine fluorescence are used to establish criteria for admitting patients to the randomized trial. If the first two monthly visits show that the patient has followed his instructions, he is randomized; if it is evident that he has not done so, the trial-period is extended for a maximum of two additional monthly visits. To qualify for randomization the patient must show no violations on two successive visits to the clinic, including the one at which he is randomized. The pill-count technique has been a revelation to us in disclosing the frequency with which patients neglect to take their medication regularly. The detection and exclusion of many of these patients prior to entrance into the randomized trial seems to be an important step if misleading results are to be avoided.

Treatment regimen

If the patient passes all his tests during the trial-period, he is randomized and placed on one of two double-blind assigned regimens. This is accomplished by opening a numbered, sealed envelope containing a card assigning him to a code-numbered regimen. The cards are made up by the statistician from tables of random numbers. The regimens are either hydrochlorothiazide (50 mg.) plus reserpine (0.1 mg.), incorporated in a single tablet and taken twice daily, plus hydralazine (25 mg.) in a second tablet taken three times daily, or placebos of these drugs. On the next visit, if the diastolic pressure recorded in the clinic after a 15-minute rest period is above 90 mm. Hg, the dose of hydralazine is increased and maintained at 50 mg. three times daily. If it is below 90 mm. Hg, the dose is not increased. If the diastolic pressure is below 90 mm. Hg and side effects are complained of, the doses of the code-labelled drugs are reduced.

The effectiveness of this regimen on blood pressure was shown in the previous drug-oriented trials, in which these three antihypertensive agents were used alone or in combination (*6*). The antihypertensive efficacy of this triple-drug regimen was again demonstrated in the present study; the average pretreatment basal diastolic pressures in the drug- and placebo-treated groups were almost identical, whereas the first post-randomization visit shows that the diastolic pressure measured in the clinic averaged 19 mm. Hg lower in the actively treated group than in the placebo group.

Comparability of treated versus placebo groups

Although no attempt was made to match drug- and placebo-treated patients, the allocations being truly random, the two groups have thus far proved to be similar in most respects. However, in the first 200 randomized patients, slightly more of those in the 35—44 age group were randomized into the actively treated, and somewhat more in the 65-and-over age group into the placebo-treated series. It is hoped that this age discrepancy in favor of the actively treated patients will be corrected as more patients enter the study.

The two groups were practically identical with regard to the distribution of basal diastolic blood pressure. Approximately three fourths of the patients in both groups had diastolic levels averaging between 90 and 110 mm. Hg. The distribution of changes in the optic fundi was also very similar in the two groups. With respect to a history or electrocardiographic evidence of previous cardiac abnormality, such as congestive heart failure or myocardial infarction, the difference between the actively treated and placebo groups was insignificant. Similarly, enlargement of the heart as revealed by x-ray, using UNGERLEIDER's criteria, showed very little difference, the incidence of enlarged heart being insignificantly higher in the actively treated patients.

In the actively treated patients, 5% had B.U.N. levels between 25 and 50 mg.%, while in the placebo group 9% had such elevations. The slight differences, however, are constantly shifting as more patients enter the randomized trial.

Reduction of bias

The double-blind procedure is not easily maintained when the active drugs produce such wide differences in blood pressure as compared with placebos. In some, but not all, patients, it is apparent to the participating physicians that active drugs are being used. This is an admittedly undesirable feature of the trial, but one that would be difficult, if not impossible, to avoid. The effectiveness of the antihypertensive drug regimen admittedly introduces an element of bias into the study. The participating physicians may be more willing to overlook minor morbid events in a patient whose blood pressure is well controlled than in one who exhibits an elevated blood pressure. Since two other physicians, the chairman and his associate, as well as the biostatisticians scrutinize all reports, this source of bias is somewhat diminished. To further reduce the occurrence of such bias, the morbid events have been subdivided into three classes:

Class A comprises morbid events that require the patient's removal from the protocol. They include signs of accelerated hypertension, such as hemorrhages, cotton-wool exudates, or papilledema, in the optic fundi, congestive heart failure persisting despite routine treatment, dissecting aneurysm, subarachnoid or cerebral hemorrhage, acute hypertensive encephalopathy, 50% or more elevation of B.U.N. to levels above 60 mg.%, and persistent elevation of clinic diastolic pressures to 140 mm. Hg or higher.

Class B morbid events are those which require only temporary discontinuation of protocol treatment, but represent complications which can be objectively demonstrated, such as congestive heart failure with overt signs responding to routine treatment, myocardial infarction confirmed by transaminase and/or E.C.G. changes, cerebrovascular thrombosis with paresis or paralysis persisting for one day or longer, atrial fibrillation, bundle-branch block, etc., and the appearance of significant proteinuria. Some of these objective changes will be revealed during the physical and laboratory examinations which are carried out annually.

Class C complications include subjective changes, such as angina or dyspnea on exertion, without objective evidence of infarction or congestive heart failure, persistent occipital headaches, or other neurological complaints not demonstrable by neurological examination.

Only Class A and B changes are counted as significant morbid events. Class C changes are regarded as complications of questionable significance for use in the final analysis. Since it is difficult to overlook or discount morbid events of Classes A and B, it is hoped that such bias as may occur will be limited primarily to the Class C complications.

The tablet counts and urine-fluorescence tests are continued during the post-randomization period. The uncooperative patients thus revealed, who failed to take their pills regularly, actually represent a third group intermediate between the fully treated and placebo-treated patients. It is planned to include the morbid events occurring in this group, because their exclusion following randomization could bias the results. The uncooperative patients are defined as those who are shown to be guilty of one or more violations in either the pill-count or the urine-fluorescence test on each of three visits to the clinic in any one-year period. Thus far, they represent 5% of the randomized patients, but their number will most probably increase as the study proceeds.

In the previous cooperative studies we found that the protocol-assigned treatment was occasionally altered by the physicians for inadequate reasons. This was due to thoughtlessness or to lack of familiarity with the protocol on the part of some of the participants. Prompt referral of all records to the chairman has done much to correct this source of error. As an additional precaution, a system of referees has been established. Each referee is responsible for five or six different hospitals. Whenever protocol-assigned treatment is discontinued, whether because of morbidity, severe side effects, drop-out, or other reasons, a "Loss to Protocol" report must be made out and sent to the referee along with the patient's records. The referee then decides whether the patient can legitimately be dropped or whether further efforts should be made to maintain or return him to the randomized treatment. Since these precautions were adopted, unjustified losses to protocol have been eliminated.

Is this study feasible? It appears to be, providing the limitations already imposed are accepted and a continuous check is made on the performance of the participants. Will the study yield valid results? This will depend in a large measure on the number of drop-outs and pill-count violations. Thus far, the drop-out rate has been very low. The number of pill-count violations has been higher, even with the selectivity used, but not enough to jeopardize the study so far. Within these limitations we are hopeful that useful data will be collected.

Summary

The design of a multiclinic therapeutic trial in primary hypertension is described. Results are judged on the basis of incidence of hypertensive and atherosclerotic morbid events which can be objectively demonstrated. Various precautions are taken against potential drop-outs as well as patients who fail to take medication regularly. The importance of prompt review of all records by a single responsible physician is stressed.

Zusammenfassung

Der Versuchsplan einer gleichzeitig an mehreren Kliniken vorgenommenen therapeutischen Studie bei primärem Hochdruck wird beschrieben. Die

Resultate werden auf der Basis der Häufigkeit von Hochdruck- und objektiv nachweisbaren atherosklerotischen Komplikationen beurteilt. Verschiedene Vorsichtsmaßnahmen sind notwendig, sowohl gegenüber möglichen Ausfällen von Patienten als auch gegenüber Patienten, welche die vorgeschriebene Medikation nicht regelmäßig nehmen. Die Bedeutung einer unverzüglichen Kontrolle aller Aufzeichnungen durch einen einzelnen verantwortlichen Arzt wird unterstrichen.

Résumé

On décrit le plan d'une expérimentation thérapeutique dans l'hypertension essentielle, menée conjointement dans plusieurs centres hospitaliers. Les résultats sont jugés sur la base de l'incidence des accidents hypertensifs ou athéroscléreux objectivement constatés. Diverses précautions sont prises contre les défections éventuelles et contre les malades qui ne prennent pas régulièrement leurs médicaments. On souligne l'importance d'une revue rapide de toutes les observations par un seul médecin responsable.

References

1. HODGE, J. V., E. G. MCQUEEN, and F. H. SMIRK: Brit. Med. J. 1961/I, 1. — 2. LEISHMAN, A. W. D.: Brit. Med. J. 1959/I, 1361. — 3. HAMILTON, M., E. N. THOMPSON, and T. K. M. WISNIEWSKI: Lancet 1964/I, 235. — 4. ARMSTRONG, M. L. et al.: Arch. Int. Med. **106**, 81 (1960). — 5. ARMSTRONG, M. L. et al.: Arch. Int. Med. **110**, 126 (1962). — 6. ARMSTRONG, M. L. et al.: Arch. Int. Med. **110**, 134 (1962). — 7. SMIRK, F. H.: N. Zealand Med. J. **63**, 413 (1964).

Prognosis in retinal Grade I and II patients

By

F. H. Smirk

We have been able to show that the basal blood-pressure level and the presence or absence of certain complications are of great value in assessing the prognosis in hypertension. In the present study, some conclusions will be drawn with regard to the influence of treatment on the prognosis in hypertensive patients without Grade III or Grade IV changes in the retina.

Some 25 years ago, my colleague Alam and I (*1*) carried out a series of very frequent and regular blood-pressure measurements and found that blood pressures fell considerably when the patients were kept under very quiet conditions. In healthy young adult males, blood-pressure levels of 90–100 mm. Hg systolic, or less, were not uncommon under such conditions. Later (*2*) it was found that blood pressures would fall to even lower levels if the following measurement techniques were used:

1. The patient is assured that there will be no frightening procedures.
2. The patient is admitted to hospital on the evening before the test and is given 100–200 mg. pentobarbitone to ensure a night's rest.
3. In the morning, bladder and bowels are emptied if desired and, if the patient is not sleepy, a further 100 mg. pentobarbitone are given.
4. A technician or doctor then enters the single room in which the patient has been sleeping and, without conversation, measures the blood pressure regularly at half-minute intervals for 10–15 minutes.

It is important that no other persons should enter the room while the measurements are in progress. Throughout the test, the observer should sit quietly by the patient, who should have been asked not to speak but to relax as completely as possible, physically and mentally.

The lowest blood pressure obtained by this technique is known as the *basal blood pressure*. To signify the blood pressure ordinarily measured in hospital or consulting room without special precautions we suggested that the term *casual blood pressure* might be used. The difference between the casual blood pressure and the basal blood pressure is referred to as the *supplemental blood pressure*.

Although the level of the casual blood pressure varies in the same person from day to day, under the unstimulating conditions described the blood pressure usually fell to a level which in normotensives was almost a physiological constant for the individual at the time. This observation was confirmed by the more exact methods used by KILPATRICK (*3*).

The rise in basal pressure with advancing age is much more consistent than the rise in supplemental pressure (*4*). In hypertensive patients, the basal blood pressure is a little more variable than in normotensives, but much more constant than the casual blood pressure.

The supplemental blood pressure, therefore, represents the variable or labile aspect of the blood pressure and is determined multifactorially, being dependent upon the state of physical, emotional, and probably also metabolic activity at the time of measuring.

ALSTAD and I happened to be engaged on a prospective study of the prognosis in hypertension before hexamethonium became available. Following the introduction of this drug in 1950, the preliminary investigation of patients referred to our hypertensive clinic for treatment still followed closely the same lines as the earlier prospective study on the prognosis in untreated patients (*5*).

For our comparative study of the prognosis in patients with Grade I and Grade II eyegrounds, we now have 199 untreated, or virtually untreated, and 270 treated hypertensive patients of ages ranging from 40 to 69 years. All have had basal as well as casual blood pressures recorded, and all have been followed up at least to the fifth anniversary of their initial clinical investigation.

Usually the first casual blood pressure measured on making contact with the patient was the one recorded; the supplemental blood pressure was obtained by calculating the difference between the casual and basal blood pressures. Results are expressed in terms of mortality over a period of five years.

A follow-up study of the untreated patients five years after the initial measurements of the basal and supplemental blood pressures showed a strong positive correlation between the original height of the basal blood pressure and the subsequent mortality rate, which was much higher in patients with high basal blood pressures (systolic or diastolic) than in those whose basal blood pressures were low. There was, however, no such correlation between the height of the supplemental blood pressure (systolic or diastolic) and mortality. In other words, the outlook in patients with high supplemental blood pressures was as good as in those whose supplemental blood pressures were low.

A comparison of the supplemental blood pressures of untreated patients who survived an eight-year follow-up period and of those who did not, can be seen in Table 1. There is no appreciable difference between the systolic pressures and very little difference between the diastolic pressures in the two groups, although diastolic pressures tend to be slightly higher among the survivors. This applies to males and females.

Table 1. *Comparison of the supplemental blood pressures in patients who survived an eight-year follow-up period and those who did not*

40—69 years	Numbers at eight years		Supplemental blood pressures					
			Systolic mm. Hg			Diastolic mm. Hg		
	Dead	Alive	Dead	Alive	Diff.	Dead	Alive	Diff.
Females . . .	43	51	57	58	+ 1	23	20	— 3
Males	47	22	55	56	+ 1	30	23	— 7
Females and males . . .	90	73	56	57	+ 1	26	21	— 5

The relationship between the percentage mortality after five years and the basal and supplemental pressures in patients with Grade I and Grade II eyegrounds is shown in Fig. 1. There is a close correlation between high basal blood pressure and mortality, but no clear-cut relationship between the supplemental blood-pressure level and mortality.

Thus, over a period of five or even eight years, the supplemental blood pressure shows no tendency to influence the prognosis adversely.

When we speak of supplemental pressures in this way, it is important to remember that the ones referred to are those measured in a clinical setting and not the supplemental pressures which may exist under conditions of physical exertion or prolonged emotional stress.

It is now generally accepted that mortality in patients with Grade III and Grade IV eyegrounds is reduced by treatment, but there has been some dispute about whether the same applies to patients with Grade I and II eyegrounds. It was decided, therefore, to compare treated and untreated patients in these retinal grades. Once again, the results were expressed in terms of mortality over a period of five years from the initial investigation. Variations in the duration of exposure to risk were thus eliminated.

The treatment involved the use of modern drugs, starting with hexamethonium. The aim throughout was to reduce the blood pressure to levels as near normal as could be attained without

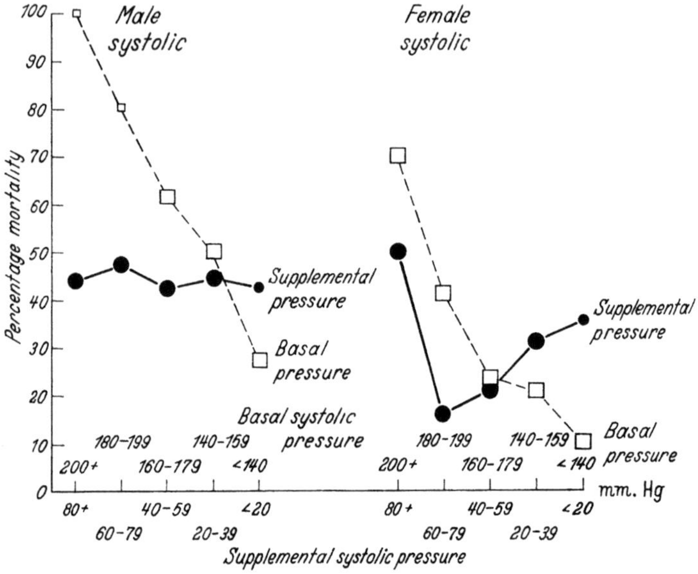

Fig. 1. Relationship between the percentage mortality over a period of five years and the initial levels of basal and supplemental blood pressure.

causing distress. The results in treated patients are compared with the results in untreated patients to which reference has already been made (*5*).

The patients in the untreated group as a whole were milder cases, none having been rejected as being too mild for treatment, whereas the treated group contained only those patients whom we thought should be treated.

The relationship between basal blood pressure and the five-year mortality in treated and untreated males can be seen in Fig. 2. At each basal blood-pressure level, systolic and diastolic, the mortality rate is appreciably higher in the untreated than in the treated patients. The reduction in the mortality rate achieved by treatment is more pronounced when the basal blood pressure is high than when it is low.

The mortality in treated and untreated persons is also influenced considerably by the presence or absence of certain complications at the beginning of the period of investigation (Table 2). The complications referred to are: congestive heart failure, minor strokes,

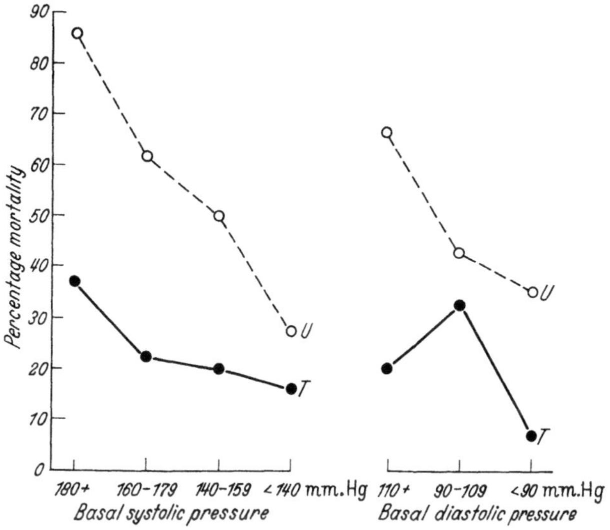

Fig. 2. Relationship between mortality and basal blood pressure in treated (T) and untreated (U) males aged 49—69.

major strokes, substantial renal excretory defects, and evidence of coronary arterial disease. It will be seen that in both treated and untreated males and females the mortality rate is lowest when no

Table 2. *Relationship between the percentage mortality over five years and the number at the outset of certain specified complications*

	0 Complication			1 Complication			2 Complications		
	Dead	Total	%	Dead	Total	%	Dead	Total	%
Females									
Treated	5	65	7.7	8	54	14.8	8	26	30.8
Untreated	10	42	23.8	3	37	24.3	9	11	81.8
Males									
Treated	3	27	11.1	13	40	32.5	4	12	33.3
Untreated	8	16	50.0	7	12	58.3	7	10	70.0

such complications were present at the beginning of the follow-up period, but higher when one of the above-mentioned complications was present, and higher still when two of them were present. Mortality was consistently lower in the treated than in the untreated group (Table 2).

In the treated group, both the proportion of patients with high pressures, whether casual or basal, systolic or diastolic, and the incidence at the outset of such complications as stroke, heart failure, coronary disease, or substantial renal defect were higher than in the untreated group. There were, however, more young people in the treated group. In order to compensate for this we have deleted a corresponding number of the results obtained in young persons in the treated group, thus increasing the mortality rate among the remaining patients in this group. Despite this adjustment, the mortality rate after five years is still significantly lower in the treated than in the untreated group. All the corrections exert a negative influence on the evaluation, and in the corrected results the various factors mentioned as affecting prognosis adversely are either present to an equal degree in the treated and untreated groups or more pronounced in the treated group.

In some of the following tables, an adjustment has been made in respect of the age distribution; in others, the methods of analysis used eliminate the need for such an adjustment. For example, Table 3 shows the results obtained in all males with basal systolic blood pressures of 140 mm. Hg or more; the left-hand side of the table contains the uncorrected data. It will be seen that the mortality in each age group and in the age groups combined is appreciably higher in untreated than in treated males. The difference is highly significant ($P < 0.001$). The general degree of hypertension in the untreated group was less severe than in the treated, but there was a higher proportion of persons in the 40–49 age group among the treated hypertensives. To correct for this, the number of persons in the treated group between the ages of 40 and 49 years was scaled down from 21 to 16, maintaining the same percentage mortality. After correction, the age distribution is now very slightly adverse to the treated group. The difference in the mortality rates remains significant ($0.025 > P > 0.01$). Similar tables have been drawn up to show the results obtained in males with diastolic pressures of 90 mm. Hg or more, females with systolic pressures of 140 mm. Hg or more, and females with diastolic pressures of 90 mm. Hg or more. Any corrections made reduce the difference between the mortality rates in treated and untreated hypertensives, which, however, remains significant.

Table 3. *Mortality in treated (T) and untreated (U) male patients corrected by deduction of surplus patients in the various age groups*

Age		Male basal systolic 140 + mm. Hg						% Distribution	Male basal diastolic 90 + mm. Hg						% Distribution
		Uncorrected			Corrected				Uncorrected			Corrected			
		Dead	Total	%	Dead	Total	%		Dead	Total	%	Dead	Total	%	
60—69	T	7	22	31.8	7	22	31.8	29.7	7	21	33.3	7	21	33.3	27.6
	U	14	21	66.7	5.33	8	66.7	30.8	9	13	69.2	7	11	63.6	28.9
50—59	T	10	36	27.8	10	36	27.8	48.6	10	35	28.6	10	35	28.6	46.1
	U	6	13	46.2	5	12	41.7	46.1	7	15	46.7	7	15	46.7	39.5
40—49	T	3	21	14.3	2.29	16	14.3	21.6	4	20	20.0	4	20	20.0	26.3
	U	4	6	66.7	4	6	66.7	23.1	5	12	41.7	5	12	41.7	31.6
40—69	T	20	79	25.3	19.29	74	26.1	99.9	21	76	27.6	21	76	27.6	100.0
	U	24	40	60.0	14.33	26	55.1	100.0	21	40	52.5	19	38	50.0	100.0
		$X^2 = 12.2598$ $P < 0.001$			$X^2 = 6.031$ $0.025 > P > 0.01$				$X^2 = 5.9816$ $0.025 > P > 0.01$			$X^2 = 4.6264$ $0.05 > P > 0.02$			

In the case of males, the removal from the untreated group of some or all of the persons with three or more complications is justified by the fact that there are no treated males with as many as three complications; furthermore, all three untreated males with three or more complications died, and inclusion of these deaths in the untreated group would be favourable to the eventual conclusion.

A proportional deduction is made from the 60—69 age group which is in excess. The deduction leaves the corrected tables as follows:

Basal systolic treated group has:

1. Similar age distribution
2. 0.82 complications per person (0.81 in untreated)
3. Higher blood pressures in treated group

Basal diastolic treated group has:

1. Slightly older ages
2. 0.75 complications per person (0.66 in untreated)
3. Higher blood pressures in treated persons

Table 4. *Mortality in treated (T) and untreated (U) patients (male and female) with basal systolic blood pressures of 140 mm. Hg or more*

Patients having at the outset none of the specified complications

Age		Dead	Total	% Mortality	% Distribution uncorrected	Corrected numbers for age Dead	Corrected numbers for age Total	% Mortality	% Distribution corrected
60—69	T	3	15	20.0	16.30	3	15	20.0	18.1
	U	7	20	35.0	34.48	3.5	10	35.0	20.8
50—59	T	3	41	7.3	44.57	3	41	7.3	49.4
	U	6	20	30.0	34.48	6	20	30.0	41.7
40—49	T	2	36	5.6	39.13	1.5	27	5.6	32.5
	U	5	18	27.8	31.03	5	18	27.8	37.5
40—69	T	8	92	8.7	100.00	7.5	83	9.04	100.0
	U	18	58	31.0	99.99	14.5	48	30.2	100.0

In the corrected figures, sex ratio, age distribution, blood pressure distribution, and the incidence of electrocardiographic abnormalities and other cardiac manifestations all favour longer survival in the untreated than in the treated group.

Corrected by deduction $X^2 = 8.29969$ $0.01 > P > 0.001$

Note:

Sex ratio: female/male treated 65/27 = 2.41; female/male untreated 42/16 = 2.63.

Table 5. *Mortality in treated (T) and untreated (U) female and male patients in relation to the basal diastolic blood pressure and the number of specified complications*

	Diastolic pressures		0 Complication 110 +			0 Complication 90—109			1 Complication 110 +			1 Complication 90—109			2 Complications 110 +			2 Complications 90—109			0 + 1 + 2 Complications 110 +			0 + 1 + 2 Complications 90—109		
			1 D	2 T	3 %	4 D	5 T	6 %	7 D	8 T	9 %	10 D	11 T	12 %	13 D	14 T	15 %	16 D	17 T	18 %	19 D	20 T	21 %	22 D	23 T	24 %
a	60	T	0	1	0	1	5	20	2	6	33	2	8	25	1	3	33	2	5	40	3	10	30	5	18	28
b	69	U	2	5	40	1	4	25	2	4	50	1	4	25	2	2	100	1	3	33	6	11	55	3	11	27
c	50	T	1	10	10	2	20	10	1	8	13	2	10	20	0	1	0	1	5	20	2	19	11	5	35	14
d	59	U	1	3	33	3	11	27	2	7	29	2	9	22	4	4	100	1	1	100	7	14	50	6	21	29
e	40	T	1	10	10	0	17	0	0	8	0	0	8	0	1	4	25	0	3	0	2	22	9	0	28	0
f	49	U	2	6	33	1	10	10	0	2	0	0	5	0	0	0	0	1	1	100	2	8	25	2	16	13
g	40	T	2	21	10	3	42	7	3	22	14	4	26	15	2	8	25	3	13	23	7	51	14	10	81	12
h	69	U	5	14	36	5	25	20	4	13	31	3	18	17	6	6	100	3	5	60	15	33	45	11	48	23
i	60	T	0	2	0	2	6	33	2	5	40	2	7	29	0	0	0	1	1	100	2	7	29	5	14	36
j	69	U	0	1	0	3	5	60	2	2	100	2	3	67	1	1	100	0	0	0	3	4	75	5	8	62
k	50	T	0	5	0	0	4	0	3	10	30	5	11	45	1	3	33	1	2	50	4	18	22	6	17	35
l	59	U	1	4	25	1	2	50	1	1	100	1	5	20	1	1	100	0	0	0	3	6	50	2	7	29
m	40	T	0	4	0	2	6	33	0	3	0	1	5	20	1	2	50	0	0	0	1	9	11	3	11	27
n	49	U	2	3	67	1	6	17	0	0	0	0	1	0	1	1	100	1	1	100	3	4	75	2	8	25
o	40	T	0	11	0	4	16	25	5	18	28	8	23	35	2	5	40	2	3	67	7	34	21	14	42	33
p	69	U	3	8	38	5	13	38	3	3	100	3	9	33	3	3	100	1	1	100	9	14	64	9	23	39
q	F 40	T	2	32	6	7	58	12	8	40	20	12	49	24	4	13	31	5	16	31	14	85	16	24	123	20
r	+ M 69	U	8	22	36	10	38	26	7	16	44	6	27	22	9	9	100	4	6	67	24	47	51	20	71	28

The results (males and females combined) in patients who at the start of the follow-up period presented none of the specified complications are shown in Table 4. There is an important and significant decrease in mortality among the treated patients.

In Table 5 the results are presented in a way which eliminates the need for correcting age distribution. In each compartment of the table, the untreated and treated persons are all alike in respect of retinal grade (I or II), sex, age group, number of complications, and basal blood-pressure range. All have been followed up for five years from the date of their first clinical investigation. The compartments are marked with a horizontal bar if the mortality rate was lower in the treated persons, with a vertical bar if the opposite applies, and with both if the mortality rates in treated and untreated cases were the same. Tables of the same type, using basal systolic pressures, casual systolic and casual diastolic pressures, show essentially similar results.

In the table based on diastolic pressures in males and females, the results shown in 22 compartments indicate that treatment was helpful, those in four that treatment was disadvantageous, and those in one that there was no difference. Statistically, these results are highly significant ($P < 0.001$) and support the view that treatment had a beneficial effect. The results are similar when patients are subdivided according to their basal systolic pressures.

Casual pressures are a less satisfactory guide to prognosis, but yield similar results. In a table based on casual systolic blood pressures set out in the same way, but subdivided into three blood-pressure levels, the number of compartments favouring the view that treatment was beneficial is 26, as compared with ten against; the results shown in two compartments are not indicative. Here again, the difference is significant: ($X^2 = 6.7368, 0.01 > P > 0.001$). If comparison is restricted to persons with casual systolic blood pressures of 200 mm. Hg or more, the results are: 22 favourable, four unfavourable, one equal ($X^2 = 12.0$, $P < 0.001$). Another table subdivided into three levels of casual diastolic pressure shows very similar results (20 favourable, three unfavourable, one equal).

In patients with a history of stroke, heart failure, or coronary arterial disease at the outset of the follow-up period, the mortality rate was lower if they were treated than if they remained untreated (Table 6).

I should like to refer very briefly to the statistics for all retinal grades relating to New Zealand, since much attention has been devoted to the treatment of high blood pressure in that country.

Table 6. *Mortality in treated (T) and untreated (U) patients with basal systolic pressures of 140 mm. Hg or more in relation to the presence at the outset of various complications*

		Female			Male			Female and Male		
		Dead	Total	%	Dead	Total	%	Dead	Total	%
Angina alone	T	3	13	23	2	10	20	5	23	22
	U	4	14	29	2	3	67	6	17	35
Angina with and without other complications	T	8	34	24	3	13	23	11	47	23
	U	8	18	44	9	13	69	17	31	55
Major stroke with or without minor strokes	T	1	11	9	3	7	43	4	18	22
	U	3	8	38	1	3	33	4	11	36
Minor stroke without major stroke	T	0	17	0	5	11	45	5	28	18
	U	1	4	25	0	1	0	1	5	20
Major and minor strokes with other complications	T	8	24	33	1	3	33	9	27	33
	U	5	8	63	6	6	100	11	14	79
All strokes including those with other complications	T	9	52	17	9	21	43	18	73	25
	U	9	20	45	7	10	70	16	30	53
Heart failure only	T	5	13	38	2	11	18	7	24	29
	U	2	11	18	3	4	75	5	15	33
Heart failure with other complications	T	5	21	24	3	6	50	8	27	30
	U	7	9	78	7	10	70	14	19	74
All heart failure	T	10	34	29	5	17	29	15	51	29
	U	9	20	45	10	14	71	19	34	56
Advanced renal disease with and without other complications	T	4	8	50	3	9	33	7	17	41
	U	0	2	0	2	2	100	2	4	50

The mortality due to high blood pressure in females of various age groups is shown in Fig. 3, from which it is evident that the fall in mortality affects the 70—75 age group and the 75—80 age group as well as the lower ones. A rather similar reduction in the mortality due to cerebrovascular accidents can be seen in Fig. 4. In males, mortality due to hypertension is reduced, but the New Zealand national statistics reveal no fall in the mortality due to cerebrovascular disease in males between 1950 and 1964.

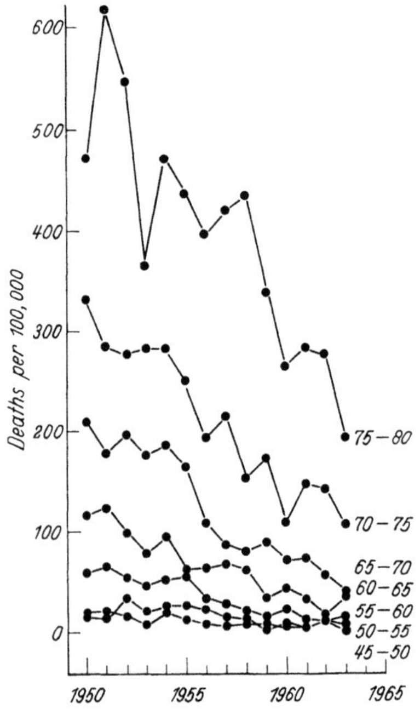

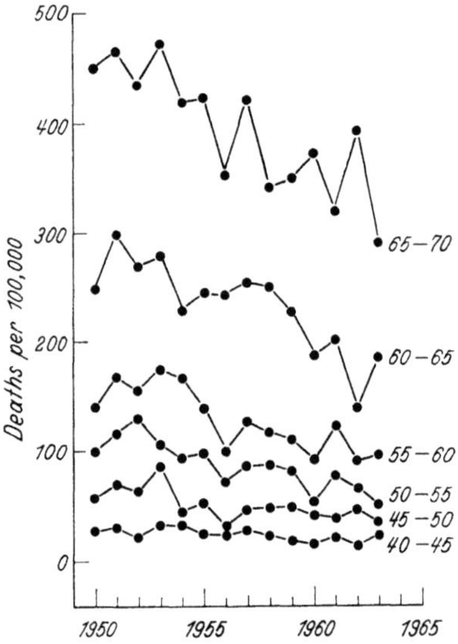

Fig. 4. Mortality due to cerebrovascular accidents in New Zealand females (330—334).

Fig. 3. Mortality due to hypertension in New Zealand females (440—447).

There are now many reports of clinical improvements, including reduced mortality, brought about by lowering the blood pressure. Improvement does not depend to any great extent upon which of the many antihypertensive drugs is used, provided the blood pressure is reduced. The preventive treatment of early cases is important.

Summary

1. Prognosis for survival in both untreated and treated hypertensive patients with Grade I and Grade II eyegrounds is strongly influenced by all of the following factors: age, sex, and the presence at the outset of such

associated complications as heart failure, minor stroke, major stroke, defect of renal excretory function, and coronary arterial disease. The presence of two or more such complications implies a worse prognosis than when one only is present.

2. In untreated hypertensive patients of the same retinal grades, the five-year mortality is closely related to the height of the basal systolic and diastolic blood pressures and to the basal pulse pressure. The supplemental pressure, i.e. the labile aspect of the casual blood pressure, is, however, of little or no value in assessing the five-year mortality.

3. The five-year mortality among adequately treated patients is reduced considerably below that of comparable or milder hypertensives who remain untreated.

The degree of reduction in the mortality, as one might expect, is greater when the basal blood pressure is high than when it is only moderately elevated.

4. The reduction in mortality affects groups of patients with a history of heart failure, stroke, or coronary disease before the start of treatment, but in such patients the regimen must be very carefully supervised.

5. Even so, in patients receiving effective treatment, the five-year mortality is still strongly influenced by the presence of hypertensive disabilities at the time of the initial assessment. In contrast, as one might expect, the adverse influence of a high initial basal blood pressure can be greatly lessened by treatment.

6. Standards of normality applicable to casual blood pressures do not apply to basal pressures. The five-year mortality is higher than normal in women with basal systolic pressures of about 150 mm. Hg or basal diastolic pressures of 90 mm. Hg and in men with corresponding figures of 140 and 90 mm. Hg, or less.

7. HODGE and I (7) have examined the pattern of mortality in our treated hypertensive patients and found that it has changed greatly, the figures for the last six years in patients with Grade I and II eyegrounds being as follows: coronary arterial disease, together with sudden cardiac death probably, but not definitely, due to coronary disease: 42%; strokes: 22.5%; non-hypertensive disorders: 18%; heart failure: 6%; uraemia: 9.5%.

8. The five-year mortality of patients with Grade I and Grade II eyegrounds and high basal pressures, but with few or no objective complications of the types mentioned, is improved by antihypertensive drug treatment. In my view the preventive treatment of early cases is important.

Zusammenfassung

1. Die Prognose für das Überleben von behandelten und unbehandelten Hochdruckpatienten mit Augenhintergrundsveränderungen der Grade I und II wird weitgehend durch die folgenden Faktoren beeinflußt: Alter, Geschlecht sowie Komplikationen, die mit der Grundkrankheit in Zusammenhang stehen, wie Herzinsuffizienz, leichte oder schwere Apoplexie, verschlechterte Nierenleistung und Erkrankung der Koronararterien. Liegen zwei oder mehr dieser Komplikationen gleichzeitig vor, so ist die Prognose schlechter als wenn nur eine von ihnen vorhanden ist.

2. Bei unbehandelten Hochdruckpatienten mit einem gleichen Grad von Retinaveränderungen ist die Fünfjahressterblichkeit eng mit der Höhe des basalen systolischen und diastolischen Blutdruckes sowie mit dem basalen Pulsdruck korreliert. Der supplementäre Druck, als Ausdruck des labilen

Anteils des ohne besondere Maßnahmen unter üblichen Bedingungen gemessenen Blutdruckes, ist dagegen nur von geringer oder ohne Bedeutung für die Bestimmung der Fünfjahresmortalität.

3. Die Fünfjahressterblichkeit bei angemessen behandelten Patienten liegt beträchtlich unter derjenigen unbehandelter Patienten mit gleich schwerem oder leichterem Hochdruck.

Wie zu erwarten, nimmt die Sterblichkeit bei hohem basalem Blutdruck stärker ab als bei mäßig erhöhtem.

4. Die Abnahme der Mortalität betrifft auch Gruppen von Patienten, in deren Vorgeschichte Herzinsuffizienz, Schlaganfall oder Koronarerkrankungen auftreten, ehe die Behandlung einsetzt. Bei solchen Patienten ist der Behandlungsplan besonders sorgfältig zu überwachen.

5. Selbst dann wird bei Patienten, die eine wirksame Behandlung erhalten, die Fünfjahresmortalität durch das Vorliegen von Hochdruckkomplikationen zum Zeitpunkt der ersten Beurteilung noch stark beeinflußt. Dagegen kann, wie erwartet, der ungünstige Einfluß eines anfänglich hohen basalen Blutdruckes durch die Behandlung erheblich vermindert werden.

6. Der Standard für die Norm des üblichen Blutdruckes hat keine Gültigkeit für den basalen Blutdruck. Die Fünfjahressterblichkeit ist höher als normal bei Frauen mit basalem systolischem Druck von ungefähr 150 mm Hg oder basalem diastolischem Druck von 90 mm Hg und bei Männern mit entsprechenden Werten von 140 und 90 mm Hg oder weniger.

7. Bei der Untersuchung der Todesursachen unserer Hochdruckpatienten fanden Hodge und ich (7), daß sich die Verhältnisse erheblich geändert haben. Die Zahlen für die letzten sechs Jahre bei Patienten mit Augenhintergrundsveränderungen der Grade I und II waren die folgenden: arterielle Koronarerkrankungen zusammen mit plötzlichem Herztod, wahrscheinliche aber nicht sichere Folge einer Koronarerkrankung: 42%; Schlaganfall: 22,5%; nicht auf Hochdruck zurückzuführende Störungen: 18%; Herzinsuffizienz: 6%; Urämie: 9,5%.

8. Die Fünfjahressterblichkeit von Patienten mit Augenhintergrundsveränderungen der Grade I und II und hohen basalen Drucken, aber mit nur geringen oder keinen objektiv nachweisbaren Komplikationen der erwähnten Art, wird durch die medikamentöse Blutdrucksenkung verbessert. Meiner Meinung nach ist die frühzeitige präventive Therapie des Hochdrucks wichtig.

Résumé

1. Le pronostic de survie des hypertendus avec un fond d'oeil au stade I ou II, traités ou non traités, est fortement influencé par chacun des facteurs suivants: âge, sexe, existence au début de complications associées telles qu'insuffisance cardiaque, accident cérébral majeur ou mineur, insuffisance rénale, maladie coronarienne. L'existence de deux ou davantage de ces complications implique un plus mauvais pronostic que lorsqu'il n'en existe qu'une seule.

2. Chez des malades hypertendus non traités de même stade au fond d'oeil, la mortalité dans les cinq ans est étroitement liée au niveau des pressions systolique, diastolique et différentielle de base. La «pression supplémentaire», c'est-à-dire la portion labile de la «pression accidentelle» (celle trouvée lors d'une mesure faite d'emblée, sans précautions spéciales), n'a que peu ou pas de valeur pour l'évaluation de la mortalité dans les cinq ans.

3. La mortalité dans les cinq ans chez les malades correctement traités est considérablement inférieure à celle observée chez les malades non traités porteurs d'hypertensions comparables ou plus modérées.

Le degré de réduction de la mortalité, comme on pouvait s'y attendre, est plus grand lorsque la pression artérielle de base est très élevée que lorsqu'elle ne l'est que modérément.

4. La réduction de mortalité intéresse aussi des groupes de malades présentant avant le début du traitement des antécédents d'insuffisance cardiaque, d'accident cérébral ou d'affection coronarienne; le traitement doit être tout particulièrement surveillé chez des malades de ce genre.

5. Même ainsi, chez les malades traités efficacement, la mortalité dans les cinq ans est encore fortement influencée par l'existence lors du premier examen de complications hypertensives. Au contraire, comme on pouvait s'y attendre, l'influence péjorative d'une pression artérielle de base initialement élevée peut être fortement réduite par le traitement.

6. Les normes applicables aux «pressions accidentelles» ne s'appliquent pas aux pressions de base. Le taux de mortalité dans les cinq ans est plus élevé que la normale chez les femmes ayant une pression systolique de base d'environ 150 mm Hg ou une pression diastolique de base de 90 mm Hg et chez les hommes ayant des chiffres correspondants de 140 et 90 mm Hg, ou moins.

7. HODGE et moi (7) avons examiné le type de mortalité de nos malades hypertendus traités et trouvé qu'il s'est beaucoup modifié, les chiffres des six dernières années chez les malades avec fond d'oeil de stade I et II étant les suivants: affection coronarienne et mort cardiaque subite probablement, mais non certainement, liée à une maladie coronarienne: 42%; attaques cérébrales: 22,5%; troubles non hypertensifs: 18%; insuffisance cardiaque: 6%; urémie: 9,5%.

8. La mortalité dans les cinq ans de malades avec fond d'oeil aux stades I et II et pression artérielle de base élevée, mais avec peu ou pas de complications objectives des types mentionnés, est améliorée par le traitement médicamenteux antihypertenseur. A mon avis, le traitement préventif des cas précoces est important.

Acknowledgement

Thanks are due to the Medical Research Council of New Zealand, who defrayed the expenses of the research.

References

1. ALAM, G. M., and F. H. SMIRK: Brit. Heart J. 5, 152 (1943). — 2. SMIRK, F. H.: Brit. Heart J. 6, 176 (1944). — 3. KILPATRICK, J. A.: Brit. Heart J. 10, 48 (1948). — 4. SIMPSON, F. O., and F. H. SMIRK: unpublished. — 5. SMIRK, F. H., A. M. O. VEALE, and K. ALSTAD: N. Zealand Med. J. 58, 711 (1959). — 6. SMIRK, F. H.: N. Zealand Med. J. 63, 413 (1964). — 7. HODGE, J. V., and F. H. SMIRK: unpublished.

Analysis of mortality and survival in actively treated hypertensive disease

By

B. Hood, M. Aurell, T. Falkheden, and S. Björk

The material on which this analysis is based comprises about 1,000 hypertensive patients who were admitted to hospital and were below the age of 66 when first submitted to active antihypertensive treatment between September 1st, 1950, and December 31st, 1960. The treatment was essentially a combination regimen, and the use of a single drug, such as reserpine or a saluretic, was considered as active treatment only in the few instances in which the blood pressure could be brought down to normal levels in this way, making the addition of a second drug unnecessary. Treatment was also regarded as active if any of the drugs were used in such conditions as advanced uraemia, malignant hypertension, or acute massive cerebrovascular lesions with very high diastolic blood-pressure levels. In other words, all patients except those who were moribund upon admission to hospital have been included in the series.

The subjects have been collected in two co-operating university departments in Göteborg and Uppsala. After the initial period of hospitalisation, the patients have been treated within the ordinary out-patient facilities available in these departments. Thus, no special hypertension clinics have been set up. To us, a clinic devoted entirely to one disease is a research tool, which, though suitable as such, may in some respects have drawbacks. Certainly this policy of ours has increased the number of patients defaulting from active treatment and thus the number of failures. However, the launching of large-scale attacks on major disorders is not a task which can be left to the resources of a small group of specialists. At a fairly early stage, we came to the conclusion that wider circles of physicians should be encouraged to participate in active work with antihypertensive regimens.

As to pharmacological details, our policy has been flexible; this study has not been a prolonged clinicopharmacological experiment. We have used combination treatment with ganglionic blockers, followed successively by guanethidine and bethanidine, together with hydralazine, as the backbone of the regimen. Reserpine and thiazide have been important adjuncts. Our policy has closely resembled the one followed by SCHROEDER and his group (for reference see SCHROEDER and PERRY, 1960), although our attempts to achieve strict normotension have perhaps not been pursued in such an uncompromising way. We have usually pushed the treatment to the point where side effects have appeared and then allowed a short respite.

The material includes cases of cryptogenetic hypertension, malformation of the kidney, and chronic pyelonephritis with hypertension as the predominant symptom. It can now be said that a good number of undiagnosed cases of renal artery stenosis must certainly be involved as well. Not included, however, are cases of chronic glomerulonephritis, polycystic kidney, coarctation of the aorta, tuberculosis of the kidney, diabetic glomerulopathy, and initially normotensive, chronic pyelonephritis with hypertension appearing as a late, progressive phenomenon.

We have put forward the following problems for consideration:

1) Have long-term results changed successively during the first decade of active treatment?

2) Has active treatment changed the picture of the population of hypertensives as it appears at admission to hospital?

3) Have the major causes of death in hypertensive disease shifted during this period of active treatment? Can the analysis of pre- and post-mortem records contribute to an understanding of our failures and help in planning new lines of attack?

4) Has active treatment become wide-spread and efficient enough to influence the major causes of death in the general population?

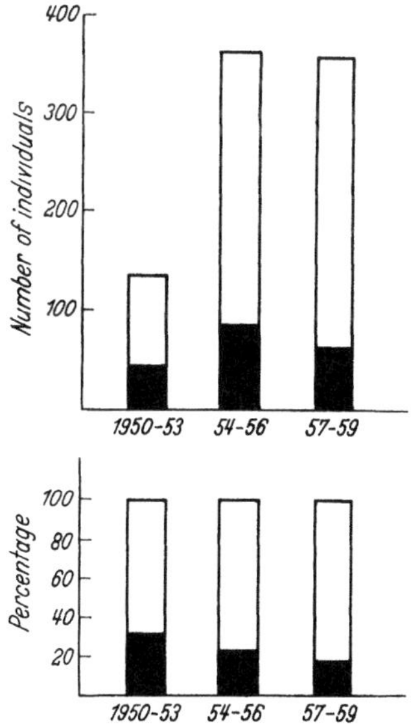

Fig. 1. Five-year survival and mortality in relation to the period when active antihypertensive treatment was started. □: Alive; ■: Dead within 60 months.

Results

1. Survival rate

In Fig. 1, five-year survival and mortality have been summarised in three groups of patients, i.e. those starting treatment in the early fifties

(1950—1953), middle fifties (1954—1956), and late fifties (1957—1959). The obvious objection that these results might only reflect the inclusion of successively greater numbers of less advanced cases has been analysed in different ways.

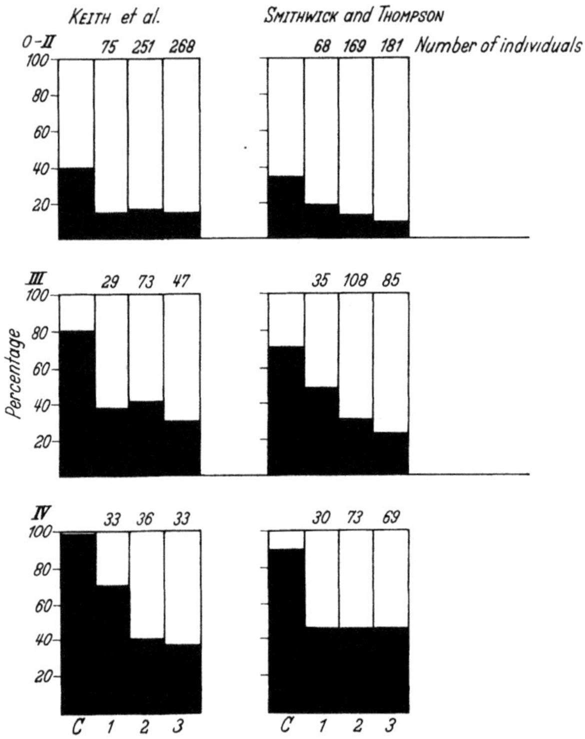

Fig. 2. Five-year survival and mortality in relation to the period when active antihypertensive treatment was started. Comparison with earlier material. □: Alive; ■: Dead within 60 months. C: According to Keith et al. (1939) and to Smithwick and Thompson (1953) respectively. Own material 1950—1959. 1: 1950—1953; 2: 1954—1956; 3: 1957—1959.

The material has been subdivided according to the most comprehensive systems of prognostic classification available, i.e. the systems of Keith et al. (1939), Smithwick and Thompson (1953), Palmer et al. (1948), and Hammarström and Bechgaard (1950). This information is summarised in Figs 2 and 3. It seems that in all the sub-groups, regardless of the classification system used, there has already been a striking improvement in survival in those patients who began active treatment in the early fifties. In the two following periods, there has been a further, though less dramatic, improvement, particularly in the more severe grades. However, in SMITHWICK's Grade IV and KEITH's Grade III there was no further change after the considerable increase in five-year

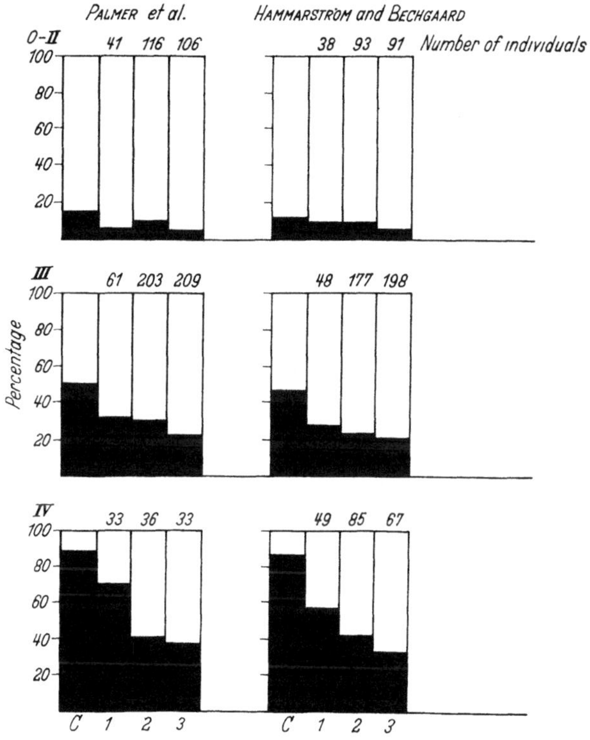

Fig. 3. Five-year survival and mortality in relation to the period when active antihypertensive treatment was started. Comparison with earlier material. □: Alive; ■: Dead within 60 months. C: According to PALMER et al. (1948) and to HAMMARSTRÖM and BECHGAARD (1950) respectively. Own material 1950—1959. 1: 1950—1953; 2: 1954—1956; 3: 1957—1959.

survival obtained in the early fifties. In view of the substantial contribution of advanced cerebrovascular and coronary pathology and advanced renal impairment, especially in SMITHWICK's Grade IV, this finding seems in no way surprising.

2. Patients admitted to hospital

The second question, i.e. whether the population of hypertensives admitted to hospital has undergone any change, may be answered in part by the analysis we have made in the Göteborg material from 1950–1960 of all in-patients below 66 years of age in whom hypertension was registered (Fig. 4). The upper series of

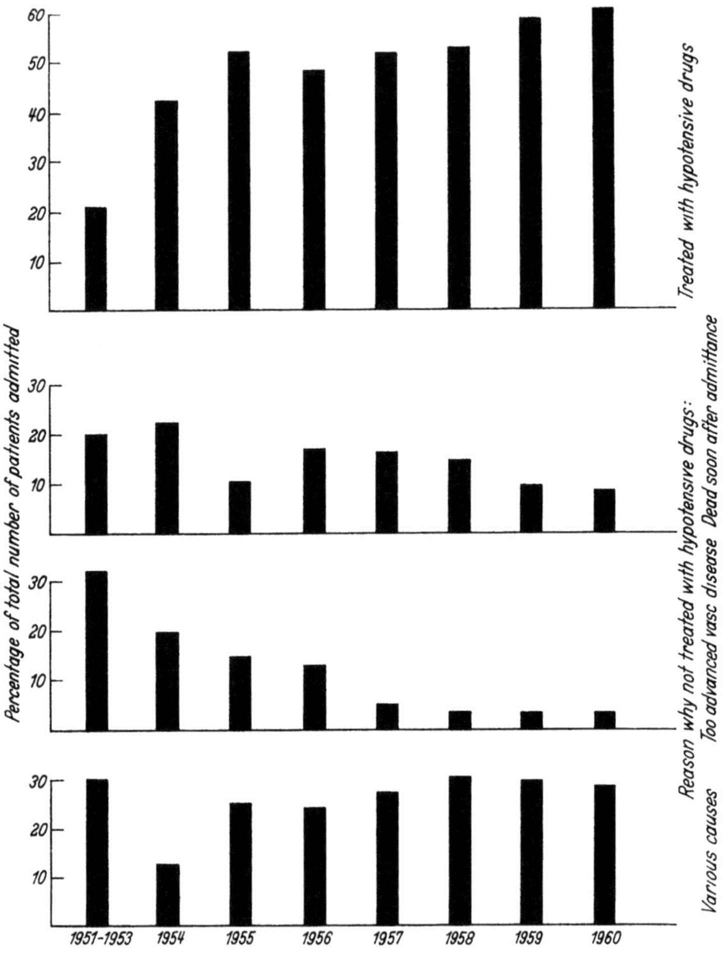

Fig. 4. Successive change in the proportion of hypertensive patients put on treatment with hypotensive drugs. Reasons for refraining from treatment.

columns shows the successive increase in the number of hypertensive patients below the age of 66 years receiving active treatment between 1951 and 1960. The second row of columns shows the steady decline (from about 20% to 8%) in the number of hypertensives not treated owing to the fact that they were in a sub-final state at the time of admission to hospital, usually dying within a few days from cerebrovascular lesions or myocardial infarction. The third line indicates the number of patients who were not actively treated because of severe vascular disease, i.e. fresh massive cerebrovascular lesions, severe cerebral deterioration, fresh myocardial infarction, and advanced uraemia. The decline in this group from 32% to 3% of the total admitted material has presumably been caused by a number of factors. We have certainly tended more and more to apply active treatment to all but the dying. The number of cases admitted for diagnostic work-up or for active treatment on a tentative basis has increased steeply. This has led to a decrease in the relative proportion of cases in which the hospital was used merely to provide care and accommodation for the sub-finally advanced or dying. There is, however, also some evidence — which we shall discuss later — that the actual number of severe complications of hypertensive disease might have been reduced in the general population. Finally, the fourth row of Fig. 4 shows that the number of cases not submitted to active treatment for various reasons – such as too mild hypertension and severe co-existing disease, e.g. malignant tumours – seems to have remained fairly constant during this decade.

3. Analysis of the deaths

The total number of deaths occurring before May 1st, 1965, in the group in which active treatment was begun between September 1st, 1950, and December 31st, 1960, was 323. The distribution of the various causes of death is shown in Table 1. Bronchopneumonia and peptic-ulcer bleeding are considered to bear a certain relation to hypertensive disease, the argument being that death from these causes is exceedingly rare – except in the very old – if there is no serious underlying disease.

The age at death from the four major causes can be seen in Fig. 5. Mortality due to cerebrovascular lesions reaches its peak in the 50–60 age range and that due to myocardial infarction not until the 60–70 range. Even in these subjects with serious hypertensive disease, death below the age of 50 from myocardial infarction is rare. The deaths at an early age due to uraemia occur predominantly in females with hypoplasia of the kidney and/or chronic pyelonephritis. The limited importance and rather late appearance of death from congestive heart failure is evident. The single instance of death from this cause below the age of 40 occurred in a woman with a large adrenocortical adenoma, intractable hypertension, and congestive heart failure.

An attempt has been made to discover whether the major causes of death have shifted in the cases starting treatment during the various periods under study, and whether there has been any

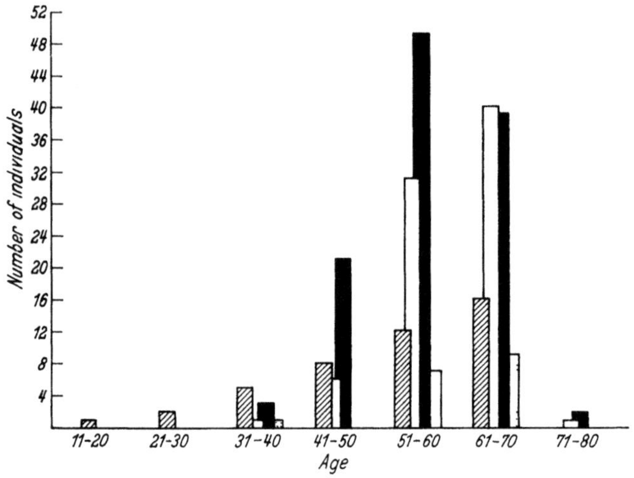

Fig. 5. The age at death from the four major causes in hypertensive disease. ▨. Uraemia; □: Myocardial infarction; ■: Cerebrovascular lesion; ⊡: Congestive heart failure.

change in the age at death. The relevant figures are given in Tables 2 and 3. For obvious reasons, only deaths occurring during the first five years after the introduction of active treatment have been included in these tables. Owing to the difference in the size of the groups starting treatment in the three periods, the mortality figures have been recalculated as percentage values of the entire population at risk for the period in question. Thus, the percentage figures are not based on age-matched groups.

As might be expected, the proportion of deaths due to congestive heart failure, which was initially low, dwindled during the late fifties to insignificance. Deaths due to uraemia were somewhat more frequent in the early fifties. In all age groups, and particularly among patients below 50 years, the percentage of deaths due to cerebrovascular lesions decreased progressively in the three consecutive periods. No corresponding reduction in the number of deaths due to myocardial infarction was found.

Table 1. *Causes of death in 990 cases submitted to active antihypertensive treatment*

Deaths due to the four major causes		
Cerebrovascular lesions	115	
Myocardial infarction	79	
Congestive heart failure	17	
Uraemia	44	
Chronic pyelonephritis 22		
Other 22		
	255	255
Deaths from other vascular and cardiac manifestations		
Vascular		
Dissecting aortic aneurysm	7	
Pulmonary embolism	2	
Thrombosis of coeliac artery	2	
Cerebral aneurysm	1	
Thrombosis of femoral artery (op.)	1	
	13	13
Valvular disease (mitral and aortic)	3	3
Deaths indirectly related to the hypertensive disease		
Pneumonia	18	
Gastric haemorrhage	1	
	19	19
Deaths related to the regimen used		
"Hexamethonium lung"	1	
Suicide (reserpine)	1	
Pentolinium poisoning	1	
Hypopotassaemia (respiratory failure)	1	
Paralytic ileus (Mevasine)	1	
	5	5
	Sum	295
Deaths with no relation to the hypertensive disease		
Tumours	19	
Various causes, accidental deaths, etc.	6	
	25	25
Incomplete records	3	3
	Total	323

Table 2. *Age at death and causes of death in relation to the period when active treatment was started. Five-year mortality*

Period	I (1950—1953) n = 137				II (1954—1956) n = 367				III (1957—1959) n = 359			
Age	≦50	51—60	≧61	Sum	≦50	51—60	≧61	Sum	≦50	51—60	≧61	Sum
Cerebrovascular lesion												
number . .	10	8	2	20	9	22	9	40	1	12	13	26
percentage.	7.3	5.8	1.5	14.6	2.5	6.0	2.5	11	0.3	3.3	3.6	7.2
Myocardial infarction												
number . .	1	5	1	7	4	9	8	21	2	9	8	19
percentage.	0.7	3.6	0.7	5.0	1.1	2.5	2.2	5.8	0.6	2.5	2.2	5.3

Table 3. *Age at death and causes of death in relation to the period when active treatment was started. Five-year mortality*

Period	I (1950—1953) n = 137				II (1954—1956) n = 367				III (1957—1959) n = 359			
Age	≦50	51—60	≧61	Sum	≦50	51—60	≧61	Sum	≦50	51—60	≧61	Sum
Uraemia												
number . .	4	5	2	11	3	3	2	8	6	3	3	12
percentage.	2.9	3.7	1.5	8.1	0.8	0.8	0.5	2.1	1.7	0.8	0.8	3.3
Congestive heart failure												
number . .	1	1	2	4	0	5	3	8	0	1	2	3
percentage.	0.7	0.7	1.5	2.9	0	1.4	0.8	2.2	0	0.3	0.6	0.9

As regards deaths due to uraemia, Fig. 6 shows the length of survival, eyeground alterations, and some morphological changes of the kidneys in the 40 patients – out of a total of 44 who died – in whom treatment was started between 1950 and 1959. It can be seen that males predominated among the cases with arteriolar sclerosis, and that the age at death was more uniformly advanced. Eyegrounds at the beginning were with few exceptions Grade IV. Survival was generally very short.

In the group starting treatment in the late fifties, those who survived for less than eight months were – with one exception – long-distance referrals who arrived in a severe uraemic state. The cases of chronic pyelonephritis on the right (black) constitute only that part of a large group of subjects with chronic pyelonephritis in which hypertension figured as the predominant symptom from the beginning. Survival was generally longer and eyegrounds were less consistently advanced. Marked abuse of analgesics was evident in those cases in which close questioning on this subject was reported in the records.

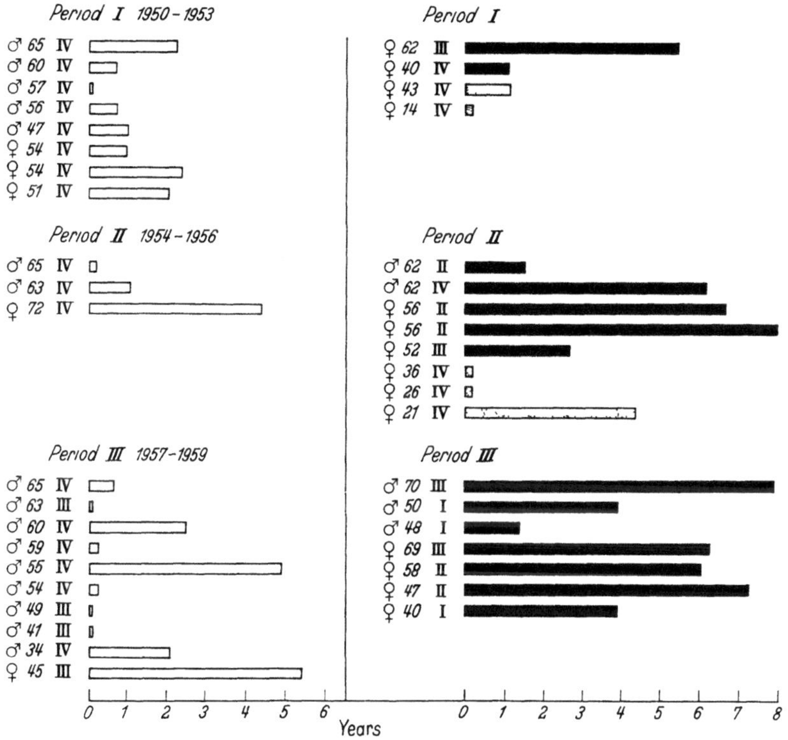

Fig. 6. Sex, age, eyegrounds, and length of survival in the uraemic patients in relation to the underlying disorder. □: Arteriolar sclerosis and arteriolar necrosis; ■: Chronic pyelonephritis; ▤: Malformation of the kidney.

The generally short survival and the lower age at death in the patients with malformed kidneys are apparent. Since 1957 we have had a slowly increasing number of cases with malformed kidneys and severe hypertension, and among these patients there has not been a single death.

The analysis of the state of therapy at death naturally creates many difficulties. As all the records for the present series have not yet been completed in this respect, we have resorted here to a study made two years ago on the same material, covering about two thirds of the deaths (218 as against 323). Tables 4 and 5 show the result of this analysis of the four major causes of death. As has been pointed out earlier, our group of cerebrovascular deaths contains a

Table 4. *State of antihypertensive therapy in the deaths from the four major causes*

	Continuous therapy Degree of B.P. control				Therapy abandoned	Long breaks in therapy	Un-known		
	Normalised or diastolic lowered by > 35 mm.	Diastolic lowered by 20—35 mm.	Diastolic lowered by 0—20 mm.	Sum				Sum	Total
Cerebrovascular lesion	2	16	9	27	46	4	6	56	83
Myocardial infarction . . .	15	13	2	30	21	—	2	23	53
Congestive heart failure	—	2	2	4	9	—	—	9	13
Uraemia	3	4	5	12	21	—	—	21	33

Table 5. *Major reason for abandoning therapy*

	Continuous therapy abandoned 1—60 days before death		Continuous therapy abandoned > 60 days before death			Long breaks in therapy	Un-known
	Physician's responsibility	Patient's responsibility	Too severe vascular disease	Physician's responsibility	Patient's responsibility		
Cerebrovascular lesion	11	5	5	5	20	4	6
Myocardial infarction . . .	1	2	5	2	11	—	2
Congestive heart failure	—	—	5	3	1	—	—
Uraemia	—	—	10	3	8	—	—

collection of our worst therapeutic failures, the majority of these being patients who defaulted from treatment, particularly during the early years. There were only a few patients in whose case treatment was known to have been adequate and efficient up to the time of the last examinations before death.

This is in sharp contrast with the situation in cases of myocardial infarction, where treatment was well maintained in the majority of cases and blood-pressure control was excellent or good in at least half of the subjects who died. In renal insufficiency we have, of course, often been forced to diminish or withdraw treatment, owing either to the initially advanced state or to progressive, chronic pyelonephritis. As to the degree of blood-pressure control and progression into uraemia, we have earlier differed in opinion from the Cleveland group with regard to the occurrence of what they have called "delayed uraemia" in malignant hypertension. More than half of the subjects in our series who died of uraemia originally had severely impaired renal function with serum creatinine above 3 mg. %. If the serum creatinine was initially below 3 mg. %, progression into uraemia was always associated either with lack of control or with progressive pyelonephritis. We have as yet failed to observe progression into uraemia in patients in whom renal function was initially well maintained or only moderately decreased, blood-pressure control good, and chronic pyelonephritis absent.

Finally, in congestive heart failure, the majority of the patients had abandoned treatment for a variety of reasons. The patients who received continuous treatment up to the time of death were in the minority. These cases initially had either congestive heart failure of long standing or advanced coronary sclerosis, or both.

The over-all picture presented by the autopsy records is a grim one; the predominant features are advanced and extensive atherosclerosis or chronic progressive parenchymatous disease of the kidney. One very strong impression left by our studies is that any advances which ensure smooth control of the blood pressure will have only a limited effect and that measures of another type, which can be instituted at an earlier stage, will have to be introduced if any real progress is to be made in the treatment of this group of diseases.

4. Effect of treatment on causes of death

Has active treatment had any effect on the incidence and severity of any of the major causes of death in the general population? W.H.O. statistics for many European countries and local statistics for Sweden show a decline in mortality due to cerebrovascular disorders during recent years. At least in the Swedish statistics, however, it seems that the mortality curves already began to show a downward trend in the early fifties, particularly in females. It may safely be said that antihypertensive treatment at that time can neither have been wide-spread enough nor efficient enough in most hands to have made any impact. It seems more reasonable to assume that greater numbers of patients with occlusive cerebrovascular disease survived as a result of general improvement in care and the use of antibiotics.

As massive cerebral haemorrhage is nearly always lethal, the number of autopsy-proven cases should approximate very closely to the actual number of these haemorrhages occurring. In Göteborg, we have analysed the autopsy records from the main General Hospital and the Hospital for Chronic Diseases as well as from the

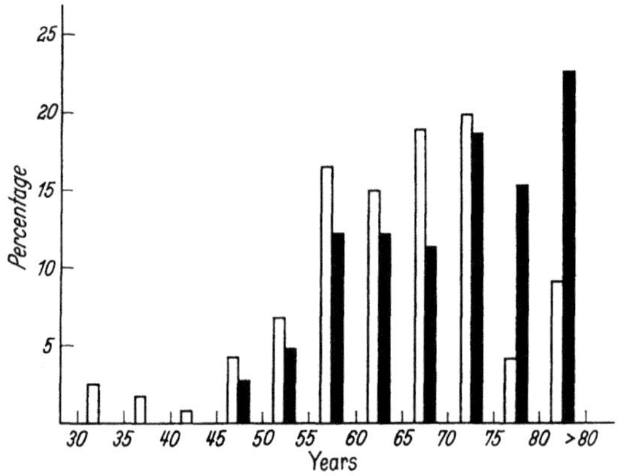

Fig. 7. Percentage distribution in 5-year brackets of all individuals with lethal cerebral haemorrhage. □: 1948 + 1949; ■: 1960 + 1961.

Coroner's Office for two two-year periods, 1948/49 and 1960/61 (Table 6). Our clinical impression that cerebral haemorrhage had become rare in age groups below 50 years was substantiated. Up to the age of 75 years, the absolute number of cerebral haemorrhages in terms of the population at risk in the various age brackets had decreased. The proportion of cerebral haemorrhages occurring in the age groups beyond 75 had increased steeply (Fig. 7). An analysis of the pre-mortem records of the patients aged 65 and below who died in 1960 and 1961 from cerebral haemorrhage showed that almost half were unaware of their hypertension and that active treatment had been rare and generally inefficient (Table 7). There was not a single case among those who died of cerebral haemorrhage in which a record of consistent and adequate antihypertensive treatment was found.

Our interpretation of these findings and the analysis of the cerebrovascular lesions in our actively treated subjects is that cerebrovascular lesions, and especially cerebral haemorrhage, occurred, with very few exceptions, in patients whose blood pressure was poorly controlled and in those who escaped entirely from treatment. It seems evident that adequate antihypertensive treatment offers good protection against cerebrovascular lesions and particularly so against cerebral haemorrhage. We also conclude that antihypertensive treatment has become prevalent and efficient enough to affect mortality due to cerebral haemorrhage in the general population, at least in some regions.

Table 6. *Cerebral haemorrhage in autopsies at Sahlgren's hospital*

Cerebral haemorrhage		1948 + 1949	1960 + 1961
Number of cases	patients < 65 years of age	57	47
Number of autopsies . . .		1,566	2,806
Percentage of all autopsies		3.4	1.7
Percentage of cerebral haemorrhage — all ages		48	32

Table 7. *Analysis of patients dying of cerebral haemorrhage in 1960 and 1961. Age 65 and below*

	Total number	Hypertensive disease not known	Hypertensive disease known			
			No.	Active treatment		
				Definitely tried	Not known	Not tried
Males . . .	23	13	10	1	1	8
Females . .	27	6	19	2	10	7
Total . . .	50	19	29	3	11	15

As early as 1951 and 1952 two things had become absolutely clear: firstly, that it was possible to effect a dramatic improvement and even normalise the blood pressure and clinical manifestations in malignant hypertension; secondly, that severe cerebrovascular and coronary disease as well as renal impairment, if advanced, were obstacles which effectively blocked further progress. We then thought, as we still do, that the interrelations between atherosclerosis and hypertension as well as between chronic kidney disease and hypertension should be regarded as being the most important from the practical clinical standpoint of keeping more people in better health. The obvious advantages to be derived from a fuller understanding of the basic mechanisms governing hypertension, from pharmacological advances in the field of antihypertensive drugs, and from more efficient dissemination of the technical knowledge relevant to treatment, tremendously important as they are, would then take second place from the clinician's point of view.

In relation to the treatment of hypertensive disease, a more aggressive approach should be adopted towards other recognisable high-risk factors in coronary disease. Likewise, modern concepts of nephrology should be more consistently put into practice.

Summary

1. Survival and mortality have been analysed in the first 1,000 patients with hypertensive disease who began to receive active treatment between 1950 and 1959. The backbone of the treatment has been a successive combination of ganglionic blockers, guanethidine, and bethanidine with hydralazine. Reserpine has played a minor transitory role and thiazides a larger and continuous role as additional drugs.

2. Regardless of the classification system used, there was an over-all progressive improvement in the five-year survival figures for groups starting treatment in the early, middle, and late fifties. The exceptions to this were the patients in Smithwick's Grade IV, in whose case the striking increase in survival from the early fifties could not be further improved upon.

3. The percentage five-year mortality in congestive heart failure, cerebrovascular lesions, and uraemia decreased successively, while the five-year mortality in myocardial infarction remained unchanged.

4. In deaths due to uraemia, the emphasis has shifted from essential Grade IV hypertension and short duration to chronic pyelonephritis with superimposed Grade III or Grade IV hypertension with a more prolonged course.

5. In Göteborg a definite decrease in the incidence of massive cerebral haemorrhage (verified by autopsy) in age groups below 75 years was evident when the two-year period 1960/61 was compared with the period 1948/49.

6. Our main conclusion is that, although technical improvements in drugs and their use will continue to improve results, the major break-throughs in the future must involve simultaneous tackling of other recognisable high-risk factors in coronary disease. In uraemia, the early detection of a moderate decrease in filtration as well as the elimination of analgesic abuse seem promising as lines of approach.

Zusammenfassung

1. Überlebensrate und Sterblichkeit werden für die ersten 1000 Patienten mit Hochdruck analysiert, bei denen während der Jahre 1950 bis 1959 eine aktive medikamentöse Behandlung begonnen wurde. Die Grundlage der Behandlung war eine aufeinanderfolgende Kombination von Ganglienblockern, Guanethidin und Bethanidin mit Hydralazin. Reserpin hat lediglich eine geringe und nur vorübergehende Rolle gespielt, die Thiazide waren dagegen als zusätzliche Präparate von größerer und anhaltender Bedeutung.

2. Ungeachtet der verwendeten Einteilung der Hypertension ergab sich insgesamt eine fortschreitende Verbesserung in der Fünfjahresüberlebensrate für die Gruppen, welche die Behandlung zu Beginn, in der Mitte oder gegen Ende der Periode von 1950 bis 1959 begannen. Ausnahmen davon waren die Patienten mit schweren Augenhintergrundsveränderungen (Grad IV), bei denen die bemerkenswerte Verbesserung der Überlebensrate, die in der frühen Behandlungsgruppe erreicht wurde, später nicht weiter gesteigert werden konnte.

3. Die prozentuale Fünfjahresmortalität an Herzinsuffizienz, cerebrovaskulären Störungen und Urämie nahm nach und nach ab, während die Fünfjahresmortalität infolge Herzinfarkt unverändert blieb.

4. Bei den Todesfällen infolge Urämie verschob sich das Gewicht von der essentiellen Hypertonie Grad IV von kurzer Dauer zur chronischen Pyelonephritis mit aufgepfropftem Hochdruck Grad III oder IV von langer Dauer.

5. In Göteborg fand sich bei einem Vergleich der Zweijahresperiode 1960/61 mit derjenigen von 1948/49 eine deutliche Abnahme der Häufigkeit massiver zerebraler Blutungen (kontrolliert durch Sektionen) in der Altersgruppe unter 75 Jahren.

6. Die wesentliche Schlußfolgerung ist, daß — wenn auch Verbesserungen der Pharmaka und ihrer Anwendung zu noch günstigeren Resultaten führen mögen — entscheidende künftige Fortschritte gleichzeitig auch andere erkennbare hohe Risikofaktoren bei der Erkrankung der Koronarien einbeziehen müssen. Bei der Urämie dürfte die frühzeitige Erkennung einer mäßigen Abnahme des Filtrates ebenso wie die Ausschaltung des Mißbrauches von Analgetika Aussicht auf Erfolg versprechen.

Résumé

1. On présente une analyse des taux de mortalité et de survie chez 1.000 hypertendus ayant commencé à être traités entre 1950 et 1959. La base du traitement a été une association, successivement: de ganglioplégiques, de guanéthidine, de béthanidine, à l'hydralazine. Quant aux traitements complémentaires, la réserpine n'a joué qu'un rôle secondaire et transitoire, tandis que les thiazides ont été plus largement utilisés et de façon plus soutenue.

2. Si l'on fait abstraction du système de classification utilisé, on a observé dans l'ensemble une amélioration successive des chiffres de survie de cinq ans dans les trois groupes ayant commencé le traitement soit au début, soit dans le milieu, soit vers la fin de cette période 1950/59. Firent exception les malades au stade IV de Smithwick, chez qui l'importante amélioration de la survie obtenue dans le début de cette période n'a pu s'accentuer par la suite.

3. Le pourcentage de mortalité dans les cinq ans par défaillance cardiaque, affections vasculaires cérébrales, urémie a successivement diminué, tandis que la mortalité dans les cinq ans par infarctus du myocarde est restée inchangée.

4. Quant aux décès par urémie, leur maximum de fréquence s'est déplacé de l'hypertension essentielle stade IV et de courte durée à la pyélonéphrite chronique hypertensive stade III ou IV d'évolution plus prolongée.

5. On a constaté de façon évidente à Göteborg, par comparaison entre la période de deux ans 1960/61 et la période 1948/49, une diminution de la fréquence de l'hémorragie cérébrale massive (vérifiée par autopsie) dans les groupes au dessous de 75 ans d'âge.

6. Notre conclusion essentielle est que si les progrès techniques dans les médicaments et leur maniement continueront à améliorer les résultats, les efforts essentiels devront comprendre également à l'avenir la mise en oeuvre des moyens de détection des facteurs de haut risque dans les maladies coronariennes. Dans l'urémie le dépistage précoce d'une faible diminution de la filtration ainsi que la suppression de l'abus des analgésiques semblent ouvrir des débouchés prometteurs.

References

HAMMARSTRÖM, S., and P. BECHGAARD: Amer. J. Med. 8, 53 (1950). — KEITH, N. M., H. P. WAGENER, and N. W. BARKER: Amer. J. Med. Sc. **197**, 332 (1939). — PALMER, R. S., D. LOOFBOUROW, and C. R. DOERING: N. England J. Med. **239**, 990 (1948). — SCHROEDER, H. A., and H. M. PERRY, Jr.: In: Essential Hypertension. An International Symposium. Ed. by K. D. BOCK and P. T. COTTIER. Springer, Berlin, 1960, p. 307. — SMITHWICK, R. H., and J. E. THOMPSON: J. Amer. Med. Ass. **152**, 1501 (1953).

Discussion

PUDDU: There is no doubt that in recent years useful new drugs have been developed with which hypertension can be combated, nor that we have obtained factual evidence of a favourable modification in the long-term evolution of many cases rationally treated. I should like to make a few comments on the criteria of evaluation of long-term treatment.

When we compare the fates of treated and untreated cases, we consider groups of patients that are as homogeneous as possible. In this respect we take into account pressure values, age, sex, and grade of abnormalities of eyeground, kidney, and heart; but very often we disregard heredity. Now heredity is a tremendously important factor as far as resistance to disease is concerned — not only to the development of the disease, but also to its evolution. Very often, we see cases of hypertension that are comparable in every respect, except as regards inheritance, but show a very different pattern of behaviour over the years.

The fate of the hypertensive patient is dominated by complications — renal, cerebral, and cardiac complications. Besides hypertension *per se*, many other factors, such as atherosclerosis, metabolic disorders, etc., are involved in the development of these complications. These associated diseases — above all metabolic disorders — are very sensitive to changes in nutritional habits, physical activity, body weight, etc. How is the influence of these factors taken into account in the evaluation of the natural history of hypertension and in the comparison between treated and untreated population groups?

Finally, I should like to hear the views of this distinguished gathering on the problem of stress and hypertension. As perhaps Dr. HOOD and Dr. HUMERFELT remember, during our Bucharest meeting last March, Dr. MYASNIKOV spoke at length on the question of stress as a factor in hypertension and on the importance of relaxation in the treatment of the disease. Our Eastern European colleagues frequently publish the good results they have obtained in their special relaxation clinics or spas. If I remember correctly, we were a little sceptical about the degree of importance that Dr. MYASNIKOV attached to this factor. However, I should be very pleased to hear the opinions of this group.

HOOD: I should only like to say that if you eliminate stress in a person — which presumably was done if he or she were treated for a while in hospital in the days when no active drugs were available — and plot his long-term records, you see all that can be achieved by a nice spell in hospital that brings the pressure down to normal values. If you have a good, complete follow-up, the small indentations do not appear in the general pressure curve. You have, let's say, four periods of one month or six weeks each, during which pressure drops to near normal values; but within a few weeks it has risen again, and this does not do very much towards achieving long-term control of the pressure throughout the year.

REUBI: That is certainly true, and I believe every one of us can confirm this statement.

PICKERING: I think that all the papers this afternoon have been faced with the difficult problem of trying to make like patients like and unlike unlike — in other words, classification — and of getting a series of values which you can measure. I believe Dr. PUDDU is quite right to mention that many factors that are very difficult to measure are probably involved. Inheritance is one. I don't quite know what is meant by stress, because so many people use the term in different ways, but I do know that people experience very different degrees of unhappiness and frustration, and various kinds of situation that concern the mind and cause pleasure or displeasure. I think that SMIRK's attempt to get reproducible pressures by using what he calls basal pressure is a step in the right direction. I have always had some difficulties with this. The first is that some basal pressures are more basal than others. ADDIS I think it was, who first started it; he took the pressures in the early morning, just like a basal metabolic rate. I think SMIRK's method has run to three editions since then, and I am sure edition three is very much better than edition one.

Our difficulty is that it's very hard to get the necessary personnel to do the measuring. HAMILTON et al.[1] started on hypertensive patients in our St. Mary's family studies. But going into a London hospital at half past five in the morning isn't the thing that you want to do very often. I had Dr. RICHARDSON working with me in Oxford on this sleep business. Americans, as you know, are absolute gluttons for punishment, and one would have thought that RICHARDSON would have hurried off to be there early in the morning to measure the blood pressures under basal conditions in our patients, but instead he took the easy way and chose Mark I of the SMIRK basal pressures — the one which SMIRK, quite rightly, says wasn't the best. In other words, I think basal pressure is fine if you have got the drive and the personnel to do it, as SMIRK has; I never have had, and so I have never used it.

I think perhaps the casual pressure is a little bit underrated; I find it is quite useful, and all the studies have shown that it bears a relationship to the causal and consequential factors in hypertension. I am not sure that the supplemental pressure is of any value. As far as I know, SMIRK invented it and SMIRK has now castigated it. I should never have suspected that it would be much good, because it is of course the effect of the circumstances in which the casual is taken. I know, for example, that if I have an out-patient sent to me with some questions about blood pressure, I am worth about 30 mm. Hg as compared with one of my assistants, so that a large quota of the supplemental pressure has nothing to do with the patient.

Then about the retinal changes: — I think the Keith-Wagener classification was outmoded when they produced it. They hadn't read FOSTER MOORE's[2] paper on the different retinal appearances of what subsequently have become the benign and malignant phases. There are two kinds of exudate in hypertension; the large woolly ones mean one thing, the sharply defined ones mean another. And so Grade III comprises two conditions of totally different prognosis. Grades I and II are absolutely useless. One of the striking things is the way in which one's students or one's house-officers will tell one that the patient has Grade I or II. If the pressure is elevated, they imagine the rest.

---

[1] HAMILTON, M., G. W. PICKERING, J. A. F. ROBERTS, and G. S. C. SOWRY: Clin. Sc. **13**, 11 (1954).

[2] MOORE, R. F.: Quart. J. Med. **10**, 29 (1917).

Now Dr. Freis had three entries on his card; one was segmental spasm, which Dollery clearly showed us was a figment of the imagination. Another one was copper wire. I have never been able to see this in the retina. I have looked at copper wire a lot of times, but I have never seen a retinal artery that looks like copper wire. The third was silver wire. I have an eminent opponent in affairs of hypertension, and I used to examine with him. His views about silver wire were quite different from mine. I have the same difficulty with my interns. I say to them: "If I sent you out for some silver wire and you brought me back something like this, I should never send you out to shop for me again." — So I am very doubtful whether some of these small changes in retinal arteries are anything more than subjective judgements. I doubt whether they are very helpful in determining the goodness or badness of the patient's prognosis.

Brod: My first question concerns Dr. Smirk's paper. He was one of the members at the meeting of experts in Geneva which proposed a new W. H. O. classification of hypertension; it was also suggested at this meeting that studies which would determine the prognosis of Stage I as defined at that W. H. O. meeting would be useful. I wonder whether Dr. Smirk has any data in this respect, because the patients he discussed were obviously already out of Stage I, as defined in Geneva, since this stage involves no retinal changes at all and certainly no angina pectoris, etc. Are these patients going to develop anything serious, and are we doing them any good with our treatment or not? This is not only a medical, but also an economic and social problem.

My second question is addressed to Dr. Hood. I should like to know whether all his patients with chronic pyelonephritis were patients diagnosed at *post mortem*. How many of these patients were recognised *in vivo*? How many of them were adequately treated? Our own impression is that patients with pyelonephritis are the best ones from the point of view of treatment, and you can, even if they are far progressed, maintain their residual renal function if you keep the urinary infection under control.

Wilson: I should like to emphasise this question of the classification of hypertension which was agreed upon in Geneva. In the natural history of essential hypertension, there are patients with high blood pressure but without any evidence of cardiovascular hypertrophy. We then have the group with evidence of cardiovascular hypertrophy but without any evidence of arterial degeneration, and, finally, the group with vascular disease. There are various criteria on the basis of which these three grades can be fairly well separated. Such a separation is important, not only from the point of view of the natural history of hypertension in the same patient, but also because we may be dealing with different disorders. A classification which is based on already existent vascular damage omits two of the most common forms of hypertension. From the therapeutic point of view we need to know whether it is possible to prevent patients in Grade I from developing cardiovascular hypertrophy and patients in Grade II from developing vascular degeneration. In the terminology used by Dr. Smirk, does the patient who has a normal basal pressure but a high supplemental pressure pass into the grade with a high basal pressure? This is a more realistic classification (since it is based on the natural history of the disease) than one which is based on eyeground changes, which, apart from papilloedema, have a very uncertain prognostic value.

Freis: I agree with Dr. Pickering on the retinal grading. We have some participants who send in a great number of positive reports of silver wire and others who send in none. I am sure that we shall find many criteria in our study that are absolutely useless. But still I think it's probably valuable to gather them to see which ones are helpful and which ones are not. I am sure that both silver-wire appearance and segmental spasm can occur, although they are admittedly rare.

SMIRK: I was very much in agreement, I think, with pretty well everything that Dr. PICKERING just said. So far as retinal Grades I and II are concerned, we lump them together for the reason that we have found variations in the assigning of these grades by our clinic doctors, and even a shift over the years affecting the clinic as a whole. We can recognise something that is clearly more advanced than what has usually been called Grade I, but the border line between Grades I and II is most indefinite.

There was not enough time to mention other things which concern the prognosis of hypertension; for example, we are not concerned only with the blood pressure, but also with the susceptibility of the individual to the blood pressure. We see that there is a big difference between people in Japan and people in the United States as regards the occurrence of disabilities secondary to hypertension. Differences between males and females in the capacity to tolerate hypertension are well known.

I was asked about patients in whom the various disabilities that we referred to (stroke, heart failure, renal excretory defect, coronary artery disease) were not found. I have further subdivided this group into patients who, when they presented, had some cardiac impairment, such as breathlessness, heart enlargement, or some electrocardiographic defect, and those who had none of these. The mortality among patients with breathlessness or some such cardiac manifestation was appreciably higher than among those who were altogether free from such disorders. In the last group, which was the mildest one, none out of 32 females died among the treated, and six out of 49 females died among the untreated. They all had basal diastolic pressures of 90 mm. Hg or more. Of the males, four out of 16 died among the treated, and four out of 24 among the untreated. The results are similar if we study all persons with basal systolic pressures of 140 mm. Hg or more.

Regarding basal blood pressure, I agree that some are more basal than others. If you take a series of four to six basal blood pressures in the same person, as KILPATRICK[1] did, and if you make it a laboratory investigation, then you arrive at something more closely approaching the lowest sleeping pressures. Basal pressures — even the basal systolic pressures — usually behave consistently when measured repeatedly[2]. Fig. 1, showing the basal pressure measurements repeated during a five-year period in patients who were receiving little or no treatment, indicates that the figures are pretty consistent.

The first basal blood pressure is shown on the abscissa and the second, taken in the same individual within five years, on the ordinate. Points lying above the line drawn at 45° represent rises, those below falls in the basal blood pressure. There are few large changes. If you do the same for the supplemental systolic pressures (Fig. 2), they are all over the place. Within five years the casual blood-pressure variations are usually due mainly to variations in the supplemental pressure.

If, however, we repeat measurements of the basal systolic pressure in untreated persons who have survived for between five and 16 years, it will be seen that there has usually been a rise in the basal blood pressure (Fig. 3).

---

[1] KILPATRICK, J. A.: Brit. Heart J. **10**, 48 (1948).

[2] SIMPSON, F. O., and F. H. SMIRK: unpublished.

All these persons had high casual blood pressures, so that those starting with low basal systolic blood pressures had high supplemental pressures.

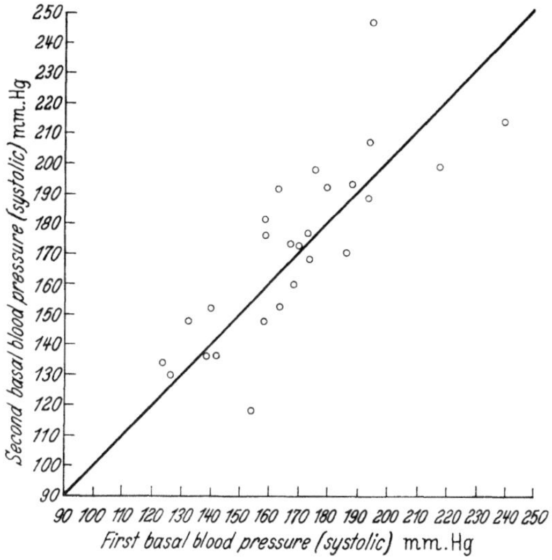

Fig. 1. Measurements of basal blood pressure in untreated patients, repeated within five years.

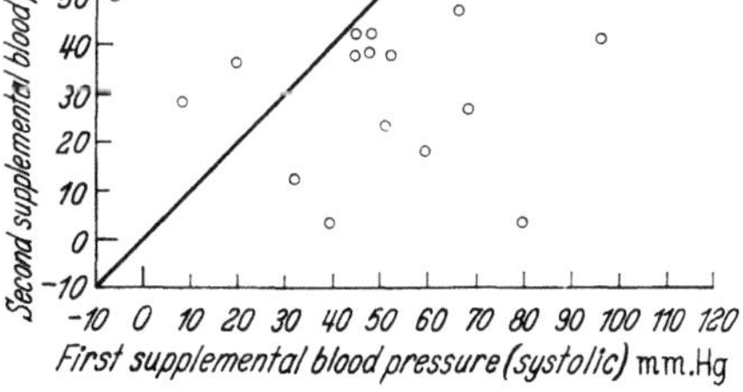

Fig. 2. Measurements of supplemental blood pressure in untreated patients, repeated within five years.

Now the question of whether supplemental pressures which are frequently high lead on to high basal pressures after some long period of time is a subject we are investigating.

The patients studied were not treated, either because of a comparatively low basal blood pressure or because treatment was declined. They are also a selected group, for they do not include persons who later returned and were treated. Within five years, 15 showed some rise and 11 some fall in basal systolic pressure; only five falls, but nine rises, exceeded 10 mm. Hg. The patients in whom measurement of the basal blood pressure was repeated after five to 16 years did not include any with initial basal systolic pressures above 190 mm. Hg and only two with levels above 170 mm. Hg, almost

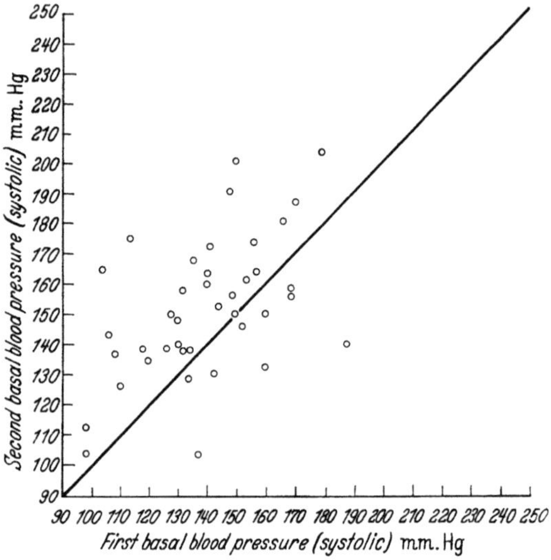

Fig. 3. Measurements of basal blood pressure in untreated patients, repeated after five to 16 years.

certainly because few would have survived the first five years[1]. Nine basal systolic pressures had fallen, 30 had risen. Five falls and 22 rises in pressure were in excess of 10 mm. Hg systolic. In a follow-up study of this duration, there is reason to believe that rapid rises in the basal pressure to high levels will be underestimated, as death abstracts most such patients from a follow-up study.

Hood: I disagree emphatically with Dr. Pickering about eyegrounds. When we, 25 years after Keith et al.[2], put together material showing the same degrees of hypertension as theirs, we got exactly the same 99% mortality within five years in those not actively treated. Grade III is still very serious if you understand by Grade III patients who have cotton-wool exudates and not simply those with only hyaline exudates. As regards the low grades, I lumped them together into one single group, as Smirk has been doing, but I think it is still possible for a good ophthalmologist,

[1] Smirk, F. H.: N. Zealand Med. J. **63**, 413 (1964).

[2] Keith, N. M., H. P. Wagener, and N. W. Barker: Amer. J. Med. Sc. **197**, 332 (1939).

without knowing whether hypertension is present or not, to single out practically every patient who has got hypertension as measured by the internist afterwards. The signs are undoubtedly there for those who have eyes to see them, though they may perhaps be rather hazy for the average internist.

As to Dr. Brod's question, the chronic pyelonephritis cases dying, which I referred to, were all confirmed at autopsy. All of them received first-class treatment; they were in the hands of experts. How big a material did they come from? As I said, the condition for being included in this material was that they should present with hypertension as the dominant feature from the outset. They have, in other words, been taken from a much bigger group of chronic pyelonephritis patients who were normotensive or very mildly hypertensive at the outset, with hypertension appearing as a late phenomenon. These were not included. The number of pyelonephritic cases involved in this study was about 70, which makes about 50 survivors at the present time.

The present status of symptomatic surgical treatment for arterial hypertension

By

P. Tcherdakoff, J. Vaysse, M. Lacombe, P. Oudea, J. Mourad, F. Tarrette, and P. Milliez

As progress continues to be made in the medicinal treatment of hypertension, there are two main questions which arise with regard to surgical therapy: firstly, how effective is such therapy and, secondly, what role is it still capable of playing in the management of hypertension? It is these two questions which we shall now attempt to answer in the light of our own experience.

Interventions confined to the adrenals only

Since we have not had any personal experience of this type of surgical intervention, we shall merely summarise the data given by authors who have employed it.

The oldest form of symptomatic surgical treatment for arterial hypertension is subtotal adrenalectomy, in which the adrenal is completely removed on one side, together with all but 10 to 15% of the adrenocortical tissue on the other side. This type of operation has now been abandoned. The most recent paper devoted to it is that of Wolferth et al. (*20*), which appeared in 1953 and refers to 12 cases. The findings in nine of the patients, who were followed up over a period of 11 to 20 years, were as follows:

Assessed in terms of the effect on the blood pressure, there were four complete failures, two moderately successful responses, and three cases in which the pressure reverted to normal. The blood pressure does not decline unless the operation results in adrenal insufficiency; in cases where adrenal insufficiency is achieved, the pressure sometimes decreases and sometimes remains elevated.

Two of the patients were suffering from cardiac insufficiency prior to the operation; in both cases, the signs of heart failure disappeared after surgery, and the heart diminished in size.

Renal failure is the major contra-indication to subtotal adrenalectomy; the operation should never be performed if Van Slyke's test yields values of less than 40%, since in this case it produces little improvement in renal function.

Examination of the eyegrounds usually reveals a distinct improvement.

Referring to this same study again in 1957, WOLFERTH et al. (*21*) conclude that the operation is more likely to be successful if combined with sympathectomy.

Total bilateral adrenalectomy has only been possible since adrenal hormones suitable for substitution therapy became available. It was GREEN et al. (*6*) in 1950 who first attempted this type of intervention. The literature published since then contains references only to a few isolated cases or small groups of patients upon whom the operation was performed [HANLEY (*7*), MORSE et al. (*11*), and VAN'T HOFF (*19*)]. All the patients in question were suffering from malignant hypertension. Usually, the operation is carried out in two stages, and occasionally in one. Substitution therapy is already initiated a few days prior to the intervention; high doses are administered during the immediate postoperative period and can later be progressively reduced to a final level of 37.5–75 mg. cortisone daily. The following results have been obtained with interventions of this kind:

All authors agree that the operation does not affect the blood-pressure levels. A reduction in blood pressure can be achieved only by diminishing the doses of cortisone administered, i.e. by eliciting a state of adrenal insufficiency.

It exerts a remarkably beneficial effect on exertional dyspnoea and on signs of cardiac failure; the size of the heart also decreases.

It has far less influence on renal function, which undergoes little change. The intervention is, moreover, strictly contra-indicated in the presence of renal insufficiency. It should also be noted that any attempt to lower the dosage of corticosteroids given as replacement therapy provokes acute uraemia coupled with renal insufficiency.

Marked relief from headache is obtained, and examination of the eyegrounds reveals disappearance of papilloedema.

The operation appears to have a favourable effect on the patient's life expectancy; some of the patients treated by HANLEY, although suffering from malignant hypertension, were still alive four or even five years after the operation.

It would thus seem that, although these surgical interventions confined to the adrenals produce little improvement in the blood-pressure levels, they do exert a beneficial influence on the vascular complications of malignant hypertension. They are not widely resorted to, however, because they entail substitution therapy of indefinite duration and call for rigorous surveillance of the patient.

Interventions on the splanchnic and sympathetic nerves, with or without subtotal adrenalectomy

Between 1948 and 1964, we have carried out sympathectomy – with or without subtotal adrenalectomy – on 231 of our hypertensive patients. It is upon these 231 cases that the present study is based. We propose now to examine the features presented by this group of patients prior to surgery, to describe the different types of operation performed, and, finally, to outline the immediate and long-term results obtained.

1. Cases treated

a) Age. The ages of the 231 patients were as follows:

Under 20 years	6
20—29 years	26
30—39 years	77
40—49 years	99
50—59 years	22
60 years and over	1

From the above list it will be seen that the majority were between the ages of 30 and 49 years.

b) Sex. The proportion of males and females was almost identical, i.e.:

Women	116
Men	115

c) Lapse of time between the diagnosis of hypertension and the date of the operation.

Less than 5 years	91
5— 9 years	67
10—14 years	45
15—19 years	18
20 years and over	6
Impossible to determine	4

These figures purporting to show the duration of the hypertension have very little significance. Many of the patients did not realise that they were suffering from hypertension until the symptoms of the disease finally induced them to consult a doctor; in such cases, the disease may well already have been present for years without giving rise to any symptoms. On the other hand, since 1949, thanks to the introduction in France of systematic medical examinations undertaken by the *Médecine du Travail* and to the fact that doctors have become increasingly aware of the dangers of hypertensive disease, more and more cases of incipient hypertension are now being discovered. However, the fact that the working population consists predominantly of males means that latent hypertension tends to be diagnosed more frequently in men than in women.

Once again, then, it should be pointed out that figures for the duration of hypertensive disease in a patient must be regarded with extreme scepticism.

d) Complications recorded in the patients' case histories. Complications from which the patients had already suffered at some time prior to surgery were as follows:

Regressive hemiplegia and meningeal haemorrhages	60
Amaurosis	11
Retinal haemorrhages	5
Scotomas	5
Acute pulmonary oedema	16
Congestive heart failure	5
Coronary accidents	3

There was thus quite a high incidence of prior complications in our group of patients, particularly since in some instances more than one of the complications listed had occurred in one and the same patient.

e) Blood-pressure levels prior to surgery (in mm. Hg).

Systolic	
Below 180	10
180—200	48
Above 200	172
Unknown	1
Diastolic	
Below 100	4
100—120	70
Above 120	153
Unknown	4

Most of the patients had very high blood pressure. Those who were operated upon although their blood pressure was only moderately elevated either had already suffered from repeated complications or comprised cases in which serious disorders affecting the viscera had developed; a few of them were women who had repeatedly aborted and were desirous of carrying a pregnancy to term.

f) Ocular findings.

Condition of the eyegrounds (according to the classification of KEITH and WAGENER)

Normal	16
Grade I	39
Grade II	62
Grade III	52
Grade IV	57
Unknown	5

Diastolic pressure in the central retinal artery (in cm. H_2O)

Below 35	2
35—60	52
61—90	83
Above 90	50
Unknown	44

Almost half the patients (109) showed signs of hypertensive retinopathy (Grades III and IV), and in a further 57, the eyeground findings were consonant with malignant hypertension. In more than half of the patients (133), the diastolic pressure in the central retinal artery was higher than 60 cm. H_2O.

g) Cardiac findings. The extent to which the hypertension had already affected the heart was assessed by reference to the electrocardiographic recordings:

Normal	55
Left ventricular hypertrophy (L.V.H.) only	123
Myocardial ischaemia only	4
L.V.H. plus left ventricular strain	27
L.V.H. plus myocardial ischaemia	9
Complete left bundle-branch block	1
Unknown	12

In roughly two thirds of the cases (164), the hypertension had already exerted deleterious effects on the heart.

h) Renal findings. In most of our patients, a thorough study of renal function was carried out prior to surgery, the state of renal function being assessed on the basis of the results yielded by Van Slyke's test. Among the first patients upon whom we operated there were some cases in which we merely measured the blood urea concentrations. The findings obtained were as follows:

Van Slyke	
60% or higher	152
40—59%	43
Below 40%	9

Blood urea

Below 0.45 g./l.	23
0.45 g./l. or higher	1
Unknown	3

The majority of our patients showed minimal renal involvement; only in nine of them did the Van Slyke test yield a figure of less than 40% and only in one case was the blood urea higher than normal. We shall refer to this fact later.

The studies carried out in this group of patients thus revealed that the vast majority were suffering from severe hypertension, as confirmed by their very high, fixed blood-pressure levels, by the occurrence of grave complications in their case histories, or by marked signs of cardiac or ocular involvement. On the evidence of papilloedema alone, 57 out of the total of 231 can be considered as cases of malignant hypertension.

2. Type of operation performed

During the first few years of the period covered by this study, i.e. between 1948 and 1954, we carried out thoracolumbar sympathectomy of the SMITHWICK type (from T 8–9 to L 3), together with splanchnicectomy, in 26 patients. The operation was undertaken in two stages, the interval between the first and second stage being at least one month, but usually three months; occasionally, i.e. where the patient had failed to report back at the proper time, the interval was anything up to two years.

From 1954 onwards, this type of intervention was combined with bilateral adrenalectomy – total on the one side and subtotal (removal of all but about 10% of adrenal tissue) on the other. The number of patients subjected to this procedure was 173.

To these two groups of cases must be added a further 10 patients who underwent only the first stage of the operation and died before the second could be performed.

Finally, it should be mentioned that one of us (J. VAYSSE) has recently perfected a single-stage surgical method comprising subtotal adrenalectomy, bilateral splanchnicectomy, and bilateral sympathectomy which – involving as it does a more limited segment (from T 12 to L 3) – renders thoracotomy unnecessary; 21 patients have been operated on in this way.

In one of our cases we have been unable to trace the records of the operation and cannot therefore specify precisely which type of intervention was carried out.

3. Results

a) Complications and deaths attributable to surgery. Included in this category are all accidents and deaths occurring within one month of the operation. Table 1 lists the nature and incidence of the postoperative complications encountered. The total of 68 complications involved 54 out of 134 patients (from the over-all total of 231 patients covered by this study, one must subtract 21 operational deaths, which will be discussed later, as well as 76 patients about whose immediate postoperative course we have no information). The high incidence of complications reflects the fact that the operation is a serious one; when considering the cause of these accidents, there are three main points to be borne in mind:

Table 1. *Complications following symptomatic surgical treatment for hypertension. The total of 68 complications involved 54 out of 134 patients*

Regressive hyperazotaemia	6
Urinary-tract infections	21
Incontinence of urine	1
Regressive circulatory collapse	6
Acute pulmonary oedema	1
Cardiac arrhythmia	1
Congestive heart failure	1
Acute ischaemia of the lower extremities	1
Regressive hemiplegia	2
Epileptic crisis	1
Status lacunaris	1
Phlebitis of the legs	7
Pulmonary embolism	5
Pleural effusions	6
Haemothorax	1
Acute pulmonary focus	1
Retroperitoneal haematoma	1
Haematoma of the psoas muscle	1
Acute renal insufficiency	4
Total	68

Certain of the complications, such as phlebitis or pulmonary embolism, are of a type liable to occur as a sequel to any operation.

Others, such as renal, cardiac, or neurological accidents, can be ascribed to the hypertensive disease itself, for — as we have seen — the majority of the patients were suffering from severe arterial hypertension. Incidentally, it is also interesting to note the comparative frequency of postoperative urinary-tract infections.

These infections can presumably be accounted for by reference to the surgical technique employed. The cases of collapse resulted from the sympathectomy and adrenalectomy. Pleural effusions occurred only among cases in which thoracotomy had been carried out. Acute adrenal insufficiency was obviously due to the adrenalectomy and should be prevented by systematic administration of corticosteroids before, during, and after the operation.

The mortality worked out at 9.9%, i.e. 21 deaths among 231 patients; of these 21 patients, ten died after the first stage of the operation and the remaining 11 after having undergone a bilateral intervention. The causes of death were as follows:

Cardiac arrest during the operation	1
Irreversible collapse	2
Myocardial infarction	1
Uraemic coma	3
Cerebrovascular accident	3
Retroperitoneal haemorrhage	3
Acute adrenal insufficiency	1
Pulmonary embolism	2
Delirium tremens	1
Cause of death unknown	4

Apart from the case of delirium tremens, the same remarks apply to the causes of death as to those of the reversible complications:

Embolism is a risk inherent in any form of surgery.

The cardiac, renal, and cerebral accidents are a consequence of the hypertensive disease.

Retroperitoneal haematomas are a hazard peculiar to this type of surgery.

The case of acute adrenal insufficiency calls for a few comments: the patient in question died after the first stage of the operation, which had consisted of subtotal adrenalectomy; the subsequent autopsy revealed congenital absence of the contralateral adrenal. It was our ignorance of this anomaly which caused the accident, since systematic administration of corticosteroids was not undertaken at the time of the first stage of the operation, because it was naturally assumed that the patient still had an intact contralateral adrenal.

Does the type of operation performed have any bearing on the mortality? The 11 deaths occurring as a sequel to bilateral surgery took place in two of the following three groups:

Sympathectomy without adrenalectomy	0 deaths among 26 patients
Sympathectomy with adrenalectomy performed in two stages	9 deaths among 173 patients (5.2%)
Sympathectomy with adrenalectomy performed in a single operation	2 deaths among 21 patients (9.5%)

The size of the three groups is, in fact, too disparate to permit of any conclusions in this connection.

Does the severity of the hypertension play any role? Leaving aside the patient who died in delirium tremens after the operation, an impression of the gravity of the hypertension in the patients who died can be gained from Table 2. It will be seen that all but a few of the fatalities occurred among patients suffering from very severe forms of hypertension. It is precisely in such cases that surgery is most frequently indicated, and one must therefore reckon with a fairly high mortality rate.

Table 2. *Data showing the severity of hypertensive disease in 20 patients who failed to survive symptomatic surgical treatment*

Blood pressure	
Systolic (mm. Hg)	
Below 180	1
180—200	1
Above 200	18
Diastolic (mm. Hg)	
Below 100	1
100—120	2
Above 120	17
Eyeground findings	
Normal	1
Grade I	1
Grade II	8
Grade III	1
Grade IV	8
Unknown	1
Pressure in the central retinal artery (cm. H_2O)	
Below 35	0
35—60	1
61—90	5
Above 90	8
Unknown	6
Electrocardiographic findings	
Normal	2
Left ventricular hypertrophy (L.V.H.)	12
L.V.H. plus left ventricular strain	2
L.V.H. plus ischaemia	2
Unknown	2
Van Slyke	
60% or higher	14
40—59%	1
Below 40%	1
Blood urea less than 0.45 g./l.	4

b) Survival rates and later deaths. Apart from the 21 deaths occurring immediately after surgery and the 31 patients who could not be traced, the time elapsing between the operation and the date of the surviving patients' last consultation is as follows:

Between 6 and 12 months	30
1—5 years	84
6—10 years	34
11—15 years	16
Over 15 years	1

The number of later deaths, i.e. deaths not attributable to surgery itself, is 14, and the causes are as follows:

Renal insufficiency, with or without anuria	4
Myocardial infarction	1
Acute pulmonary oedema	1
Cardiac insufficiency	1
Cerebrovascular accident	1
Cerebral oedema	1
Perforated peptic ulcer	1
Ruptured arterial aneurysm	1
Cause of death unknown	3

Of the 11 deaths in which the cause was known, nine were due to an accident attributable to the hypertensive disease.

c) Effect of surgery on the hypertensive disease.

α) *Effect on the blood pressure.* Apart from the 29 patients who died following the operation or whose postoperative blood-pressure readings are not known, the postoperative blood-pressure levels (in mm. Hg) were as follows:

Systolic	
145 or below	134
Above 145	68
Diastolic	
95 or below	128
Above 95	70
Unknown	4

Assuming that a decrease in diastolic pressure of 20 mm. Hg or more can be regarded as constituting an improvement, the results obtained were as follows:

Improvement	167
No improvement	31
Died, or blood pressure unknown	33

At first sight these figures would appear to be highly encouraging; unfortunately, however, they present far too optimistic a picture. What frequently happens is that in due course the blood pressure rises again, rather than showing any further decrease. One has to wait 6—12 months before one can make any final assessment of the success of the operation as regards the blood-pressure levels; after this period, the blood pressure seems to become stable. Comparing the immediate postoperative blood-pressure recordings with those measured at the patient's last consultation, the findings are as follows:

No subsequent rise in B.P.	84
Subsequent rise in B.P.	52
Subsequent fall in B.P.	6
Doubtful (rise less than 20 mm. Hg diastolic)	23

The same pattern is reflected particularly clearly in the percentages showing systolic and diastolic pressures before, immediately

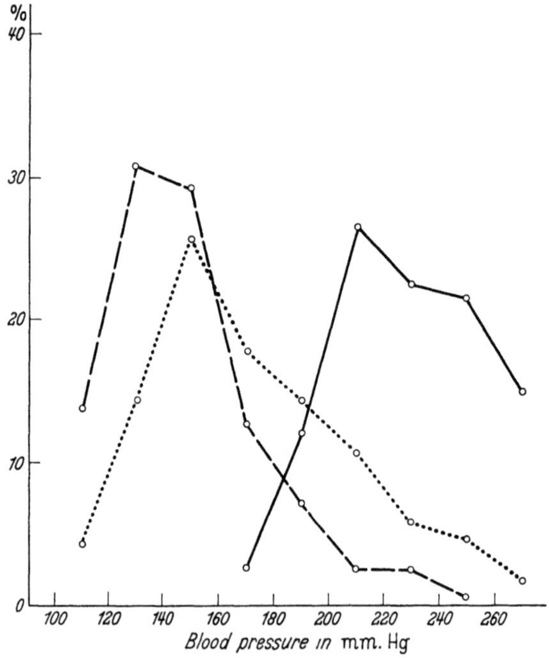

Fig. 1. Systolic blood-pressure levels recorded before (———), immediately after (– – –), and one year or more after (· · · · · ·) symptomatic surgical treatment in 165 hypertensive patients.

after, and one year or more after surgery (Figs 1 and 2). Here it can be seen that the distribution curve for the blood-pressure levels shifts sharply to the left (i.e. towards the lower levels) immediately after the operation, but subsequently swings back towards the right, the curve for the pressures recorded one year or more after surgery being situated between that of the preoperative and immediate postoperative blood-pressure recordings.

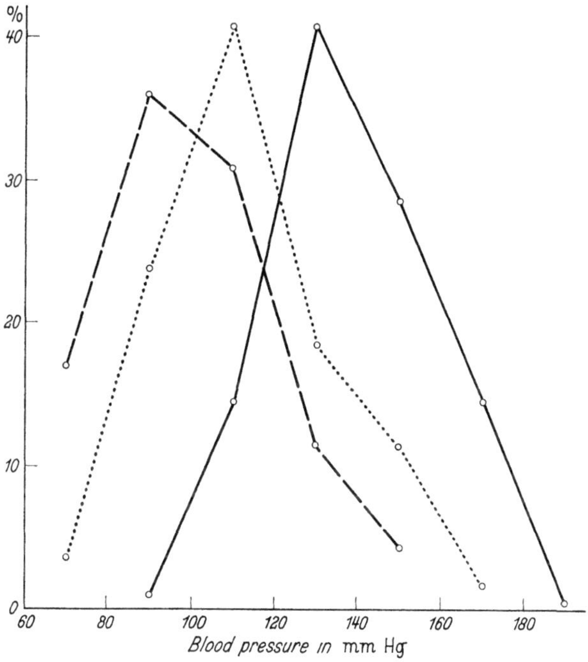

Fig. 2. Diastolic blood-pressure levels recorded before (———), immediately after (– – – –), and one year or more after (· · · · ·) symptomatic surgical treatment in 165 hypertensive patients.

Of the total of 231 patients, 66 either died or were lost trace of; when the blood pressure of the remaining 165 was measured after a due lapse of time following the operation, 46 (27.9%) still had diastolic levels of 95 mm. Hg or below.

Postural hypotension is frequently encountered immediately after surgery. A certain prognostic value is sometimes ascribed to this phenomenon, on the grounds that postural hypotension — even if only transitory — may be regarded as auguring well for the long-term evolution of the patients' blood pressure.

Below is a statistical analysis of the results assessed at least one year after surgery, based on the following criteria: postural hypotension = decrease in systolic and diastolic pressure of 20 mm. Hg or more; normalisation of blood pressure = decrease to at least 145 mm. Hg systolic and 95 mm. Hg diastolic; improvement = decrease in diastolic pressure of 20 mm. Hg or more.

	Postural hypotension	No postural hypotension
Cured	9 (16.3%)	7 (14%)
Improved	31 (56.3%)	25 (50%)
No improvement	15 (27.3%)	18 (36%)
Totals	55	50

From these figures it will be seen that, in cases where postural hypotension occurs postoperatively, the percentage of long-term successes is a little higher and that of the failures somewhat lower; but no reliable conclusions can be drawn from this observation.

β) *Effect of surgery on retinal lesions and blood pressure in the central retinal artery.* Since 21 patients died during the period immediately after the operation and a further 43 failed to report back or were not examined beforehand, the number in whom it was possible to examine the eyegrounds before and some time after surgery amounted to 167. The findings in these 167 cases were as follows:

Improvement	101
No improvement	57
Eyegrounds normal before and after surgery	9

Fig. 3 indicates the status of the eyegrounds in 226 cases before, and in 169 patients one year or more after, surgery.

The number of patients with Grade III and IV eyegrounds diminished greatly, i.e. from 109 to 17; but these figures should not be taken at their face value, because it is possible that many of the patients who did not have their eyes examined some time after the operation may still have had Grade III or IV eyegrounds.

Far more significant is the fact that the number of patients with normal or only slightly pathological eyegrounds (Grades 0 and I) rose from 55 to 97.

Measurement of the blood pressure in the central retinal artery, which was carried out in 120 patients before and some time after surgery, also yielded encouraging findings:

Improvement (decrease by at least 10 cm. H_2O)	77
No improvement	42
Normal before and after surgery	1

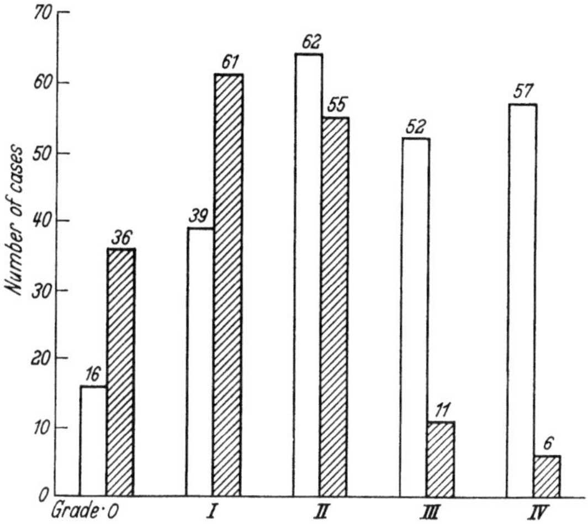

Fig. 3. Status of the eyegrounds in hypertensive patients before (□), and one year or more after (▨), symptomatic surgical treatment. Classification according to KEITH and WAGENER.

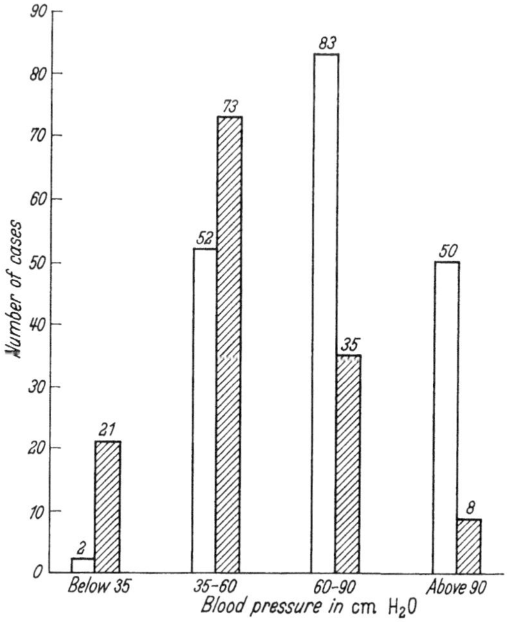

Fig. 4. Retinal arterial pressure before (□), and one year or more after (▨), symptomatic surgical treatment.

Fig. 4 shows the retinal artery pressures of 187 patients before surgery and 137 patients one year or more after surgery.

The number of patients with pressures exceeding 60 cm. H_2O diminished from 133 to 43, but the same criticism applies to these figures as to those for the Grade III and IV eyegrounds.

The number of patients with pressures of less than 60 cm. H_2O increased from 54 to 94 — a fact to which much more importance can be attached.

The effect of the operation on the retinal lesions and the pressure in the central retinal artery was thus satisfactory.

γ) *Effect of surgery on the electrocardiographic findings.* Electrocardiograms, taken before and one year or more after the operation, are available in respect of 135 cases. The picture revealed by these electrocardiograms is as follows:

Improvement	59
No improvement	35
Aggravation	10
Normal before and after surgery	31

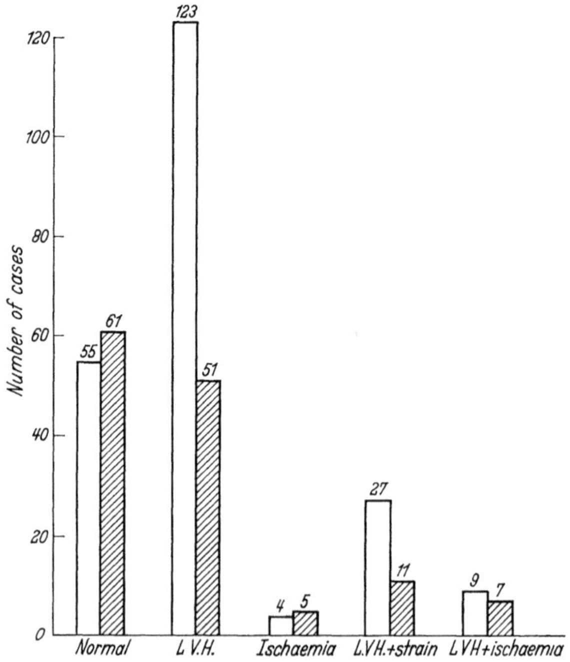

Fig. 5. Electrocardiographic findings before (□), and one year or more after (▨), symptomatic surgical treatment in hypertensive patients.

Shown in Fig. 5 are the electrocardiographic findings for 218 patients before surgery and for 135 patients one year or more after surgery. One has much more difficulty in interpreting these results than, for example, those for the eyegrounds as outlined in Fig. 3, because it is virtually impossible to quantitate the degree of left ventricular hypertrophy or, for that matter, of any other electrocardiographic anomaly. This means, for instance, that, although the electrocardiogram of a patient with left ventricular hypertrophy may reveal some improvement in response to surgery, it will still have to be included among the electrocardiograms indicating persistence of L.V.H. after the intervention. Nevertheless, the number of normal electrocardiograms rose from 55 out of 218 before surgery (25.2%) to 61 out of 135 after surgery (45.2%); but, here again, the percentages are suspect, because it is quite possible that a fair proportion of the 83 patients for whom no postoperative electrocardiograms are available may still have shown pathological E.C.G. findings after surgery. Much the same criticism applies to the figures for the pathological electrocardiograms, i.e. 163 out of 218 before surgery (74.8%), as compared to 74 out of 135 after surgery (54.8%).

δ) *Effect of surgery on renal function.* The Van Slyke test was performed in 113 cases before, and some time after, surgery. The results obtained were as follows:

Improvement	15
No improvement	34
Normal before and after surgery	29
Mild aggravation (decrease of less than 20%)	30
Severe aggravation or death from renal failure	5

The influence of surgery upon renal function thus appears to be far less favourable than in the case of the other parameters studied. The operation produced an improvement in only 15 out of 113 patients, whereas mild to severe aggravation was observed in 35 cases.

The figures yielded by the Van Slyke test in 204 patients prior to surgery and in 113 patients after surgery differ too widely to be of much significance. Before the operation, 152 out of the 204 patients (74.5%) had values exceeding 60%, and 52 (25.4%) values below 60%. After the operation, those with values above 60% totalled 76 out of 113 (67.2%), as compared with 36 (31.8%) showing values below 60%. These figures are subject to the same criticisms as already applied to the results for the eyeground and E.C.G. examinations. What is more, the number of patients with blood urea levels of over 0.45 g./l. rose from one prior to surgery to seven after the operation.

The effect of surgery on renal function was thus much less favourable than in the case of the other parameters, and may indeed even have been frankly unfavourable.

ε) Over-all results of surgery. The over-all results of surgery, assessed after at least six months following the operation, were classified according to the following criteria:

Cured:

Blood pressure reduced to 145/95 or below.

Eyegrounds of Grade 0 or I, with pressure in the central retinal artery 35 cm. H_2O or below.

Electrocardiogram normal.

Van Slyke's test 60% or more.

Improved:

Improvement in the pathological condition as revealed by one or more of the above-mentioned parameters.

Decrease in diastolic pressure of at least 20 mm. Hg as compared with pre-operative levels.

Improvement in the eyegrounds, in the central retinal artery pressure, or in the electrocardiogram, with stabilisation or improvement in renal function, despite the absence of any significant decrease in systemic blood pressure.

Failure:

No improvement in any of the above listed parameters.

Among the 133 patients in whom it was possible to study all the parameters referred to, there were 11 cases cured (8.3%), 80 improved (60.1%), and 42 failures (31.6%). These figures undoubtedly present an over-optimistic picture, because they do not include the 35 deaths occurring either immediately or some time after the operation, nor do they allow for the fact that among the other patients not included there may perhaps have been more failures than successes.

Are there any specific factors which influence the results obtained?

An analysis of the results, classified according to the type of operation employed, reveals the following:

	Operation in two stages without adrenalectomy	Operation in two stages with adrenalectomy	Operation in one stage
Cured	3	8	0
Improved.	12	56	12
Failure	8	23	11

The differences in the numbers of patients in each group are too great to permit of any valid conclusions, although the figures do appear to suggest that the one-stage operation yields poorer results.

Analysed by reference to the degree of severity of the renal arteriolar lesions as determined by biopsy prior to surgery, and graded 0—IV, the results were as follows:

	0	I	II	III	IV
Cured	0	1	3	1	1
Improved	2	4	19	18	2
Failure	0	2	10	6	0

Here, once again, no reliable conclusion can be drawn, because the number of cases involved is too small; it is nevertheless interesting to note that, even in a patient with Grade IV lesions, it is possible to achieve a cure, whereas, on the other hand, failures were encountered in patients with only Grade I lesions.

Another possibility is that the success of surgical treatment might conceivably depend on whether the patient is suffering from so-called essential hypertension or from hypertension secondary to renal disease. Analysed on this basis, the results were as follows:

	Essential hypertension	Secondary hypertension
Cured	11	0
Improved.	72	8
Failure.	41	1

Again, the figures for the patients suffering from hypertension due to renal lesions are not comparable with those for the patients with essential hypertension, because the difference in the size of the two groups is too great; but the results do at least indicate that an improvement is possible even in patients suffering from hypertension of renal origin.

To sum up – apart from the fact that operations restricted to sympathectomy plus subtotal bilateral adrenalectomy, and performed in one stage, appear to yield less satisfactory results – neither the type of operation, nor the anatomopathological stage reached by the disease, nor the cause of the hypertension seems to have any clear bearing on the postoperative course. The fact remains, however, that complete failures occurred in only one third of the total number of patients operated upon, and that two thirds of the patients were either cured or improved. The results obtained are comparable with those observed by us during the period 1949–1963 in hypertensive patients who had undergone nephrectomy (Table 3).

Table 3. *Results obtained in response to nephrectomy in patients suffering from hypertension*

No. of cases	Cured	Improved	No improvement
75	26 (35%)	23 (30%)	26 (35%)

Discussion

We propose here to confine our remarks to interventions involving the sympathetic nervous system, since operations on the adrenals alone are virtually no longer performed.

It is difficult to evaluate the over-all results of operations entailing sympathectomy and splanchnicectomy, with or without adrenalectomy, because the opinions of the various authors differ very considerably.

Regarding the effect of such surgery on the blood pressure itself, most authors [HOOBLER et al. (*8*), LEISHMAN (*10*), and NEWCOMBE et al. (*12*)] agree with our findings: in other words, a decrease in blood pressure immediately after the operation has very little significance, and to judge the final results one must wait for at least one year. According to LEISHMAN (*10*) and WOLFERTH et al. (*21*), the occurrence of postoperative postural hypotension indicates that the operation is likely to prove successful as regards the long-term effect on the patient's blood-pressure levels; NEWCOMBE et al. (*12*), on the other hand, consider that postural hypotension such as is frequently encountered during the first few weeks following surgery has little long-term prognostic value, and our own results appear to confirm this view. Assessments differ as to the long-term effects of surgery on the blood-pressure levels: EVELYN et al. (*4*) claim that the blood pressure shows a significant decrease in roughly one third of cases, and HOOBLER et al. (*8*) report similar results; BLAKEMORE et al. (*1, 2*) obtained significant improvements in 37% of patients undergoing operations without adrenalectomy, and in 55% of those cases in which the operation also included adrenalectomy; finally, among 31 patients who survived from a total of 143 operated on for malignant hypertension, PEET and ISBERG (*13*) observed significant decreases in blood pressure in 11 cases.

Our own results (improvements in 68.4% of patients) appear at first sight to be more encouraging, but it must be remembered, firstly, that they do not include those patients who died, or those who could not be traced afterwards, or those who did not receive a sufficiently thorough examination at the time of their last consultation and, secondly, that they do include patients in whom, though there was no significant reduction in blood pressure, the condition of the visceral organs nevertheless showed an improvement. Be that as it may, the fact remains that the operation does lead to a significant decrease in blood pressure in quite a considerable number of cases.

Most authors [EVELYN et al. (*4*), LEISHMAN (*10*), NEWCOMBE et al. (*12*), and WOLFERTH et al. (*20, 21*)] agree that surgery has a beneficial effect on the eyeground lesions. The papilloedema and retinopathy appear to respond more favourably than the arteriopathic lesions. According to NEWCOMBE et al. (*12*), the eyeground lesions may still show an improvement even in cases where the blood pressure rises again some time after the operation – a claim which also seems to be borne out by our own experience.

BLAKEMORE et al. (*1, 2*), PEET and ISBERG (*13*), and WOLFERTH et al. (*20, 21*) report that surgery also has a favourable influence on the accompanying cardiac disorders, and, here again, our own experience bears this out. When EVELYN et al. (*4*) compared the condition of the heart in patients who had undergone surgery with that of controls in whom the disease had evolved spontaneously, they found three cases of improvement among 50 patients operated upon, whereas in the controls significant aggravation of the cardiac lesions occurred more frequently.

The effect of surgery upon renal function is more dubious; our own results in this respect do not seem particularly encouraging. According to WOLFERTH et al. (*21*), the operation produces little improvement in renal function. BLAKEMORE et al. (*2*) report that in 74% of cases renal function either improved or showed no further deterioration, whereas in the remaining 26% it worsened. EVELYN et al. (*4*), on the other hand, noted a tendency towards improvement in the operated cases as compared with controls, but the difference is not significant. However, as we shall see later, most authors regard impaired renal function as a contra-indication to surgery.

We ourselves have not made any reliable study of the influence of surgery upon survival rates; but most advocates of symptomatic surgical treatment for hypertension have presented favourable statistics in this connection. BLAKEMORE et al. (*2*), NEWCOMBE et al. (*12*), PEET and ISBERG (*13*), SMITHWICK and his collaborators (*16, 17, 18*), and KINSEY et al. (*9*) all claim that surgery definitely prolongs the patients' survival. On the other hand, in a very careful investigation in which they studied the fates of 50 operated patients and 50 non-treated controls in whom the severity of the hypertensive disease was virtually identical, EVELYN et al. (*4*) found only a minor difference in the five-year survival rate (59% as compared with 53%); among the patients who died, there was no difference between the operated cases and the controls as regards survival time, and among those who were still alive after ten years or more, the condition of the operated patients was slightly better than that of the controls, but the difference was not significant.

From these various findings it may be concluded that symptomatic surgical treatment undoubtedly proves effective in a certain number of cases of arterial hypertension; but it is anything but easy to evaluate the results in precise terms because of the difficulty in classifying the patients [the classification attempted by SMITHWICK (*16*), although one of the most unambiguous, has been searchingly criticised by EVELYN (*4*)] and because the criteria used in assessing the degree of improvement are so many and varied.

We have already raised the question as to whether the type of operation performed has any influence on the results obtained. According to HOOBLER et al. (*8*), considerable importance attaches to the level to which sympathectomy is carried; they claim that, if one goes as far as T 6 or further, good results are achieved in 50% of cases (percentage based on a total of 54 patients), whereas if one does not go beyond T 9, the proportion of good results drops to 21% (total number of patients: 43). Although our experience of operations without thoracotomy is still limited, we also have the impression that surgery of more restricted scope does not yield such good results as in cases where the sympathectomy is carried further up the sympathetic trunk. It is possible that combination with adrenalectomy may make for improved results, but we do not have sufficient data at our disposal to be able to affirm this. In point of fact, all the various types of intervention have given roughly similar results when carried out by their respective advocates.

It is very difficult to draw a comparison between the results of symptomatic surgical treatment for hypertension and the results obtained with antihypertensive drugs. Here, once again, reports on the responses elicited with drug therapy differ appreciably: the number of patients with Grade IV eyegrounds surviving for more than six years is quoted as 26% by FARMER et al. (*5*); SMIRK (*15*) reports that 34% of his patients with eyeground lesions of similar severity survived for more than five years, while the percentage of patients surviving for longer than four years is put at 64% by PERRY and SCHROEDER (*14*); these last two authors are the only ones whose statistics indicate that medicinal therapy yields better results than surgical treatment, i.e. 64% survivals as compared with the 48% reported by SMITHWICK (*16*) for patients treated surgically. In our opinion, however, it is impossible at present to make a valid comparison between the two types of treatment, for the following reasons:

Firstly, so far as we are aware, no accurate study similar to that of EVELYN et al. (*4*) has ever been undertaken to compare the results of medication with those of surgery in matched patients.

Secondly, progress in the drug treatment of hypertension is being made at a very rapid pace. One therefore cannot possibly draw a valid comparison with conservative therapy in 1948, the year in which PEET and ISBERG (*13*) wrote their paper, and in 1963, when the paper by FARMER et al. (*5*) appeared. A broad study of patients receiving symptomatic surgical treatment for hypertension must of necessity cover quite a large number of years. This means that one is not comparing the results of surgical treatment with the same data when the study is undertaken as when it has almost been completed.

The types of patient likely to benefit from surgery are approximately the same as those specified by CHAVEZ and MENDEZ in 1949 (*3*):

Mild to moderate hypertension without complications: surgery not indicated.

Severe hypertension, but with no complications and no symptoms: this is a good indication for surgery, although the patient often refuses to undergo an operation. In fact, as the situation is at present, medicinal therapy should be tried first in such cases.

Severe hypertension which has already given rise to serious disorders of the visceral organs: here, surgery is indicated, but in certain cases medical treatment should be given a trial first.

Very severe hypertension associated with renal failure, cardiac insufficiency, or marked encephalopathy: this is stated in the literature to be a contra-indication to surgery. At the moment, however, only renal failure can be regarded as a contra-indication. Patients who have suffered cardiac or neurological accidents may well benefit from surgery, provided the accident in question occurred more than three months previously.

The reason why our own study includes cases of benign hypertension, as well as patients aged over 55 years, is that it began at a time when our experience of surgery was still limited and when the antihypertensive drugs available were, to say the least, of low efficacity. But among those cases which we feel might still benefit from surgery, we should include the following:

Cases in which systematically conducted treatment with effective drugs over a period of three to six months has proved of no avail.

Cases in which, for reasons of a psychological or social nature, medicinal therapy cannot be carried out.

Cases in which one has the impression that, owing to the rate at which the disease is progressing, the patient is in really urgent need of radical treatment; in such circumstances, an attempt at medicinal therapy may, if it proves ineffective, involve a loss of precious time, with the result that — particularly in view of the risk of rapidly worsening renal insufficiency — it may then be too late to resort to surgery.

Thus, although progress in the medicinal treatment of arterial hypertension has meant that drug therapy is now gradually encroaching upon the domain of symptomatic surgical treatment, the latter — thanks to its effectiveness and rapidity of effect — still has certain precise indications. It is possible, however, that with the development of new antihypertensive agents these indications will in the future become progressively fewer.

Summary

1) As antihypertensive drugs become more effective and as research on the aetiology of hypertension succeeds in revealing in more and more cases the curable causes underlying hypertensive disease, the field of indications for the symptomatic surgical treatment of arterial hypertension is becoming narrower.

2) Symptomatic surgical treatment is still indicated in the following cases:

a) In severe hypertension which proves refractory to antihypertensive drugs and in patients not responsive to prolonged treatment.

b) In hypertensive toxaemia of pregnancy in women who are desirous of bearing a child and who, despite systematically conducted drug therapy, are unable to carry a pregnancy to term.

Zusammenfassung

1. Die symptomatische chirurgische Behandlung des Hochdrucks verliert zunehmend ihre Berechtigung, je wirksamer die blutdrucksenkenden Präparate werden und je häufiger es den ätiologischen Forschungen gelingt, eine heilbare Ursache als Grundlage des Gefäßleidens aufzudecken.

2. Eine symptomatische chirurgische Behandlung ist noch immer bei den folgenden Fällen zweckmäßig:

a) bei schwerem Hochdruck, der sich gegenüber einer Behandlung mit drucksenkenden Mitteln als refraktär erweist, und bei Patienten, die nicht auf eine langdauernde Behandlung ansprechen.

b) bei Schwangerschaftstoxikose mit Hochdruck bei Frauen, die sich ein Kind wünschen und bei denen es trotz systematisch durchgeführter medikamentöser Behandlung nicht gelingt, die Schwangerschaft zu Ende zu führen.

Résumé

1. La chirurgie symptomatique de l'hypertension artérielle perd de ses indications à mesure que les médications hypotensives sont plus actives et que les recherches étiologiques permettent de trouver plus souvent une cause curable à l'origine de l'angiopathie.

2. La chirurgie symptomatique est encore utile:

a) dans les hypertensions artérielles graves qui ne réagissent pas aux drogues, ou chez des malades indociles au traitement continu.

b) dans les toxémies surajoutées à l'hypertension artérielle chez des femmes qui, malgré un traitement médical bien conduit, ne peuvent mener à terme les grossesses qu'elles désirent.

References

1. Blakemore, W. S., H. A. Zintel, W. A. Jeffers, A. M. Sellers, A. I. Smithwick, and M. A. Lindauer: Surgery **43**, 102 (1958). — 2. Blakemore, W. S., W. A. Jeffers, A. M. Sellers, H. D. Itskovitz, D. Y. Cooper, C. C. Wolferth, and H. A. Zintel: In: Hypertension. Recent Advances. The Second Hahnemann Symposium on Hypertensive Disease. Ed. by A. N. Brest and J. H. Moyer. Lea and Febiger, Philadelphia, 1961, p. 619. — 3. Chavez, I., and L. Mendez: Amer. Heart J. **37**, 323 (1949). — 4. Evelyn, K. A., M. M. Singh, W. P. Chapman, G. A. Perera, and H. Thaler: Amer. J. Med. **28**, 188 (1960). — 5. Farmer, R. G., R. W. Gifford, and E. A. Hines: Arch. Int. Med. **112**, 118 (1963). — 6. Green, D. M., J. N. Nelson, G. A. Dodds, and R. E. Smallery: J. Amer. Med. Ass. **144**, 439 (1950). — 7. Hanley, H. G.: Brit. J. Urol. **29**, 359 (1957). — 8. Hoobler, S. W., J. T. Manning, W. G. Paine, S. G. McClellan, P. O. Helcher, H. Renfert, Jr., M. M. Peet, and E. A. Kahn: Circulation **4**, 173 (1951). — 9. Kinsey, D., G. P. Whitelaw, R. J. Walther, C. A. Theophilis, and R. H. Smithwick: J. Amer. Med. Ass. **181**, 571 (1962). — 10. Leishman, A. W. D.: Brit. Med. J. 1959/I, 1361. — 11. Morse, W. I., M. G. Criscitiello, A. E. Renold, J. H. Harrison, G. J. Dammin, and G. W. Thorn: Amer. J. Med. **26**, 31 (1959). — 12. Newcombe, C. P., H. S. Shucksmith, and W. S. Suffern: Brit. Med.

J. 1959/I, 142. — 13. PEET, M. M., and E. M. ISBERG: Ann. Int. Med. **28**, 755 (1948). — 14. PERRY, H. M., Jr., and H. A. SCHROEDER: Arch. Int. Med. **102**, 418 (1958). — 15. SMIRK, F. H.: High Arterial Pressure. Blackwell Scientific Publications, Oxford, 1957. — 16. SMITHWICK, R. H.: J. Chron. Dis. **1**, 477 (1955). — 17. SMITHWICK, R. H., R. D. BUSH, and D. KINSEY: J. Amer. Med. Ass. **160**, 1023 (1956). — 18. SMITHWICK, R. H., G. P. WHITELAW, and D. KINSEY: In: Hypertension. Recent Advances. The Second Hahnemann Symposium on Hypertensive Disease. Ed. by A. N. BREST and J. H. MOYER. Lea and Febiger, Philadelphia, 1961, p. 603. — 19. VAN'T HOFF, W.: Quart. J. Med. **26**, 149 (1957). — 20. WOLFERTH, C. C., W. A. JEFFERS, H. A. ZINTEL, J. H. HAFKENSCHIEL, and A. G. HILLS: Bull. N. Y. Acad. Med. **29**, 115 (1953). — 21. WOLFERTH, C. C., W. T. FITTS, W. A. JEFFERS, and A. M. SELLERS: Bull. N. Y. Acad. Med. **33**, 151 (1957).

Discussion

REUBI: Dr. MILLIEZ will probably be interested in knowing the present status of the indications for surgical treatment of hypertension in other countries. Has anyone from the United States a definite opinion to express on this point?

BREST: We have been utilising sympathectomy for occasional patients with severe hypertension who have not been responsive to standard antihypertensive drug therapy. We have been impressed in some cases. Certain patients will be responsive to antihypertensive drugs following sympathectomy, although they had not been before. This has been seen at times even in patients with very limited sympathectomies and occasionally in a patient who has had unilateral sympathectomy.

REUBI: What is your experience, Dr. PAGE?

PAGE: This is largely a historical account. In 1932 we began with what was known as an anterior nerve root section requiring a laminectomy about two feet long. For the first time we saw a reversal of the eyeground changes in malignant hypertension. We learned a lot from that. Then, as you know, PEET[1] performed many splanchnicectomies; after that came SMITHWICK's[2] modification, and later there was the total sympathectomy that GRIMSON[3] did. Finally, adrenalectomies were added, and that completed this first foray of the surgeons into our field. As you well know, after literally thousands of such operations had been performed, these techniques were gradually given up, and now you will find few surgeons in the United States who even remember how to do a sympathectomy. It has been said for years that even if sympathectomies are not very effective they increase the responsiveness to antihypertensive drugs. I have yet to see any substantial evidence to support this contention; no one, to my knowledge, has ever published any. But this was being used more and more as a reason for doing sympathectomy.

REUBI: Would you like to express another opinion, Dr. HOOBLER?

HOOBLER: Yes. I probably have the largest collection of sympathectomised patients in the U.S.A. under my control at the moment, except, perhaps, for the series in Boston. I have had some interesting experiences which, I think, clearly support the view that a sympathectomised patient is more sensitive to saluretic drugs, just as a person receiving hexamethonium is more responsive to a diuretic agent. In other words, a buffer mechanism is removed and the antihypertensive effect of saluresis is thereby enhanced[4]. This conclusion is based on experience with patients after the PEET type of sympathectomy. It has been very impressive how small doses of diuretic agents can lower their blood pressure and keep it at low-to-normal levels for many years after the sympathectomy. The reduction in pressure is very much greater than the average response to a thiazide, and I am quite convinced of this difference. When it comes to subjecting a patient to sympathectomy, I may say that Dr. EDGAR KAHN in Ann Arbor can still do them;

[1] PEET, M. M.: Amer. J. Surg. **75**, 48 (1948).
[2] SMITHWICK, R. H.: Arch. Surg. **49**, 180 (1944).
[3] GRIMSON, K. S.: Ann. Surg. **114**, 753 (1941).
[4] WELLER, J. M., and S. W. HOOBLER: Ann. Int. Med. **50**, 106 (1959).

I think he does about one a year. It is probably not advisable, except in a few cases where it is extremely hard to control the pressure owing to the unreliability of the patient; but because of the enhanced antihypertensive action of diuretics after sympathectomy I am not sure that, if I had very serious hypertension, I wouldn't rather take the gamble of having the sympathectomy and then taking only a diuretic agent for the rest of my life than take guanethidine all my life in addition to a diuretic agent. I know a few physicians who have chosen this alternative in the past few years, and they are doing very well. However, it is hard to tell a patient that you can lower blood pressure with drugs and then expect him to choose an operation. This is the only honest statement you can give to the patient, because you can usually lower his blood pressure either way. And the patient will naturally prefer drug treatment to an operation.

Reubi: What is the British experience on this problem?

Wilson: In the past we have performed about 100 sympathectomies at the London Hospital, and the last I can recall was done about seven years ago. The patient concerned refused to take hypotensive drugs regularly. After sympathectomy, her blood pressure rose again to the pre-operative level. I think sympathectomy is still indicated for the patient with malignant hypertension who refuses drug therapy.

Reubi: Now from another part of the Commonwealth, Dr. Smirk.

Smirk: As far as I know, although hypertensive patients are referred directly to the surgeon if the doctor wants that, we have not had a sympathectomy for hypertension in the Dunedin Hospital for something like 14 years; but we did have a series of patients who had undergone sympathectomies before this, and, although our experience was not very wide, we thought that these patients responded more vigorously to hexamethonium. May I offer the suggestion that anything which stimulates the homoeostatic mechanisms to increase sympathetic activity makes a person more susceptible to any of the ganglion blocking or peripherally acting sympatholytic drugs. And if, as in sympathectomy, much of the sympathetic is removed, homoeostasis should increase the activity of those parts of the sympathetic nervous system which remain. Similarly, after a venesection the amount of sympathetic activity is increased, and the person is made much more susceptible to hexamethonium; in other words, maintenance of the blood-pressure level becomes dependent on the sympathetic. Hexamethonium then administered removes the homoeostatic support upon which maintenance of the blood pressure has become dependent.

Reubi: May we have a voice from the Continent?

Brod: There is no doubt that the sympathectomies performed in the past were, at least in part of our hypertensives, successful, and I still have patients who were sympathectomised some 15 years ago for malignant hypertension and are alive and active today. At that time, this operation constituted a powerful weapon, at least as far as some of the patients were concerned. We have abandoned sympathectomies today almost entirely. We perform them perhaps once in two years in the odd patient who will not respond to any other treatment, and the impression remains that these patients, who were not responsive before, start to respond to drug treatment after sympathectomy. Often, the operation itself does not make the patients normotensive or even improve their blood pressure; however, it frequently makes them more susceptible to some therapeutic agents. I have mentioned this before, at a round-table conference at the Second European Congress of Cardiology in Stockholm in 1956. Dr. PATON[1] was a member of the symposium, and he offered a different explanation from Dr. SMIRK's, namely that regenerating sympathetic fibres are much more likely to respond to any sort of blocking agents than normal sympathetic fibres. He thought that this might account for the therapeutic effect observed.

I should like to make one more comment about nephrectomies, because this was the other topic discussed by Dr. MILLIEZ and Dr. TCHERDAKOFF. In unilateral kidney disease in which we consider that nephrectomy is indicated — and today we are very cautious as regards indications — we get a good response only in about 40% of the patients. We should therefore be very hesitant about recommending nephrectomy for hypertension in a patient with unilateral renal disease but with a functioning kidney.

HOOD: I think sympathectomy is not a completely dead issue. We still do it, for example, in patients who won't take drug therapy, and we also do it in those cases of renal hypertension in which we have had trouble with the medication.

Our practice in patients of this kind is to perform what I call an "insurance-policy sympathectomy"; in other words, we carry out a sympathectomy on one side — provided the patient is not a young male — and, if the result after nephrectomy is not satisfactory, we can then sympathectomise the other side. This applies, of course, only to patients in whom persistent, consequent antihypertensive treatment has failed more or less completely.

DUSTAN: I should like to make a request to Dr. HOOBLER that, if the time comes when he needs a sympathectomy, he establish his responsiveness to antihypertensive drugs very carefully prior to the operation, so that we may know whether sympathectomy truly enhances responsiveness to antihypertensive drugs. The declaration of enhanced responsiveness has been made repeatedly, and we, too, have seen chlorothiazide produce normal blood pressure in a sympathectomised patient. Unfortunately, we had no idea how the patient would have responded to this drug prior to sympathectomy, because the operation had been done before chlorothiazide was introduced. Now we also are plagued by this problem regarding surgical treatment for occlusive renal arterial disease, because the surgeons tell us that patients who fail to respond to operation become more responsive to drug therapy. To my way of thinking, such patients have not failed to respond to treatment pre-operatively, but rather have not received adequate antihypertensive drug therapy. I would urge all people who have any comparative information on drug responsiveness before and after sympathectomy to make it available, so that we can clarify this difficult and confused issue.

TCHERDAKOFF: I just want to say that the patients in whom sympathectomy appears to be indicated are those who either don't respond to correct drug therapy or are quite unwilling to take that therapy. This rules out operations on patients with normal, Grade I, or Grade II eyegrounds: such patients were operated on in 1947. As far as nephrectomy is concerned, we quite agree with Dr. HOOD. In fact, all of our patients who are subjected to nephrectomy for unilateral renal disease with hypertension simultaneously undergo sympathectomy on the same side, and eventually, if nephrectomy doesn't give satisfactory results, we perform a sympathectomy on the other side as well.

---

[1] PATON, W. D. M.: Round-table conference on Therapy of Essential Hypertension. Proc. 2nd Europ. Congress of Cardiology. Stockholm, 1956.

Potassium loss and potassium replacement during long-term diuretic treatment in hypertension

By

C. Bartorelli, N. Gargano, and G. Leonetti

1. Introduction

While investigating the mechanisms of the hypotensive action of the benzothiazides years ago (*1*, *2*), we made a few observations that stimulated our interest in potassium turnover during long-term diuretic treatment and, more generally, in the influence of the potassium ion on hypertension. The latter problem has not yet been thoroughly studied, but, to judge by the contradictory nature of the available data, it appears to be extremely complex. Indeed, modifications in the potassium balance in opposite directions, i.e. both decreased (*3*, *4*) and increased intake (*5*, *6*), seem to produce the same effect, namely a reduction in blood pressure. However, the mechanism governing the long-term hypotensive effect of the benzothiazides has also not been fully elucidated yet, nor has the role of potassium loss been adequately investigated. We should therefore like, first of all, to consider the importance of potassium loss during long-term diuretic treatment and the effects of potassium replacement in these conditions, and secondly, to deal with the more general problem of the relationship between potassium and blood pressure.

2. Potassium loss during long-term diuretic treatment

The first observations made in patients receiving short-term treatment with diuretics tended to suggest that there is a cause-and-effect relation between sodium depletion and blood-pressure decrease (*7*, *8*). Such an explanation is probably right during the first few days of diuretic treatment, when a reduction in body sodium and plasma volume can be demonstrated; but it does not hold good in the later stages of therapy, during which the hypotensive effect persists, in spite of the fact that exchangeable body sodium and plasma volume have reverted to pretreatment values (*9*, *10*, *11*).

In 33 patients we have investigated the mechanisms governing the long-term hypotensive action of the benzothiazides, continuing and extending the work of the authors referred to above. The subjects of our study were severely or moderately hypertensive patients, who, after an adequate period of control, were treated with hydrochlorothiazide in oral doses of 100 mg. per day for

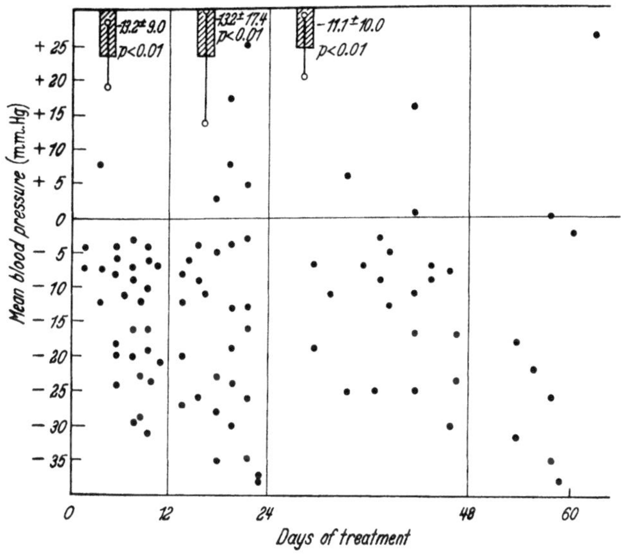

Fig. 1. Changes in mean blood pressure after treatment with hydrochlorothiazide. In this and in Figs 2—4 and 6 the hatched rectangles in the upper part of the figures show the mean changes and the vertical lines the standard deviations. The actual figures are also given; "p" shows results of analysis of variance, expressed in terms of probability.

periods ranging from 20 days to seven months. Blood pressure was recorded daily, during both the control and the treatment periods, and at different intervals measurements were taken of plasma volume (dye dilution method), exchangeable sodium and potassium (by determination of their isotopes Na^{24} and K^{42} at the 24th hour), and extracellular fluid volume (by determination of Na^{24} at the 3rd hour). Body weight and changes in serum sodium and potassium were also noted. The information thus obtained has been treated statistically by analysis of variance over arbitrary periods of time. The administration of hydrochlorothiazide caused a rapid and significant fall in blood pressure, which showed no tendency to rise again during long-term treatment with the saluretic agent (Fig. 1).

The variations in exchangeable sodium as a measure of both the extra- and intracellular sodium pool are shown in Fig. 2. The extent of the reduction in total body sodium was particularly striking during the first days of treatment, but gradually diminished as treatment was prolonged. In the first period (1st–12th day) the reduction was 220 $\pm$ 134 mEq. ($p < 0.001$); in the second (13th to 24th day) it was 142 $\pm$ 133 mEq. ($p < 0.001$). On the other hand,

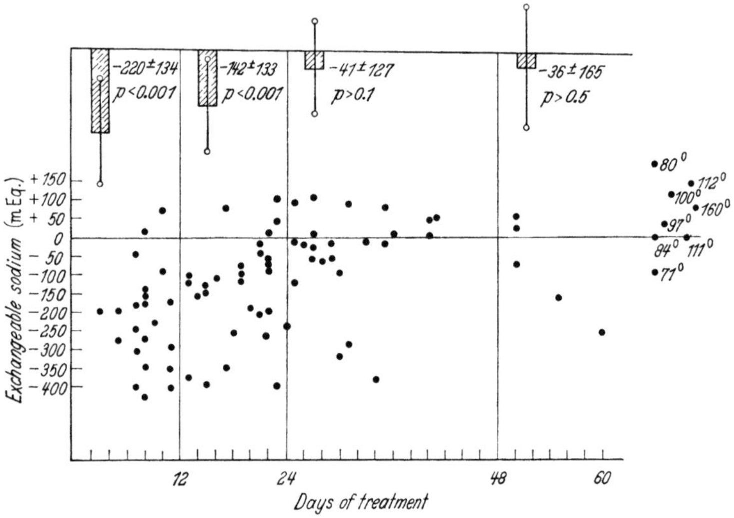

Fig. 2. Changes in exchangeable sodium after treatment with hydrochlorothiazide (for key see Fig. 1).

during the third and fourth periods the changes in total body sodium became progressively smaller, until they were no longer statistically significant. The variations in plasma volume (Fig. 3) and extracellular fluid (Fig. 4) followed a similar pattern. Both decreased during the first two periods of treatment, but gradually showed less tendency to change.

To conclude, our observations confirm those of other authors in showing that after the 24th day of treatment there is no further reduction in exchangeable sodium and that after the 48th day the plasma and extracellular fluid volumes rise to control values. At this stage there must be another cause of the persistence of blood-pressure lowering.

The influence which a deficiency in potassium caused by thiazide derivatives might have on blood pressure has, strangely enough, been overlooked, in spite of the fact that hypokalaemia

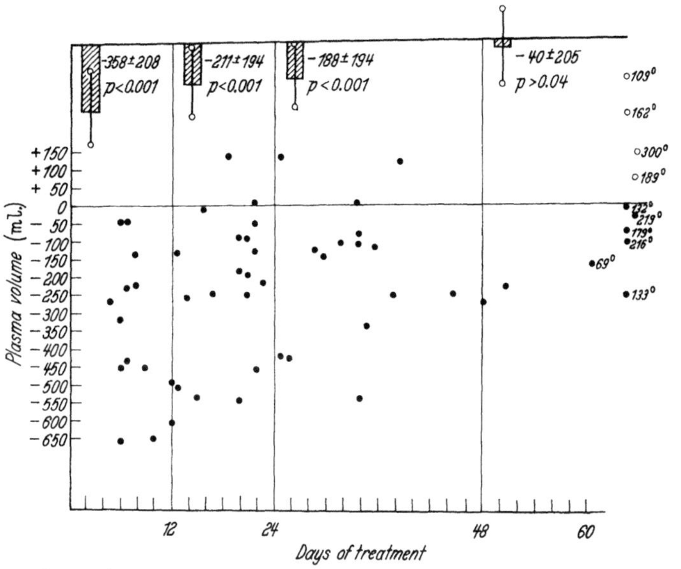

Fig. 3. Changes in plasma volume after treatment with hydrochlorothiazide (for key see Fig. 1).

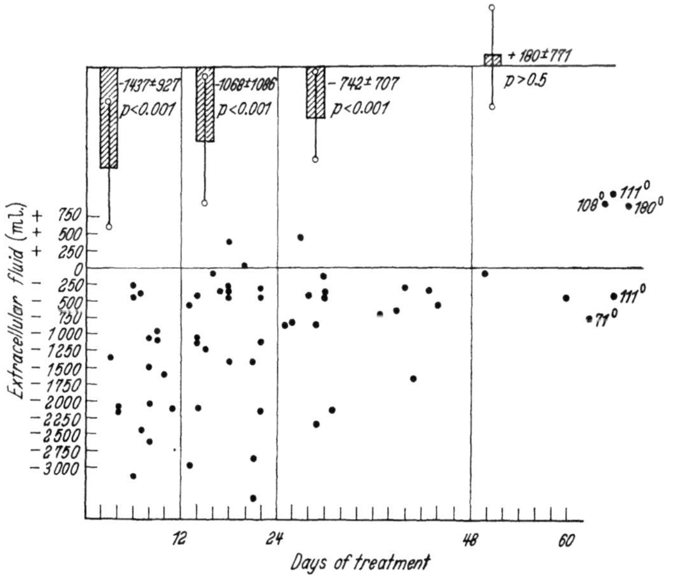

Fig. 4. Changes in extracellular fluid after treatment with hydrochlorothiazide (for key see Fig. 1).

is, we might say, a regular consequence of diuretic therapy and a reduction in exchangeable potassium has been shown since the first observations (*9*, *12*). Figs 5 and 6 emphasise the magnitude of this

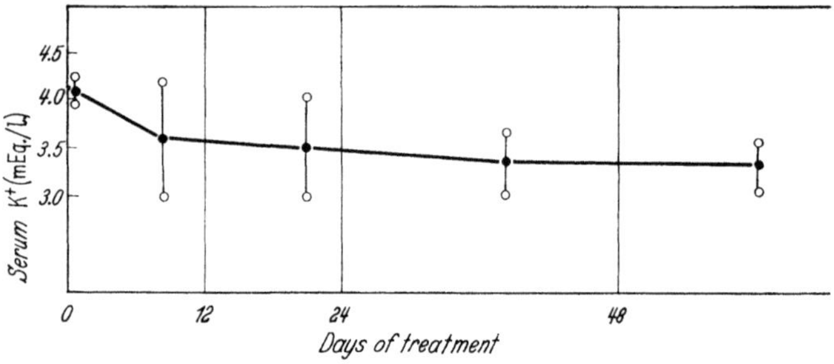

Fig. 5. Changes in serum potassium levels after treatment with hydrochlorothiazide. Mean values and standard deviations are given.

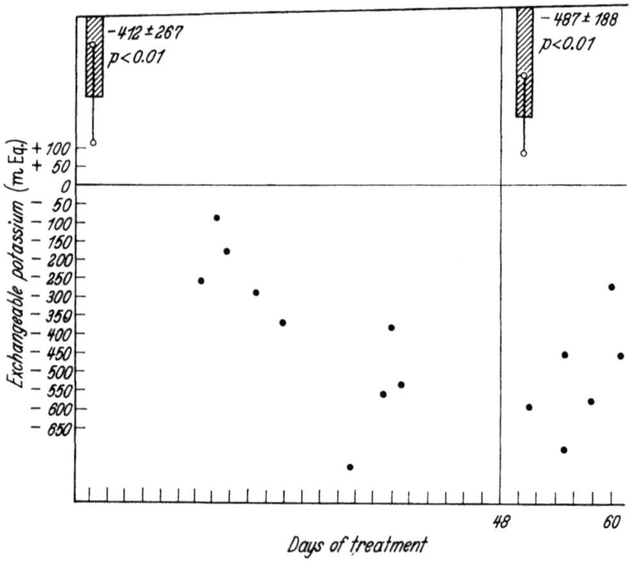

Fig. 6. Changes in exchangeable potassium after treatment with hydrochlorothiazide (for key see Fig. 1).

phenomenon. The serum potassium levels dropped from a mean value of 4.2 mEq./l. in the control period to 3.5, 3.4, and 3.3 mEq./l. during the different periods of diuretic therapy considered. The reduction in total body potassium – 412 mEq. in patients studied up to the 48th day of diuretic therapy and 487 mEq. in those studied for a longer period – was highly significant (Fig. 6). The amount of potassium lost may thus be considered as being equal to between one sixth and one fifth of the total body potassium. In our patients, this phenomenon was more pronounced than what has been observed by other authors (*9*, *12*), probably because our observations were carried out in hospitalised patients following a diet with a rather low potassium content (30–40 mEq. per day).

3. Potassium replacement during long-term diuretic treatment

The significance of potassium depletion in relation to the long-term hypotensive effect of thiazide derivatives should be proved by a rise in blood pressure after potassium replacement. In this sort of experiment, the well-known natriuretic effect of potassium

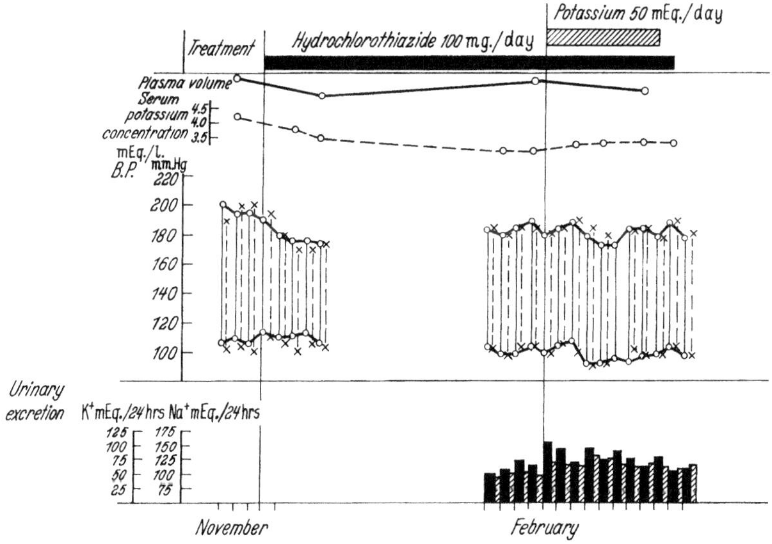

Fig. 7. Effects of chronic replacement of potassium in a patient undergoing long-term treatment with hydrochlorothiazide.

salts creates a serious difficulty (*13*). The administration of small amounts of potassium (50 mEq. per day) for many days did not modify blood pressure to any considerable degree. This is exemplified in Fig. 7; the patient in question had been treated with thiazide compounds for about two months, and therapy was continued during potassium replacement. It is interesting to note, however, that kaliuresis rose in comparison with that found on the days preceding potassium administration, from which we may assume that the increase in potassium stores was very moderate. Furthermore, it should also be noted that potassium replacement activated natriuresis and caused a slight reduction in plasma volume, as if the hypotensive mechanisms generally regarded as being active during the first days of diuretic therapy had again been stimulated into activity. This explains why even those who suggest, as we do, that potassium loss may be one of the mechanisms which play a part in the long-term hypotensive effect of diuretics have no objection to the use of daily potassium supplements to the diet of hypertensive patients undergoing benzothiazide therapy.

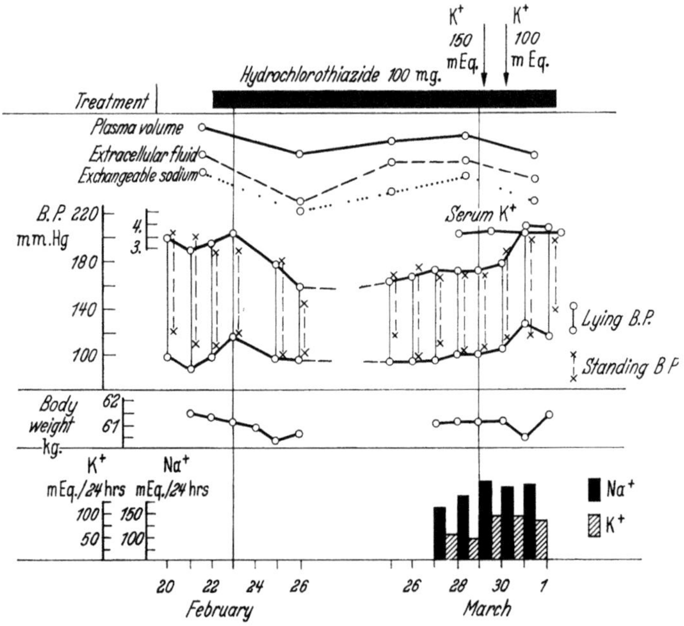

Fig. 8. Effects of acute replacement of potassium in a patient undergoing long-term treatment with hydrochlorothiazide.

More significant data on the hypotensive role of potassium loss were obtained when another method of potassium replacement was used. This study involved 11 patients who had been treated with hydrochlorothiazide for more than 24 days and in whom plasma volume, extracellular fluid, and exchangeable sodium had completely or almost returned to the values recorded in the control period.

Table 1. *Influence of potassium replacement on the hypotensive effect of hydrochlorothiazide on blood pressure (B.P.), plasma volume (P.V.), extracellular fluid volume (E.C.F.), and exchangeable sodium (Na^+)*

Case	Control period				Before potassium replacement				After potassium replacement			
	B.P. mm. Hg	P.V. ml.	E.C.F. ml.	Na^+ mEq.	B.P. mm. Hg	P.V. ml.	E.C.F. ml.	Na^+ mEq.	B.P. mm. Hg	P.V. ml.	E.C.F. ml.	Na^+ mEq.
B. G.	200/100	3,013	16,211	2,708	170/105	2,716	15,387	2,696	210/130	2,525	14,819	2,525
S. P.	170/95	2,477	14,200	2,238	130/80	2,613	13,936	2,176	155/100	2,347		
A. An.	210/105	2,890	17,225	2,813	160/90	2,891	17,639	2,791	180/95	2,875		
G. Gi.	230/130			2,532	175/120		15,500	2,438	200/130		15,250	2,356
F. I.	190/110	2,843		3,120	165/100	2,737		3,202	190/130			2,914
B. U.	200/105			2,789	170/100			2,854	130/100			
C. P.	210/110	2,654	18,120	2,758	180/110		17,806	2,781	210/110		17,200	2,529
S. P.	180/90	2,716	15,376	2,383	155/80	2,569			170/110	2,538		
B. M.	230/100	2,548	18,225	2,879	180/95	2,464			195/105	2,462		
F. A.	200/90	2,503	13,036	2,190	160/80	2,225	13,108	1,993	190/100	2,006		
C. M.	210/100	2,755	16,348	2,767	180/110	2,746	16,037	2,644	200/110	2,273	15,429	2,538

Within a period of two days they were given 250 mEq. of potassium ions, partly by intravenous injection (100 mEq. on the first and 50 mEq. on the second day) and partly by mouth (50 mEq. on both the first and second day). A typical case is shown in Fig. 8. The blood pressure, which had been lowered by treatment with hydrochlorothiazide, rose to the control-period values. The serum potassium level returned to normal values. It should be stressed that simultaneously there was a reduction in both extracellular fluid and exchangeable sodium. All the results relating to the cases studied are summarised in Table 1. It can be seen that, in spite of the natriuretic effect accompanied by a reduction in exchangeable sodium and extracellular fluid, this method of potassium replacement consistently caused an increase in blood pressure in ten patients, although the magnitude of this rise varied from subject to subject. Therefore, the rise in blood pressure to the values recorded in the control period cannot be ascribed to expansion of plasma volume and is probably attributable to a direct circulatory effect of the replacement of potassium. In support of this opinion it may be said that in the only patient in whom the administration of potassium did not cause a rise in blood pressure, but a striking hypotension, the administration of potassium was followed by pronounced natriuresis (300 mEq. in one day with a reduction of 1 kg. in body weight).

4. Potassium administration in untreated hypertensive and normotensive subjects

It was precisely this last observation, and the fact that the literature contains reports indicating that the administration of potassium may have a hypotensive effect (*14, 15*), that prompted us to investigate the opposite aspect of the problem, namely changes in blood pressure and electrolyte balance caused by a large dose of potassium in hypertensive patients who had not undergone hypotensive or diuretic therapy, and in normotensive patients serving as a control group.

These effects were studied in seven patients with moderate or severe hypertension in whom there were no signs of cardiac failure and renal function was good (renal blood flow greater than 400 ml./min.). 100 mEq. of potassium ions were given intravenously in 350 ml. of a 5 % glucose solution; the rate of infusion was 0.42 ml./min., and the whole procedure lasted four hours. The infusion caused a slight rise in the serum concentration of potassium (from 4.2 to 4.5 mEq./l.), a transient increase in serum sodium (from 143 to 150 mEq./l.), and a striking increase in the urinary excretion of sodium to about five times the values recorded in the control period (Fig. 9). The excretion of chloride was less striking and the excretion of potassium only slightly increased. Plasma volume was

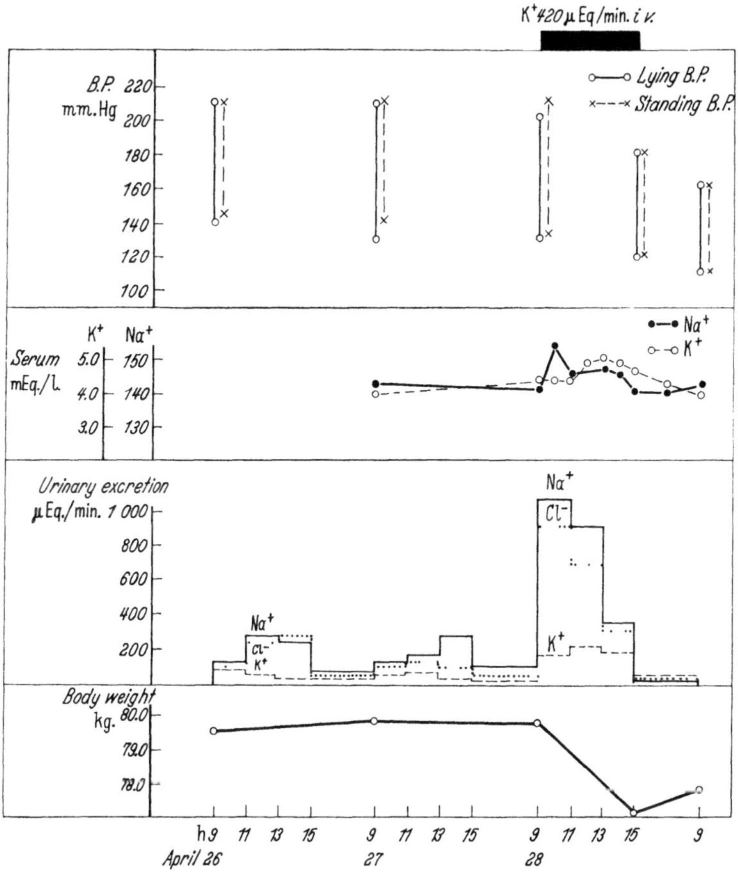

Fig. 9. Effects of an acute load of potassium on blood pressure and urinary and plasma electrolytes in an untreated hypertensive patient.

consistently reduced by 200—300 ml. in those hypertensive patients in whom it had been checked. In all subjects, blood pressure was significantly lowered at the end of the infusion and to a more conspicuous degree on the subsequent day. In normotensive subjects the potassium infusion did not cause any definite change in blood pressure, and the increase in sodium excretion was also scarcely significant, its mean value (52 mEq.) being approximately half that observed in hypertensive patients (107 mEq.).

5. Discussion

The results we have reported illustrate the complexity of the influence exerted by potassium on the regulation of blood pressure, but may also help to explain the mechanisms involved. Our last group of experiments confirms the findings of Addison and Clark (*14*) and Priddle (*15*) in man and of other authors in different forms of experimental hypertension (*5*, *6*), i.e. that the administration of large amounts of potassium has a hypotensive effect. According to our observations, there is no doubt that the sodium loss and consequently the reduction in plasma volume play an important part in causing this hypotension. More complicated mechanisms, however, related to a modified excitability of the muscle fibres of small arteries and therefore to a decreased peripheral resistance, should also be considered. Indeed, it is well known from experiments on striated muscle fibres and on nerve cells or axons that the excitability of cellular membranes is, at least within certain limits, inversely proportional to the membrane potential. This is fundamentally owing to the ratio K_i/K_e (according to Nernst's equation). In other words, the greater the negative intracellular potential, the less excitable is the cell; on the other hand, the less the resting potential, the greater is the excitability and the lower the threshold of excitation. If a large dose of potassium is administered, the mild and transient rise in the serum concentration of this ion, as well as the slight increase in its urinary excretion, suggests that the greater part of the administered potassium rapidly penetrates the cells, causing an increase in the K_i/K_e ratio and in the membrane potential and a reduction in the excitability of arterial smooth muscle.

It is conceivable that this hypothesis might also account for the reduction in peripheral resistance shown by many authors to be the cause of blood-pressure lowering during diuretic treatment. As Seller et al. (*16*) showed very recently, after a long-term treatment with hydrochlorothiazide the intracellular potassium (at least inside red blood cells) is only slightly and inconsistently reduced, whereas the reduction in the serum potassium concentration is much more marked. In our studies, the average decrease of 480 mEq. in exchangeable potassium corresponds to a percentage reduction of 14%, while the reduction of 1 mEq. of serum potassium is equivalent to 25% of extracellular potassium. As a consequence of this, the K_i/K_e ratio should be increased. If we bear in mind the fact that long-term treatment with diuretics may cause a loss of intracellular water (*11*), there should be a further rise in the intracellular concentration of potassium and a further increase in the K_i/K_e ratio. An increase in the intracellular concentration of potassium is also indicated by the direct measurements of VILLAMIL et al. (*17*) in biopsy material from hypertensive patients treated with thiazides.

However, before concluding that changes in the potassium distribution are responsible for changes in vascular excitability in arterial hypertension, and even before accepting the more limited assumption that a disturbance of the potassium balance constitutes the main mechanism of the long-term hypotensive action of diuretics, we must remember that membrane excitability is controlled by the state of equilibrium of several different ions and that SELLER et al. (*16*) have clearly shown that prolonged administration of hydrochlorothiazide induces alterations in magnesium metabolism, besides the changes in potassium distribution referred to above. Our studies have shown that changes in the potassium balance can hardly be induced without consequent alterations in sodium excretion. Our results therefore cannot be taken as a definitive answer to any of the questions raised in the introduction to this paper, but rather as a contribution towards the solving of a complicated, though important, problem which seems worthy of further study.

Summary

In 33 patients with arterial hypertension, hydrochlorothiazide (100 mg. daily) was administered for periods ranging from 20 days to seven months, and the consequent fall in blood pressure was correlated with changes in plasma volume, extracellular fluid volume, exchangeable body sodium, and potassium. Although during the first weeks of treatment the hypotensive effect was associated with significant decreases in plasma and extracellular fluid volumes, and in exchangeable sodium, in a later period all these values returned to pretreatment levels, and beyond the seventh week of diuretic therapy the persistent hypotensive effect could only be correlated with a growing depletion in potassium stores.

In this period, protracted oral administration of small amounts of potassium (50 mEq. per day) failed to restore blood pressure to pretreatment levels and was associated with increased natriuresis and a fall in plasma volume, thus reinstating the hypotensive mechanism active during early periods of diuretic therapy. Only after acute (mainly intravenous) administration of large amounts of potassium (250 mEq. within two days) did blood pressure return to pretreatment values, provided the natriuretic effect was not too large.

Similarely, acute administration of potassium to hypertensive patients whose potassium stores had not been depleted previously by prolonged diuretic therapy was followed by a striking increase in the urinary excretion of sodium and by a consistent decrease in blood pressure. No blood-pressure change was observed in normotensive subjects, but their sodium excretion was scarcely affected by potassium administration.

The role of the potassium ion in regulating vascular excitability in hypertensive patients, either untreated or treated with diuretics, is discussed.

Zusammenfassung

Dreiunddreißig Patienten mit Hochdruck erhielten während Perioden von 20 Tagen bis zu sieben Monaten 100 mg Hydrochlorothiazid täglich. Der während dieser Behandlung auftretende Blutdruckabfall wurde in Beziehung gesetzt zu Änderungen des Plasmavolumens, des extrazellulären Flüssigkeitsvolumens, des austauschbaren Körpernatriums und des Kaliums. Obwohl während der ersten Wochen der Behandlung die Blutdrucksenkung mit signifikanter Abnahme des Plasma- und des extrazellulären Flüssigkeitsvolumens sowie mit einer Verminderung des austauschbaren Natriums verbunden war, kehrten zu einem späteren Zeitpunkt alle diese Werte auf die vor der Behandlung gemessenen zurück. Nach der siebenten Woche der diuretischen Therapie war der anhaltende drucksenkende Effekt lediglich mit einer zunehmenden Verminderung des Kaliumgehaltes zu korrelieren.

Zu dieser Zeit war es nicht möglich, den Blutdruck durch langfristige orale Gabe kleiner Kaliummengen (50 mÄq pro Tag) auf die Werte vor Beginn der Behandlung einzustellen; dagegen kam es zu Natriurese und Abnahme des Plasmavolumens und damit zu einem gleichen hypotensiven Mechanismus wie in der Frühphase der diuretischen Behandlung. Nur nach akuter (vorwiegend intravenöser) Gabe großer Mengen von Kalium (250 mÄq während zwei Tagen) kehrte der Blutdruck auf die Ausgangswerte vor der Behandlung zurück, vorausgesetzt, daß der gleichzeitig auftretende natriuretische Effekt nicht zu stark war.

Bei Hochdruckpatienten, deren Kaliumspeicher nicht durch eine vorhergehende langdauernde Therapie mit Diuretika vermindert waren, folgte der akuten Gabe von Kalium ebenfalls ein erheblicher Anstieg der Natriumausscheidung und ein entsprechender Blutdruckabfall. Bei normotensiven Personen ließ sich keine Blutdruckänderung beobachten, aber auch die Natriumausscheidung war kaum durch die Kaliumgabe beeinflußt.

Die Rolle des Kaliumions bei der Regulation der Gefäßerregbarkeit von Hochdruckpatienten, entweder ohne Behandlung oder während der Gabe von Diuretika, wird besprochen.

Résumé

Trente-trois malades hypertendus ont reçu de l'hydrochlorothiazide (100 mg par jour) pendant des périodes allant de 20 jours à sept mois. Les baisses de pression artérielle qu'ils ont présentées se sont accompagnées de modifications du volume plasmatique, du volume des liquides extracellulaires, du sodium et du potassium échangeables. Bien qu'au cours des premières semaines du traitement l'effet hypotenseur se soit accompagné d'une diminution notable du volume du plasma, des liquides extracellulaires et du sodium échangeable, plus tard tous ces trois paramètres retournèrent à leurs valeurs primitives antérieures au traitement, et au-delà de la septième semaine du traitement diurétique l'effet hypotenseur toujours présent ne s'accompagnait plus que d'une déperdition croissante de potassium.

De petites doses orales de potassium (50 mEq par jour) ont alors été administrées de façon prolongée et n'ont pas fait remonter la pression artérielle à ses valeurs antérieures; elles ont provoqué un accroissement de la natriurèse et une chute du volume plasmatique, réinstallant ainsi le mécanisme hypotenseur intervenu à la période initiale du traitement diurétique. Ce n'est qu'après l'administration aiguë (surtout intra-veineuse) de grandes quantités de potassium (250 mEq en deux jours) que la pression artérielle est remontée à ses valeurs antérieures au traitement, à condition toutefois que l'effet natriurétique n'ait pas été trop intense.

Une même administration aiguë de potassium chez des hypertendus dont les réserves en potassium n'avaient pas été préalablement diminuées par un traitement diurétique prolongé, a été suivie d'une augmentation frappante de l'excrétion urinaire du sodium et d'une diminution correspondante de la tension artérielle. Aucune modification tensionnelle n'a été observée chez les sujets normotendus, mais leur excrétion de sodium a été à peine influencée par l'administration de potassium.

Le rôle de l'ion potassium dans la régulation de l'excitabilité vasculaire chez les malades hypertendus, traités ou non par les diurétiques, est discuté.

References

1. Bartorelli, C., N. Gargano, and A. Zanchetti: Arch. stud. fisiopat. ricambio **25**, 234 (1961). — 2. Bartorelli, C.: In: Essential Hypertension. An International Symposium. Ed. by K. D. Bock and P. T. Cottier. Springer, Berlin, 1960, p. 283. — 3. Freed, C. S., and M. Friedman: Proc. Soc. Exper. Biol. Med. **78**, 74 (1951). — 4. Perera, G. A.: J. Clin. Invest. **32**, 633 (1953). — 5. Rosenman, R. H.: Proc. Soc. Exper. Biol. Med. **78**, 77 (1951). — 6. Rosenman, R. H., C. S. Freed, and M. Friedman: Circulation **5**, 412 (1952). — 7. Freis, E. D., A. Wanko, I. M. Wilson, and A. E. Parrish: Ann. N. Y. Acad. Sc. **71**, 450 (1958). — 8. Tapia, F. A., H. P. Dustan, R. A. Schneckloth, A. C. Corcoran, and I. H. Page: Lancet 1957/II, 831. — 9. Hollander, W., and A. V. Chobanian: J. Clin. Invest. **37**, 902 (1958). — 10. Aleksandrow, D., W. Wyszacka, and J. Gayewski: N. England J. Med. **260**, 51 (1959). — 11. Lauwers, P., and J. Conway: J. Laborat. Clin. Med. **56**, 401 (1960). — 12. Winer, B. M.: Circulation **23**, 211 (1961). — 13. Pitts, R. F.: The Physiological Basis of Diuretic Therapy. Thomas, Springfield, Ill., 1959. — 14. Addison, W. L. T., and M. B. Clark: Canad. Med. Ass. J. **15**, 913 (1925). — 15. Priddle, W.: Canad. Med. Ass. J. **25**, 5 (1931). — 16. Seller, R. H., O. Ramirez-Muxo, A. N. Brest, and J. H. Moyer: J. Amer. Med. Ass. **191**, 654 (1965). — 17. Villamil, M. F., N. Yeyati, M. A. Enero, C. Rubianes, and A. C. Taquini: Amer. Heart J., **65**, 294 (1963).

Disturbances in carbohydrate and uric-acid metabolism during diuretic treatment

By

F. HARTMANN and V. HEIMSOTH

Since the introduction of thiazide diuretics into the long-term treatment of hypertension, a number of metabolic disorders have become known, the most frequently encountered and the most important of which is hypokalaemia (Table 1) (*1–46*, *48–110*).

Table 1. *Various metabolic changes produced by treatment with saluretics*

Hypokalaemia
Hyponatraemia
Hypochloraemic alkalosis with tetany
Hyperammonaemia → hepatic coma in patients with liver cirrhosis
Increase in non-protein nitrogen (N.P.N.) → uraemic coma in patients with diseases of the kidneys
Hyperuraemia → gout attack
Hyperglycaemia → diabetic coma

No common biochemical or biophysical denominator for these effects has yet been found. We have seen two cases of hypochloraemic tetany, in both of which the plasma calcium level was normal. In the first case, tetanic episodes occurred during treatment with 100 mg. hydroflumethiazide; potassium fell to 2.15 mEq./l. and the chloride concentration came down to 82 mEq./l. In the other case, a hypochloraemia of 84.5 mEq./l. developed after intravenous administration of 100 mg. ethacrynic acid, and the patient became tetanic; all other serum electrolytes remained unaffected.

Although saluretic treatment can produce hyperammonaemia and precipitate hepatic or uraemic coma in cases with pre-existing liver or kidney damage, we have never encountered this in patients receiving long-term treatment in our special out-patient clinic for hypertension (*47*). I should like to present our experiences with disturbances in carbohydrate and uric-acid metabolism under two headings:

1. Glucose tolerance and uric-acid levels in the plasma before and immediately after a single intravenous injection of a saluretic drug.

2. Blood glucose, glycosuria, tolbutamide test, insulin requirement, and uric-acid levels during long-term treatment with saluretics.

Acute experiments. We selected 57 patients between 21 and 79 years of age, with hypertension. In 11 of them we determined the fasting blood glucose over a period of two hours, before and after intravenous doses of 100 mg. ethacrynic acid. Although diuresis started about 20 minutes after the injection, no significant changes in blood glucose could be observed. This means that haemoconcentration does not necessarily increase the blood sugar level.

In 46 patients we tested glucose tolerance following an oral load of 0.80 g./kg. some days before and immediately after intravenous injection of 200 mg. hydrochlorothiazide, or 100 mg. ethacrynic acid, or 100 mg. furosemide. We compared statistically the highest blood glucose concentrations reached after glucose loading (expressed as percentages of the fasting blood glucose).

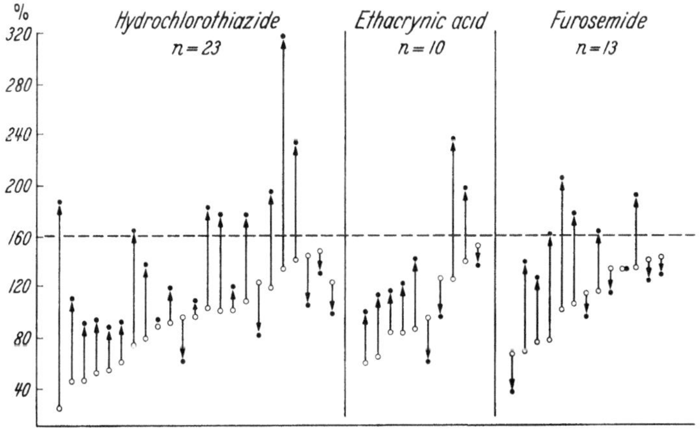

Fig. 1. Maximum increase in blood sugar after oral load of glucose (0.80 g./kg.). Ordinate indicates percent of blood glucose level before applying the load (control value = 0). ● after, ○ before intravenous diuretics.

As Fig. 1 shows, glucose tolerance was diminished in 14 cases – i.e. rose above the upper normal limit of 160% – irrespective of which diuretic agent was given. In the case of hydrochlorothiazide the result is significant ($p = 0.017$). The average age in this group was

47 years. The average age of the patients with decreased tolerance in the three groups together was 52 years, and that in the group not influenced by diuretics, 47 years.

We found no correlation between the reduced glucose tolerance and the concentrations of potassium, sodium, and calcium in the serum, the latter being enhanced significantly after hydrochlorothiazide and ethacrynic acid. Hence, the effect of diuretics on carbohydrate metabolism is independent of the electrolyte balance or the excretion of electrolytes. No rise in the uric-acid level in the serum was observed in the acute experiments.

We were also unable to demonstrate a correlation between serum creatinine elevation and glucose tolerance. In response to intravenous injection of hydrochlorothiazide and ethacrynic acid, but not of furosemide, serum creatinine increased significantly ($p < 0.001$).

The reasons for the change in glucose tolerance remain uncertain. The findings cannot be explained in terms of haemoconcentration followed by accelerated absorption of glucose from the intestine. We think that the cause may be a diminution in glucose utilisation, perhaps in the effect of insulin on it, as was suggested by DOLLERY et al. (*25*), KÖNIGSTEIN and MÄHR (*53*), and WOLFF (*102*) and supported by the experiments on rats made by FORMANEK (*32*). We also investigated the responsiveness of blood glucose to 0.1 unit of insulin per kg. body weight after the injection of diuretics. Only in the eight patients in the hydrochlorothiazide group in whom glucose tolerance was reduced were we able to demonstrate a significant diminution in the insulin effect ($p = 0.035$).

Long-term treatment. The results described below were obtained in a group of 113 hypertensive patients receiving long-term diuretic treatment (average duration 18.3 months) with average doses of chlorothiazide, hydrochlorothiazide, hydroflumethiazide, thiabutazide, chlorthalidone, or ethacrynic acid equivalent to 88.4 mg. hydrochlorothiazide. In 73 of our patients there was no familial history of diabetes and neither the tolbutamide test nor the glucose tolerance (Staub-Traugott) test revealed any evidence of latent diabetes. Three of these patients, aged 46, 62, and 64 years and all overweight, developed imbalance in carbohydrate metabolism, two of them in a clinically manifest form. In the two latter cases, latent diabetes necessitating dietary regulation remained after saluretic therapy was discontinued; hyperglycaemia and glycosuria disappeared immediately (Fig. 2). The precipitation of the diabetes in these cases did not depend on the daily dose of the saluretic nor on the duration of treatment. If we look at the blood glucose distribution curve (Fig. 3), the impression is strengthened that only a small group of patients is predisposed to a "diabetogenic"

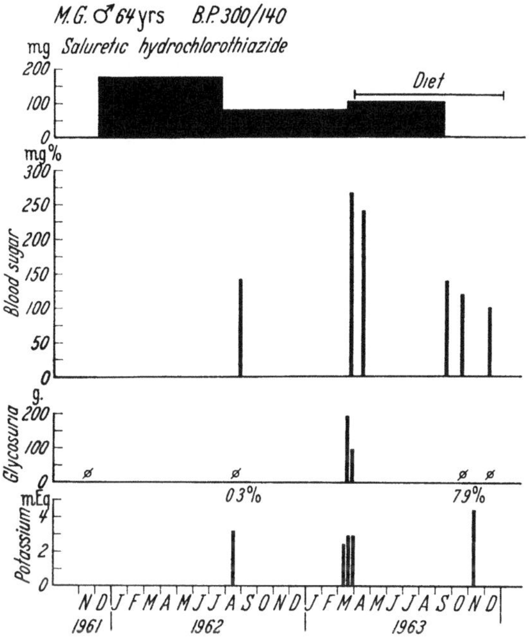

Fig. 2. Blood sugar, glycosuria, and potassium excretion in a diabetic hypertensive patient before, during, and after treatment with hydrochlorothiazide.

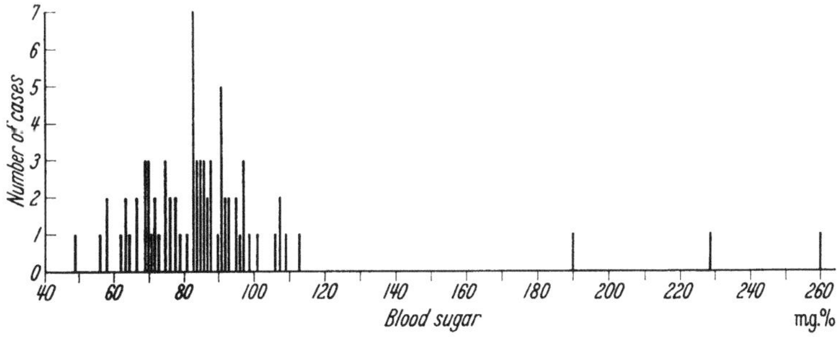

Fig. 3. Fasting blood sugar in 113 hypertensive patients treated with saluretics.

response to saluretics. This group is smaller than the number of diabetics within the whole group of 1,092 hypertensive patients followed up in our out-patient clinic, which comprises about 32% manifest and 30% latent cases.

The same special sensitivity of a small number of patients to the diabetogenic action of saluretics was observed in the groups with potential, latent, and manifest diabetes. Only one of our six patients who displayed no diabetic symptoms but in whose family there was a history of diabetes developed a manifest and irreversible diabetes, which at first responded to sulphonylurea, but later required treatment with insulin and the interruption of saluretic therapy. There have been reports in the literature to the effect that carbohydrate metabolism may be influenced in the course of treatment with saluretics in about 55% of patients with latent diabetes; in our series, such an effect was evident in only three out of 12 cases.

Seven of our 22 diabetic patients who were treated for one and a half years with saluretics decompensated; none of them developed diabetic coma and all responded very satisfactorily to antidiabetic treatment, even if saluretic therapy had to be continued. One case, (Fig. 4), well compensated by sulphonylurea and dietary measures, decompensated immediately after the onset of saluretic treatment. Insulin treatment became inevitable, and the patient demanded continued insulin treatment even after the saluretics were withdrawn.

Other cases recompensate immediately, as did, for instance, the one shown in Fig. 5. In four patients we had to switch from treatment with sulphonylurea to insulin, and in one case from a diet to sulphonylurea. One 71-year-old woman with hypertension of 240/125 mm. Hg and diabetes well controlled by insulin showed decompensation with elevation of blood glucose, increased daily glucose loss in the urine, and need of additional insulin a few days after beginning antihypertensive treatment with 60 mg. furosemide daily (Fig. 6). We were unable to demonstrate a quantitative correlation between the dose and the "diabetogenic" action of a saluretic drug, although it must be borne in mind that in a number of cases the dose of insulin or sulphonylurea needed decreases or the diabetes disappears after withdrawal of the saluretics.

From these observations we conclude that if a patient requires saluretic antihypertensive and antidiabetic treatment, he should be given both, except in the few cases in which the diabetes is difficult to control during saluretic treatment.

If a diabetic patient, after a short period of tentative treatment with saluretics, does not decompensate, it is improbable that he will do so later. After receiving saluretic treatment for more than

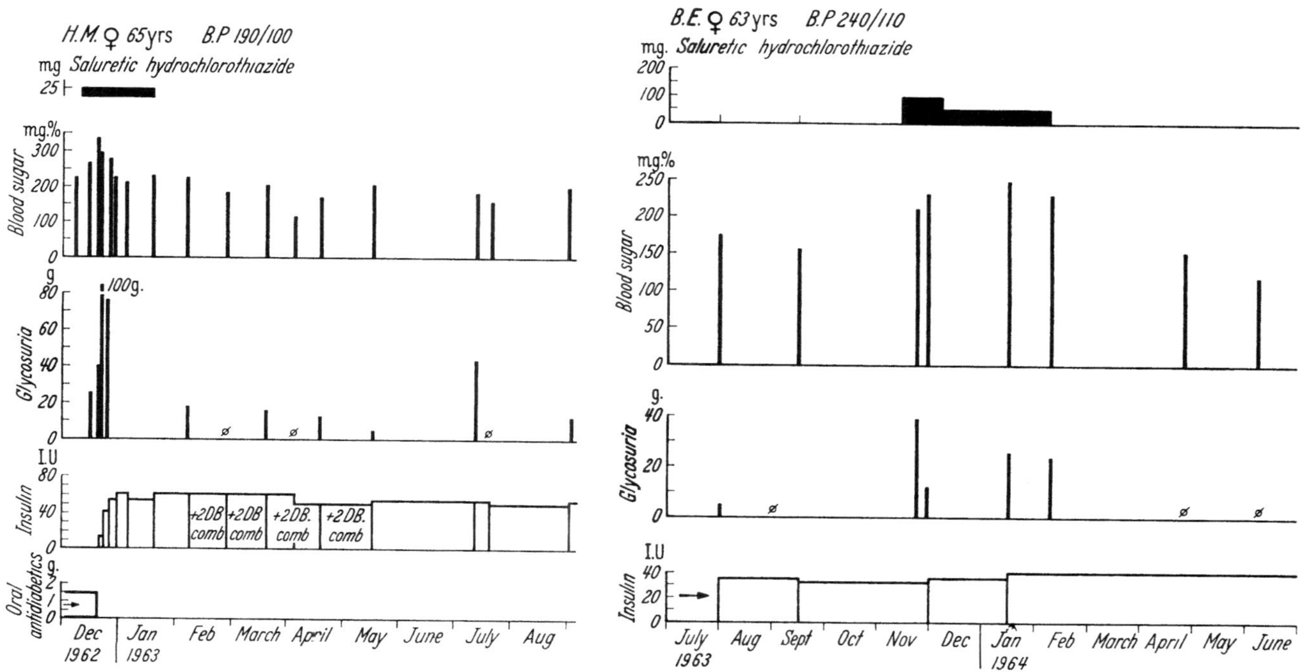

Figs 4 and 5. Blood sugar, glycosuria, and insulin dose in two diabetic hypertensive patients before, during, and after treatment with hydrochlorothiazide.

two years, 15 of our diabetic patients exhibited no signs of progressive disturbance in their carbohydrate metabolism. This means that not even all diabetics are liable to show a deterioration in the metabolic imbalance in response to saluretic therapy.

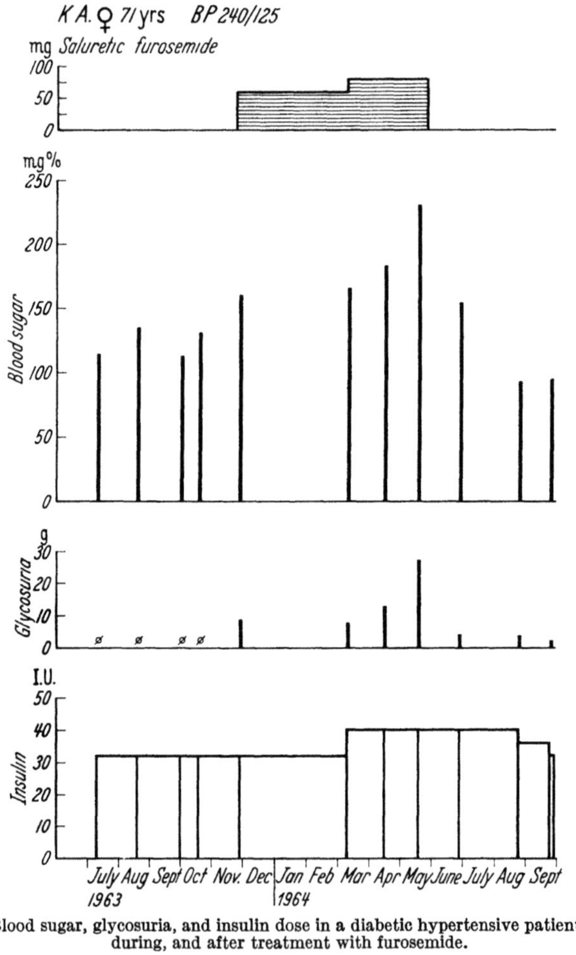

Fig. 6. Blood sugar, glycosuria, and insulin dose in a diabetic hypertensive patient before, during, and after treatment with furosemide.

It should be remembered, however, that either the spontaneous manifestation of, or a spontaneous deterioration in, diabetes is a common occurrence in hypertensive patients in the fifth and sixth decades of life.

The problems associated with hyperuricaemia are in some respects comparable with those raised by hyperglycaemia. Only a small number of patients develop hyperuricaemia. If at all, it

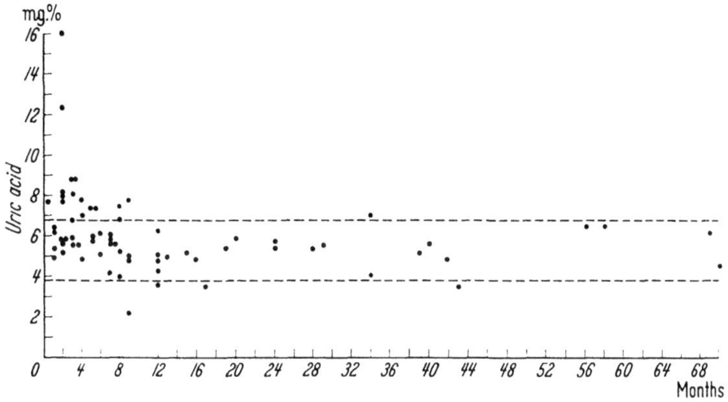

Fig. 7. Concentration of uric acid in the serum of 69 hypertensive patients treated with saluretics for varying periods.

appears immediately (Fig. 7) after the beginning of saluretic treatment, independently of the duration of this treatment. However, within a certain range, there seems to be a correlation between

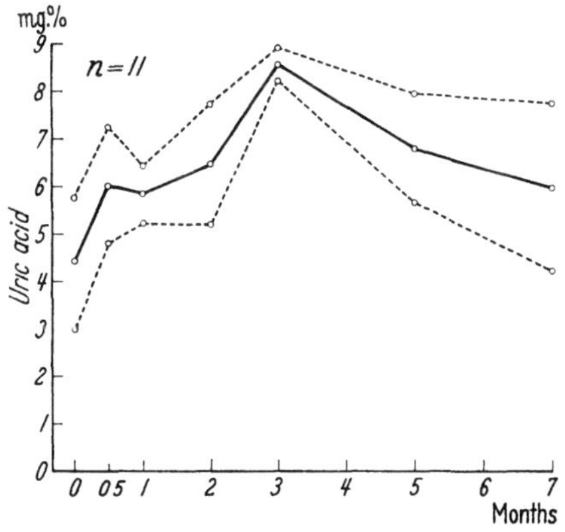

Fig. 8. Concentration of uric acid in serum during long-term therapy with saluretics.

the dose of saluretics given and the incidence and degree of hyperuricaemia. The highest levels of uric acid are reached in the second and third months of saluretic treatment — a phenomenon which cannot be reproduced in acute experiments. The fact that after this time the uric acid level comes down again (Fig. 8), often to normal concentrations, whether saluretic treatment is withdrawn or not, might shed some light on the pathogenic mechanisms which lead to hyperuricaemia. Some adaptation mechanism, probably of an enzymatic nature, that may be localised in the renal tubule, seems to be involved. In two cases an attack of gout occurred during saluretic treatment; one of the patients was already known to suffer from the disease.

The most important metabolic disturbances which may be provoked by saluretic treatment are summarised in Table 2.

Table 2. *Metabolic effects of saluretics*

	Acute experiment	Long-term treatment	Reversibility after interruption of treatment	Progression with continued treatment
Uric acid . . .	—	+	+	—
Carbohydrates .	+	+	(+)	+
Potassium. . .	+	+	+	+

Summary

1. Acute loading with saluretics may produce hypokalaemia, hyperglycaemia, and glycosuria, but not hyperuricaemia.

2. During long-term saluretic treatment, hyperglycaemia and hyperuricaemia may occur in addition to hypokalaemia, but independently of the latter and of each other. Hyperuricaemia is fully reversible, even — in many cases — if treatment is continued. In our series, attacks of gout were precipitated in one gouty patient and in one with normal uric-acid metabolism. Diabetes may develop or, if already present, may deteriorate if special but still unknown conditions, probably of a genetic nature, create a predisposition. In general, the disturbance of carbohydrate metabolism produced by saluretics is either reversible if saluretic treatment is stopped, or can be controlled by antidiabetic therapy even if saluretic treatment is continued.

Zusammenfassung

1. Akute Belastung mit Saluretika kann Hypokaliämie, Hyperglykamie und Glykosurie hervorrufen, jedoch keine Hyperurikämie.

2. Während langdauernder Behandlung mit Saluretika kann eine Hyperglykàmie und eine Hyperurikämie zusätzlich zu einer Hypokaliämie auftreten, und zwar unabhängig von der letzteren und auch unabhängig voneinander. Die Hyperurikämie ist voll reversibel, in vielen Fällen sogar wenn die Behandlung fortgesetzt wird. In unserer Untersuchungsreihe traten Gichtanfälle nur bei einem Patienten auf, der bereits an Gicht litt, und bei einem zweiten mit normalem Harnsäurestoffwechsel. Ein Diabetes kann ausgelöst oder — wenn bereits vorhanden — verschlechtert werden, wenn auf Grund besonderer, bisher noch unbekannter Bedingungen, wahrscheinlich genetischer Natur, eine Prädisposition vorliegt. Im allgemeinen geht die

Storung des Kohlenhydratstoffwechsels, die durch Saluretika verursacht wird, zurück, wenn man die Präparate absetzt, oder sie kann durch eine antidiabetische Behandlung unter Kontrolle gehalten werden, und zwar auch dann, wenn weiterhin Saluretika gegeben werden.

Résumé

1. L'administration aiguë de salidiurétiques peut conduire à l'hypokaliémie, à l'hyperglycémie et à la glycosurie, mais non pas à l'hyperuricémie.

2. Au cours des traitements salidiurétiques prolongés, en plus de l'hypokaliémie peuvent survenir hyperglycémie et hyperuricémie, mais indépendamment l'une de l'autre ainsi que de l'hypokaliémie. L'hyperuricémie est complètement réversible, même — dans beaucoup de cas — si l'on poursuit le traitement. Dans notre série, des attaques de goutte n'ont été déclenchées que chez un goutteux et chez un malade présentant un métabolisme normal de l'acide urique. Un diabète peut apparaître, ou s'aggraver s'il existe déjà, si des conditions spéciales mais encore inconnues, probablement de nature génétique, créent un terrain prédisposé. En général, le trouble du métabolisme des hydrates de carbone provoqué par les salidiurétiques est soit réversible avec leur interruption, soit curable par le traitement antidiabétique si l'administration des salidiurétiques est maintenue.

References

1. Aronoff, A.: N. England J. Med. **262**, 767 (1960). — 2. Aronoff, A., and H. Barkum: Canad. Med. Ass. J. **84**, 1181 (1961). — 3. Ayrazian, J. H., and L. F. Ayrazian: J. Clin. Invest. **40**, 1961 (1961). — 4. Bartorelli, C., N. Gargano, G. Leonetti, and A. Zanchetti: Circulation **27**, 895 (1963). — 5. Bompiani, G. D., and C. Pavino: Clin. terap. **23**, 1125 (1962). — 6. Borhni, N. O.: Ann. Int. Med. **53**, 342 (1960). — 7. Bowlus, W. E., and H. G. Langford: Clin. Pharmacol. Therap. **5**, 708 (1964). — 8. Brahms, O., and K. Kühns: Medizinische **25**, 1213 (1959). — 9. Brest, A. N.: J. Amer. Med. Ass. **185**, 679 (1963). — 10. Brest, A. N., G. Onesti, G. Sekine, R. Seller, and S. H. Moyer: Geriatrics **17**, 752 (1962). — 11. Bryant, J. M., T. F. Yü, L. Berger, N. Schwartz, S. Torosday, L. Fletcher, H. Fertig, M. S. Schwarz, and R. B. F. Quan: Amer. J. Med. **33**, 408 (1962). — 12. Buchborn, E.: Paper read at the 16. Ärztlicher Fortbildungskurs, April 3—4, 1965, Bad Kissingen. — 13. Carliner, N. H., J.-L. Schelling, R. Patterson-Russell, R. Okun, and M. Davis: J. Amer. Med. Ass. **191**, 535 (1965). — 14. Chart, J. J., A. A. Renzi, W. Barrett, and H. Sheppard: Schweiz. med. Wschr. **89**, 325 (1959). — 15. Chase, P. H., and S. L. Wallace: Metabolism **10**, 372 (1961). — 16. Christen, P., and W. Siegenthaler: Praxis **53**, 152 (1964). — 17. Cornish, A. L.: Antibiot. Med. Clin. Therapy **5**, 310 (1958). — 18. Cornish, A. L., J. T. McClellan, and D. H. Johnston: N. England J. Med. **265**, 673 (1961). — 19. Cospite, M., and M. Palazzoadriano: Clin. terap. **25**, 337 (1963). — 20. Cottier, P.: Therap. Umschau **19**, 182 (1962). — 21. Curchod, B.: Diabète **5**, 201 (1960). — 22. D'Addabbo, A., G. Seybold, and E. Kallee: Zschr. exper. Med. **138**, 105 (1964). — 23. Dettli, L., and P. Spring: Dtsch. med. Wschr. **86**, 2327 (1961). — 24. Dollery, C. T., H. Duncan, and G. Schumer: Brit. Med. J. 1960/II, 83. — 25. Dollery, C. T., B. L. Pentecost, and N. A. Samaan: Lancet 1962/II, 735. — 26. Edson, J. N., and J. Schluger: Amer. Heart J. **60**, 641 (1960). — 27. Esch, A. F., I. M.

WILSON, and E. D. FREIS: Med. Ann. District of Columbia 28, 9 (1959). — 28. FERGUSON, M. J.: Amer. J. Cardiol. 7, 568 (1961). — 29. FIELD, J. B., and S. MANDELL: Metabolism 13, 959 (1964). — 30. FINNERTY, F. A., Jr.: In: Hypertension. The First Hahnemann Symposium on Hypertensive Disease. Ed. by J. F. Moyer. W. B. Saunders Company, Philadelphia, 1959, p. 653. — 31. FINNERTY, F. A., Jr., and J. H. BUCHHOLZ: Circulation 18, 718 (1958). — 32. FORMANEK, K.: Wien. klin. Wschr. 75, 211 (1963). — 33. FREEMAN, R. B., and G. G. DUNCAN: Metabolism 9, 1107 (1960). — 34. FREIS, E. D.: In: Hypertension. The First Hahnemann Symposium on Hypertensive Disease. Ed. by J. F. Moyer. W. B. Saunders Company, Philadelphia, 1959, p. 652. — 35. FREIS, E. D.: J. Amer. Med. Ass. 187, 462 (1964). — 36. GEHLE, W.: Med. Klin. 57, 890 (1962). — 37. GOLDNER, M. G., and S. I. BLEICHER: Ärztl. Forsch. 19, 170 (1965). — 38. GOLDNER, M. G., H. ZAROWITZ, and S. AKGUN: N. England J. Med. 262, 403 (1960). — 39. GRANDJEAN, L. C.: Uskr. Laeger 123, 848 (1961). — 40. GREENBERG, S. R., R. G. KLOTZ, P. ROEDIGER, and C. M. ELKINS: Amer. J. Med. Sc. 243, 574 (1962). — 41. GREENBERG, S. R., M. DRESNER, and R. GORCZYCA: Amer. J. Med. Sc. 246, 329 (1963). — 42. GRONBAEK, P., and E. SECHER-HANSEN: Uskr. Laeger 124, 1605 (1962). — 43. HALPRIN, H.: J. Med. Soc. N. Jersey 57, 254 (1960). — 44. HAUMANN, R. L., and J. M. WELLER: Clin. Res. 9, 180 (1961). — 45. HEALEY, L. A., G. J. MAGIT, and J. L. DECKER: N. England J. Med. 261, 1362 (1959). — 46. HEGE, H.: Med. Welt 1962/II, 598. — 47. HEIMSOTH, V., H. DEICHER, D. GÖDECKE, and F. HARTMANN: Dtsch. med. Wschr. 90, 1209 (1965). — 48. HODGE, J. V., F. O. SIMPSON, and G. F. SPEARS: N. Zealand Med. J. 61, 258 (1962). — 49. HOLLIS, W. C.: J. Amer. Med. Ass. 176, 947 (1961). — 50. JOHNSTON, D. H., and A. L. CORNISH: J. Amer. Med. Ass. 170, 2054 (1959). — 51. JONES, M. F., and J. R. CALDWELL: N. England J. Med. 267, 1029 (1962). — 52. KÖNIGSTEIN, R. P.: Wien. med. Wschr. 113, 354 (1963). — 53. KÖNIGSTEIN, R. P., and G. MÄHR: Wien. med. Wschr. 112, 83 (1962). — 54. LAKIN, M., and I. ZEYTINOGLU: J. Amer. Med. Ass. 173, 353 (1960). — 55. LANE, P.: Brit. Med. J. 1960/II, 1383. — 56. LANGDON, R. G., and F. W. WOLFF: Brit. Med. J. 1962/II, 926. — 57. LARAGH, J. H., H. O. HEINEMANN, and F. E. DEMARTINI: J. Amer. Med. Ass. 166, 145 (1958). — 58. LYON, A. F., and A. C. DEGRAFF: Amer. Heart J. 68, 710 (1964). — 59. MACH, R. S., and R. C. DESOUSA: Schweiz. med. Wschr. 93, 1256 (1963). — 60. MARCH, J. F.: Wisconsin Med. J. 62, 257 (1963). — 61. MASSZI, F., and P. VARGA: Zschr. inn. Med. 18, 602 (1963). — 62. MEHNERT, H., H. STÜDLEIN, and H. FÖRSTER: Klin. Wschr. 42, 1099 (1964). — 63. MENG, K., and G. KRONEBERG: Arch. exper. Path. Pharmak. 247, 351 (1964). — 64. MONROE, K. E., L. H. GRANT, A. A. SASAHARA, and D. LITTMANN: N. England J. Med. 261, 290 (1959). — 65. NAIMARK, A., and T. W. FYLES: Canad. Med. Ass. J. 83, 819 (1960). — 66. NICOLAY, K.: Medizinische 43, 2078 (1959). — 67. NICOLE, J. C., and W. PULVER: Helvet. med. acta 29, 556 (1962). — 68. OKUN, R., W. R. WILSON, and M. D. GELFAND: J. Chron. Dis. 17, 31 (1964). — 69. OLIVIER, C.: Presse méd. 72, 1631 (1964). — 70. OREN, B. G., M. RICH, and M. S. BELLE: J. Amer. Med. Ass. 168, 2128 (1958). — 71. RAPOPORT, M. I., and H. F. HURD: Arch. Int. Med. 113, 405 (1964). — 72. REUTTER, F., and A. LABHARDT: Helvet. med. acta 28, 487 (1961). — 73. REUTTER, F., and F. SCHAUB: Dtsch. med. Wschr. 89, 1101 (1964). — 74. RICHTERICH, R.: Klin. Wschr. 37, 355 (1959). — 75. ROEDIGER, P. M., and J. C. HUTCHINSON: Med. Times 92, 1172 (1964). — 76. RUNYAN, J. W., Jr.: N. England J. Med. 267, 541 (1962). — 77. SAMAAN, N. A., C. T. DOL-

LERY, and R. FRASER: Lancet 1963/II, 1244. — 78. SAUDAN, Y., D. MASSON, and B. CURCHOD: Praxis **50**, 45 (1961). — 79. SCHAEFER, H. F.: Med. Welt 1964/I, 922. — 80. SCHLUGER, J., D. RATNER, and J. N. EDSON: Monogr. Therap. **5**, 19 (1960). — 81. SCHÖNDUBE, W., and P. COLLISCHONN: Therap. Gegenw. **100**, 82 (1961). — 82. SCHREIBER, W.: Med. Welt 1963/II, 2146. — 83. SCHWAB, R. H., J. K. PERLOFF, and R. L. PORUS: Arch. Int. Med. **111**, 465 (1963). — 84. SHANKLIN, D. R.: N. England J. Med. **266**, 1097 (1962). — 85. SHAPIRO, A. P., T. G. BENEDEK, and J. L. SMALL: N. England J. Med. **265**, 1028 (1961). — 86. SHELBURNE, P. F., F. A. SASSEN, and E. S. ORGAIN: Amer. J. Med. Sc. **247**, 307 (1964). — 87. SHERLOCK, S.: In: Diuresis and Diuretics. An International Symposium. Ed. by E. BUCHBORN and K. D. BOCK. Springer Verlag, Berlin, 1959, p. 258. — 88. SIEGEL, I. A., and A. DUBIN: Obstet. Gynecol. **15**, 226 (1960). — 89. SMILO, R. P., W. R. BEISEL, and P. H. FORSHAM: N. England J. Med. **267**, 1225 (1962). — 90. SUGAR, S. J. N.: J. Amer. Med. Ass. **175**, 618 (1961). — 91. VEHERANTA, T.: Suom. lääk. aikakausl. **19**, 1569 (1964). — 92. VERBOV, J. L., and N. E. DUDLEY: Brit. J. Clin. Pract. **19**, 29 (1965). — 93. VEYRAT, R.: Méd. et hyg. (Genève) **18**, No. 470, 505 (1960). — 94. VON ROMELING, G.: Münch. med. Wschr. **104**, 2333 (1962). — 95. WARSHAW, L. J.: J. Amer. Med. Ass. **172**, 802 (1960). — 96. WEISSBECKER, L.: Therap.woche **13**, 269 (1963). — 97. WEISSEL, W.: Wien. Zschr. inn. Med. **43**, 389 (1962). — 98. WEISSEL, W., and E. ZIMMERMAN: Wien. klin. Wschr. **76**, 414 (1964). — 99. WETZEL, H.: Med. Klin. **57**, 167 (1962). — 100. WILKINS, R. W.: Schweiz. med. Wschr. 88, 745 (1958). — 101. WILKINS, R. W.: Ann. Int. Med. **50**, 1 (1959). — 102. WOLFF, F. W.: J. Amer. Med. Ass. **185**, 679 (1963). — 103. WOLFF, F. W., and R. G. LANGDON: J. Chron. Dis. **17**, 585 (1964). — 104. WOLFF, F. W., and W. W. PARMLEY: Lancet 1963/II, 69. — 105. WOLFF, F. W., and W. W. PARMLEY: J. Amer. Med. Ass. **188**, 473 (1964). — 106. WOLFF, F. W., and W. W. PARMLEY: Diabetes **13**, 115 (1964). — 107. WOLFF, F. W., W. W. PARMLEY, K. WHITE, and R. OKUN: J. Amer. Med. Ass. **185**, 568 (1963). — 108. ZATUCHNI, I., and F. KORDASZ: Amer. J. Cardiol. **7**, 565 (1961). — 109. ZÖLLERN, N.: Erg. inn. Med. **14**, 334 (1960). — 110. ZWEIFFLER, A. J., and G. R. THOMPSON: Circulation **30**, Suppl. **3**, 181 (1964).

Comparison of long-term effects of saluretics and of anabolic steroids on renal functions

By

A. S. Dontas, N. T. Papanicolaou, and C. S. Cottas

Introduction

The benzothiadiazine diuretics are used by persons with varying degrees of reduced renal function over long periods, often without close medical supervision. It would therefore be of considerable practical value to determine whether their long-term use depresses any of the main renal functions.

As long ago as 1959, Corcoran et al. reported an average decrease in glomerular filtration rate of 29 % in a group of eleven hypertensives treated with 2.0 g. chlorothiazide daily for three to 14 days. Subsequently, Cottier (1960) and Reubi (1961) reported decreases in glomerular filtration rate of 4.9 % and 7.5 % respectively in hypertensives treated with 1.0 g. chlorothiazide daily for four weeks. The changes in renal plasma flow observed by both investigators were not consistent.

These and more recent reports (Reubi, 1963) stress the variability of individual responses to long-term saluretic treatment. According to Reubi's textbook (1961), for instance, the changes in $C_{In.}$ after therapy range from $+31\,\%$ to $-33\,\%$ of the control values. Other reports (e.g. Fairbairn, 1965) indicate that variable azotaemia occurs in about 50 % of non-uraemic patients treated with saluretics; increased urea levels may be present up to three to five years after the initiation of treatment.

Since the renal adjustments to the chronic administration of saluretics might be modified by the course of the underlying disease, it has seemed advisable to study the renal responses in subjects with reduced but stable renal functions. As such, elderly subjects offer several advantages, since in selected cases the impairment of function is due solely to atherosclerosis and not to primary inflammatory processes. Furthermore, homoeostatic mechanisms operate much more slowly in advanced age; thus, any impairment of renal functions will remain evident for longer periods.

On the other hand, the protein-sparing effect of anabolic steroids has been used to achieve a positive nitrogen balance in renal failure (THAYSEN, 1962) and potassium balance in elderly persons (DYMLING et al., 1962). This method of potassium sparing might offer certain advantages over the continuous oral administration of potassium salts in long-term saluretic therapy. There have been no reports on the improvement of specific renal functions in subjects without renal failure. We should therefore like to describe the effects of long-term administration of saluretics and of anabolic steroids on an ambulant basis to two groups of elderly subjects.

Methods

The subjects were selected from a group of 850 ambulant residents of the Athens Home for the Aged. These persons, aged over 60, were clinically healthy upon admission. Their renal plasma flows ranged from one half to two thirds of the accepted normal levels for healthy adults. We chose subjects whose previous history was negative and in whom physical examination revealed no abnormal findings, apart from "arteriosclerotic" hypertension. Their urines showed low-normal Addis counts and bacteria levels and no more than a trace of protein. The males either had no prostatic enlargement or had been operated for it in the past and presented no mechanical obstructions at the time of the study.

Hydrochlorothiazide was administered as sole agent to 42 of these subjects, in a dosage of 50 mg. daily, for as long as possible during the autumn of 1964. The subjects underwent one or two complete renal function tests before the outset of treatment and were studied again three to six months after uninterrupted administration. Only 20 subjects completed the entire cycle; the remainder either discontinued treatment because of hypotension or weakness, or refused to be subjected to a post-therapy renal function test. During the same period, 12 residents of the Home were studied before and after treatment with a total of 150 mg. methandrostenolone (seven subjects) or nandrolone phenylpropionate, administered intramuscularly over a period of one and a half months. No dietary or drug supplements of any kind were used while either study was in progress.

Results

1. Distribution of clearances in our material

The distribution of the clearances of inulin and P.A.H. in our subjects, as compared with the range of "normal" clearance values for healthy adults as given by REUBI, is shown in Fig. 1. It is evident that both clearances, and especially that of P.A.H., are markedly reduced; thus, the filtration fractions are generally high and tend to scatter to the right of the accepted upper normal limit of 0.233. The relatively larger reduction in renal plasma flow is to be expected in subjects with renal vascular sclerosis. In none of the

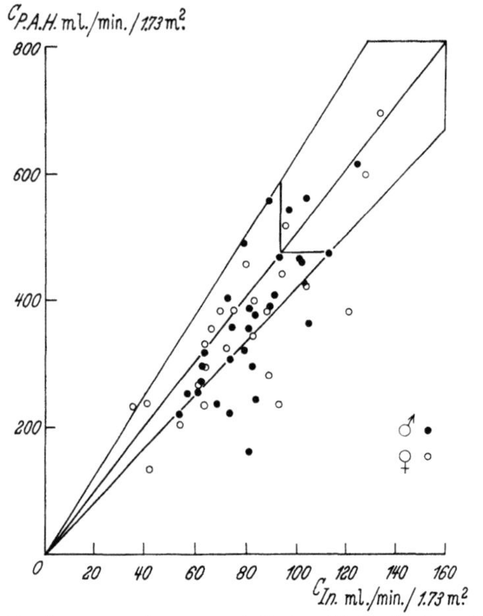

Fig. 1. P. A. H. and inulin clearance in a group of elderly subjects. The framed area corresponds to the range of "normal" clearance values (according to REUBI, 1961).

subjects was the clearance of inulin and P.A.H. less than 35 and 138 ml./min./1.73 m.² respectively. Serum creatinine and blood urea values were normal at the outset of the study.

The relations between simultaneously determined clearances of endogenous, non-chromogen creatinine and of inulin in the same 54 subjects are given in Fig. 2. There is a satisfactory correlation between the two clearances, and the regression line relating the clearance of inulin to that of creatinine is

$$C_{In.} = 5.16 + 0.91 \times C_{Creat.}$$

The correlation coefficient (r) is 0.842, and the standard error of estimate 11.5. In contrast to other authors (REUBI, 1961), we have observed no systematic deviation of the ratio of the two clearances at either end of the distribution of glomerular filtration rates.

Fig. 3 shows the distribution of $T_{m\,P.A.H.}$ values in our subjects in relation to age and indicates that in 30% of these subjects

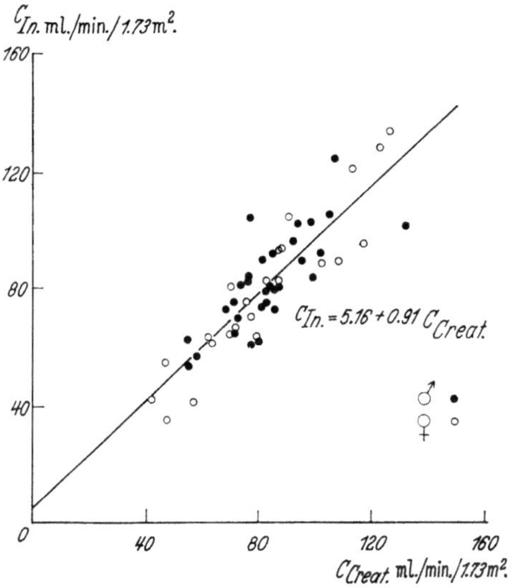

Fig. 2. Correlation between inulin clearance and creatinine clearance in the same subjects as in Fig. 1.

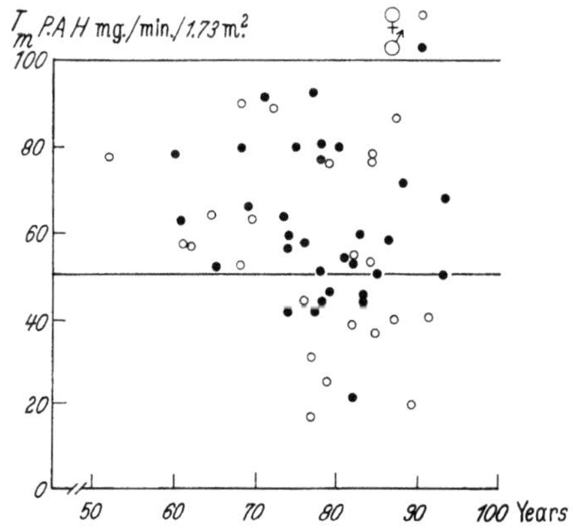

Fig. 3. Tubular secretion of P.A.H. in relation to age in the same group of elderly subjects as in Figs 1 and 2. 50 mg./min./1.73 m.² (horizontal line) is taken as the lower normal limit.

tubular excretory mass was less than the accepted lower normal limit (50 mg./min./1.73 m.²) for middle-aged persons.

2. Changes after saluretic therapy

a) Blood pressure. Mean recumbent blood-pressure values determined during the clearance periods decreased significantly after hydrochlorothiazide to 84.7 % of the control values (Table 1).

Table 1. *Renal haemodynamic effects of prolonged saluretic therapy*

	Control values			Treatment values		
	M.B.P. mm. Hg	$C_{P.A.H.}$ ml./min./ 1.73 m.²	R.R. dyn./sec./ cm.⁻⁵	M.B.P. mm. Hg	$C_{P.A.H.}$ ml./min./ 1.73 m.²	R.R. dyn./sec./ cm.⁻⁵
Means:	133.1	405.2	13.853	112.9	348.8	12.830
S. D.:	23.4	97.1	4.629	23.2	75.1	4.411
(n = 20)				(84.7%)	(86.1%)	(92.6%)
				$p < 0.001$	$p < 0.05$	N. S.

R.R.: renal resistance; S. D.: standard deviation; N. S.: not significant

This fall is equal to that observed by FREIS (1960), but somewhat lower than the levels reported by COTTIER (1960). The difference is probably related to the particular type of hypertension in our elderly group. Five of our subjects were normotensive before treatment, with mean arterial pressures of less than 110 mm. Hg. The average post-treatment mean pressure in these subjects was 84.1 % of the control levels, i.e. equal to that in the remaining subjects. Thus, the increased hypotensive effectiveness of hydrochlorothiazide in our group was not dependent on the presence of hypertension of the arteriosclerotic type, with wide pulse pressure.

b) Renal function. Fig. 4 indicates in graphic form the changes in glomerular filtration rate, renal plasma flow, and maximal tubular excretory capacity for P.A.H. in the 20 subjects who completed the three to six months' therapy with hydrochlorothiazide. Post-treatment values compared with control levels averaged 83.4 % for $C_{In.}$ (t : 2.65), 86.1 % for $C_{P.A.H.}$ (t : 2.04,), and 90.5 % for $T_{m\,P.A.H.}$ (t : 1.15) (Table 2). The reductions in $C_{In.}$ and $C_{P.A.H.}$ were significant at the 1 % and 5 % levels respectively. As a result of the differential decreases of G.F.R. and R.P.F., the mean value of the filtration fraction decreased by 5.5 %. It is of interest to note that the changes in T_m tend to fall into two groups: although the majority evidenced minor changes or definite decreases, marked increases in tubular activity were observed in certain subjects.

The possibility that there might be a correlation between these changes and serum electrolyte changes was investigated. The mean pretreatment and post-treatment levels of serum sodium were almost identical, at 142.5 ± 1.7 and 141.3 ± 1.6 mEq./l. In contrast, serum potassium levels decreased consistently and significantly (mean pretreatment level: 4.86 ± 0.14, post-treatment

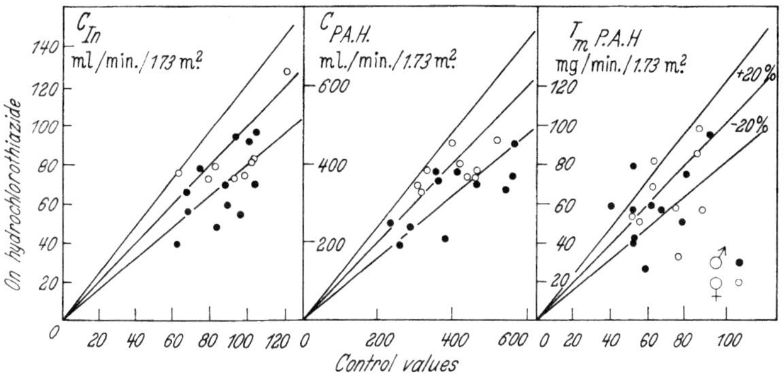

Fig. 4. Renal-function changes after prolonged therapy with hydrochlorothiazide in 20 elderly subjects who completed the experiment. Abscissa: control values; ordinate: values during hydrochlorothiazide treatment.

level: 4.40 ± 0.16 mEq./l.; t : 4.38, $p < 0.001$). If the recorded differences in $C_{In.}$, $C_{P.A.H.}$, and $T_{m\,P.A.H.}$ values are plotted against the difference in serum potassium levels before and after therapy,

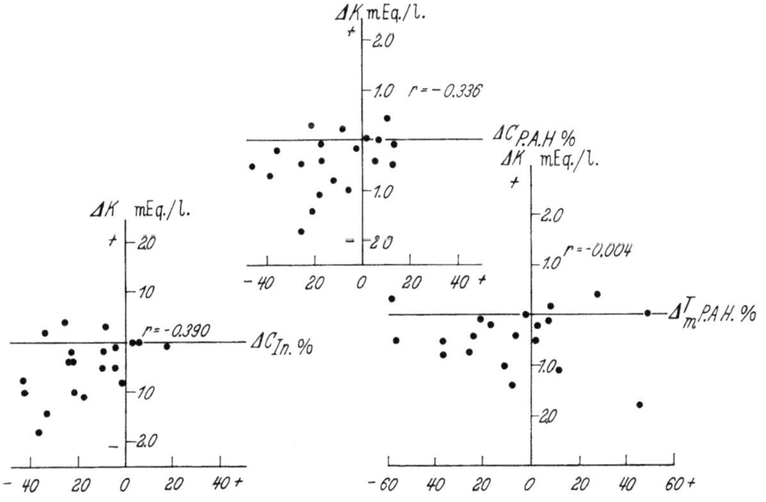

Fig. 5. Correlations between differences in serum potassium levels before and after hydrochlorothiazide treatment, and variations in inulin clearance, P.A.H. clearance, and $T_{m\,P.A.H.}$

Table 2. *Renal functions after prolonged saluretic therapy*

	Control values					Treatment values				
	$C_{Creat.}$	$C_{In.}$	$C_{P.A.H.}$	F.F.	$T_{mP.A.H.}$ mg./min./1.73 m.²	$C_{Creat.}$	$C_{In.}$	$C_{P.A.H.}$	F.F.	$T_{mP.A.H.}$ mg./min./1.73 m.²
	ml./min./1.73 m.²					ml./min./1.73 m.²				
Means:	90.1	89.3	405.2	0.229	67.3	76.1	74.5	348.8	0.217	60.9
S. D.:	16.7	15.4	97.1		15.1	19.1	18.8	75.1		19.1
(n = 20)						(84.5%)	(83.4%)	(86.1%)	(94.5%)	(90.5%)
						$p < 0.01$	$p < 0.01$	$p < 0.05$		N. S.

Explanations as in Table 1

Table 3. *Renal functions after anabolic treatment*

	Control values					Treatment values				
	$C_{Creat.}$	$C_{In.}$	$C_{P.A.H.}$	F.F.	$T_{mP.A.H.}$ mg./min./1.73 m.²	$C_{Creat.}$	$C_{In.}$	$C_{P.A.H.}$	F.F.	$T_{mP.A.H.}$ mg./min./1.73 m.²
	ml./min./1.73 m.²					ml./min./1.73 m.²				
Means:	71.4	70.4	326.6	0.216	40.8	89.5	78.6	398.6	0.199	60.6
S. D.:	19.8	21.4	103.1		14.0	29.7	22.7	126.6		19.4
(n = 12)						(125.5%)	(111.7%)	(122.1%)	(92.1%)	(148.6%)
						$p < 0.01$	$p < 0.01$	N. S.		$p < 0.001$

Explanations as in Table 1

it becomes apparent that there is a low correlation in the case of $\Delta C_{In.}$ and $\Delta C_{P.A.H.}$, but no correlation between $\Delta T_{m\,P.A.H.}$ and ΔK (Fig. 5). The correlation coefficients are 0.390 ($\Delta C_{In.}/\Delta K$), 0.336 ($\Delta C_{P.A.H.}/\Delta K$), and 0.004 ($\Delta T_{m\,P.A.H.}/\Delta K$). None of these r-values is statistically significant.

Total renal resistances, calculated according to Gomez's formula, as given by HOMER SMITH, are indicated in Table 1, along with the changes in mean blood pressure and plasma flow. The mean drop in total renal resistance was 7.4 %. Since cardiac output is not altered during long-term saluretic therapy (CONWAY and LAUWERS, 1960; VILLARREAL et al., 1962a), and since the decrease in mean blood pressure exceeded that of renal resistance in our subjects, vasodilatation must have occurred in other vascular beds.

3. Changes after anabolic therapy

In contrast to the above changes of a generally negative nature, the administration of the two anabolic hormones brought about varying increases in all three renal functions, in addition to the marked feeling of well-being commented upon by our subjects. The changes in $C_{In.}$, $C_{P.A.H.}$, and $T_{m\,P.A.H.}$, observed after six weeks of anabolic therapy, are given in Fig. 6. The mean increase in $C_{In.}$, as

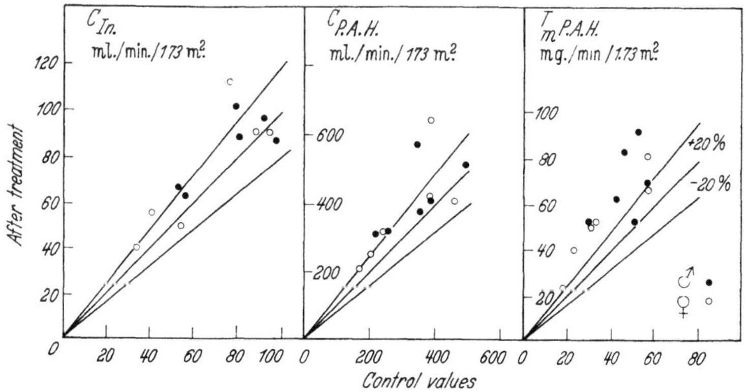

Fig. 6. Effect of anabolic steroids on various renal functions. Abscissa and ordinate as in Fig. 4.

compared with the control values, averaged 11.7 % (t: 2.87, $p < 0.01$), that in $C_{P.A.H.}$ 22.1 % (t: 1.53, $p < 0.2$), and that in $T_{m\,P.A.H.}$ 48.6 % (t: 9.19, $p < 0.001$) (Table 3). As the blood pressure was unaltered by this treatment, total renal resistance fell by an average of 20.6 % (Table 4). The subjects who received anabolic therapy were chosen from one group with relatively high, and a second group with very low, basal renal plasma flow values; thus, the changes in mean R.P.F. and renal resistance were not significant. No difference in the incremental response of R.P.F. was evident between subjects with low and those with high initial R.P.F. values.

Table 4. *Renal haemodynamic effects of anabolic treatment*

	Control values			Treatment values		
	M.B.P. mm. Hg	$C_{P.A.H.}$ ml./min./ 1.73 m.^{2}	R.R. dyn./sec./ cm.$^{-5}$	M.B.P. mm. Hg	$C_{P.A.H.}$ ml./min./ 1.73 m.^{2}	R.R. dyn./sec./ cm.$^{-5}$
Means:	107.6	326.6	13.790	109.2	398.6	10.950
S. D.:	26.6	103.1	6.100	25.3	126.6	4.580
(n = 12)				(101.4%)	(122.1%)	(79.4%)
				N. S.	N. S.	N. S.

Explanations as in Table 1

In two of the subjects receiving anabolic steroids the response to saluretics had been studied, and they continued to receive hydrochlorothiazide throughout the period of anabolic treatment. Apart from a further decline in the $C_{P.A.H.}$ in one of the two, the remaining functions in both subjects returned to, or exceeded, the levels recorded during their pre-diuretic periods.

4. Changes in the ratio of $C_{Creat.}$ to $C_{In.}$ under saluretic and anabolic therapy

The mean value of the $C_{Creat.}/C_{In.}$ ratio in our entire material was 1.04 ± 0.02. In the 20 subjects receiving saluretics, the mean ratio was 1.020 before, and 1.033 at the end of, therapy; this change was not significant. The mean level of serum creatinine in the same subjects increased from 0.85 ± 0.07 mg.% to 0.97 ± 0.07 mg.% in the post-treatment test; this increase was not significant (t: 1.34). However, two subjects with pretreatment serum creatinine levels of 1.05 mg.% and 1.45 mg.% showed elevations to 1.60 mg.% and 1.80 mg.% at the end of treatment.

In contrast, treatment with the two anabolic steroids led to a moderate increase in the $C_{Creat.}/C_{In.}$ ratio in nine of the 12 subjects (1.026 to 1.126), but this change is also not significant (t : 1.97). The serum creatinine levels were not affected by the anabolic therapy (0.95 ± 0.08 mg.% before, 0.93 ± 0.08 mg.% after treatment).

Discussion

This report on the prolonged effects of saluretics on renal haemodynamics is purposely biased as regards the selection of patients and the scope of the end results. As indicated, most of our subjects were elderly hypertensives in no need of therapy, and this study was conducted with the sole aim of testing their capacity to accept saluretic treatment for as long as possible.

More than half of the subjects did not complete the minimum period of treatment with hydrochlorothiazide. In contrast, not a single person among those receiving anabolic therapy withdrew from the programme. The reasons for the interruption of the saluretic treatment were: 1) a rapid decrease in blood pressure to low levels in hypertensives and normotensives, accompanied by occasional spells of dizziness in both; 2) complaints of weakness, irrespective of blood-pressure changes, after more than a few weeks' therapy; these necessitated the reduction of the daily dose of hydrochlorothiazide to less than 25 mg., or intermittent administration; 3) refusal of the subjects to undergo another renal function test at the end of the treatment.

Untoward effects of prolonged diuretic therapy on renal functions can be brought about by three different mechanisms: 1) a direct toxic effect on renal parenchyma; 2) the production of electrolyte disorders, which may induce *per se* glomerular or tubular cell damage; and 3) depression of renal blood flow and glomerular filtration rate by reduction of cardiac output, or its redistribution at the expense of the renal vascular bed.

It has been demonstrated that the direct toxicity of the usual saluretics is very low (Peck et al., 1958; Renzi et al., 1959).

The second mechanism, i.e. drug-induced electrolyte disturbances which by themselves affect renal function, bears some resemblance to the nephropathy of chronic diarrhoeal syndromes (Relman and Schwartz, 1956). Functional impairment paralleling the decreases in serum potassium may be detected if undiscriminating tests, such as the "approximate urea clearance", are used, even in persons receiving potassium supplements (Cranston et al., 1963).

To prevent this potential imbalance, it has become common practice to supplement the saluretic therapy with fixed daily doses of potassium chloride. This practice is not without danger, as discussed earlier in this symposium, quite apart from the fact that kaliuresis is deficient in patients with severely reduced glomerular filtration rates (Reubi and Cottier, 1961). As a result, simultaneous administration of thiazides and potassium salts may lead to rapid increases in serum potassium levels in persons with only moderately reduced glomerular filtration rates (Cottas et al., 1963).

Our present data indicate that severe reduction of one or more of the renal functions may occur without significant hypopotassaemia. The correlation between the decreases in primarily vascular functions, such as G.F.R. or R.P.F., and those in serum potassium is low; furthermore, there is no correlation between the changes in renal tubular cell activity and those in serum potassium. Thus, electrolyte disturbances of the reported magnitude are probably not the cause of the decreases in renal function, but rather a parallel indicator of a common circulatory disturbance.

The third mechanism of renal impairment by saluretics is worthy of closer consideration, since the acute and the chronic effects of saluretics on systemic haemodynamics are prominent and are exerted on different targets.

It has long been known that the acute haemodynamic effects of the saluretics in man are a reduction in plasma volume, cardiac output (Wilson and Freis, 1959; Dustan et al., 1959), and glomerular filtration rate levels (Crosley et al., 1960; Villarreal et al., 1962b). In contrast, after chronic administration, plasma volume and cardiac output are not affected, whereas total peripheral resistance is grossly reduced (Conway and Lauwers, 1960; Villarreal et al., 1962a). It is also accepted that hypotension will occur only in hypertensive, but not in normotensive persons (Freis et al., 1958; Freis, 1960; Wilkins et al., 1958).

Most of these data have been obtained in young or middle-aged hypertensives with normal cardiac outputs. With advancing age, however, resting cardiac output is significantly reduced (Brandfonbrener et al., 1955), and, in addition, the recovery of most functions following any stress is delayed. Thus, the basic differences between our subjects and those of previous studies are a lower initial cardiac output and a tendency to recover more slowly following the early phase of diuretics. As a result, our elderly normotensives showed reductions in resting blood pressures equal to those found in the elderly hypertensives. Orthostatic decreases in pressure exceeding those observed during the clearance period were quite common in our subjects; these decreases were the principal cause of the refusal of the majority of the subjects to carry on with thiazide therapy.

Various investigators have reported varying degrees of reduction in renal haemodynamics after prolonged chlorothiazide treatment (Corcoran et al., 1959; Cottier, 1960; Reubi, 1961). The reported mean decrements in G.F.R. range from 5 % (Cottier) to

29 % (CORCORAN et al.) of the control values. There is no doubt that the length of treatment, the daily dosage, and the age of the subjects determine the final extent of renal impairment as well as the subsequent progress of the disease. In acute studies (CROSLEY et al., 1960; VILLARREAL et al., 1962b) and the shorter "long-term" studies (CORCORAN et al., 1959), the reductions in G.F.R. are larger than those observed in the longer "long-term" studies (COTTIER, 1960). The present data indicate that several months of saluretic therapy in elderly hypertensives will decrease the G.F.R. by amounts equal to those observed in short-term studies in middle-aged adults; furthermore, that significant decreases in renal plasma flow and in tubular activity will be present in individual patients, not necessarily in those persons with the highest initial plasma flow levels. Serial clearances of creatinine should be of help as a warning indicator, in view of their high correlation with the clearance of inulin and the ease with which they can be carried out.

The equal decrease in blood pressure and renal plasma flow in our subjects indicates that renal homoeostatic adjustments are virtually absent and that the reduction in total peripheral resistance due to saluretics is brought about by way of other vascular beds.

In contrast to hydrochlorothiazide, the two anabolic agents increased all renal functions by varying degrees in a smaller group of elderly subjects, without affecting their blood pressures. To our knowledge, this is the first group of substances shown to cause long-lasting increases in all three renal functions. T_m values in particular have been most strikingly and consistently enhanced. The improved tubular function is also evidenced by the small increase in the ratio of $C_{Creat.}$ to $C_{In.}$. This agrees with recent experimental findings made by O'CONNELL et al. (1962) in male dogs or in female dogs treated with testosterone; in these animals, peak stop-flow creatinine U/P over inulin U/P ratios increased after testosterone, indicating creatinine secretion. Such observations offer an explanation for the discrepant reports in the literature on the validity of the clearance of creatinine as an indicator of glomerular filtration rate in man.

Simultaneous administration of enteric-coated potassium chloride and saluretics has aroused criticism lately for a variety of theoretical and practical reasons. Since anabolic agents can achieve positive potassium balance in the aged (DYMLING et al., 1962) and have been shown herein to improve the over-all renal functional status, they could be used beneficially as a supplement to long-term saluretic treatment. Of course, these agents should be used on subjects in whom the potential androgenic effects of the steroids do not create a problem.

Summary

In a group of 20 elderly hypertensive and normotensive residents of a Home for the Aged, renal functions were studied before and after three to six months of therapy with 50 mg. hydrochlorothiazide daily. These subjects had renal plasma flows (R.P.F.) averaging 60% and glomerular filtration rates (G.F.R.) averaging 70% of those of middle-aged persons.

Blood pressure was reduced in all subjects, including the few normotensives who completed the period of treatment. At the end of treatment, $C_{In.}$ and $C_{P.A.H.}$ were significantly decreased to means of 83.4% and 86.1% of the respective control values, while $T_{m\,P.A.H.}$ decreased — though not significantly — to 90.5%. A moderate hypopotassaemia developed in all subjects, but no significant correlation between it and the decrease in $C_{In.}$ or $C_{P.A.H.}$ was present. Tubular functional mass changes were quite unrelated to changes in serum potassium.

Since the average reduction in mean blood pressure (—15.3%) equalled that of renal plasma flow, whereas total renal resistance was not consistently reduced (—7.8%), decrease in vascular resistance must have occurred in beds other than the renal.

Diametrically opposite renal functional responses were obtained by administration of 150 mg. methandrostenolone or nandrolone phenylpropionate over a six-week period to 12 subjects, two of whom were simultaneously receiving hydrochlorothiazide. Significant increases in G.F.R. and $T_{m\,P.A.H.}$ were observed; R.P.F. and renal resistance increased and decreased respectively, but these changes were not significant. Anabolic treatment did not affect blood pressures or the serum levels of sodium and potassium. The possibility that anabolic steroids could be used in long-term saluretic therapy to forestall renal functional impairment might be worthy of clinical trial.

Zusammenfassung

Bei einer Gruppe von 20 hypertonen und normotonen Insassen eines Altersheimes wurde die Nierenfunktion vor und nach einer drei bis sechs Monate langen täglichen Behandlung mit 50 mg Hydrochlorothiazid untersucht. Im Vergleich zu Personen mittleren Alters hatten die Probanden eine Nierendurchblutung von ungefähr 60% und ein Glomerulumfiltrat von durchschnittlich 70%.

Der Blutdruck nahm bei allen Versuchspersonen ab, auch bei den wenigen normotonen, die die Behandlungsperiode beendeten. Bei Abschluß der Behandlung waren die C_{In} und die $C_{P.A.H.}$ signifikant vermindert auf Mittelwerte von 83,4% und 86,1% der betreffenden Kontrollwerte, während die $T_{m\,P.A.H.}$ nur in nicht signifikanter Weise auf 90,5% abnahm. Bei allen Personen trat eine mäßige Hypokaliämie auf, jedoch bestand keine eindeutige Korrelation zwischen ihr und der Abnahme von C_{In} oder $C_{P.A.H.}$. Die Änderungen der tubulären Gesamtfunktion standen in keinem Verhältnis zu den Änderungen im Plasmakalium.

Da die durchschnittliche Verminderung des mittleren Blutdruckes (—15,3%) gleich war wie diejenige der Nierendurchblutung, während der Gesamtnierenwiderstand nicht wesentlich abnahm (—7,8%), muß der Gefäßwiderstand in anderen Gefäßgebieten als in der Niere zurückgegangen sein.

Diametral entgegengesetzte Nierenfunktionsänderungen ergaben sich bei 12 Versuchspersonen unter der Gabe von 150 mg Methandrostenolon oder Nandrolon-phenylpropionat während einer Periode von sechs Wochen. Zwei von ihnen erhielten gleichzeitig Hydrochlorothiazid. Glomerulumfiltrat und

$T_{m\ P.A.H.}$ stiegen signifikant an; die Nierendurchblutung nahm leicht zu, der Nierenwiderstand etwas ab, beide jedoch nicht in signifikanter Weise. Die Behandlung mit anabolen Steroiden beeinflußte weder den Blutdruck noch die Plasmakonzentration von Natrium oder Kalium. Die Möglichkeit, anabole Steroide während einer Langzeittherapie mit Saluretika anzuwenden, um einer Verschlechterung der Nierenfunktion vorzubeugen, ist eines Versuches wert.

Résumé

Les fonctions rénales d'un groupe de 20 sujets âgés, hypertendus et normotendus, pensionnaires d'une maison de vieillards, ont été étudiées avant et après un traitement de trois à six mois de 50 mg d'hydrochlorothiazide par jour. Ces sujets avaient un flux plasmatique rénal et une filtration glomérulaire en moyenne de 60% et 70%, respectivement, de ceux des personnes d'âge moyen.

La tension artérielle a diminué chez tous les sujets, y compris les quelques normotendus qui suivirent le traitement. A la fin du traitement, les C_{In} et $C_{P.A.H.}$ ont été abaissées de façon significative jusqu'à 83,4% et 86,1%, respectivement, des valeurs initiales de contrôle, tandis que le $T_{m\ P.A.H.}$ a diminué — bien que de façon non significative — jusqu'à 90,5%. Une hypokaliémie modérée s'est installée chez tous les sujets, mais aucune corrélation significative n'a été trouvée entre cette hypokaliémie et la diminution de la C_{In} ou de la $C_{P.A.H.}$. Les modifications de la masse tubulaire fonctionnelle ont été sans aucune relation avec les modifications du potassium sérique.

Puisque la diminution dans l'ensemble de la pression artérielle moyenne (—15,3%) s'est montrée égale à celle du flux plasmatique rénal, tandis que la résistance rénale totale n'a pas notablement diminué (—7,8%), c'est qu'une diminution de la résistance vasculaire s'est certainement développée dans des territoires autres que le territoire rénal.

Des réponses diamétralement opposées de la fonction rénale ont été obtenues après administration de 150 mg de méthandrosténolone ou de phénylpropionate de nandrolone pendant six semaines chez 12 sujets, dont deux recevaient simultanément de l'hydrochlorothiazide. Une augmentation significative de la filtration glomérulaire et du $T_{m\ P.A.H.}$ a été observée; le flux plasmatique rénal et la résistance rénale ont, le premier augmenté, la seconde diminué, mais de façon non significative. Le traitement anabolisant n'a pas modifié la pression artérielle ni les taux de sodium et de potassium sériques. La possibilité d'utilisation d'un stéroide anabolisant avec le traitement salidiurétique prolongé en vue de prévenir l'altération des fonctions rénales mériterait d'être expérimentée cliniquement.

Acknowledgements

This work was supported in part by grants from the World Health Organization and the Royal Hellenic Research Foundation. Dr. Nathan W. Shock, Baltimore City Hospitals, kindly supplied all inulin and sodium para-aminohippurate used. Dr. George Michalis, CIBA Athens, provided valuable support.

References

Brandfonbrener, M., M. Landowne, and N. W. Shock: Circulation **12**, 557 (1955). — Conway, J., and P. Lauwers: Circulation **21**, 21 (1960). — Corcoran, A. C., C. Macleod, H. P. Dustan, and I. H. Page: Circulation **19**,

355 (1959). — COTTAS, C. S., N. T. PAPANICOLAOU, and A. S. DONTAS: J. Geront. **18**, 155 (1963). — COTTIER, P. T.: Helvet. med. acta **27**, Suppl. **34** (1960). — CRANSTON, W. I., B. E. JUEL-JENSEN, A. M. SEMMENCE, R. P. C. HANFIELD JONES, J. A. FORBES, and L. M. M. MUTCH: Lancet 1963/II, 966. — CROSLEY, A. P., Jr., R. C. CULLEN, D. WHITE, J. F. FREEMAN, C. A. CASTILLO, and G. G. ROWE: J. Laborat. Clin. Med. **55**, 182 (1960). — DUSTAN, H. P., G. R. CUMMING, A. C. CORCORAN, and I. H. PAGE: Circulation **19**, 360 (1959). — DYMLING, J.-F., B. ISAKSSON, and B. SJÖGREN: In: Protein Metabolism. An International Symposium. Ed. by F. GROSS. Springer, Berlin, 1962, p. 412. — FAIRBAIRN, J. F.: In: Cardiovascular Drug Therapy. The Eleventh Hahnemann Symposium. Ed. by A. N. BREST and J. H. MOYER. Grune and Stratton, New York, 1965, p. 24. — FREIS, E. D.: In: Essential Hypertension. An International Symposium. Ed. by K. D. BOCK and P. T. COTTIER. Springer, Berlin, 1960, p. 179. — FREIS, E. D., A. WANKO, I. M. WILSON, and A. E. PARRISH: Ann. N. Y. Acad. Sc. **71**, 450 (1958). — O'CONNELL, J. M. B., J. A. ROMEO, and G. H. MUDGE: Amer. J. Physiol. **203**, 985 (1962). — PECK, H. M., S. E. McKINNEY, J. E. BAER, E. C. McMANUS, and K. H. BEYER: J. Pharmacol. Exper. Therap. **122**, 60 (1958). — RELMAN, A. S., and W. B. SCHWARTZ: N. England J. Med. **255**, 195 (1956). — RENZI, A. A., J. J. CHART, and R. GAUNT: Toxicol. Appl. Pharmacol. **1**, 406 (1959). — REUBI, F. C.: Néphrologie Clinique. Masson et Cie, Paris, 1961. — REUBI, F. C.: Clearance Tests in Clinical Medicine. Thomas, Sprinfield, Ill., 1963. — REUBI, F. C., and P. T. COTTIER: Circulation **23**, 200 (1961). — THAYSEN, J. H.: In: Protein Metabolism. An International Symposium. Ed. by F. GROSS. Springer, Berlin, 1962, p. 450. — VILLARREAL, H., J. E. EXAIRE, A. REVOLLO, and J. SONI: Circulation **26**, 405 (1962a). — VILLARREAL, H., A. REVOLLO, J. C. EXAIRE, and F. LARRONDO: Circulation **26**, 409 (1962b). — WILKINS, R. W., W. HOLLANDER, and A. V. CHOBANIAN: Ann. N. Y. Acad. Sc. **71**, 465 (1958). — WILSON, I. M., and E. D. FREIS: Circulation **20**, 1028 (1959).

Discussion

Reubi: Before we proceed to the discussion of the papers on diuretics, I'd like to ask Dr. Mach to make some remarks.

Mach: I should like to illustrate briefly two side effects encountered during short-term treatment with saluretic agents. After having observed

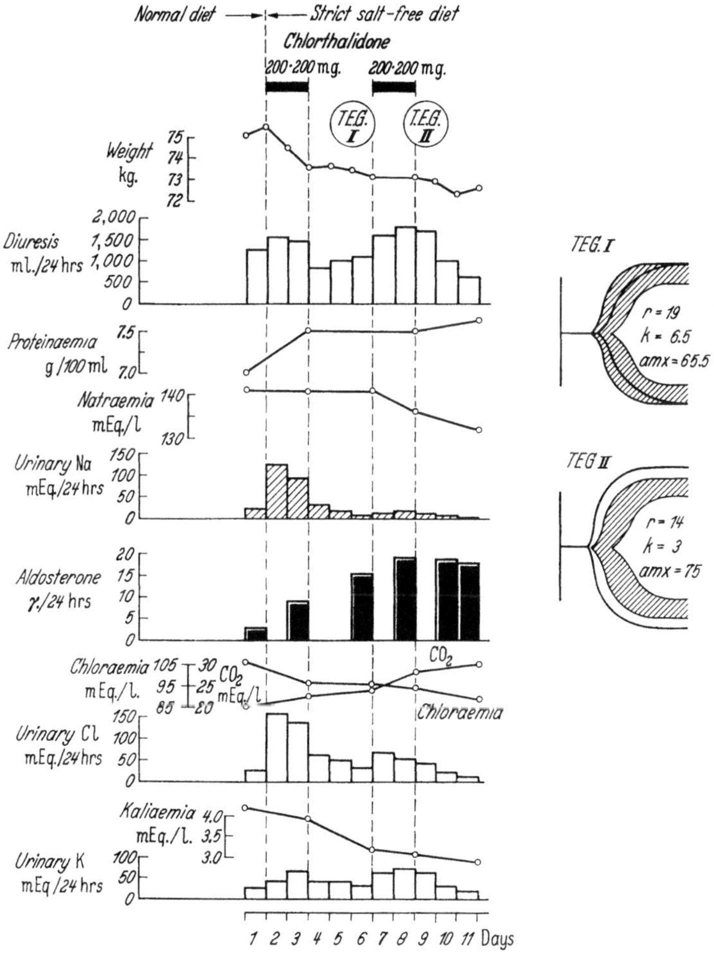

Fig. 1. Effect of the administration of a saluretic (chlorthalidone) in a healthy 55-year-old female subject during sodium-restricted diet. T.E.G. (thrombelastogram) is given on the right side of the figure.

two cases of cerebral thrombosis during acute administration of saluretics, we studied, together with Dr. VEYRAT, the effects of these agents on haemodynamic and coagulation factors. Fig. 1 shows the effects of the administration of a saluretic agent to a normal subject. There is a loss of weight, an

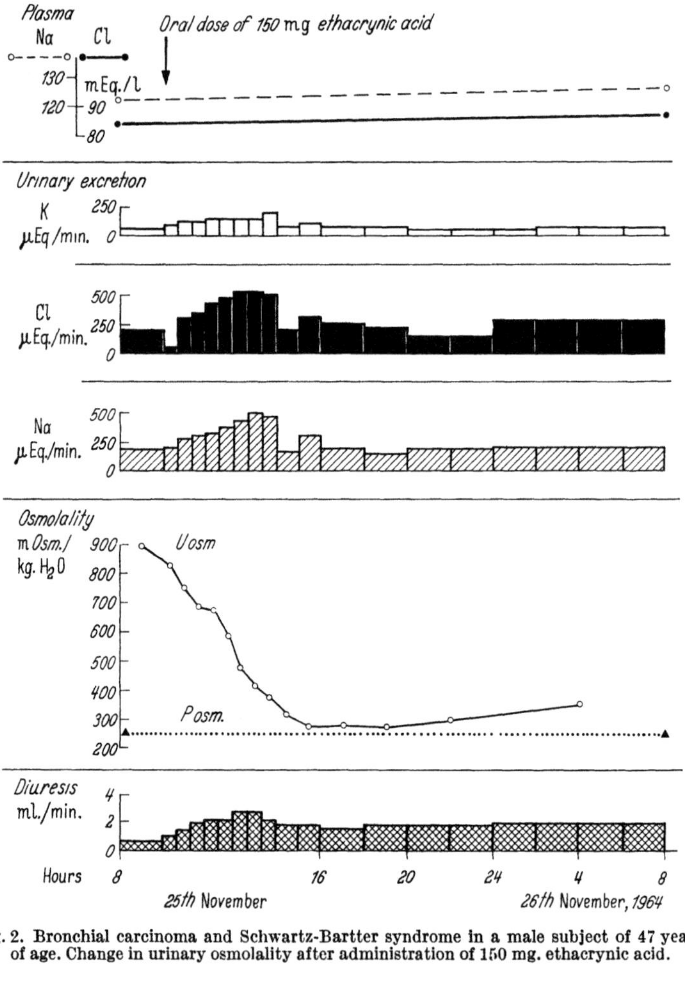

Fig. 2. Bronchial carcinoma and Schwartz-Bartter syndrome in a male subject of 47 years of age. Change in urinary osmolality after administration of 150 mg. ethacrynic acid.

increase in serum protein, an enhanced natriuresis and kaliuresis with hypokalaemia, an increase in aldosterone excretion, alkalosis, and changes in the thrombelastogram which have a relative value but show clearly a decrease in the reaction time. We think there may be a danger, in older patients, in producing by means of such a powerful agent an excessively acute and massive reduction of extracellular fluid, with all its consequences as regards the coagulation factors.

The second point I should like to stress is the clinical importance of hyponatraemia and its correction in patients with hypertension and congestive heart failure. In such patients, the aim of treatment is not to remove salt but to increase free water clearance. Of the many diuretic agents we have studied, the only one we have found effective in correcting hyponatraemia and in decreasing urinary osmotic concentration is ethacrynic acid. We have recently had the opportunity to study, together with DE SOUSA and JENNY, two cases of Schwartz-Bartter syndrome due to lung carcinoma with inadequate secretion of antidiuretic hormone. Hyponatraemia was corrected by administering ethacrynic acid, leading to an increase in free water clearance (Fig. 2). This aspect of hyponatraemia and water intoxication resulting from abusive administration of potent saluretic agents remains a major problem at the present time. It is a clear indication for the orientation of our research efforts.

REUBI: I should now like to ask Dr. BARTORELLI or Dr. LEONETTI how they visualise the problem of potassium substitution in thiazide-treated patients. This was not absolutely clear to me from their conclusions.

LEONETTI: I touched on this problem in my paper but I am grateful to have the opportunity to stress the point again. In our Fig. 7 we have shown that daily oral potassium supplements of 50 mEq., although they increase the potassium stores slightly, activate natriuresis and reduce plasma volume; no change in blood pressure ensues. It seems that the reduction of one hypotensive factor, the chronic one, i.e. potassium loss, is effectively counterbalanced by the reinstitution of the acute hypotensive factors, sodium loss and plasma volume decrease. Therefore there is no reason why one should not give potassium to a hypertensive subject receiving benzothiazides, if one wants to correct the annoying symptoms of hypopotassaemia; blood pressure will be kept down by the subsequent activation of natriuresis.

COTTIER: Dr. LEONETTI, did you perform any studies with regard to the intensity of intestinal potassium reabsorption in various degrees of hypopotassaemia?

Another question to the experts of this meeting: — How does it come about that hypopotassaemia is usually well tolerated by hypertensive patients on prolonged saluretic therapy?

LEONETTI: I think the answer to the first question is no. We never tried to see how fast and complete potassium reabsorption is. However, we are going to perform some experiments of this type very soon, giving potassium to patients under long-term diuretic treatment and measuring the rate of potassium disappearance from serum.

As to the second question, we don't know why, but some patients are able to have a serum potassium level as low as 2.5 or 2.8 or perhaps lower, without any complaints.

PETERS: I wish to comment briefly on Dr. HARTMANN's findings with regard to carbohydrate metabolism. The so-called diabetogenic effect of thiazide diuretics appears to correspond to three different phenomena. One is an increase in blood sugar in individuals given a single, large dose of a diuretic: rather unexpectedly, it does not seem to be related to dehydration. The decrease in glucose tolerance observed in a large fraction of non-diabetic patients after some days or weeks of treatment is quite a different effect. It is not comparable to "pre-diabetes", since it is always completely reversible. Another fundamental difference may be reflected in the "typical" insulin-like activity of the blood, which is high in a majority of pre-diabetics but appears to be low in some of the patients treated with thiazides. This latter finding needs confirmation. The third phenomenon would be an acute increase in blood sugar in the hours following a single, very large oral dose of a diuretic. This type of hyperglycaemic response was first found in rats after diazoxide[1], but also to a lesser extent after thiazide diuretics. We could not reproduce it with reasonably high doses of hydrochlorothiazide. The intraperitoneal dose of hydrochlorothiazide necessary for inducing a significant rise in blood sugar in the rat within an hour has recently been found to be 320 mg./kg.[2]

Dollery: I should like to comment on Dr. Hartmann's paper and Dr. Peters' gloss on it. I do not entirely agree with Dr. Hartmann's findings concerning uric acid. We have measured the uric acid in our patients on thiazides over a period of some years and found that about 65% of them have serum uric-acid levels above 7 mg.%.

The second point I wish to raise concerns the diabetogenic effects of thiazides. Recently we have completed a study of 32 patients who have been on thiazides continuously for more than three years. Eleven of these patients were diabetic, as judged by a blood sugar of more than 120 mg./100 ml. two hours after a 50 g. glucose load. This incidence is twice as high as would be predicted from the number of diabetics discovered in normal populations by survey techniques. Furthermore, some of these patients are improving after withdrawal of diuretics.

Nine of the 11 patients have higher than normal levels of insulin in their blood, as measured either by the immunochemical assay or a bio-assay. This is the same pattern as that seen in obese diabetics, but only one of these patients was obese. Two patients with more severe diabetes (blood sugars over 200 mg./100 ml. at two hours) had low levels of insulin in their blood, as measured by both methods, and the insulin concentration failed to rise in response to the glucose load.

Another six patients who had developed symptomatic diabetes on thiazides but were not studied during this survey also had low levels of insulin in their blood. Our present hypothesis concerning the diabetogenic effects of thiazides is that they first interfere with the peripheral action of insulin and that later some of the patients exhaust their pancreas and develop more severe diabetes.

Reubi: I should like to add one comment to Dr. Peters' remark. There is, I think, a fourth possibility as regards decreased glucose tolerance in such cases, namely that it is simply due to chronic hypokalaemia. Chronic hypokalaemia of any origin may produce a diminished glucose tolerance. However, I am sure that in most cases being treated with diuretics there is no marked hypokalaemia. Thus, this factor is probably not very important.

I should like to ask Dr. Hartmann whether he has any experience with furosemide, because it has been asserted that furosemide does not decrease glucose tolerance and does not cause diabetes.

---

[1] Wolff, F. W., and W. W. Parmley: Diabetes **13**, 115 (1964).

[2] Tabachnick, I. I. A., A. Gulbenkian, and A. Yannell: Life Sc. **4**, 1931 (1965).

Smirk: I should like to know whether Dr. Dollery's cases were hypertensives or normotensives.

Dollery: The control data were based on a population survey carried out by Dr. Butterfield of Guy's Hospital.

Smirk: We have found an appreciable incidence of impairment in the glucose tolerance test in hypertensive patients who are not receiving thiazides.

Hartmann: Among our 1,092 patients with hypertension, 32% had manifest diabetes and, in addition, 30% latent diabetes. There is a very high incidence of latent diabetes in patients with hypertension. We couldn't find a correlation between the potassium level and glucose tolerance.

Reubi: Glucose tolerance is impaired only in cases with chronic hypokalaemia.

Hartmann: We saw one case of diabetes which deteriorated under treatment with furosemide and a decreased glucose tolerance in three or four cases in acute experiments.

Reubi: Was it a clear-cut case?

Hartmann: I think so.

Reubi: Is there no doubt about it?

Hartmann: No.

Reubi: Has anybody else observed such cases after furosemide?

Lagerlöf: Large doses of thiazides may be accompanied by increased serum amylase values, indicating pancreatitis. Necroses are also seen in the gland. As disturbances of the carbohydrate metabolism are common in pancreatitis, this mechanism could be responsible for decreased glucose tolerance.

Brest: I should like to comment on the effect of diuretics on electrolyte excretion and on relating the effect of electrolyte changes upon parameters such as blood pressure, renal function, and the like. I think it is very difficult to speculate on such effects unless one can look at the total electrolyte spectrum. Most studies have dealt mainly with sodium and potassium. However, magnesium is also a major intracellular ion. Our studies indicate that diuretics cause a significant magnesuria. This results in significant changes in blood magnesium as well as magnesium concentration in red blood cells. These alterations must be taken into account when considering the effect of ionic changes on vascular reactivity.

Diagnosis and treatment of renovascular and other forms of renal hypertension

Diagnosis of renal artery stenosis

By

W. S. PEART

The diagnosis of renal artery disease can be approached from a number of directions, and many of these are to be discussed in detail by subsequent speakers. I should like to take this opportunity, therefore, to make some preliminary dogmatic utterances.

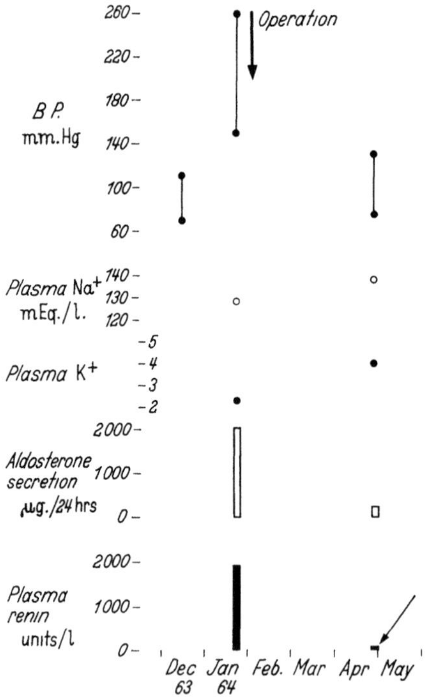

Fig. 1. Findings in a patient with the development of acute hypertension due to renal artery stenosis, cured by surgery. Note the low plasma sodium and potassium pre-operatively.

Clinical manifestations

There are very few clinical manifestations which enable the diagnosis to be made with any certainty, either from the history or from examination of the patient. The occasional abrupt onset of malignant hypertension with severe retinal changes and heavy proteinuria, associated with a history of weakness, polyuria and cramps due to both sodium and potassium loss in the urine, may make the diagnosis of acute renal artery stenosis more certain (Fig. 1) (DEMING, 1954; FITZGERALD et al., 1957; DOLLERY et al., 1959; FITZ and ARMSTRONG, 1964). In some cases, infarction of the kidney is heralded by pain in the loin, but on the whole there is little to distinguish those hypertensive patients with renal artery stenosis from those without it. The presence of an upper abdominal murmur, while often due to a renal artery stenosis (PEART and ROB, 1960), is often not so associated, and it could not be labelled as a certain diagnostic sign.

Special investigations

1. Pyelogram. This is of the greatest help, and about 75% of cases of definitely proven renal artery stenosis in our series at St. Mary's Hospital have had diagnostic pyelograms (BROWN et al., 1960). It is important to realise that the pyelogram must be carried out without lower abdominal compression, since one is looking for differences in urine flow and dye intensity between the two kidneys. The conventional compression pyelogram can obscure the picture. On the whole, the ordinary type of pyelogram with dehydration after overnight fasting suffices to show the characteristic picture, which is based on the fact that reduction in renal blood flow leads to increased water reabsorption and increased concentration of filtered, non-reabsorbed substances, such as the dyes used in pyelography. With very low blood flow, there is a delay in the appearance of the pyelogram in films taken at one, three, and five minutes (Fig. 2a), and in the later films, the size of the collecting system is smaller and the concentration of dye more intense (Fig. 2b). When the dye is slow to appear, the kidney is always small, since the stenosis is very tight. Although the kidney is usually smaller, this may not always be easily discernible, even in the presence of an increased concentration of dye, showing that a functional change is present. Sometimes, of course, a difference in the concentration of dye is due to disease in one kidney, leading to a failure of water reabsorption, e.g. pyelonephritis, and this is not always easy to diagnose on the pyelogram. Manipulation of the pyelographic appearances can be carried out by water-loading, which, by increasing the urine flow more in the normal kidney, will wash out the picture, leaving the kidney with the stenosed artery standing out clearly (Fig. 3a and b). On the whole, like the delayed appearance, this is a frill which does not add much more to the ordinary pyelogram.

2. Isotopic renogram. Since this technique was introduced by TAPLIN et al. (1956), it has been widely used and subsequently modified to give greater precision (WINTER et al., 1961). It is obviously a subjective technique made semi-quantitative and is capable of yielding false positives and negatives. The difficulty clearly lies in the aiming of the collimated tubes collecting the counts from the kidneys. Development of the scintiscanning renogram (MCAFEE and WAGNER, 1960) promises to add a little more

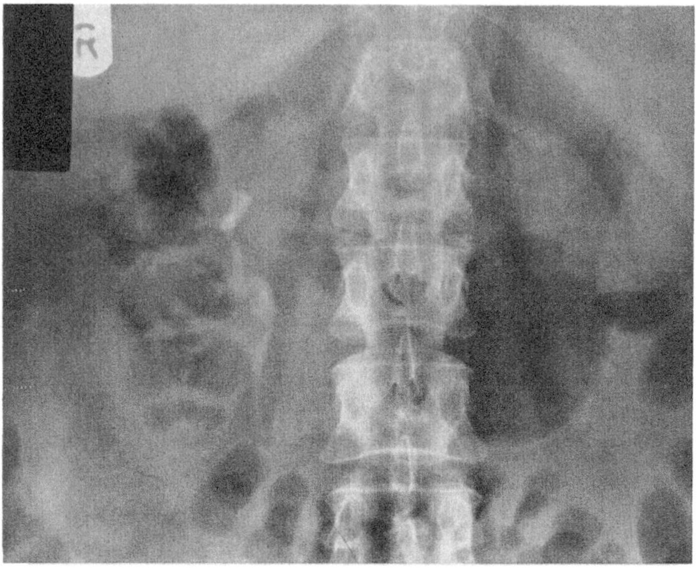

a

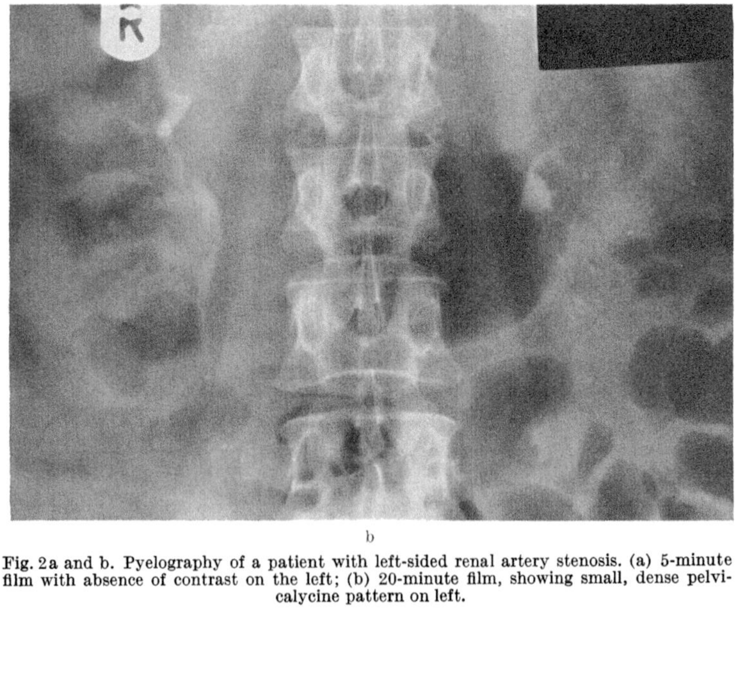

b

Fig. 2a and b. Pyelography of a patient with left-sided renal artery stenosis. (a) 5-minute film with absence of contrast on the left; (b) 20-minute film, showing small, dense pelvi-calycine pattern on left.

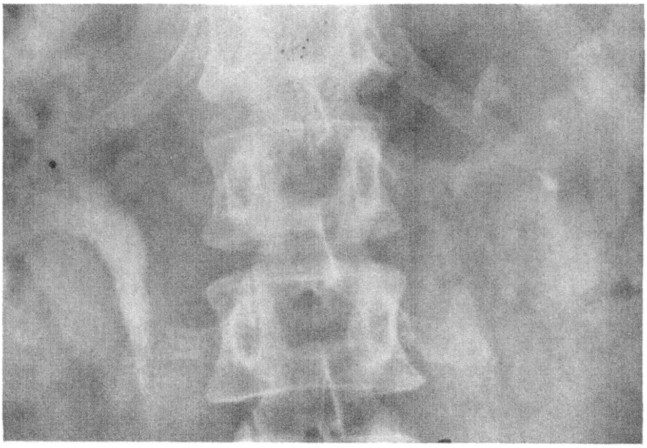

a

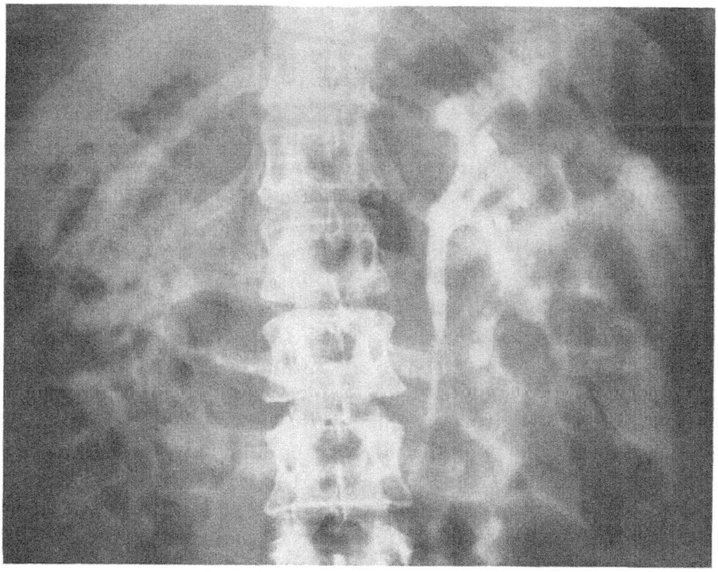

b

Fig. 3a and b. Pyelogram of a patient with left renal artery stenosis. (a) Dehydrated. Small pelvi-calycine system on left; (b) After water-load. Pyelogram on right washed out and on left (stenosis) standing out clearly.

quantitation, but this process is not yet ideal (Fig. 4). Both these techniques will probably be superseded by the gamma camera which gives simultaneous scans of both kidneys (ANGER, 1958; MALLARD and MYERS, 1963).

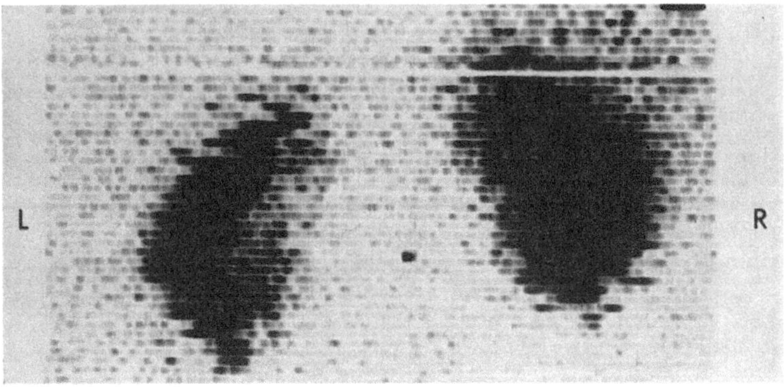

Fig. 4. Renal scintigram — Neohydrin Hg. 203. Left kidney smaller than right. Left-sided renal artery stenosis.

3. Arteriography. Various techniques, each with its own advantages and disadvantages, are used (BROWN et al., 1960; SUTTON, 1962), but the main principle to be observed is that arteriography should not be undertaken with any technique unless the blood pressure is first brought down specially, so as to avoid morbidity, which usually takes the form of bleeding from catheter or needle holes in big vessels. If necessary, 1—2.5 mg. pentolinium intramuscularly will lower the lying pressure satisfactorily for this procedure in most patients. The next important point is that, as far as is possible, by rotation and other forms of manoeuvring, the whole course of all the renal arteries to both kidneys should be visualised. It also seems to be an advantage in some patients to take the pictures in full inspiration or with the patient standing, so as to straighten out tortuosities which simulate stenoses in this region. Some cases of what would otherwise be labelled as fibromuscular hyperplasia may well disappear with this technique. The various characteristic appearances, ranging from the atheromatous block with dilatation beyond the stenosis to fibromuscular hyperplasia, usually occurring in the middle or peripheral part of the artery, are shown in Figs 5a, b, and 6. Fibromuscular hyperplasia is very difficult to diagnose arteriographically, since the multiple indentations in the wall, which in themselves are sufficient to cause quite a big pressure drop across the artery, do not necessarily distort the column of dye very much (Fig. 7). Rather grosser changes, such as polar atrophy, are usually well shown by any technique.

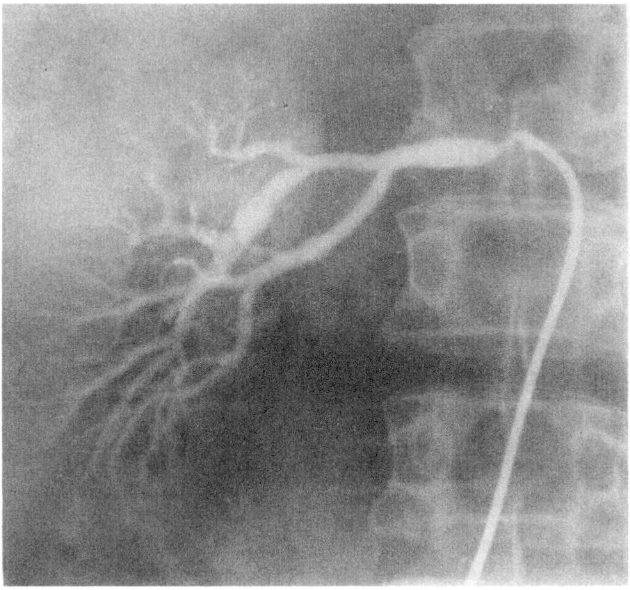

Fig. 5a. Arteriography, selective. Atheromatous block at origin of right renal artery with post-stenotic dilatation.

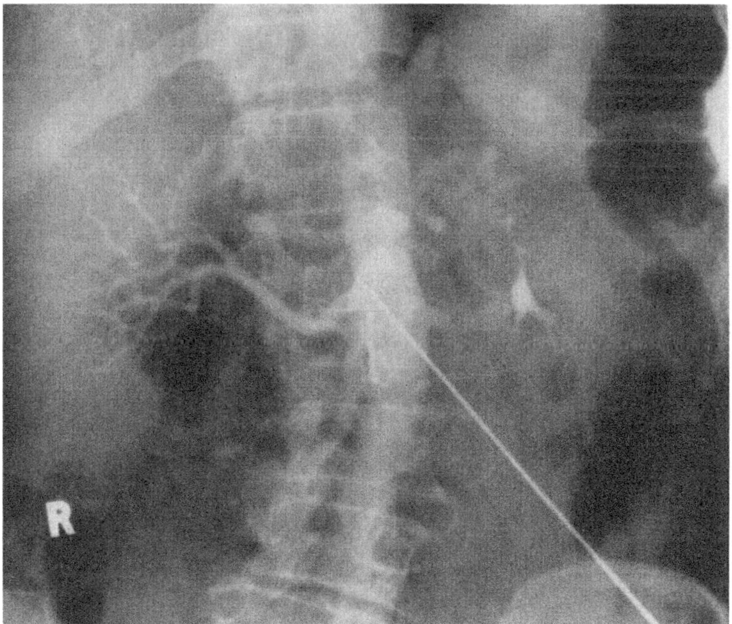

Fig. 5b. Aortography. Atheromatous block mid-renal artery, showing in addition typical, dense pyelogram.

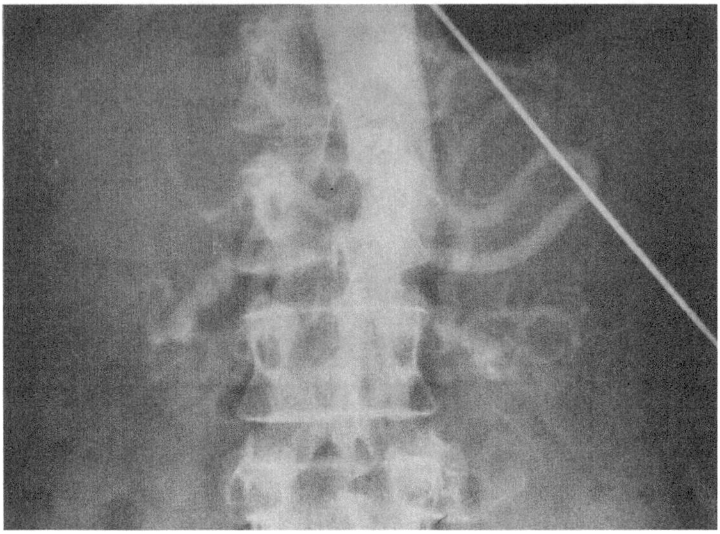

Fig. 6. Aortography. Fibromuscular hyperplasia right renal artery, best shown at border of vertebral body.

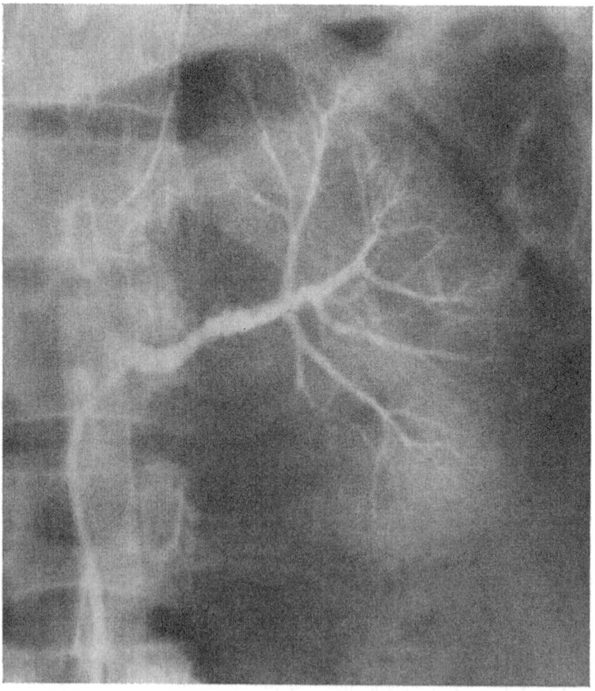

Fig. 7. Arteriography, selective. Fibromuscular hyperplasia middle third left renal artery.

4. Divided renal function studies. So far no technique has been devised which allows the same degree of diagnostic certainty as this technique. Many have abandoned it because of technical difficulties or supposed morbidity, but it works well, given experience and a surgeon who is vitally concerned in the technique (BROWN et al., 1960). The functional basis, resting as it does on the work of SELKURT (1951), who first showed that lowering the renal artery pressure caused reduction in glomerular filtration rate and increased sodium and water reabsorption, has been repeatedly confirmed (HOWARD et al., 1954; POUTASSE, 1956; DE CAMP and BIRCHALL, 1958; BROWN et al., 1960; DUSTAN et al., 1961), and, in our experience, the technique of STAMEY and GOOD (1961) works best. The figures of a typical study are shown in Table 1. As was first pointed out by CONNOR et al. (1957), the increased sodium reabsorption can be seen clearly and – which is of greater importance – is

Table 1. *Divided right and left renal function studies in stenosis of the right main renal artery. Typical reduction in urine volume, sodium concentration, and creatinine and P.A.H. clearances, with increase in the creatinine and P.A.H. concentrations on the stenosed right side*

	Period	R	L
Urine volume (ml./min.)	8	0.25	3.7
	9	0.17	4.5
	10	0.15	5.5
Sodium (mEq./l.)	8	45.0	100.0
	9	67.0	135.0
	10	115.0	144.0
Chloride (mEq./l.).	8	19.0	86.0
	9	32.0	123.0
	10	58.0	130.0
Urine P.A.H. concentration (mg.%)	9	752	167
	10	2,160	173
Urine creatinine conc. (mg.%) . .	9	81.6	12.4
	10	128.6	11.6
P.A.H. clearance (ml./min.) . . .	9	40	234
	10	98	288
Creatinine clearance (ml./min.) . .	9	17.0	65.0
	10	23.0	70.0

complemented by increased water reabsorption. Since the dyes used in pyelography are filtered and not reabsorbed, they behave like creatinine or inulin and become more concentrated as water reabsorption increases, giving the typical pyelographic appearances. Branch stenoses are obviously much more difficult to diagnose, but differences can be perceived in carefully conducted studies of such patients. The key to success from the technical point of view is the use of large catheters with high urine flows induced by the osmotic

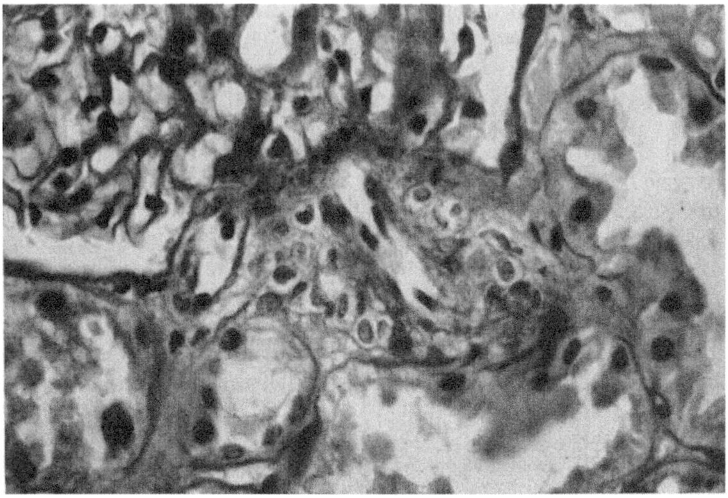

Fig. 8a. Juxtaglomerular apparatus. Base of glomerulus top left. Hypertrophied cells round the afferent arteriole (centre) as it enters the glomerulus.

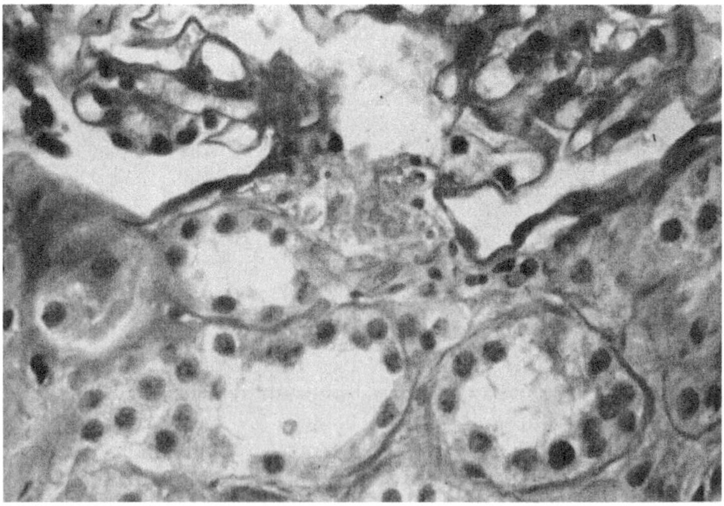

Fig. 8b. Opposite, normal side showing small apparatus.

diuresis and of prophylactic antibacterial drugs afterwards. Morbidity has been low.

5. Renal biopsy. Because interference with blood supply leads to tubular atrophy and hypertrophy of the juxtaglomerular apparatus, the possibility of using this in diagnosis and in the prognosis of operations has been investigated. Attempts to put the degree

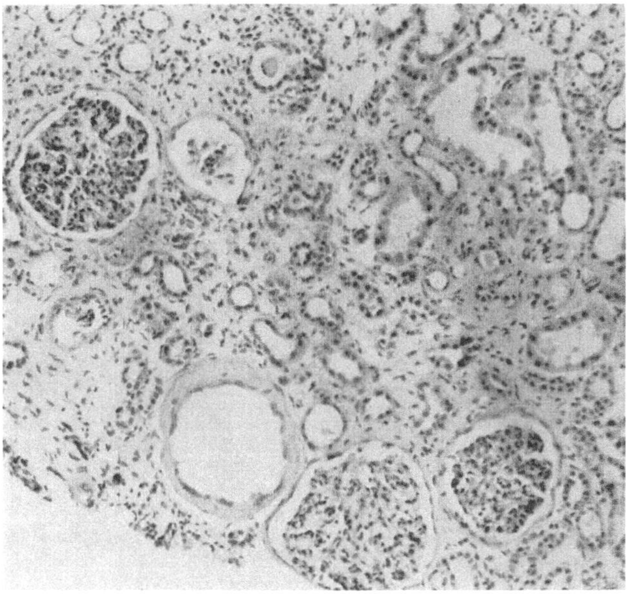

Fig. 9a. Renal cortex beyond renal artery stenosis. Artery next to glomerulus shows no intimal or medial hypertrophy. Atrophy of tubules marked.

of granulation in the juxtaglomerular apparatus on a quantitative basis have been made (HARTROFT, 1963; TOBIAN, 1963). There is no doubt that increased size of the cells and granulation within occurs with stenosis, and that in the opposite, normal kidney the converse usually applies (Fig. 8a and b). In addition, the arterial wall beyond the stenosis may be protected from the effects of raised blood pressure and show much less change than the opposite arteries, which are exposed to a higher pressure (Fig. 9a and b). As an isolated investigation, it will be difficult to put complete reliance on the appearances, and more correlation of the fate of patients operated on and the other variable metabolic factors existing in them, such as are known to affect renin levels, is necessary.

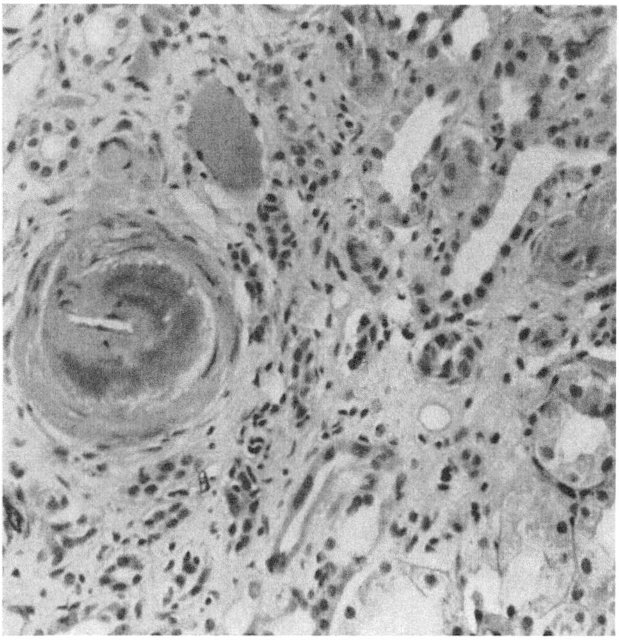

FIG. 9b. Kidney, opposite side to one with renal artery stenosis. Shows fibrinoid necrosis in hypertrophied arterial intima.

Blood changes

The electrolytes in the blood may be helpful in the sense that the presence of a lower than normal sodium and potassium is more often associated with renal artery stenosis than not. Cases of this type were earlier reported (DEMING, 1954; FITZGERALD et al., 1957; DOLLERY et al., 1959; FITZ and ARMSTRONG, 1964). The reason for the low potassium is presumably the high rate of aldosterone secretion often present in such patients, which is probably induced by the action of the renin-angiotensin system. The concomitantly low sodium is less readily explained and in some cases it may be due to the action of the sudden elevation of pressure, leading to sodium loss by the normal kidney; the sodium deficit itself may cause increased aldosterone secretion, either directly (BLAIR-WEST et al.,

1963) or via the renin-angiotensin system (Fig. 1) (Brown et al., 1964b). The presence of a low potassium alone is usually related only to the severity of the hypertension and not necessarily to the presence of a stenosed artery.

Renin and angiotensin

It is not clear how helpful the levels of renin in the plasma will be in the diagnosis of renal artery stenosis or in renal artery stenosis definitely causing hypertension. One of the most pressing needs in this field is to be able to tell which renal artery stenoses actually cause hypertension and which are secondary to atheromatous disease consequent upon previous hypertension. From the earlier reports of Morris and Robinson (1964) and Helmer and Judson (1963), based on estimations of "angiotensin and renin activity", it seems entirely possible that this prediction could be

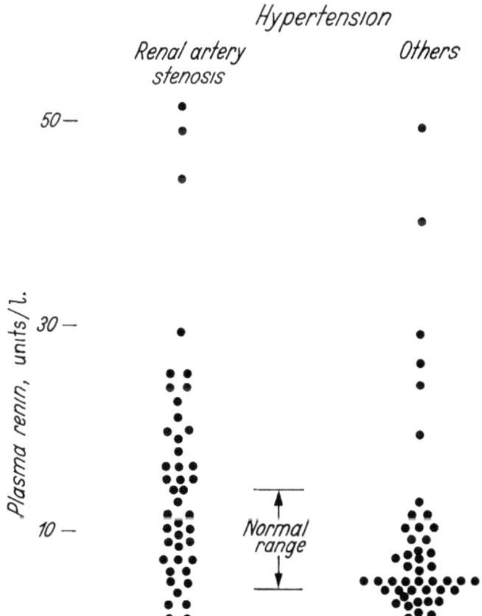

Fig. 10. Plasma renin values in patients with and without renal artery stenosis and hypertension.

fulfilled. However, as seen in Fig. 10, it is possible to have a proven renal artery stenosis with a renin level which ranges from normal, or even below normal, to well above normal levels (Brown et al., 1963; 1964c). The presence of malignant hypertension is usually associated with increased levels of renin, and it is certainly not possible to state that renal artery stenosis is associated with any particular level of plasma renin. There seems to be a better correlation with plasma sodium levels (Fig. 11) than with any other parameter yet measured, as in other cases of hypertension (BROWN et al., 1965). All the factors known, and some as yet unknown, will

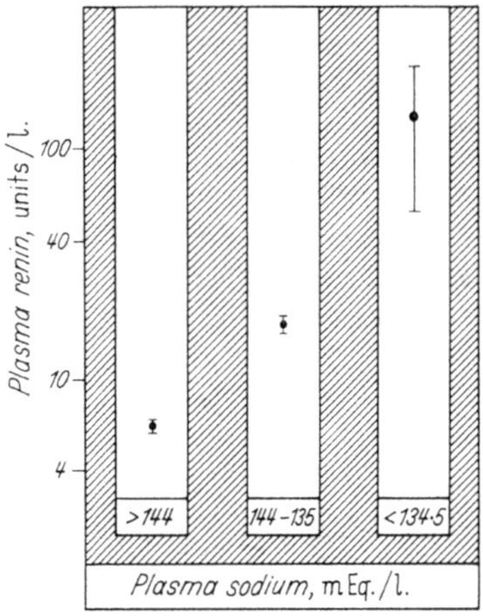

Fig. 11. Relation in hypertensive patients between plasma renin levels and plasma sodium. The lower the sodium, the higher the renin value.

have to be considered. It is probably true to say that the chance of a surgical cure in a patient with a lower than normal renin level is not good. In interpreting the particular value of renin and, of course, also of angiotensin, great attention has to be paid to sodium, the ion most intimately concerned with renin plasma levels (BROWN et al., 1964b; PEART, 1965). The patient whose levels are shown in Fig. 1 had a high aldosterone secretion rate, a very high plasma renin level, and low levels of plasma sodium and potassium. All parameters were returned to normal by successful reconstruction of the stenosed renal artery. The part played by sodium in the aldosterone and renin levels of this patient has to be conjectural. However, aldosterone secreted from a tumour is capable of depressing plasma renin levels, perhaps by alteration in sodium balance (Fig. 12) (BROWN et al., 1964a; CONN et al., 1964). It may therefore be expected that interpretation of a particular plasma renin level in a patient with a stenosed renal artery will not be completely straightforward, but it may ultimately turn out to be helpful diagnostically.

To diagnose the presence of renal artery stenosis is now relatively easy; to forecast whether reconstruction of the renal artery, or even nephrectomy, will produce a surgical cure is very difficult, and our ability to do so falls well behind our diagnostic ability.

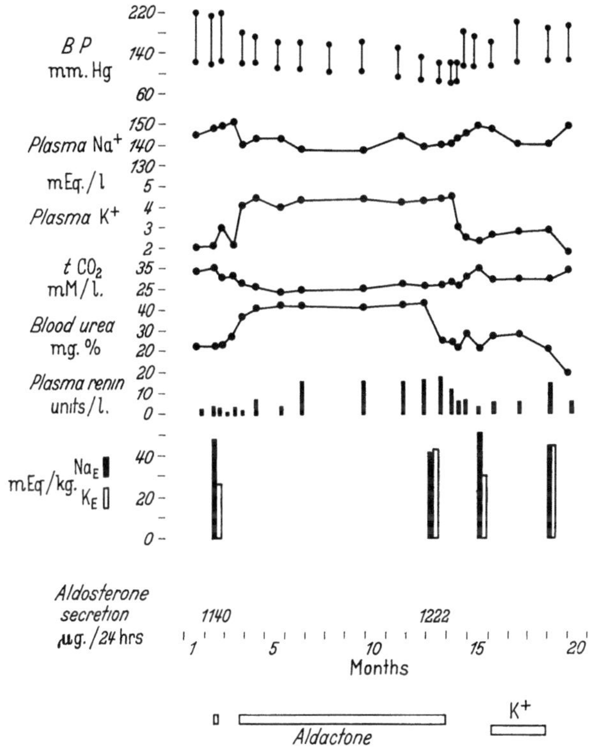

Fig. 12. The effect of Aldactone in lowering the blood pressure of a patient with a Conn's tumour. The high plasma sodium and low potassium were associated with a lower than normal plasma renin. All these figures were returned to normal with Aldactone and became abnormal off treatment. A tumour was subsequently removed from this patient with cure of the condition. Note that, as the plasma sodium dropped and plasma potassium rose, the plasma renin increased, even though the aldosterone secretion rate was unchanged.

Summary

The presence of a renal artery stenosis can be diagnosed in various ways, although it is not possible in any particular case to be certain that the stenosis is actually causing the raised arterial pressure. Clinically, there are no absolute diagnostic manifestations, although the abrupt onset of malignant hypertension, with sodium and potassium depletion due to urinary excretion, may occur. The intravenous pyelogram is very helpful, and the delayed excretion with subsequent increased concentration of dye in a small collecting system is diagnostic. Isotopic renography is sometimes a helpful adjunct. Various forms of arteriography will show up the different types of stenosis. It is easy to miss some cases of fibromuscular hyperplasia without very good arteriograms. The precise diagnosis of arterial obstruction may be made by divided renal function studies, and they are still the best for this purpose, although small branch stenoses may not be demonstrated and the arterial obstruction is not necessarily in the main renal artery but may be intrarenal. Renal biopsy shows that on the side of the stenosis there is hypertrophy of the juxtaglomerular apparatus and tubular atrophy, in contrast to the opposite, normal side. In addition, the arterial wall beyond the stenosis may be protected from the effects of high blood pressure, whereas the exposed, normal side may suffer. Estimation of plasma renin shows that this may be normal or higher than normal in proven cases of renal artery stenosis. Malignant hypertension is usually associated with increased levels of renin. It is not yet clear whether the level of plasma renin can be used in a prognostic sense for the results of reconstructive surgery.

Zusammenfassung

Das Vorliegen einer Nierenarterienstenose kann auf verschiedene Weise diagnostiziert werden, obgleich es nicht möglich ist, in jedem einzelnen Falle sicher festzustellen, daß die Stenose tatsächlich für den erhöhten Blutdruck verantwortlich ist. Klinisch gibt es keine absoluten diagnostischen Zeichen, obwohl plotzlich ein maligner Hochdruck mit Natrium- und Kaliumverarmung infolge Ausscheidung dieser Elektrolyte im Harn auftreten kann. Das intravenöse Pyelogramm ist sehr nützlich, und die verzögerte Ausscheidung mit anschließender vermehrter Farbstoffkonzentration in einem kleinen Nierenbecken ist von diagnostischer Bedeutung. Das Isotopen-Renogramm ist gelegentlich ein wertvolles Hilfsmittel. Verschiedene Formen der Arteriographie können die verschiedenen Arten der Stenose aufzeigen. Falle von fibromuskularer Hyperplasie sind leicht zu übersehen, wenn die Arteriogramme technisch nicht gut sind. Die genaue Diagnose des arteriellen Hindernisses kann durch getrennte Nierenfunktionsprüfungen erfolgen. Sie eignen sich noch immer am besten dafür, obwohl damit Stenosen in kleinen Nierenarterienästen nicht nachweisbar sind. Arterienverschlüsse betreffen nicht immer die Hauptarterie, sondern konnen intrarenal liegen. Die Nierenbiopsie zeigt, daß auf der Seite der Stenose eine Hypertrophie des juxtaglomerulären Apparates und eine tubuläre Atrophie vorliegt im Gegensatz zur kontralateralen, normalen Seite. Außerdem kann die Arterienwand jenseits der Stenose vor der Einwirkung eines erhöhten Blutdruckes geschützt sein, während die dem Hochdruck ausgesetzte, normale Niere geschädigt sein kann. Bestimmungen des Plasmarenins ergaben normale oder erhöhte Werte bei Fallen, bei denen eine Nierenarterienstenose nachzuweisen war. Maligner Hochdruck geht gewöhnlich mit erhöhten Reninwerten einher. Es ist noch nicht anzugeben, ob die Reninkonzentration im Plasma von prognostischer Bedeutung für die Resultate der operativen Behandlung von Nierenarterienstenosen ist.

Résumé

Le diagnostic de sténose de l'artère rénale peut être établi de différentes façons, bien qu'il soit impossible dans chaque cas particulier d'affirmer que la sténose est réellement la cause de l'hypertension. Il n'existe pas cliniquement de signes pathognomoniques, bien que l'apparition brutale d'une hypertension maligne avec pertes de sodium et de potassium urinaires soit évocatrice. L'urographie intra-veineuse apporte une aide précieuse au diagnostic en montrant le retard à l'excrétion avec augmentation de la concentration du produit de contraste dans les petits calices. La rénographie isotopique est parfois un utile examen d'appoint. Plusieurs techniques d'artériographie peuvent mettre en évidence les différents types de sténose. Il est facile de méconnaître certains cas d'hyperplasie fibromusculaire si les radiographies ne sont pas d'excellente qualité. Le diagnostic précis d'obstruction artérielle peut être fait par l'étude séparée des fonctions rénales, et c'est encore le meilleur moyen, bien que des sténoses des petites branches peuvent passer inaperçues et que l'obstruction artérielle ne siège pas nécessairement sur le tronc de l'artère rénale, mais peut être intra-rénale. La biopsie rénale montre que du côté de la sténose il existe une hypertrophie de l'appareil juxta-glomérulaire et une atrophie tubulaire, contrastant avec le côté opposé normal. De plus, la paroi artérielle au-delà de la sténose peut être protégée des effets de l'hypertension artérielle, tandis que du côté normal les artères exposées peuvent présenter des lésions. Le taux de rénine dans le plasma peut être normal ou plus élevé que la normale dans des cas démontrés de sténose de l'artère rénale. L'hypertension maligne s'accompagne habituellement de taux élevés de rénine. On ne sait pas encore bien clairement si le taux plasmatique de rénine peut être pris comme élément pronostique quant aux résultats de la chirurgie plastique.

Acknowledgements

Thanks are due to Butterworth & Co. Ltd., British Medical Journal, and the University of Leyden for permission to publish certain figures and the table. I am grateful to Dr. R. A. PARKER for Fig. 8a and b.

References

ANGER, H. O.: Rev. sc. instr. **29**, 27 (1958). — BLAIR-WEST, J. R., J. P. COGHLAN, D. A. DENTON, J. R. GODING, M. WINTOUR, and R. D. WRIGHT: In: Hormones and the Kidney. Mem. Soc. Endocr. No. 13. Ed. by P. C. WILLIAMS. Academic Press, London and New York, 1963, p. 341. — BROWN, J. J., D. L. DAVIES, A. F. LEVER, and J. I. S. ROBERTSON: In: Boerhaave Course on Hypertension. Ed. by J. DE GRAEFF. University of Leyden, 1963, p. 44. — BROWN, J. J., D. L. DAVIES, A. F. LEVER, W. S. PEART, and J. I. S. ROBERTSON: Brit. Med. J. 1964a/II, 1636. — BROWN, J. J., D. L. DAVIES, A. F. LEVER, and J. I. S. ROBERTSON: J. Physiol. **173**, 408 (1964b). — BROWN, J. J., D. L. DAVIES, A. F. LEVER, and J. I. S. ROBERTSON: Canad. Med. Ass. J. **90**, 201 (1964c). — BROWN, J. J., D. L. DAVIES, A. F. LEVER, and J. I. S. ROBERTSON: Brit. Med. J. 1965, in press. — BROWN, J. J., K. OWEN, W. S. PEART, J. I. S. ROBERTSON, and D. SUTTON: Brit. Med. J. 1960/II, 327. — CONN, J. W., E. L. COHEN, and D. R. ROVNER: J. Amer. Med. Ass. **190**, 213 (1964). — CONNOR, T. B., M. BERTHRONG, W. C. THOMAS, and J. E. HOWARD: Bull. Johns Hopkins Hosp. **100**, 241 (1957). — DE CAMP, P. T., and R. BIRCHALL: Surgery **43**, 134 (1958). — DEMING, Q. B.: Arch. Int. Med. **93**, 197 (1954). — DOLLERY, C. T., R. SHACKMAN, and J. SHILLINGFORD: Brit. Med. J. 1959/II, 1367. — DUSTAN, H. P., E. F. POUTASSE, A. C. CORCORAN, and I. H. PAGE: Circulation **23**, 34 (1961). — FITZ, A. E., and M. L. ARMSTRONG: Circulation **29**, 409 (1964). — FITZGERALD, M. G., P.

Fourman, A. H. James, and H. Scarborough: Scott. Med. J. **2**, 473 (1957). — Hartroft, P.: In: Angiotensin Systems and Experimental Renal Diseases. The Fourteenth Annual Conference on the Kidney sponsored by National Kidney Disease Foundation. Ed. by J. Metcoff. Churchill Ltd., London, 1963, p. 5. — Helmer, O. M., and W. E. Judson: Circulation **27**, 1050 (1963). — Howard, J. E., M. Berthrong, D. M. Gould, and E. R. Yendt: Bull. Johns Hopkins Hosp. **94**, 51 (1954). — McAfee, J. G., and H. N. Wagner, Jr.: Radiology **75**, 820 (1960). — Mallard, J. R., and M. J. Myers: Phys. Med. Biol. **8**, 183 (1963). — Morris, R. E., and P. R. Robinson: Bull. Johns Hopkins Hosp. **114**, 127 (1964). — Peart, W. S.: Recent Progr. Hormone Res. 1965, in press. — Peart, W. S., and C. Rob: Lancet 1960/II, 219. — Poutasse, E. F.: Circulation **13**, 37 (1956). — Selkurt, E. E.: Circulation **4**, 541 (1951). — Stamey, T. A., and P. H. Good: In: Hypertension. Recent Advances. The Second Hahnemann Symposium on Hypertensive Disease. Ed. by A. N. Brest and J. H. Moyer. Lea and Febiger, Philadelphia, 1961, p. 189. — Sutton, D.: Arteriography. Livingstone, Edinburgh, 1962. — Taplin, G. V., O. M. Meredith, H. Kade, and C. C. Winter: J. Laborat. Clin. Med. **48**, 886 (1956). — Tobian, L.: In: Angiotensin Systems and Experimental Renal Diseases. The Fourteenth Annual Conference on the Kidney sponsored by National Kidney Disease Foundation. Ed. by J. Metcoff. Churchill Ltd., London, 1963, p. 17. — Winter, C. C., R. A. Nordyke, and M. Tubis: J. Urol. **85**, 92 (1961).

The diagnostic value of renal biopsy in renovascular and other forms of renal hypertension

By

PRISCILLA KINCAID-SMITH

Renal biopsy is one of the investigations which can provide an accurate diagnosis in cases of renal hypertension. In young patients with severe hypertension and those with other evidence of renal disease, such as proteinuria, the cause is likely to be renal, and it is in such patients that renal biopsy is usually performed. Impairment of renal function suggests that diffuse disease is present, and where this is accompanied by an excess of red cells and casts in the urine, renal biopsy is particularly likely to be of diagnostic value.

To introduce the subject and to demonstrate some points about the diagnostic and prognostic value of renal biopsy, I should like to cite three clinically similar patients. All had malignant hypertension with papilloedema, moderate proteinuria, normal-sized kidneys radiologically, and some impairment of renal function.

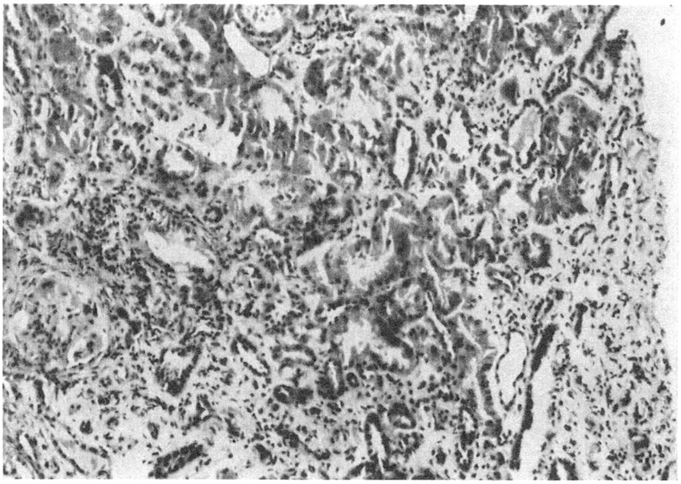

Fig. 1. Chronic, active glomerulonephritis. The glomerulus on the left shows active destructive disease within the glomerular tuft. There is wide-spread tubular atrophy and fibrosis (haematoxylin and eosin × 100).

The first was a young football-player who had felt perfectly well and complained only that he could not see the ball clearly. In spite of the fact that his blood urea was only 60 mg.%, renal biopsy showed a chronic, active glomerulonephritis in which most of the glomeruli had already been destroyed (Fig. 1). As a result of the biopsy findings, his parents were told that he was unlikely to live longer than a year or two, and this prognosis, which proved to be correct, prevented them from taking steps which could have involved serious financial loss.

The second patient was clinically similar, but his blood urea was 150 mg.%, and on clinical grounds one would therefore give a worse prognosis. However, his biopsy showed nephrocalcinosis (Fig. 2), a reversible condition, and with treatment of his previously unsuspected hypercalcaemia both his hypertension and renal disease vanished.

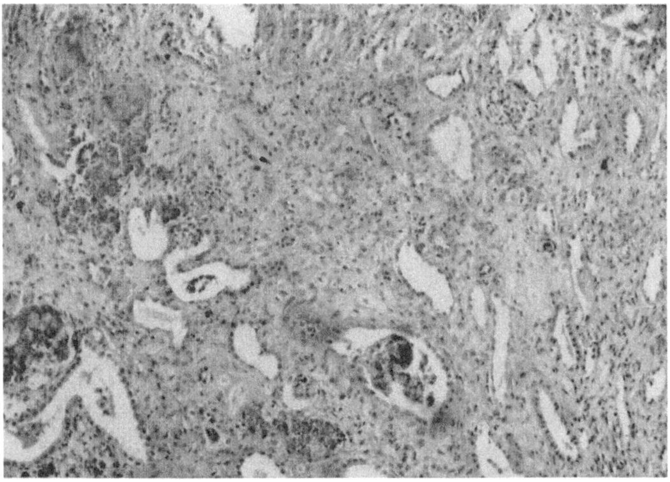

Fig. 2. Nephrocalcinosis showing calcified material within tubules and in the interstitial tissue and a great increase in interstitial tissue (haematoxylin and eosin; × 100).

The third patient had a blood urea of only 40 mg.%, but her renal biopsy showed that she had a type of malignant hypertension which still warrants the name malignant. This type of lesion is characterised by marked narrowing of interlobular arteries (Fig. 3) and resultant ischaemic atrophy in the renal parenchyma, and in such patients, even if the blood urea is normal or only slightly elevated at the time of diagnosis, one can predict a fulminating progression and a uraemic death within a period of weeks.

This type of course, which was familiar before hypotensive drugs were available, is now rare and seems to occur only in patients in whom interlobular artery narrowing is advanced when they first

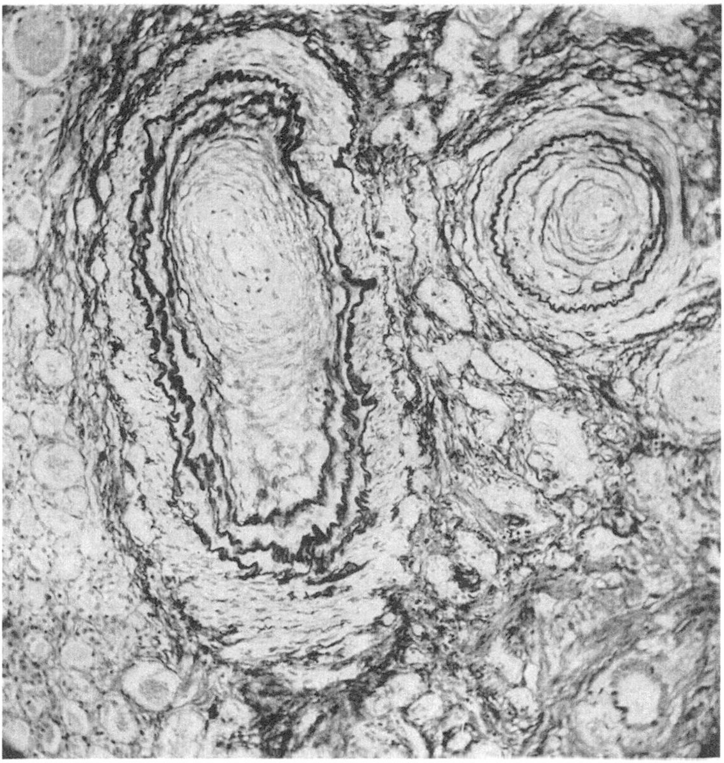

Fig. 3. Extreme narrowing of interlobular arteries by cellular intimal hyperplasia which indicates a poor prognosis in malignant hypertension, even if the blood urea is not elevated at the time of biopsy (Weigert's elastic, haematoxylin, and Van Gieson; × 130).

present. Most of these patients already have a raised blood urea, but even if it is normal, hypotensive drugs are of no avail, because this type of vessel lesion is not reversible (HARINGTON et al., 1959). If, however, interlobular artery narrowing is slight or moderate, arteriolar fibrinoid necrosis, even if it is fairly extensive, does not necessarily indicate a poor prognosis, as this change is rapidly reversed by treatment.

1. Renovascular hypertension

I shall confine my comments about renovascular hypertension to lesions of the renal arterial tree, although renal vein thrombosis may also cause hypertension.

Regardless of the level at which narrowing is present in the renal arterial system, the parenchymal lesion is the same, namely ischaemic tubular atrophy or partial infarction (Fig. 4). Although a needle biopsy may show ischaemic renal tissue, it is unlikely to

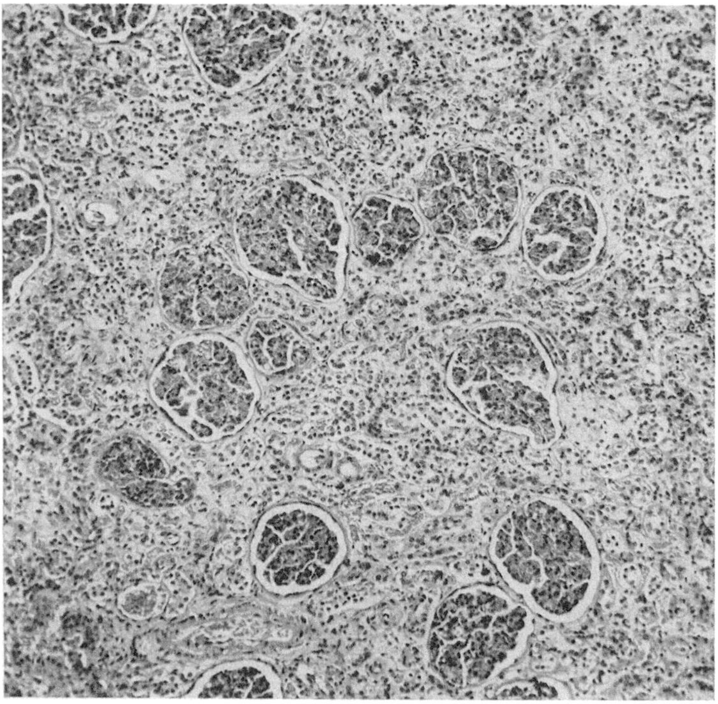

Fig. 4. Partial infarction or ischaemic tubular atrophy. The tubules are small and often have no lumen, and the glomeruli are crowded together (× 105).

reveal the cause of the vascular obstruction, except in such conditions as malignant hypertension, where the most distal branches of the arterial tree are narrowed.

It is very unlikely that a needle biopsy would permit distinctions to be made between such conditions as chronic pyelonephritis

(Fig. 5) and branch stenosis of the renal artery (Fig. 6), where the area of ischaemic scarring may be identical and in which the diagnosis may be difficult even when a large section of the kidney tissue is available. Similarly, in other conditions which cause ischaemic atrophy, such as polyarteritis nodosa, renal biopsy often fails to demonstrate the specific vascular lesions which may involve

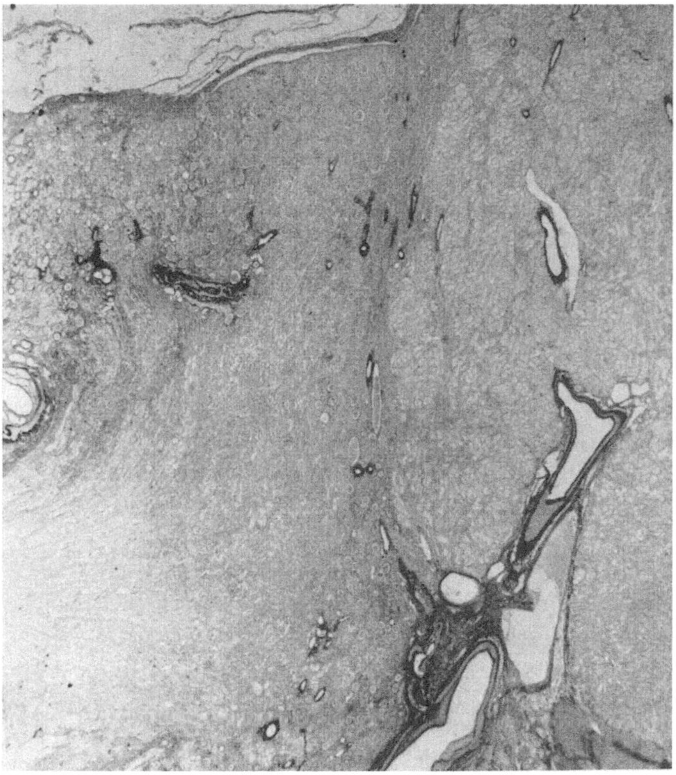

Fig. 5. An area of ischaemic scarring in pyelonephritis showing a sharp line of demarcation between normal and ischaemic tissue. A recanalised artery is seen on the extreme left-hand side of the figure, and the vessels within the scarred area are also abnormal, whereas those entering the adjacent normal parenchyma are patent (Weigert's elastic, haematoxylin, and Van Gieson; × 10).

interlobular or even larger arterial branches.

Percutaneous renal biopsy is not therefore of great value in renal ischaemia; however, as this session is largely devoted to renovascular hypertension, I shall comment upon the histological findings in renal artery stenosis on the basis of 20 biopsies taken from the ischaemic and non-ischaemic kidney at the time of operation. Unless there has been considerable reduction in the size of a kidney distal to an arterial stenosis, the histological differences

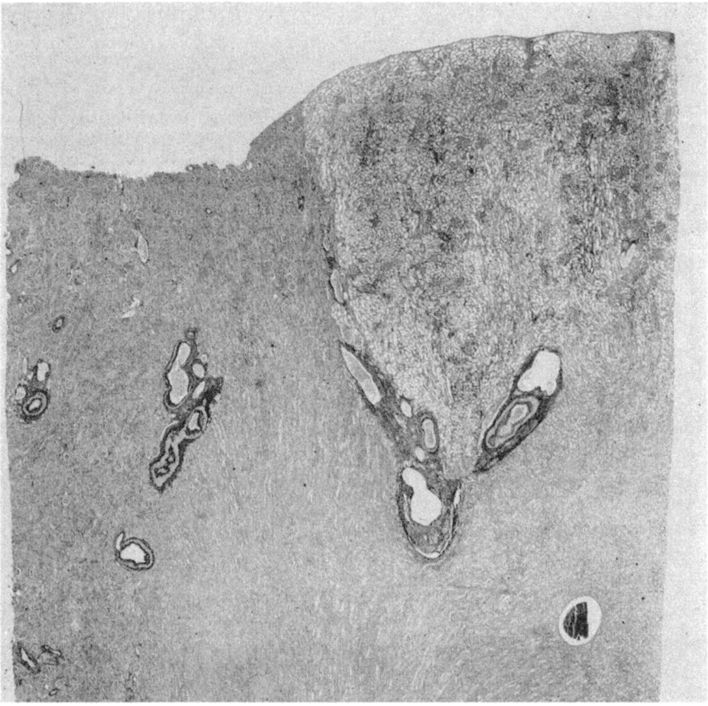

Fig. 6. An area of ischaemic scarring almost identical to that seen in Fig. 5. The cause of this area of ischaemic atrophy was a block in a major branch of the renal artery, and the arteries seen entering both the ischaemic and the normal parenchyma are patent (Weigert's elastic, haematoxylin, and Van Gieson; × 8).

between the ischaemic and non-ischaemic kidney are not striking. The shrunken kidney distal to a stenosis shows the lesion of ischaemic tubular atrophy (Fig. 4).

Vessels. The vessels show interesting differences, but these are not as clear-cut as those reported in animals. One expects to find normal "protected" vessels distal to a stenosis of the renal artery, and in view of this it is surprising that, at first sight, the vessels may appear more abnormal on the ischaemic than on the non-ischaemic side. The greater the degree of ischaemic atrophy, the more obvious are the changes, and in a small kidney the thickness of the walls of interlobular arteries is greatly increased in proportion to the size of the lumen (Fig. 7). At first, it seemed that this appearance might be due to mechanical factors, such as contraction or collapse of the

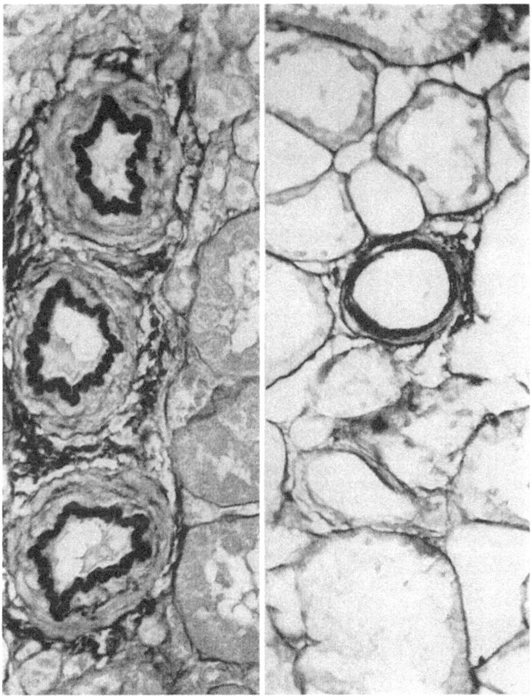

Fig. 7. The interlobular arteries on the left show the thickened wall and greatly convoluted internal elastic lamina in a shrunken ischaemic kidney distal to a main renal artery stenosis. The interlobular artery on the right shows hypertensive damage with thinning and fibrosis of the wall and reduplication of a stretched internal elastic lamina. The latter vessel is from the kidney with a patent renal artery in a case of unilateral renal artery stenosis (Weigert's elastic, haematoxylin, and Van Gieson, × 250).

vessel wall as a result of the shrinkage of the kidney together with reduction of the pressure within the lumen. The deeply convoluted internal elastic lamina (Fig. 7) suggests that such mechanisms play a part, and the normal appearance of the media, which does not show any fibrosis, supports this. In some vessels, however, there is intimal proliferation within the internal elastic lamina, so that factors other than mechanical ones appear to contribute to the thickness of these artery walls.

Arterioles distal to a main renal artery stenosis are usually relatively normal; however, in spite of the protection which the stenosis should provide, fibrinoid necrosis may be present distal to severe stenosis. In one patient in whom total occlusion of the main

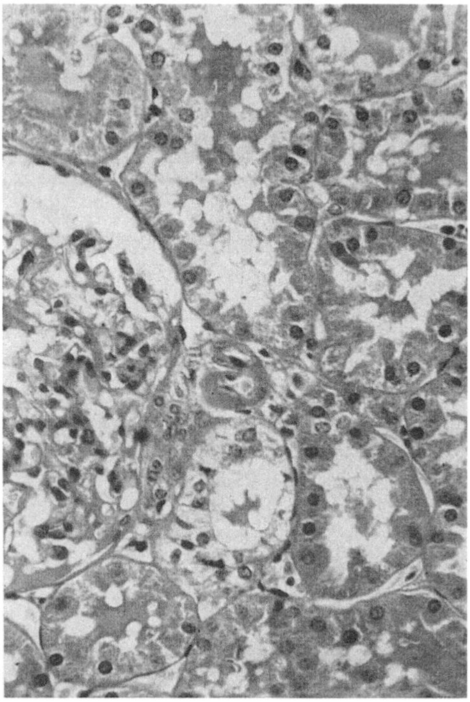

Fig. 8. Biopsy from a kidney distal to an occluded renal artery showing fibrinoid necrosis in the afferent arteriole together with hypertrophy of the juxtaglomerular apparatus (haematoxylin and eosin; × 250).

renal artery was confirmed at operation, the unusual combination of arteriolar fibrinoid necrosis and hypertrophied juxtaglomerular cells was found in the ischaemic kidney (Fig. 8).

In this group of surgical biopsies, interlobular arteries in the kidney whose main renal artery was patent differed from those in the ischaemic kidney. Interlobular arteries and arterioles showed varying degrees of hypertensive damage, usually in the form of fibrosis and hyalinisation of their walls. In contrast to the thick wall and convoluted elastic on the ischaemic side, the interlobular arteries sometimes showed apparent thinning of their walls and a stretched internal elastic lamina (Fig. 7).

Increased cellular or fibrous intimal tissue may be present, and one patient with malignant hypertension showed extreme narrowing of interlobular arteries due to cellular intimal proliferation. The renal parenchyma distal to these severely narrowed interlobular arteries showed ischaemic atrophy, and it is not surprising that removal of the opposite kindey was followed by progressive uraemia and that there was no fall in the blood pressure (KINCAID-SMITH, 1961).

Juxtaglomerular apparatus. In spite of all that has been written about the juxtaglomerular apparatus, I have not found that the changes in these cells are of particular value in the assessment of individual patients with renal artery stenosis. Where there has been a dramatic and long-lasting fall in the blood pressure following removal of an ischaemic kidney, the juxtaglomerular apparatus may not appear very prominent.

On the other hand, the most striking hypertrophy of the juxtaglomerular apparatus and the presence of large, pale, heavily granulated cells do not guarantee a satisfactory fall in the blood pressure when an ischaemic kidney of this type is removed in a case of renal artery stenosis.

The juxtaglomerular apparatus may also be prominent in the non-ischaemic kidney in patients with unilateral renal artery stenosis and in biopsies from other hypertensive and normotensive patients. In general, however, if the juxtaglomerular apparatus is easily seen in about one third of glomeruli, and if an ordinary section through the juxtaglomerular apparatus shows ten or more cells, it is likely that an ischaemic renal lesion is present.

2. The value of renal biopsy in other renal diseases

To determine the range of underlying renal disease in patients with hypertension, I went through our last 600 renal biopsies. In 216 of these 600 patients, hypertension was a significant clinical feature, and Table 1 shows the different underlying conditions in these 216 patients. This gives an idea of the relative frequency of different disorders, but also reflects our special interests and hence the large number in whom pregnancy hypertension was studied.

In this talk I can only deal in detail with one or two of these conditions. I would draw your attention to the group with focal glomerulonephritis, which is the largest group when the 12 cases discovered in relation to pregnancy hypertension are included.

Focal glomerulonephritis includes several different conditions, and one of the most interesting of these has been a type of familial glomerulonephritis. This disease has appeared in five generations of a family and has a dominant mode of inheritance. It is of interest

Table 1. *Aetiological factors in hypertension. Renal biopsies in 216 patients*

Post-streptococcal glomerulonephritis	35
Hypertension during or after pregnancy (focal glomerulonephritis 12)	29
Focal glomerulonephritis	25
Benign essential hypertension	20
Malignant essential hypertension	18
Papillary necrosis	12
Chronic proliferative glomerulonephritis	10
Diabetes	7
Membranous glomerulonephritis	7
Nephrocalcinosis	6
Pyelonephritis	6
Gouty nephropathy	6
Fibrinoid glomerulonephritis	6
Renal artery stenosis	5
Polyarteritis nodosa	4
Renal homotransplants	4
Lipoid nephrosis (also nephrotic)	3
Disseminated lupus	3
Scleroderma	2
Renal vein thrombosis	2
Henoch Schönlein purpura	2
Amyloid	2
Cortical necrosis	1
Wegener's granulomatosis	1
	216

because of its relation to hypertension and also because it is similar in some respects to the so-called auto-immune nephritis which occurs in New Zealand mice (HICKS, in preparation). In both mice and patients vascular lesions accompany the glomerular lesions.

The disease is almost invariably fatal in males before the age of 35, and the mode of death is that of fulminating malignant hypertension. Females, on the other hand, in spite of long-standing proteinuria and histologically proven renal disease, may have a normal life-span. An interesting sex difference has also been reported in mice, where females are more seriously affected than males.

The typical glomerular lesions are focal in that they involve some glomeruli and not others and, within a glomerulus, often involve only part of the tuft (Fig. 9). In early lesions, abnormal material appears to be spreading in from the hilum of the glomerulus and it often also involves arterioles and less frequently interlobular arteries.

We have demonstrated vascular lesions of this type in young men years before the onset of hypertension, and very striking hypertrophy of juxtaglomerular cells may also be present before hypertension develops.

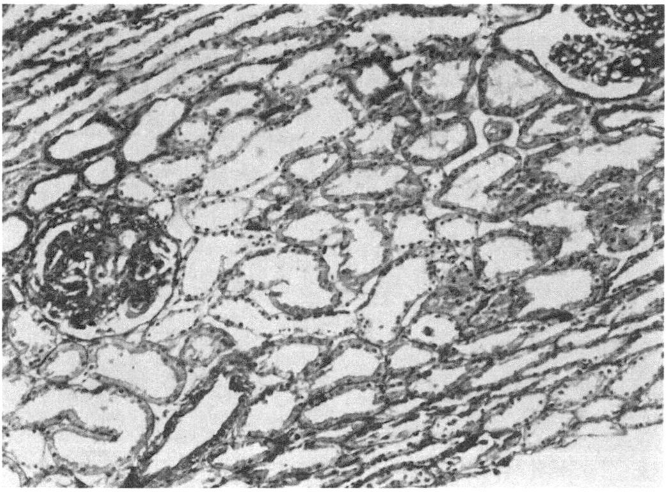

Fig. 9. Biopsy from a patient with familial glomerulonephritis. The glomerulus on the left has been almost totally destroyed by infiltration with abnormal material, and similar periodic acid Schiff-positive material is spreading in from the hilum and involving half the glomerular tuft on the right (periodic acid Schiff; × 100).

In this family and in New Zealand mice the glomerular and vascular deposits have the same staining reactions; they give a positive reaction with P.A.S. (periodic acid Schiff) and with certain fibrin stains. It is perhaps worth noting that the vascular lesions in mice and, to a lesser extent, those present in this family are similar to vascular lesions which occur at the time of rejection in homotransplants and which were for a long time attributed to hypertensive damage.

Finally, I should like to refer to a condition which may closely mimic renal artery stenosis and which is a common cause of renal hypertension in our community.

A woman aged 50, known to have had a normal blood pressure a few years previously, presented with a blood pressure of 260/

160 mm. Hg. Intravenous pyelograms showed progressive reduction in the length of the right kidney from 13.5 cm. to 9 cm. This is very suggestive of a renal artery stenosis; however, a renal biopsy showed a picture which, although not diagnostic, is very suggestive of renal papillary necrosis (Fig. 10), and the patient confirmed this diagnosis by passing several papillae down the ureter. To complete the picture, her renal arteriogram was quite normal, and she had been an analgesic addict for many years.

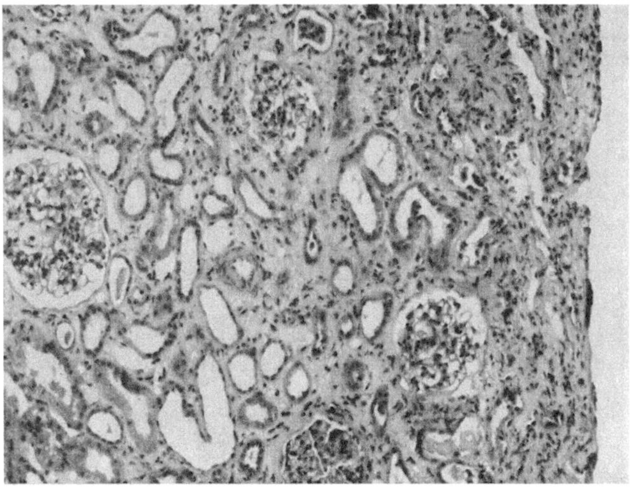

Fig. 10. A cortical biopsy from a patient with renal papillary necrosis showing characteristic atrophic tubules together with a great increase in interstitial tissue (haematoxylin and eosin, × 100).

I have tried to select some of the interesting facts which have emerged from a study of renal biopsies in hypertensive patients. In our view, percutaneous renal biopsy is a useful diagnostic method in selected cases of renal hypertension.

Summary

Renal biopsy is a useful investigation in selected patients in whom a renal cause of hypertension is likely. It is particularly useful where renal function is impaired. Patients in whom clinical features are similar may show renal lesions which have quite a different prognosis and require different forms of treatment.

In renovascular hypertension, needle biopsy is not of great value; however, surgical biopsies have revealed interesting differences between the ischaemic and non-ischaemic kidney in renal artery stenosis, and definite vascular abnormalities, including fibrinoid necrosis, have been observed distal to a stenosis of the renal artery.

The findings in 216 renal biopsies in hypertensive patients were reviewed. A form of familial focal glomerulonephritis is discussed in relation to hypertension and to "auto-immune" nephritis, which has been described in a strain of New Zealand mice.

Renal papillary necrosis associated with analgesic abuse is an important cause of hypertension in our community.

Zusammenfassung

Die Nierenbiopsie ist eine zweckmäßige Untersuchungsmethode bei ausgewählten Patienten, bei denen der Hypertension wahrscheinlich eine renale Ursache zugrunde liegt. Sie ist besonders bei verschlechterter Nierenfunktion angezeigt. Patienten mit ähnlichen klinischen Zeichen können Nierenschädigungen aufweisen, die eine ganz verschiedene Prognose haben und eine verschiedene Behandlung erfordern.

Beim renovaskulären Hochdruck ist die Nadelbiopsie nur von geringem Wert; dagegen haben chirurgische Biopsien interessante Unterschiede zwischen der ischämischen und der nicht ischämischen Niere bei Nierenarterienstenose aufgedeckt. Distal der Stenose einer Nierenarterie sind deutliche Gefäßveränderungen, eingeschlossen fibrinoide Nekrosen, beobachtet worden.

Es wird eine Übersicht über die Befunde von 216 Nierenbiopsien bei Hochdruckpatienten gegeben. Eine Form der familiären fokalen Glomerulonephritis wird in Beziehung zum Hochdruck besprochen sowie zur „autoimmunen" Nephritis, welche bei einem Stamm von Neuseelandmäusen beschrieben worden ist.

Nierenpapillennekrose in Verbindung mit Mißbrauch von Analgetika ist eine wichtige Ursache des Hochdruckes in unserer Bevölkerung.

Résumé

La biopsie rénale est un examen utile chez les malades judicieusement choisis porteurs d'une hypertension d'origine rénale vraisemblable. Elle est particulièrement indiquée quand les fonctions rénales sont altérées. Des malades présentant des tableaux cliniques identiques peuvent montrer des lésions rénales de pronostic et de traitement très différents.

Dans l'hypertension d'origine vasculaire rénale, la ponction à l'aiguille n'est pas d'un grand intérêt; cependant, des biopsies chirurgicales ont révélé des différences intéressantes entre le rein ischémique et le rein non ischémique lors de sténose de l'artère rénale, et de nettes anomalies vasculaires, y compris la nécrose fibrinoïde, ont été observées en aval d'une sténose de l'artère rénale.

Les observations de 216 biopsies rénales chez des malades hypertendus sont passées en revue. Une forme de glomérulonéphrite familiale en foyers est discutée dans ses relations avec l'hypertension et la néphrite "par auto-immunité", qui a été décrite chez une race de souris de la Nouvelle Zélande.

La nécrose papillaire au cours de l'abus d'analgésiques est une cause importante d'hypertension dans notre société.

Acknowledgements

This work has been supported by a grant from the National Health and Medical Research Council of Australia.

I am very grateful to Mr. JACK SMITH of the Department of Pathology at the University of Melbourne for help with the photomicrographs.

References

HARINGTON, M., P. KINCAID-SMITH, and J. McMICHAEL: Brit. Med. J. 1959/II, 969. — HICKS, J. D.: Submitted J. Path. Bact. — KINCAID-SMITH, P.: Australasian Ann. Med. 10, 166 (1961).

Discussion

Byrom: There is one complication of renovascular surgery which everyone seems to have overlooked. If one relieves a constriction on a renal artery, one suddenly exposes an atrophied, dilated arterial tree to excessive filling tension, and on the analogy of coarctation of the aorta this may be expected to cause arterial necrosis. I have examined this possibility experimentally and have found that if the clip is removed from the renal artery in rats with solitary kidneys and severe chronic hypertension, scattered medial necroses appear in the arteries of the kidney (Fig. 1). These lesions heal and

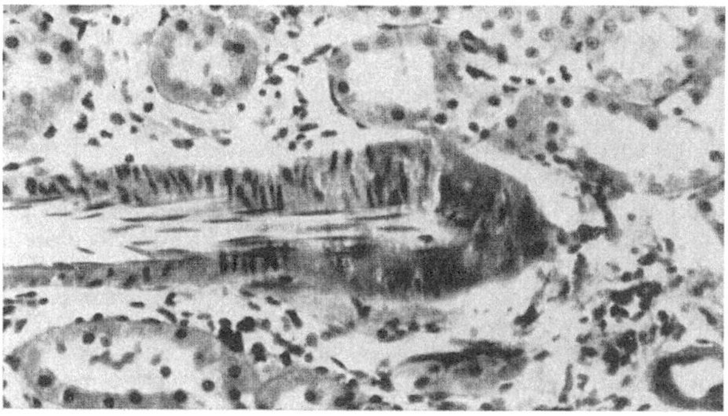

Fig. 1. Medial arterial necrosis in the solitary kidney of a renal hypertensive rat 24 hours after removing a clip from the renal artery (P.A.S.-haematoxylin; ×240).

seem to cause no permanent damage, and no doubt healing also occurs in human subjects if the operation is equally successful in abolishing the hypertension. The real danger occurs if the hypertension is arising from some source other than the constriction and persists after operation.

Tcherdakoff: As to what Dr. Peart said, I should like to insist on the variability of renin secretion in all patients, whether they are hypertensive or normotensive. In fact, we made repeated determinations in patients, standing and lying, and found that the levels differed considerably, depending upon the posture.

I should like to ask Dr. Peart whether he found the same thing as we did in a certain number of patients, that is a high renin level, while the aldosterone secretion was normal.

Regarding reduced renin in Conn's syndrome, I should like to mention that in our last patient with Conn's syndrome we had to give potassium for serious cardiac involvement due to hypokalaemia. Here we found that the renin increased definitely after potassium therapy.

With regard to Dr. Kincaid-Smith's paper, I should like to mention that in eight hypertensive patients with renal artery stenosis whom we studied carefully we performed bilateral renal biopsies. We found that in some cases the non-stenosed kidney showed serious lesions — Grade III according to SMITHWICK and CASTLEMAN — and yet two of these patients were cured by surgery. So I am not sure that needle biopsy can have a good prognostic value in selecting patients for surgery.

WILSON: I think there is very little relationship between renal biopsy findings and the effects of surgery on the blood pressure. It is common knowledge that the fulminating, perhaps malignant, hypertensive cases with unilateral renal artery disease benefit most from surgery, usually in the form of nephrectomy. It should be just these cases that develop vascular lesions in the opposite kidney. Furthermore, there is one condition in which both kidneys are exposed to severe and protracted hypertension, namely phaeochromocytoma. There are many patients in whom hypertension persists at a high level after removal of the tumour. We have done renal biopsies in these cases to see whether there is any justification for attributing the residual hypertension to renal vascular damage. The changes in the arterioles and arteries in the kidneys of these cases — even though hypertension has been severe and prolonged — have been minimal. Thirdly, increased cellularity of the juxtaglomerular apparatus is observed in hypertensive renal disease other than renal artery stenosis. In acute nephritis this may be very prominent, and there is no evidence that it is related to the severity of the hypertension.

HOOD: We can confirm the Melbourne experience. We had practically the same wall-lumen ratio on the two sides in renal artery stenosis. We tried to correlate the biopsy with various clinical features. The known duration of hypertension was the one which showed some correlation, although there were exceptions. In at least two of the cases that showed advanced arteriolar sclerosis, there was a remarkably fine reaction to surgery at postoperative appraisal after three and four years. However — to introduce a note of caution — when we performed the operative wedge biopsy in one of these cases, the tissue from the superficial layers of the kidney didn't look the same as that deeper down. As we see a lot of collateral circulation in severe renal artery stenosis, it might be possible that superficial layers of the kidney are not subject to the same pressure conditions as deeper layers.

GROSS: First of all I should like to ask Dr. PEART a question about the plasma volume in his patient with secondary aldosteronism. Did this patient have a high plasma volume, which could explain the simultaneous reduction in the sodium and potassium concentrations in the plasma? My second point is that the pressure gradient — in other words, the pressure before and after the stenosis — was not mentioned at all in your paper, and I wonder what the significance of the pressure gradient may be. You said that the clamped or stenosed kidney is protected from hypertension; but we know that the difference in pressure before and after the stenosis is often very small, and in a renal artery stenosis, which can be shown radiographically, pressure peripheral to the stenosis may not be markedly reduced. Hence, there may be factors other than lowered pressure which are responsible for the fact that the kidney behind a stenosis is protected from certain pathological changes. I should like to mention here only what Dr. PAGE and his group have recently shown, namely that in acute experiments only a very slight reduction in pressure is needed to stimulate the secretion of renin. Thus, we may have to consider factors other than purely haemodynamic ones as being perhaps responsible for this so-called protection of the kidney beyond a stenosis.

PEART: As to Dr. TCHERDAKOFF's question regarding renin and posture, LEVER et al.[1] have done some fairly recent studies on this relation, and there is no doubt that plasma renin levels do go up on standing and down again on lying. The rises are not very big. They may involve changes of the order of about 50%. They wouldn't explain anything that has been observed in most of the patients we are discussing, but they might account for some of the scatter in the normal subjects.

Now the relation between renin and aldosterone is indeed, I think, very complex because of the following observations: there is no doubt, of course, that angiotensin stimulates aldosterone production. What is interesting is the converse in Conn's syndrome, that aldosterone secretion coming from a tumour suppresses renin levels in the plasma. Whenever one talks of production, one has to be terribly careful. I am talking only of a level of an enzyme in the plasma, because this tells us nothing at the moment about turnover rate, and one has to be rather guarded about that. But at any rate, the renin level goes down with a rise in aldosterone. Now it is fairly clear, I think, that there are all sorts of grades between, because it seems to me that the effects of aldosterone, particularly on sodium — perhaps on plasma volume, too, but I think predominantly on sodium — govern the level of renin in the plasma. So I think you have a situation where, when the effects of aldosterone are being exerted very markedly, perhaps on the kidney, perhaps elsewhere, the renin level tends to go down. Thus, the renin may be very low with high aldosterone secretion and may be very high with a high aldosterone secretion. Now this, I think, is because there is more than one variable. Therefore I believe the situation you have mentioned is understandable.

In reply to Dr. WILSON's question regarding renal damage in phaeochromocytoma, I should like to say that in a series we had at St. Mary's a long time ago, two of the patients who persisted with severe hypertension had, I think, quite a lot of renal damage, and, in fact, subsequent *post mortem* examination in one of them did reveal a great deal of renal damage, so that in some cases of phaeochromocytoma at any rate, the kidneys do become damaged, but obviously it is more important to consider the ones that don't.

I think that Dr. HOOD has raised an important point about the depth of biopsy and the conclusions as to renal damage. It is my experience that the worst damage is at the periphery, and the surgeons take those nice little triangles just from the top of the kidney, and therefore they see the worst, even though two thirds of the inside of the kidney may not look all that bad. I have seen this in some ischaemic kidneys where the inside, including even the tubules, looked quite good but the outer few millimeters looked awful.

Dr. GROSS, as to the case of aldosteronism with a stenosis, I can't tell you about the plasma volume in that patient; we did not measure it.

The question of pressure gradient is, I think, very important. I disagree — not really fundamentally, but I disagree nonetheless — with your statement about pressure gradients in relation to hypertension. I should say this about it: if you consider divided renal function studies and pressure gradients in relation to what you can do surgically for a patient — in other words, to help you decide whether nephrectomy or reconstruction of the renal artery is likely to do him any good — then I would say that, if you haven't got a pressure gradient, I don't believe you'll do the patient any good. After all, we don't do so many of our patients any good, even with a

[1] LEVER, A. F., J. J. BROWN, J. I. S. ROBERTSON, and R. MCPHERSON: in press.

pressure gradient of 50 mm. Hg or more, and I think the situation in the dog, or in any other animal, is very different, for the following reason: we must not equate renin with hypertension too readily. I grant that you can increase the pressure by putting a clip on a renal artery and show, as CORCORAN and PAGE did a long time ago[1], that the pressure on either side was the same, in other words, that there wasn't a pressure gradient; and this then led, as the subsequent work by SKINNER et al.[2] showed, to the appearance of an increased amount of renin in the renal vein blood. That is not to say that in man the same procedure would lead to hypertension. There must be an obstruction. There must be a pressure gradient in that renal artery. And I think usually the pressure gradient has to be of the order of 40 or 50 mm. or more, in fact, before you could even regard it as causing renal hypertension. I don't believe anybody has removed kidneys with pressure gradients of 20 mm. Hg or less with any success, unless definite ischaemic functional changes were present.

KINCAID-SMITH: In reply to Dr. TCHERDAKOFF, Dr. HOOD, and Dr. WILSON, all of whom raised the same question about the vascular lesions in the non-ischaemic kidney, I didn't mean to convey the impression that I thought these were of particular value in relation to response to renovascular surgery. Surgical treatment may be successful when quite severe hypertensive vascular damage is present. However, I do think that where there is marked narrowing in interlobular arteries, as in one case which I discussed, one cannot expect a good result; in fact, progressive uraemia occurs very rapidly if the opposite kidney is removed in that type of case. I can certainly confirm the experience that the superficial layers of the renal cortex may be very different from deeper levels, and this is one reason why I am quite cautious about the interpretation of renal biopsies in cases of renovascular hypertension.

In relation to the question of pressure gradients, I have great difficulty in interpreting this sort of thing, but I showed you one case with very severe narrowing of the left renal artery, in which fibrinoid necrosis was present in arterioles distal to the stenosis. In this patient, careful and repeated measurements showed no pressure gradient across the stenosis.

---

[1] CORCORAN, A. C., and I. H. PAGE: Amer. J. Physiol. **135**, 361 (1941/42).

[2] SKINNER, S. L., J. W. MCCUBBIN, and I. H. PAGE: Circulation Res. **13**, 336 (1963).

Diagnostic value of selective renal arteriography in hypertension

By

A. LIBRETTI and S. GRAZI

Renal arteriography has been widely used during the past few years for the detection of occlusive diseases of the renal arteries in hypertensive patients (*1–6*). However, the fact that selective angiographic methods have recently become available has made it possible to undertake a more accurate morphological study of anatomical lesions in minor branches of the renal arterial vasculature, lesions whose detection with aortographic methods had hitherto been problematic (*7*). Furthermore, thanks to the safety of transfemoral selective renal arteriography (*8*, *9*) and to the recent introduction of angiographic contrast media which are practically devoid of nephrotoxicity (*9—12*) it is now possible to make systematic studies of the renal vasculature in hypertensive patients. With the aid of renal angiography, we have studied a group of unselected hypertensive patients, and it is upon results obtained in this study that I now propose to report.

Diagnostic classification of 90 unselected hypertensive patients

Selective renal arteriography was performed in 90 hypertensive patients, using the technique of SELDINGER (*13*) as modified by ODMAN (*14*). The patients were unselected, the only prerequisite for their inclusion in the investigation being a diastolic pressure higher than 95 mm. Hg. After selective renal angiography, the patients were classified as follows: 59 (65.6%) with essential hypertension, nine (10%) with hypertension secondary to chronic glomerulonephritis, seven (7.8%) with chronic pyelonephritis (three bilateral and four unilateral), five with stenosis of the main renal artery, and ten with miscellaneous lesions of one or both kidneys, such as hydronephrosis (three cases), polycystic kidney (two cases), horseshoe kidney (two cases), intrarenal arteriovenous fistula (one case), coarctation of the aorta (one case), and Cushing's disease (one case) (Table 1).

Table 1. *Diagnostic classification of 90 non-selected hypertensive patients*

	Number of patients	%
Essential hypertension	59	65.6
Chronic glomerulonephritis	9	10.0
Chronic pyelonephritis	7	7.8
Renal artery stenosis	5	5.6
Hydronephrosis	3	3.3
Polycystic kidney	2	2.2
Horseshoe kidney	2	2.2
Renal arteriovenous fistula	1	1.1
Coarctation of aorta	1	1.1
Cushing's disease	1	1.1
	90	100.0

Renal arteriographic pattern in essential hypertension

The 59 patients classified as cases of essential hypertension were placed in this category because no specific lesions were found which could be considered responsible for the hypertension. The renal vasculature appeared to be normal in 30 of these patients (Fig. 1),

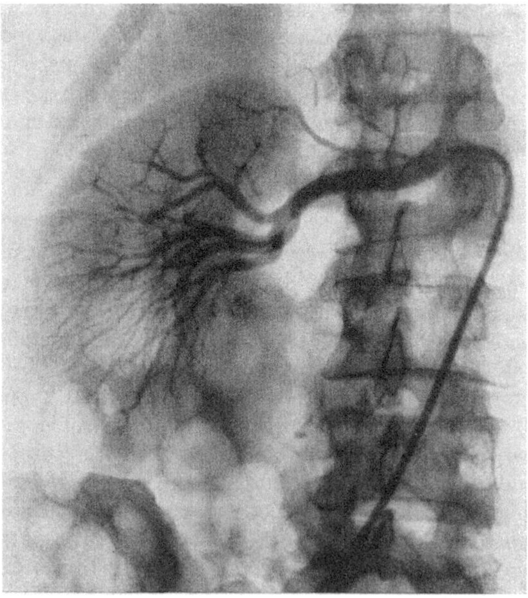

Fig. 1. Right kidney of a patient with essential hypertension. The entire renal vasculature is of normal appearance.

and the other 29 showed diffuse abnormalities. These consisted of a diffuse sclerotic appearance of the peripheral arterial vessels, which were tortuous and irregular in size and contour; the arcuate arteries, when filled, appeared distorted and tortuous; the size of both kidneys and the thickness of the cortex were not significantly altered (Fig. 2).

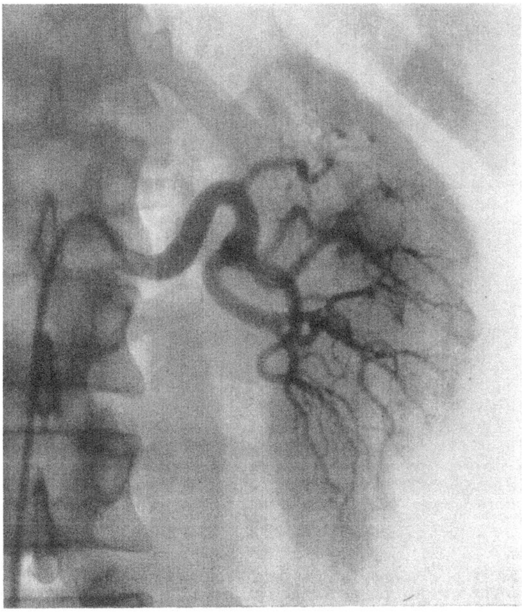

Fig. 2. Left kidney of a patient with essential hypertension. The kidney appears normal in size and contour. The intraparenchymal vessels have a tortuous appearance. The arcuate arteries are only slightly filled.

In three patients from this group, the arteriographic aspect of the renal vasculature was remarkably different and was characterised by a severe reduction in the size of both kidneys, associated with thinning of the cortical substance and a high degree of tortuosity and narrowing of the parenchymal vessels; the arcuate arteries were often not filled. In general, there was a marked reduction in the parenchymal vascularisation (Fig. 3), a feature closely resembling that observed in patients with chronic glomerulonephritis.

As is apparent from Table 2, close correlations were found in these hypertensive patients between the renal arteriographic patterns and the clinical findings. In fact, mean age, mean diastolic pressure, and duration of the hypertensive disease all appeared definitely higher in the subjects with greater vascular involvement. Renal function studies also yielded pathological results in the patients with arteriographic evidence of impaired renal vascularisation, as illustrated by the progressive decrease in the values for renal plasma flow and by the increase in the filtration fractions in

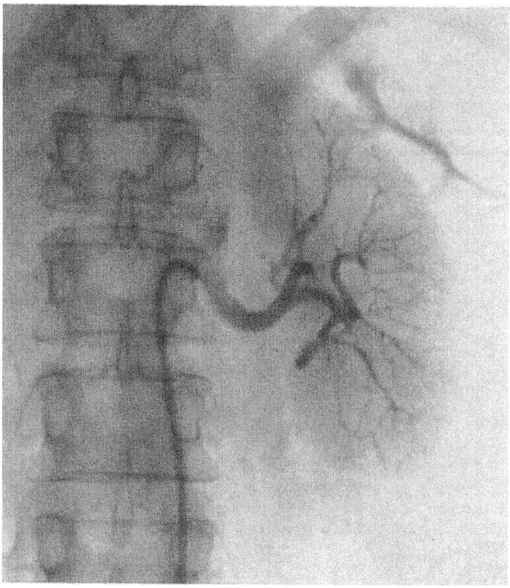

Fig. 3. Left kidney of a patient with severe essential hypertension. The kidney appears reduced in size. The intraparenchymal vessels are scanty, thin, and tortuous, and the arcuate arteries unfilled.

the more severely affected patients. Similar correlations were likewise observed with regard to the eyeground findings and the signs of left ventricular hypertrophy.

From these results it appears that selective renal arteriography is a useful aid in the diagnosis of "essential" hypertension, because it enables one to exclude – sometimes with certainty – other renal diseases as causes of the hypertension; this applies particularly to cases in which diagnosis purely on the basis of a clinical and functional evaluation is difficult. Secondly, selective renal arteriography also makes it possible to arrive at a clinical assessment of the hypertensive patient which is significantly related to the severity of renal haemodynamic impairment and to the extent of retinal and cardiac involvement. The usefulness of such an evaluation is borne out by the fact that the renal arteriographic findings in the two groups of essential hypertensives were consistently uniform, whereas the clinical data showed wide individual variations, as reflected in the high standard deviations of the mean values. Such observed correlations between angiographic morphology and

Table 2. *Clinical data and arteriographic pattern of 59 patients with essential hypertension.* n: number of patients; S.D.: standard deviation; R.P.F.: renal plasma flow; G.F.R.: glomerular filtration rate; F.F.: filtration fraction; L.V.H.: left ventricular hypertrophy

Clinical data			Arteriographic pattern	
			Normal (n = 30)	Abnormal (n = 29)
Age	(years:	mean ± S.D.)	39.9 ± 13	57.9 ± 7
Diastolic B.P.	(mm.Hg:	mean ± S.D.)	104.5 ± 18	125.4 ± 18
Duration of hypertension	(years:	mean ± S.D.)	3.6 ± 2	9.6 ± 5
R.P.F.	(ml./min.:	mean ± S.D.)	448.7 ± 98	329.4 ± 81
G.F.R.	(ml./min.:	mean ± S.D.)	92.0 ± 25	81.1 ± 19
F.F.	(%:	mean ± S.D.)	20.5 ± 1.5	27.0 ± 1.5
Blood urea nitrogen	(mg.%:	mean ± S.D.)	31.0 ± 8	37.0 ± 13
Proteinuria:	absent		27	18
	present		3	11
Sediment:	normal		28	26
	abnormal		2	3
Urography:	normal		27	18
	abnormal		3	11
Eyegrounds:	normal		13	2
	I		12	11
	II		5	11
	III		—	2
	IV		—	3
E.C.G.:	normal		25	8
	L.V.H.		5	21

functional data agree well with similar results obtained in experimental animals (*15*). However, it must be emphasised that, owing to numerous technical limitations, assessments of renal blood flow based on angiographic methods are virtually meaningless, since they relate only to the preglomerular part of the blood flow (*16*). Although some of these limitations inherent in the arteriographic method – such as the laminar flux of the contrast medium and the asymmetry of ejection from the catheter, coupled with the asymmetry of the openings of the renal arteries –

have been partly overcome by the use of the selective arteriographic technique, angiographic evaluations of renal blood flow still provide only a very approximative indication.

Renal arteriographic pattern in chronic glomerulonephritis

Nine out of the 90 hypertensive patients were clinically diagnosed as suffering from chronic glomerulonephritis. As may be seen from Table 3, their mean age was 34 years, their mean diastolic pressure 125.2 mm. Hg, and the mean duration of the hypertension four years. Renal function studies showed a marked reduction in

Table 3. *Clinical data of patients with chronic glomerulonephritis and chronic pyelonephritis.* n: number of patients; S.D.: standard deviation; R.P.F.: renal plasma flow; G.F.R.: glomerular filtration rate; F.F.: filtration fraction; L.V.H.: left ventricular hypertrophy

Clinical data			Chronic glomerulonephritis (n = 9)	Chronic pyelonephritis (n = 7)
Age	(years:	mean ± S.D.)	34.8 ± 8	49.7 ± 5
Diastolic B.P.	(mm. Hg:	mean ± S.D.)	125.2 ± 14	138.2 ± 15
Duration of hypertension	(years:	mean ± S.D.)	4.5 ± 2	4.9 ± 3
R.P.F.	(ml./min.:	mean ± S.D.)	504.3 ± 96	225.4 ± 55
G.F.R.	(ml./min.:	mean ± S.D.)	58.5 ± 15	49.5 ± 14
F.F.	(%:	mean ± S.D.)	11.6 ± 1.7	22.7 ± 1.4
Blood urea nitrogen	(mg.%:	mean ± S.D.)	68.0 ± 12	46.0 ± 9
Proteinuria:	absent		1	2
	present		8	5
Sediment:	normal		—	4
	abnormal		9	3
Urography:	normal		4	3
	abnormal		5	4
Eyegrounds:	normal		1	—
	I		2	3
	II		1	1
	III		2	2
	IV		3	1
E.C.G.:	normal		3	—
	L.V.H.		6	7

the glomerular filtration rate and no significant changes in renal plasma flow, the result being a significant decrease in the filtration fraction. The renal arteriographic patterns were characterised by a uniform and symmetrical decrease in the size of both kidneys, whose cortical thickness appeared to be extremely reduced. The interlobar arteries were thinned and stretched and the arcuate arteries almost constantly unfilled; nephrographic opacification was scanty. On the whole, the parenchymal vasculature appeared to be markedly reduced, particularly in the cortical region (Fig. 4).

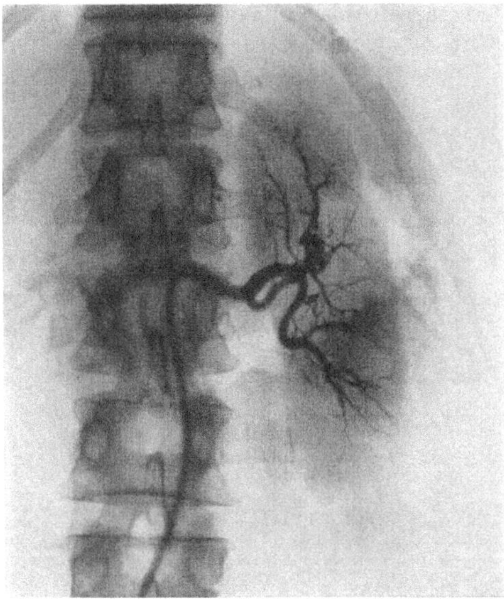

Fig. 4. Left kidney of a patient with chronic glomerulonephritis. The kidney is small in size, and the cortical substance is reduced in thickness. The intraparenchymal vessels are thin and tortuous. The appearance of an avascular area in the inferior pole of the kidney is due to a faulty filling of an inferior polar artery, as later demonstrated by aortogram.

As will be apparent from a comparison of Figs 3 and 4, the renal angiographic features of chronic glomerulonephritis were similar to, and practically indistinguishable from, those found in some patients with essential hypertension. In these cases, a clinical diagnosis could obviously only be made on the basis of the results of renal function studies. The latter, in fact, reveal characteristic differences between the two conditions, the filtration fraction being reduced in chronic glomerulonephritis and practically unchanged in essential hypertension.

Renal arteriographic pattern in chronic pyelonephritis

Chronic pyelonephritis was diagnosed in seven of our 90 hypertensive patients. In four cases, renal involvement was unilateral and in three bilateral. The pyelonephritic kidneys were smaller and showed gross alterations in contour produced by scarring retractions. Consonant with these findings was the distorted appearance of the vascular topography and the pronounced disorganisation of the pyramidal design. The cortical substance was irregular and of varying thickness, and the nephrographic opacification lacking in uniformity (Fig. 5). In three out of four patients with unilateral pyelonephritis the urogram was of normal appearance, whereas

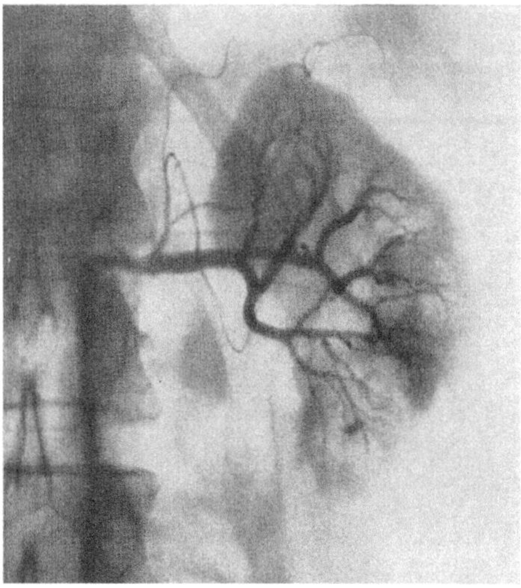

Fig. 5. Left kidney of a patient with chronic pyelonephritis. The kidney is reduced in size, and its contour shows gross irregularities. The parenchymal vascularisation is disorganised and the nephrographic opacification non-uniform.

patients with bilateral renal involvement showed inadequate elimination of the contrast medium; only in one case was clubbing of the calyces visible, a sign described by HODSON (*17*) as characteristic of pyelonephritis. The urinary sediment was normal in all four patients with unilateral pyelonephritis, and typically altered in those with bilateral involvement. Renal functional values were markedly abnormal in all the pyelonephritic patients, with a severe reduction in the values for renal plasma flow and glomerular filtration rate (see Table 3).

In the cases reported, the typical angiographic patterns of the renal vasculature enabled us to make a clear-cut diagnosis of chronic pyelonephritis, whereas a diagnosis based merely on the clinical findings would have been most uncertain.

Renal artery stenosis

In five patients, renal arteriography revealed stenosis of the main renal artery. In three cases, the stenosis was located in the proximal part of the vessel and had the appearance of a concentric atherosclerotic plaque (*4*) with a large post-stenotic dilatation (Fig. 6). In the other two cases, the occlusive lesions were situated

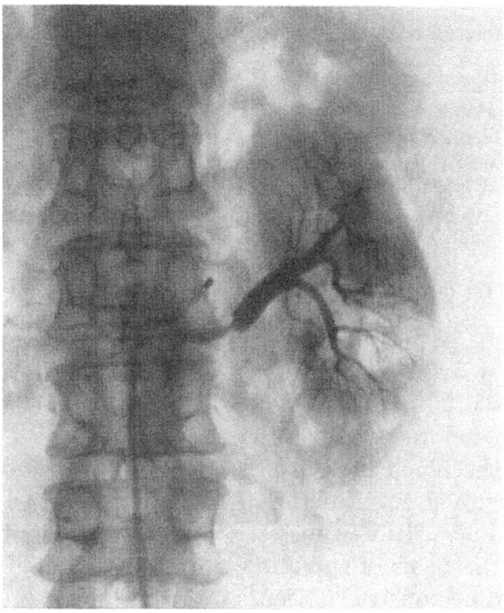

Fig. 6. Severe stenosis of the main left renal artery with a large post-stenotic dilatation. The size of this kidney was 1.5 cm. smaller than that of the contralateral kidney.

in the distal part of the renal artery, with typical patterns of fibromuscular hyperplasia (*18*); in one of these cases, the lesions were bilateral. As shown in Table 4, the case history and the physical and urographic data were not suggestive of renovascular hypertension in all these patients (*3*, *19*–*21*). The individual renal function tests were indicative of unilateral renal ischaemia in four of them (in the patient with bilateral stenosis the tests showed renal ischaemia on the side with the severer stenosis). Only in one case was the stenosis not associated with concomitant functional involvement of the affected kidney; in this case, the degree of stenosis was less than 50%, which is regarded as the minimum degree of narrowing capable of producing functional impairment (*22*).

Table 4. *Clinical data of five patients with renal artery stenosis*

	Number of patients
Absence of family history of hypertension	3
Age <20 years	—
>50 years	2
Recent onset of hypertension (within two years)	4
Recent aggravation of pre-existing hypertension	—
Flank pain	—
Generalised atherosclerosis	1
Systolic bruit	2
Hypopotassaemia	2
Urography: decrease in size of affected kidney	4
difference in "appearance time"	2
differential concentration	2
Positive Howard test	4
Positive Rapoport test	4

Miscellaneous conditions associated with arterial hypertension

Three of the hypertensive patients investigated with the aid of selective renal arteriography had vascular patterns typical of hydronephrosis (*23—25*). In one of these, surgical correction of the anomalous vessel responsible for the condition did not result in reduction of the blood pressure to normal levels.

Two patients showed angiographic abnormalities indicative of polycystic kidneys. In neither case had it been possible to make a diagnosis on the basis of the clinical and urographic data.

In two hypertensive patients the presence of a congenital horseshoe kidney had previously been suggested by urographic studies. Arteriographic examination, however, permitted a more accurate and detailed study of the malformation. In fact, selective catheterisation of each renal artery (five in one case and four in the other) revealed normal vascularisation of the renal parenchyma, with no signs of pyelonephritis, which is the most common cause of hypertension in these patients (*26*).

In one case — that of a woman aged 53 years — selective renal arteriography showed an angiomatous formation in the right kidney with an intrarenal arteriovenous fistula (Fig. 7). The presence of the arteriovenous shunt was confirmed by the finding of different degrees of oxygen saturation in the blood in the two renal veins, and its amount was calculated to be 17% of the renal blood flow. This shunt, however, was producing only limited impairment of systemic haemodynamics, as demonstrated by the fact that the values for the cardiac index were practically normal. After nephrectomy, the patient's blood pressure remained elevated – which lends support to the hypothesis that in this case the hypertension was not due to the renal arteriovenous fistula.

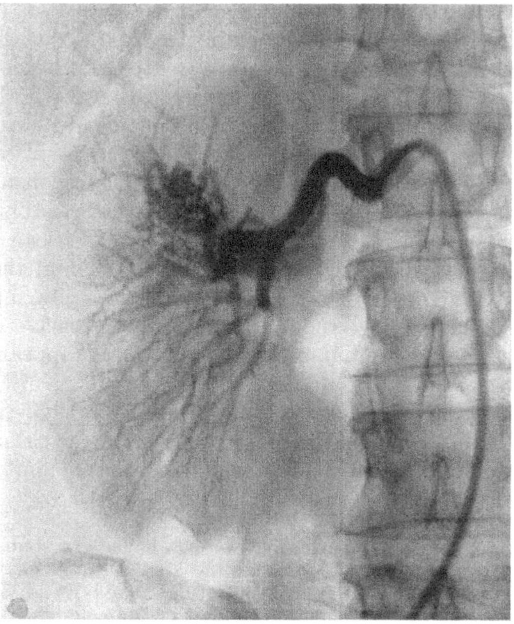

Fig. 7. Angiomatous formation in the right kidney with an intrarenal arteriovenous fistula. Note the opacification of the main renal vein and the ascending vena cava.

In two other hypertensive patients, one with coarctation of the aorta and the other with Cushing's disease, the arteriographic patterns of the kidneys appeared normal.

Conclusions

It is apparent from the results reported here that a morphological study of renal vascularisation by means of selective renal arteriography offers a useful aid by which to make an exact diagnosis in cases of hypertension. It did, in fact, enable us to confirm the diagnosis of essential hypertension in 59 out of our 90 patients and to undertake a more thorough evaluation of the renal vascular disorders present in these patients.

In the patients with chronic glomerulonephritis, no morphological alterations were observed which would have been sufficient to make it possible to differentiate this disease from very advanced essential hypertension. On the other hand, renal arteriography did prove useful in the diagnosis of chronic pyelonephritis, a condition which is sometimes difficult to distinguish from either essential hypertension or chronic glomerulonephritis.

The importance of renal arteriography in the diagnosis of renovascular hypertension is widely accepted and needs no further comment. It must be emphasised, however, that use of the selective arteriographic technique permits a more accurate study of the renal vascularisation as a whole and may also reveal evidence of lesions in the smaller vessels which could be responsible for segmentary ischaemia. Furthermore, the fact that renal angiography is free from significant complications means that it can suitably be employed in larger groups of non-selected patients; this, in turn, might provide more realistic figures regarding the incidence of occlusive diseases of the renal arteries in hypertensive patients.

Finally, arteriographic examination would appear to be an indispensable aid in the diagnosis of certain renal diseases which may be associated with hypertension (such as polycystic kidneys and renal arteriovenous fistulae) in cases where the clinical findings do not provide sufficient data on which to base a definite diagnosis.

Summary

Ninety non-selected hypertensive patients have been studied by means of selective renal arteriography. After the arteriographic examination, 59 of them (65.6%) were diagnosed as suffering from essential hypertension, nine from chronic glomerulonephritis, and seven from chronic pyelonephritis. In five, renal arteriography revealed stenosis of the main renal artery, and in the other ten, miscellaneous diseases of the kidneys, such as hydronephrosis, polycystic kidneys, horseshoe kidneys, and intrarenal arteriovenous fistula. Close correlations were found between the degree of renal vascular involvement and the clinical and functional data of the patients with essential hypertension, chronic glomerulonephritis, and chronic pyelonephritis. It is therefore concluded that the systematic use of selective renal arteriography in non-selected hypertensive patients may yield useful and sometimes unexpected results which enable one to make a more realistic causal classification of the hypertensive disease.

Zusammenfassung

Neunzig nicht ausgewählte Patienten mit Hochdruck wurden mit Hilfe der selektiven Nierenarteriographie untersucht. Nach der arteriographischen Prüfung wurde bei 59 (65,6%) von ihnen die Diagnose essentielle Hypertension gestellt, bei neun chronische Glomerulonephritis und bei sieben chronische Pyelonephritis. In fünf Fällen lag eine Stenose der Hauptnierenarterie vor und bei den anderen zehn verschiedene Nierenerkrankungen wie Hydronephrose, polyzystische Nieren, Hufeisenniere und intrarenale arteriovenöse Fisteln. Es bestand eine enge Korrelation zwischen dem Grad, in dem die Nierengefäße befallen waren, und den klinischen und funktionellen Befunden, die bei den Patienten mit essentiellem Hochdruck, chronischer Glomerulonephritis und chronischer Pyelonephritis vorlagen. Es wird geschlossen, daß die systematische Anwendung der selektiven Nierenarteriographie bei nicht ausgewählten Hochdruckpatienten zu wichtigen und oft unerwarteten Resultaten fuhren kann, die es ermöglichen, eine bessere ursächliche Einteilung der Hochdruckkrankheit vorzunehmen.

Résumé

Une artériographie rénale sélective a été systématiquement pratiquée chez 90 malades hypertendus non triés. Cet examen a permis d'établir les diagnostics étiologiques suivants: 59 (65,6%) hypertensions essentielles, neuf glomérulonéphrites chroniques, sept pyélonéphrites chroniques, cinq rétrécissements du tronc de l'artère rénale, les dix derniers cas étant représentés par des affections rénales diverses telles qu'hydronéphrose, reins polykystiques, rein en fer à cheval, anévrysme artério-veineux intra-rénal. On a pu montrer une étroite corrélation entre le degré des lésions vasculaires rénales et les signes cliniques et fonctionnels des malades présentant une hypertension essentielle, une glomérulonéphrite chronique ou une pyélonéphrite chronique. On peut donc conclure que l'utilisation systématique de l'artériographie rénale sélective chez tout malade hypertendu peut apporter des résultats utiles et parfois inattendus permettant de conduire à une classification étiologique plus exacte de la maladie hypertensive.

References

1. Poutasse, E. F., and H. P. Dustan: J. Amer. Med. Ass. **165**, 158 (1957). — 2. Brown, J. J., W. S. Peart, K. Owen, J. I. S. Robertson, and D. Sutton: Brit. Med. J. 1960/II, 327. — 3. Perloff, D., M. Sokolow, E. J. Wylie, D. R. Smith, and A. J. Palubinskas: Circulation **24**, 1286 (1961). — 4. Poutasse, E. F.: J. Amer. Med. Ass. **178**, 1078 (1961). — 5. Beall, A. C., G. C. Morris, E. S. Crawford, D. A. Cooley, and M. E. DeBakey: Surgery **49**, 772 (1961). — 6. Wilson, L. L., H. P. Dustan, I. H. Page, and E. F. Poutasse: Arch. Int. Med. **112**, 270 (1963). — 7. Meaney, T. F., and H. P. Dustan: Circulation **28**, 1035 (1963). — 8. Quin-Kong, T., T. F. Meaney, H. P. Dustan, and F. M. Sones: Amer. J. Med. Sc. **246**, 527 (1963). — 9. Grazi, S., and A. Libretti: Minerva med. **56**, 3465 (1965). — 10. Steinberg, I., and J. A. Evans: Radiology **79**, 395 (1962). — 11. Foster, J. M., E. W. Winfrey III, D. A. Killen, and R. T. Sessions: J. Amer. Med. Ass. **182**, 1009 (1962). — 12. Kanick, V., and N. Finby: Radiology **80**, 438 (1963). — 13. Seldinger, S. I.: Acta radiol. **39**, 368 (1953). — 14. Odman, P.: Acta radiol. **45**, 1 (1956). — 15. Daniel, P. M., M. M. L. Prichard, and J. N. Ward McQuald: Brit. J. Surg. **42**, 212 (1954). — 16. Stamey, T. A.: Renovascular Hypertension. Williams and Wilkins, Baltimore, 1963. — 17. Hodson, C. J.: Proc. Roy. Soc. Med. **52**, 669 (1959). — 18. Palubinskas, A. J., and E. J. Wylie: Radiology **76**, 634 (1961). — 19. Maxwell, M. H., and G. B. Prozan: Progr. Cardiovascular Diseases **5**, 81 (1962). — 20. Gilliland, P. F., J. J. Deller, and R. Hall: N. England J. Med. **264**, 659 (1961). — 21. Slaton, P. E., and E. G. Biglieri: Circulation 28, 806 (1963). — 22. Dustan, H. P., A. W. Humphries, V. G. DeWolfe, and I. H. Page: J. Amer. Med. Ass. **187**, 1028 (1964). — 23. Braasch, W. F., W. Walters, and H. J. Hammer: J. Amer. Med. Ass. **115**, 1837 (1940). — 24. Abeshouse, B. S.: Surgery **10**, 147 (1941). — 25. O'Conor, V. J.: J. Amer. Med. Ass. **120**, 579 (1942). — 26. Pickering, G. W.: High Blood Pressure. Churchill Ltd., London, 1955, p. 380.

Discussion

PAGE: I should like to say that the speakers have shown admirable restraint in presenting their material this morning. The clinical application has far outstripped the concurrent physiological and biochemical studies. The only dangerous word that I heard this morning is "ischaemia", which, as you all know, I object to. "Parameters" you can have; I have virtually abandoned my campaign against this term.

The problem of the renal arterial pressure gradients is certainly a very tricky one. SKINNER, MCCUBBIN, and I[1] found that even very slight falls in blood pressure cause the release of small amounts of renin. This is almost certainly a physiological homoeostatic mechanism. Then Dr. BUNAG[2] in our laboratory found that he could block the release of renin resulting from haemorrhage simply by anaesthetising the renal nerves or using a ganglion blocking agent. So now we have not only a physical factor, i.e. reduction in mean pressure, but apparently a neural component as well. Finally, what we showed is that if angiotensin is infused into the renal arterial blood, it suppresses renin release; so there seems to be a feed-back. There may be a great many other mechanisms responsible for the release of renin.

The term ischaemia has always bothered me, ever since HARRY GOLDBLATT first used it, because I have never been convinced that there is a relationship between renal blood flow and the height of the blood pressure. Certainly you see plenty of patients in whom there is severe ischaemia of the kidney, by which is meant a reduction in blood flow without any hypertension. My contention is simply that of course you will see ischaemic atrophy as time goes on, but I would point out that there are many patients in whom the blood pressure has come down after nephrectomy and in whom the kidney shows no ischaemic atrophy. I was delighted to see it stated that the level of plasma renin or the amount in a juxtaglomerular cell need not have any relationship to the turnover, because to assume that they do is to fall into the same trap as we fell into. Before isotopes became available, we felt that levels of things had some significance. We know now that the turnover is more important.

PEART: The reason I still use the term ischaemia, meaning a reduction in blood flow to the kidney — in the restrictive sense of the relation to what has to be called renovascular hypertension — is that I feel nobody has established any case other than that the only sort of kidney, the removal of which cures the hypertension, is a kidney with a reduced blood flow to it.

The question of pressure gradients is important, but I think you have to consider pressure gradients in relation to hypertension in man, as it is seen and as it is cured, because that is really the ultimate proof in the sense of human renovascular hypertension. Faced with disease of the renal artery or unilateral renal disease, I don't believe anybody can convincingly say at the moment which kidney is causing the hypertension in any given patient.

---

[1] SKINNER, S. L., J. W. MCCUBBIN, and I. H. PAGE: Circulation Res. **15**, 64 (1964).

[2] BUNAG, R. B., J. W. MCCUBBIN, and I. H. PAGE: The Pharmacologist **6**, 201 (1964).

This is only turning the cycle back again to what the earlier pathologists said 30 or more years ago, namely that a lot of the renal disease and a lot of the main renal artery disease was caused by the hypertension. I think there are many instances where that must be so. Our difficulty is to try and discriminate between the two things. As to the question of pressure gradients in the case Dr. KINCAID-SMITH mentioned, where there was none, I think the truth is as simple as this: if you have no blood flow distal to a stenosis, then there is no pressure gradient across it, however tight it may be, because, in fact, if there is no blood flow at all or only a very limited blood flow, the pressure across the stenosis equalises. This can be demonstrated very readily at operation if the surgeon constricts the artery distal to the stenosis by means of tapes; the pressures measured directly on both sides of the stenosis become equal. This is merely because the blood flow through tbe kidney is impeded and the pressure drop across the stenosis disappears. I should imagine that in that case mentioned, the external renal function in that kidney was very poor indeed, and that divided renal function studies would have revealed very marked ischaemia. As I see it, it is a waste of time to operate on patients, unless one has considered the divided renal function studies as well as the pressure gradients. I think those two things should be taken together.

Diagnostic significance of humoral factors in renovascular hypertension

By

J. Genest, G. Y. Tremblay[1], R. Boucher[2], J. de Champlain[1], J. M. Rojo Ortega, R. Lefebvre, P. Roy, and P. Cartier

The availability of aortography and renal angiography in many medical centres throughout the world makes it possible to obtain precise evidence of the presence or absence of renovascular lesions. Thanks to these aids, earlier necropsy findings in man reported by Blackman, showing a relationship between partial obstruction of the main renal arteries and hypertension, have been confirmed in many living hypertensive patients (*1*). But the presence of such renovascular obstructive lesions, whatever their nature, does not indicate *per se* that such lesions are the cause of the hypertensive process in a given patient.

The major problem facing the physiologist and the diagnostician is how to establish that the renal obstructive lesion is really the cause of the hypertensive process in individual patients and, by way of consequence, how to prevent unnecessary surgery. It is therefore of the utmost importance to improve and define more exactly the diagnostic criteria of true renovascular hypertension, i. e. hypertension *secondary* to an occlusive lesion of one or more renal arteries or their branches, and to be able to predict the results which adequate surgery will have on the hypertensive condition. Of all the major criteria suggested for the diagnosis of true renovascular hypertension, there are three which are based on endocrine-metabolic abnormalities and which have been proposed because they are possibly of greater importance and significance. They are: 1) the angiotensin infusion test, 2) studies of split renal function, and 3) measurement of renin activity in peripheral or in renal venous blood.

The angiotensin infusion test may be valid for the differential diagnosis of most patients with renovascular hypertension as compared with patients suffering from essential hypertension, but

[1] Medical Research Fellow of the Medical Research Council of Canada.
[2] Medical Research Associate of the Medical Research Council of Canada.

it does not appear to be as specific as originally suggested by KAPLAN and SILAH (*2*). Many patients with chronic renal parenchymatous diseases and patients with essential hypertension receiving natriuretic drugs will exhibit as much resistance to the pressor effect of infused angiotensin as patients with renovascular hypertension. The assumption on which this test is based, i. e. that the dose of angiotensin necessary to provoke an increase of 20 mm. Hg in diastolic pressure reflects the endogenous levels of circulating angiotensin, is not valid, since many normal subjects will require the same pressor dose as do some patients with renal artery stenosis. Finally, the state of the sodium balance will greatly modify vascular reactivity to the infused angiotensin, as VEYRAT has recently demonstrated (*3*).

Studies of split renal function (*4*, *5*, *6*) – involving measurement of urine volume, sodium creatinine and osmolar concentrations, glomerular filtration rate (by reference to inulin or creatinine clearance) and the percentage of sodium reabsorption, and determination of vasopressor activity, or preferably of renin activity, in the urine from each side – have much more validity and a far higher degree of metabolic significance. They are without doubt of great diagnostic value in the majority of patients with renovascular hypertension. But the performance of such split renal function studies has several disadvantages: 1) it is time-consuming (quite apart from the time required for the technical determinations of sodium osmolarity, creatinine clearances, and renin activity); 2) it carries risks of possible infection and of ureteral obstruction by blood clots; 3) it is most painful unless carried out under some form of anaesthesia (in most centres, these tests are now done under spinal anaesthesia); 4) it necessitates the enthusiastic and whole-hearted co-operation of a urologist; 5) it is not conclusive in many cases of obstruction of renal arterial branches or bilateral lesions and in patients with accessory or aberrant arteries; 6) it may be unsatisfactory because of leakage of urine around the catheter in the ureter. Notwithstanding these shortcomings, split renal function tests are of fundamental interest from the physiological point of view and prove of diagnostic importance in the majority of cases when carried out under expert supervision. The metabolic disturbances are, we believe, partly due to intrarenal haemodynamic changes and are also in part directly associated with the liberation of renin by the involved kidney and the formation of angiotensin.

Thirdly, the measurement of blood renin activity brings us to the purpose of this presentation, which is intended as a supplement to our previous report (*7*) and describes the results of studies we undertook in 37 patients in whom at least three of the following four parameters were measured: 1) systolic pressure gradient between the distal renal artery of the involved kidney and the aorta, 2) renin activity in peripheral or in renal venous blood, 3) count of the juxtaglomerular cells and measurement of their granularity, and 4) the presence or absence of arteriolar lesions in the involved kidney.

Methods and patients

The systolic pressure gradient was measured at the time of angiography in about one third of the patients by catheterisation and in the remaining two thirds during surgery. Blood renin activity was ascertained using the procedure of Boucher et al. (*8*). The renin content in renal tissue was determined after homogenisation and ultrasonification of the tissue, according to a new procedure of Boucher (*9*). Juxtaglomerular cell counts indicating the percentage of granular cells of types II and III were made in accordance with the classification of Turgeon and Sommers (*10*). Renal arteriolar changes in the kidney biopsies were graded according to the classification of Castleman and Smithwick (*11*).

Renin activity in peripheral venous blood from normal subjects varies from undetectable levels (for a total incubation time of three hours) to 32 ng./min./l.[1] of plasma with a mean of 9 $\pm$ *S. D.* 7. The mean value for renin activity in renal venous blood obtained by catheterisation in five cardiac patients with valvular disease, but without hypertension or oedema, is 37/ng./min./l. of plasma, with a range of 0 to 115. A linear correlation is obtained between renin activity in renal venous blood and granularity of the juxtaglomerular cells expressed as the total number of granular cells of types II and III per 25 juxtaglomerular apparatuses. The normal juxtaglomerular cell count is 190 $\pm$ 21 per 25 juxtaglomerular apparatuses, with a percentage of granular cells of types II and III of 4.6.

Of the large number of patients operated upon in this hospital for hypertension associated with renal artery obstruction, 37 are included in the present study, because at least three of the above parameters were measured in each case. All these patients underwent an extensive evaluation, including assessment of renal function, renal angiography, measurement of plasma electrolytes, and repeated blood-pressure readings. They were divided into four

[1] This high value exceeds three standard deviations of the mean.

groups (Table 1). The first comprises 14 patients with a significant systolic pressure gradient, a high blood renin activity, and/or a high juxtaglomerular cell count with an increased percentage of granular cells of types II and III, and absence of any renal arteriolar

Table 1. *Hypertension associated with renal artery obstruction*

Groups	No. of patients	Systolic pressure gradient	Renin activity	J.G.C. granularity	Arteriolar lesions
Group 1	14	++++	++++	++++	0
Group 2	8	++++	++++	++++	+ to ++++
Group 3	10	++++	N	N	+ or 0
Group 4	5	0	N	N	

N: normal

changes. Group 2 consists of eight patients with the same characteristics as those of Group 1, but with the presence of significant renal arteriolar changes. Group 3 is made up of ten patients with a significant pressure gradient, but without any increase either in blood renin activity at the time of blood sampling or in juxtaglomerular cell granularity. In all the patients in these three groups, the systolic pressure gradient was above 50 mm. Hg. In Group 4, there are five patients in whom no pressure gradient was found across the stenosis and who had normal renin activity and normal juxtaglomerular cell counts and granularity.

Results

The over-all results of surgery (nephrectomy or arterioplasty) in Groups 1, 2, and 3 are shown in Table 2, and data concerning each patient are given in Tables 3, 4, and 5. Two of the five patients

Table 2. *Results of surgery in patients with hypertension associated with renal artery obstruction*

Groups	No. of patients	Cured[1]	Improved[2]	Follow-up after surgery (in months)	
				average	range
Group 1	14	12	2	27	(7—84)
Group 2	8	2	0	9	(2—20)
Group 3	10	1	0	11	(1—20)

[1] B.P. below 140/90 mm. Hg.
[2] Mean decrease in diastolic pressure 25 mm. Hg.

in Group 4 were operated upon without any improvement of their hypertensive state. By "cure" we mean a fall in blood pressure after surgery to, or below, 140/90 mm. Hg, persisting without any antihypertensive medication for the entire period of observation. "Improvement" means an average fall in diastolic pressure of 25 mm. Hg or more. Of the 14 patients in Group 1, 12 have been cured and two have shown improvement over an average period of observation, following surgery, of 27 months with a range of seven to 84 months (Tables 2, 3). From this group, three patients may be selected in order to illustrate some of the studies carried out or certain specific points.

The first is a 40-year-old bus driver with a two-week history of severe hypertension at 240/140 mm. Hg. His mother was hypertensive. Angiography revealed severe constriction of the left renal artery with post-stenotic dilatation. The course of this patient is illustrated in Fig. 1. Urinary aldosterone was just slightly above

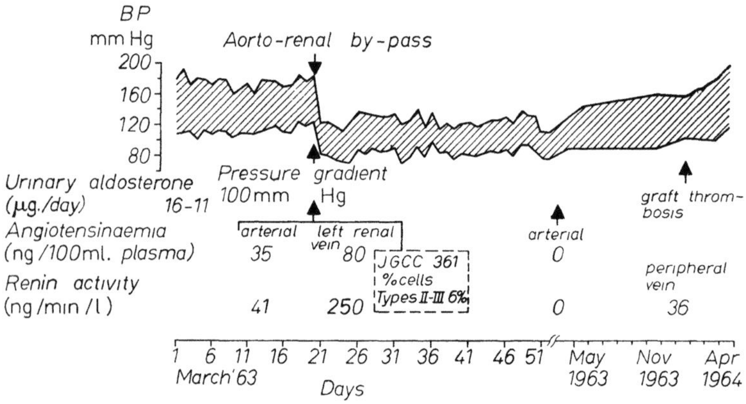

Fig. 1. 40-year-old bus driver (A. R.) with severe unilateral renal hypertension known for two weeks prior to admission. Mother hypertensive and hemiplegic. Serum potassium: 4.3 mEq./l., sodium: 142, and bicarbonates: 24. Phenolsulphonphthalein excretion: 24% in 15 min., 53% in 60 min. Creatinine clearance: 129 ml./min. No visualisation of left kidney during intravenous pyelography. Note, at the time of surgery, the high systolic gradient with the increased levels of renin activity and angiotensin in the left renal venous blood and the J.G.C.C. (juxtaglomerular cell count) of 361.

the upper limits of the normal range as determined by NOWACZYNSKI's method (*12*). The angiotensin level in the arterial blood was within the upper range of normal and was definitely excessive in the left renal venous blood. Renin activity in the blood of both arteries and in the left renal venous blood was decidedly above normal limits. At the time of operation, the systolic pressure gradient was 100 mm. Hg. Biopsy of the left kidney showed a total

Table 3. *Group 1: Significant pressure gradient, increased renin activity and/or J.G.C.C., no arteriolar changes*

Name	Age	Sex	Systolic pressure gradient	Renin activity		J.G.C.C. total	Percent types II—III	Results of surgery	Follow-up period after surgery (months)
				Renal vein	Peripheral				
L. L.	33	M	Thrombosis	525	120	250	36	Cured (partial nephrectomy)	14
J. M.	13	F	Thrombosis			427	17	Cured (partial nephrectomy)	22
R. P.	37	M	100	1,390	278	440	14	Improved (arterioplasty)	24
P. P.	39	F	Thrombosis	617	67	310	17	Improved (nephrectomy)	12
A. R.	40	M	100	250	41	361	6	Cured (arterioplasty)	24
SrA. P.	49	F	80			220	6	Cured (nephrectomy)	24
C. T.	48	M	Severe stenosis			616	30	Cured (nephrectomy)	42
F. P.	35	F	Severe stenosis			537	15	Cured (nephrectomy)	36
E. M.	46	M	Severe stenosis			225	64	Cured (nephrectomy)	60
G. T.	59	M	Severe stenosis			320	33	Cured (nephrectomy)	84
A. R.	35	M	Severe stenosis		333	258	21	Cured (nephrectomy)	7
R. M.	19	M	110	L. 310	445	216	1.5	Cured (arterioplasty)	12
				R. 840		295	20		
G. R.	36	F	107	L. 241	417	172	0	Cured (arterioplasty)	12
				R. 737		225	15		
W. R.	58	F	5—40		50			Cured (arterioplasty)	11

juxtaglomerular cell count of 361 with 6% of granular cells of types II and III. Following aorto-renal by-pass with a saphenous vein graft, the blood pressure rapidly dropped to normal levels, and both renin activity and arterial angiotensin levels fell to undetectable values. After one year of normotension, the patient's blood

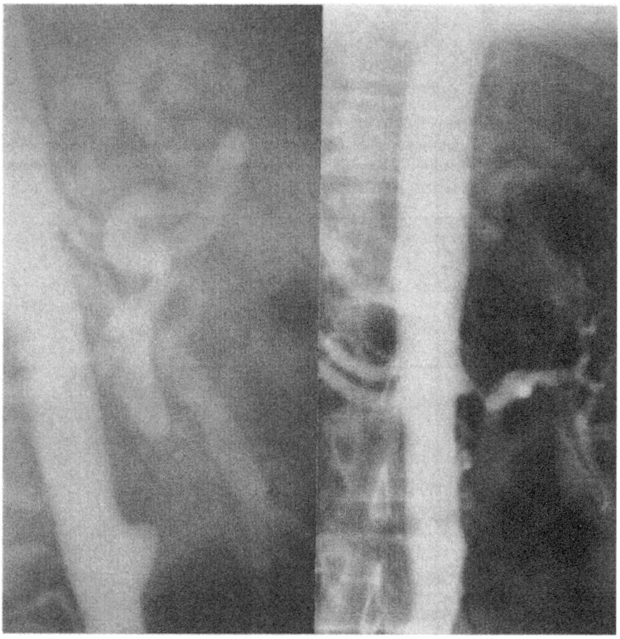

Fig. 2. Patient A. R. On the left, oblique view of the renal angiogram showing clearly the thrombosed graft by-pass. On the right, severe occlusion of the left renal artery with post-stenotic dilatation.

pressure rose again to hypertensive levels. The patient was re-admitted to hospital and, as shown in Fig. 2, renal angiography revealed a complete graft thrombosis. Peripheral venous renin activity rose again above the normal range to 36 ng./min./l. of plasma. It is of interest to emphasise that, during this year of normotension and adequate renovascular blood supply, the size of the kidney increased by 1.8×1.3 cm. One year after removal of the graft thrombus, the patient is still normotensive.

The second patient is a 39-year-old mother known to have been suffering from hypertension for the previous ten years. One year before she became aware of her hypertension, the patient presented with a history of left renal colic and haematuria. Renal angiography revealed a complete thrombosis of the middle branch of the left renal artery and a slight constriction over the lower branch (Fig. 3).

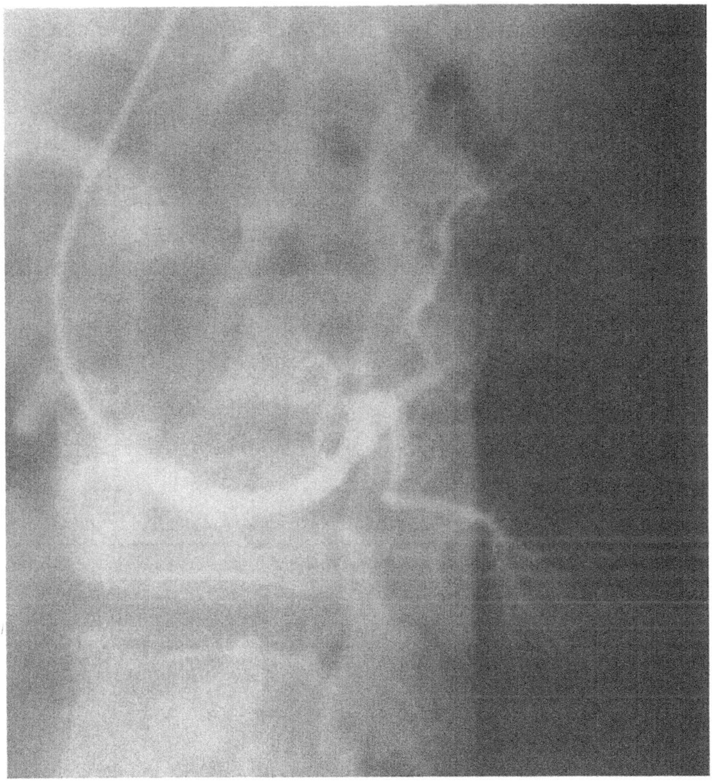

Fig. 3. Selective renal angiography of patient P. P., showing complete thrombosis of the middle branch of the left renal artery.

In response to a left nephrectomy there was a significant improvement, with an average decrease in diastolic pressure of 25 mm. Hg, which has been maintained for the last two and a half years. Fig. 4 outlines studies made on the middle infarcted region as compared with the upper and lower poles of the kidney. The middle region showed very marked and diffuse ischaemic tubular atrophy, no arteriolar lesions, a markedly increased juxtaglomerular cell count and granularity, and a very high renin activity, whereas in both upper and lower poles there were Grade II arteriolar lesions, no ischaemic tubular atrophy, a normal juxtaglomerular cell count and granularity, and a much lower renin activity in the kidney tissue. It is quite clear that the high renin activity in the renal venous blood came from the middle infarcted region. It is our assumption that the middle infarcted region – owing to complete obstruction of the middle branch of the left renal artery – was the cause of the

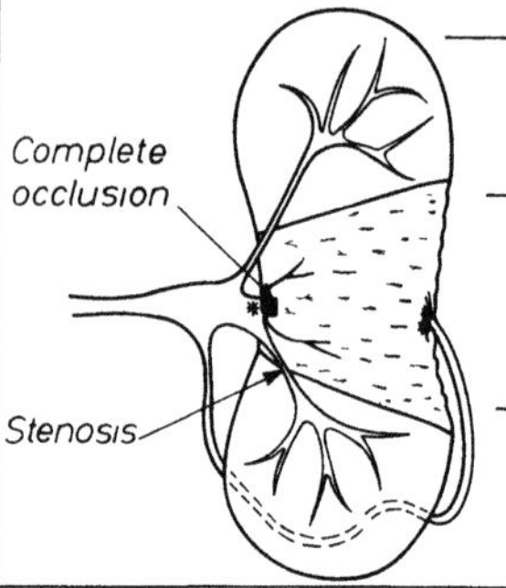

	Ischaemic tubular atrophy	Arteriolar lesions**	JGCC	%cells types II–III	Renin activity ng/min/g
	0	Gr 2	190	2	036
	++++	0	310	17	208
	0	Gr 2	208	1	057
Renin activity	renal artery 67 renal vein 617	ng/min/l plasma			

*Stenosis secondary to intimal fibrosis
**Classification of CASTLEMAN and SMITHWICK, 1943 (11)

Fig. 4. Mrs. P. P., 39 years, renovascular hypertension. Studies of the ischaemic tubular atrophy, arterioles, juxtaglomerular cell count and granularity, and renin content in the middle ischaemic part in comparison with both upper and lower poles of the left kidney. It is quite evident that the high renin activity in the peripheral and renal venous blood coincided closely with the high renin content and the hypercellularity and granularity of the middle ischaemic part of the kidney.

long-standing hypertension which, in turn, was responsible during these years for the production of arteriolar lesions in both poles of the involved kidney and, we believe, also in the contralateral kidney, and that it is these lesions which are now causing some degree of hypertension to persist in this patient.

The third patient is a 19-year-old man who had suffered from asymptomatic hypertensive disease since the age of 12. Renal angiography revealed complete obstruction of the right renal artery with marked collateral circulation (Fig. 5). The systolic pressure gradient at the time of operation was 110 mm. Hg, with very high renin activity in the renal venous blood and in the arterial blood. This was coupled with a high juxtaglomerular cell count and granularity. There was complete absence of arteriolar lesions in both kidneys. It is interesting to note that determinations of renin activity in the peripheral blood, carried out on five different days before the operation, yielded normal values (see Fig. 6

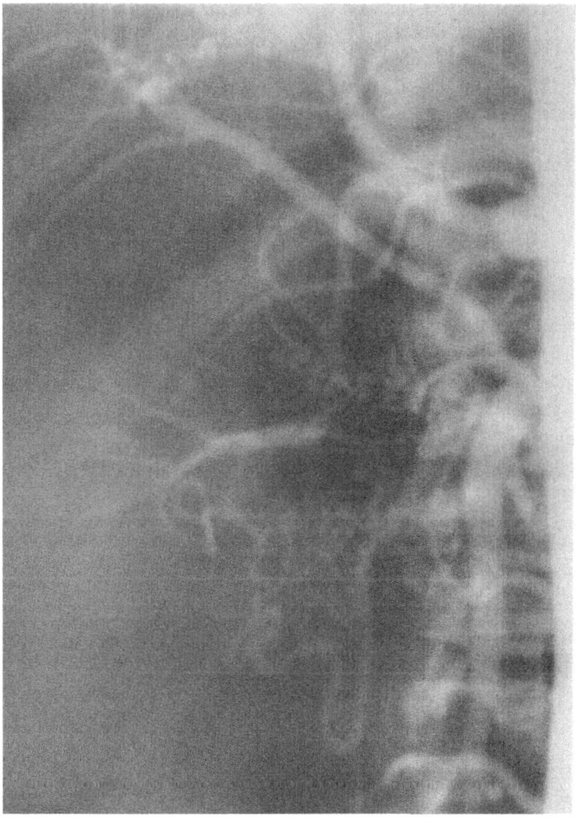

Fig. 5. Patient R. M. Angiography showing complete obstruction of the main right renal artery with marked collateral circulation.

and discussion). This patient has been normotensive for the last 12 months following aorto-renal grafting of a saphenous vein segment.

Of the eight patients in Group 2, only two were cured, the average follow-up period following surgery being ten months, with a range of two to 20 months (Table 4). The cure in these two patients was achieved despite the presence of arteriolar lesions in the involved kidney. The studies done on one of the six unsuccessful cases will be described in detail.

A 62-year-old woman (G. C.) complained at the time of her admission of severe intermittent claudication and of essential hypertension with a blood pressure of 220/120 mm. Hg, from which she

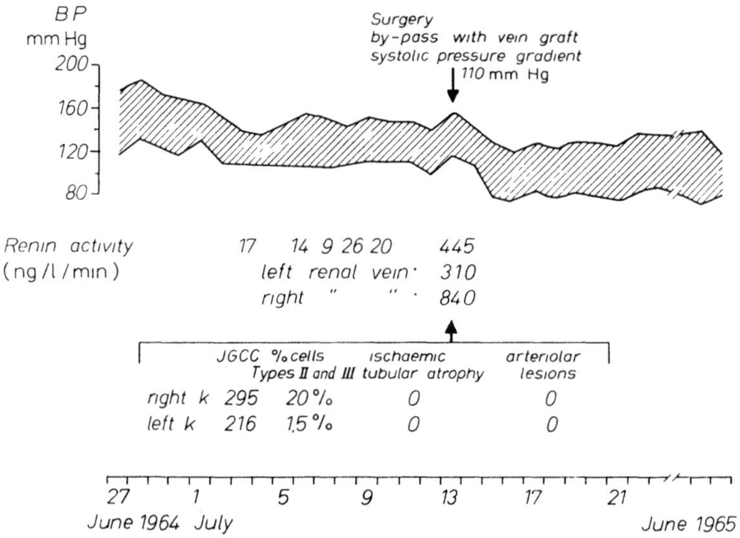

Fig. 6. 19-year-old patient R. M. with asymptomatic renovascular hypertension of seven years' duration. Normal fundi. Serum potassium was 4.3 mEq./l., sodium 140, and total CO_2 24.5. Creatinine clearance was 160 ml./min. and phenolsulphonphthalein excretion was 40% in 15 minutes and 71% in 60 minutes. On five different days prior to operation and while on a constant diet containing 135 mEq. Na and 90 mEq. K per day, peripheral blood renin activity was on each occasion within normal limits. Such a finding may occur in a patient with true renovascular hypertension and points to the necessity, in cases of this kind, of measuring renin activity in the renal venous blood as shown here and as advocated by HELMER and JUDSON (*32*) and KIRKENDALL et al. (*30*).

was known to have been suffering for the previous 15 years. In the angiotensin infusion test, 13.6 ng. of angiotensin/kg./min. were required to raise the diastolic pressure by 20 mm. Hg.

Renal angiography revealed a complete thrombosis of the main artery on the right side and the presence of a patent accessory artery over the lower pole of the same kidney (Fig. 7). This kidney was atrophic and measured 9.4 × 6 cm. on pyelographic films. Nephrectomy disclosed marked ischaemic tubular atrophy and greatly increased juxtaglomerular cell granularity over the middle and upper part of the right kidney. The renin content of this part

Table 4. *Group 2: Significant pressure gradient, increased renin activity and/or J.G.C.C., arteriolar lesions*

Name	Age	Sex	Systolic pressure gradient	Renin activity		J.G.C.C. total	Percent types II—III	Arteriolar lesions	Results of surgery	Follow-up period after surgery (months)
				Renal vein	Peripheral					
A. B.	66	F	Thrombosis	307	281	250	7	2	Failure (nephrectomy)	17
J.-C. P.	55	M	Thrombosis			310	14	2	Failure (nephrectomy)	5
A. L.	65	F	Severe stenosis			265	23	4	Cured (nephrectomy)	12
M. H.	59	F	Thrombosis	L. 78	120	L. 245[1]	13.7	2	Cured (nephrectomy)	7
				R. 117		170[2]	4.6			
						237[3]	19			
						R. 150	34	2		
M. D.	45	M	140	144	150			1	Failure (arterioplasty)	2
J. M.	52	F	Thrombosis		87	285	20	1	Failure (partial nephrectomy)	6
						193	2			
P.-E. R.	41	F	L. 105	77	85	190	4	2	Failure (arterioplasty)	20
			R. 85	274		237	3	3		
G. C.	62	F	Thrombosis, main artery	763	104	230	32[1]	2	Failure (nephrectomy)	2
			Accessory artery, lower pole			214	1[3]			

[1] Upper pole.
[2] Middle region.
[3] Lower pole.

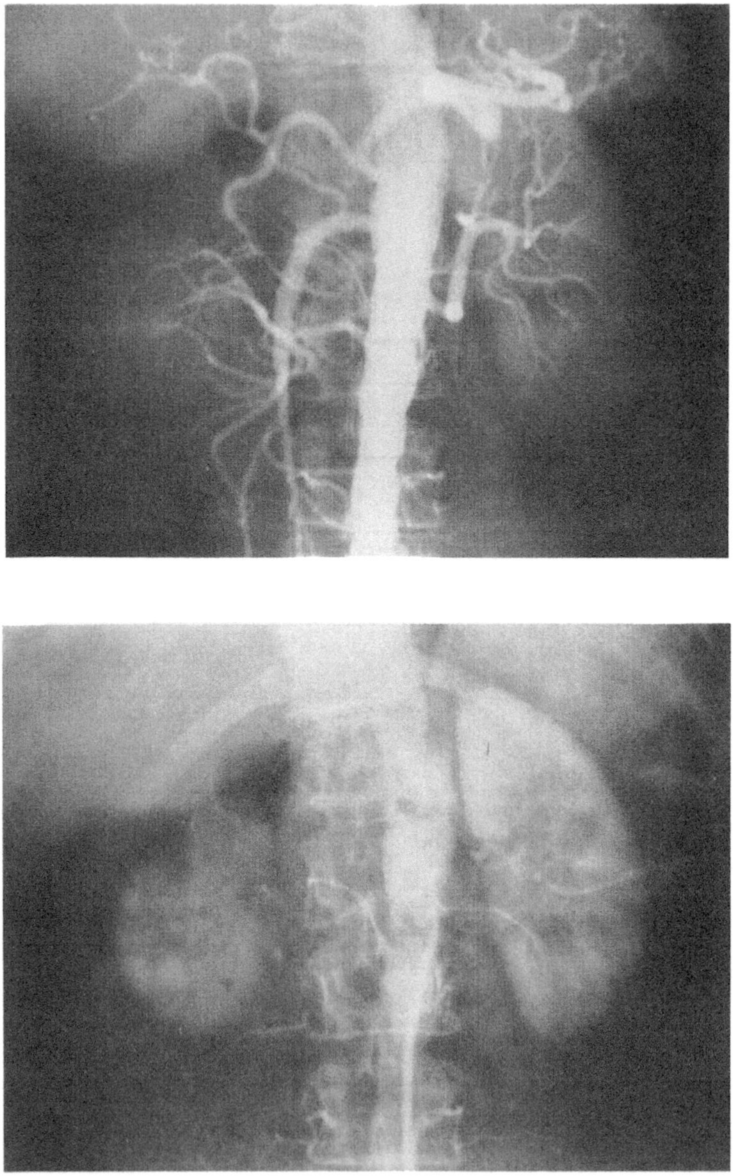

a

b

Fig. 7a and b. Patient G. C. Renal angiography showing complete thrombosis of the main right renal artery with a patent accessory artery to the lower pole.

Table 5. *Group 3: Significant pressure gradient, normal renin activity and/or J.G.C.C., arteriolar lesions, present or absent*

Name	Age	Sex	Systolic pressure gradient	Renin activity		J.G.C.C. total	Percent types II—III	Arteriolar lesions	Results of surgery	Follow-up period after surgery (months)
				Renal vein	Peripheral					
J.-P.R.	43	M	34	21				0	Failure (arterioplasty)	12
A. R.	51	F	60	22	27	250	3	1	Failure (arterioplasty)	20
H. P.	49	M	70	55	56	147	4	2	Failure (arterioplasty)	18
E. M.	60	M	90		25	L. 100	0	0	Failure (arterioplasty)	1
						R. 103	0	2		
G. B.	51	M	Severe stenosis			211	3	3	Failure (nephrectomy)	4
E. C.	57	F	Severe stenosis	9	6	235	1.5	2	Failure (nephrectomy)	3
M. B.	26	F	90	L. 82		L. 162	2	3	Failure (arterioplasty)	12
				R. 228		R. 147	4	1		
E. L.	24	M	Severe stenosis			284	1	1	Failure (nephrectomy)	12
A. W.	48	M	Severe stenosis	71	43	143	1.5	0	Failure (arterioplasty)	8
G. G.	44	M	60	L. 106	76	160	6	2	Cured (arterioplasty)	17
				R. 132						

was about 55 times higher as compared with that of the lower pole of the kidney, which had no ischaemic tubular atrophy and a low juxtaglomerular cell granularity (Fig. 8). Measurement by Dr. C. Strong of a crude fraction containing the "vaso-depressor lipid" (after extraction by chloroform-methanol and acetone precipitation of phospholipids) showed marked vasodepressor activity in

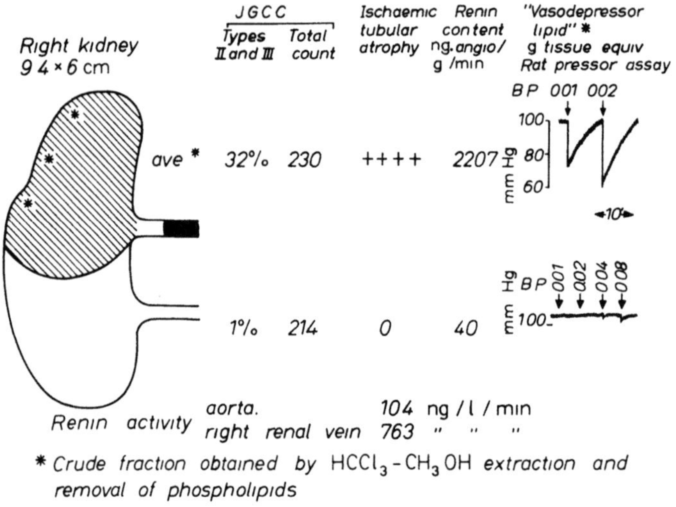

Fig. 8. 62-year-old woman G. C., admitted because of hypertension and marked intermittent claudication. Fundi showed filiform arteries. Pulsations were minimal over the left lower limb. Creatinine clearance was 77 ml./min./1.73 m.² of body surface. Phenolsulphonphthalein excretion was 24% in 15 min. and 49% in 60 min. Angiotensin infusion test required 13.6 ng./kg./min. to raise the diastolic pressure by 20 mm. Hg — a finding which suggests that the hypertensive disease is of renovascular origin. (It is worth while noting that, two months after nephrectomy, there was no improvement in the B.P.) When removed, the right kidney measured 8 × 5 × 3 cm., weighed 78 g., and showed marked atrophy of the upper pole.

the upper part of the kidney in comparison with the lower part (Fig. 8). Nephrectomy had no effect on the blood-pressure levels during a postoperative follow-up period of two months.

Of the ten patients in Group 3, only one was cured. This patient, with severe renal artery obstruction and a systolic pressure gradient of 60 mm. Hg, had a normal juxtaglomerular cell count and granularity, with only a possible slight increase in renin activity[1] in the peripheral venous blood and in the renal venous blood from the right kidney.

[1] The blood samples were obtained during surgery, and the renin activity measured in them may be within the range produced in some patients by anaesthesia alone, which has been found to provoke a slight increase in renin activity in most subjects studied.

Discussion

The very extensive reviews published by SMITH in 1943 (*13*), in 1948 (*14*), and in 1956 (*15*), and by KINCAID-SMITH in 1961 (*16*), dealing with the results of surgery for hypertension associated with unilateral renal disease, show a progressive rise in the percentage of cures (as defined according to SMITH's criteria, i. e. blood-pressure readings down to, or below, 140/90 mm. Hg for at least one year following surgery) from 9% in 1943 to 37% in 1961 (Table 6). KINCAID-SMITH emphasises in particular the marked

Table 6. *Results of surgery, since 1943, for hypertension associated with unilateral renal disease*

	No. of patients operated on	Percent success[1]
SMITH et al. (*13*) 1943	76	9
SMITH (*14*) 1948	242	19
SMITH (*15*) 1956	575	26
KINCAID-SMITH (*16*) 1961	326	37
GENEST 1965	647	60

[1] Criteria: B.P. down to, or below, 140/90 mm. Hg; one-year follow-up.

increase in the number of successfully operated cases of renal artery lesions (Table 7). Since 1961, numerous additional reports have appeared in the literature, and a survey of most of those

Table 7. *Pathological lesions in successful cases*[1]

	SMITH (*15*) 1956		KINCAID-SMITH (*16*) 1961	
	No.	%	No.	%
Chronic pyelonephritis	62	41	23	19
Renal artery lesions	19	12	78	65
Hydronephrosis	23	15	7	6
Other lesions[2]	45	30	12	10
	145 (out of 575)		120 (out of 326)	

[1] Reduction of B.P. below 140/90 mm. Hg for at least one year [SMITH's criteria (*15*)].
[2] Atrophic kidneys, renal T.B., stones [KINCAID-SMITH (*16*)].

comprising ten or more cases of hypertension associated with renal artery obstruction shows once again a further increase in the number of successfully operated cases (Table 6). Out of a total of

Table 8. *Surgical reports on renovascular hypertension, 1961—1964*

	No. of patients	Cured[1]	Improved[2]	Failures	Postoperative period of follow-up
Spencer et al. (*17*) 1961	24	12	10	2	A few months to 2 years
Wylie et al. (*18*) 1962	24	13	8	3	1 year
Hunt et al. (*19*) 1962	19	12	6	1	More than 6 months
Stewart et al. (*20*) 1962	43	17	18	8	?
Itskovitz et al. (*21*) 1963	11	3		8	Average: 6.3 months
Glenn (*22*) 1963	18	7	5	6	?
Dustan et al. (*23*) 1963	91	47	12	32[3]	1 to 6 years
Thompson et al. (*24*) 1964	29	8	18	3	Average: 16.5 months
DeBakey et al. (*25*) 1964	225	182	18	25	Average: 2 years (up to 5 years)
Poutasse (*26*) 1964	76	47	12	17	At least 1 year
Smithwick et al. (*27*) 1964	47	30	14	3	3 months to 12 years
Kirkendall et al. (*28*) 1965	40	11	14	15	?
Percent:	647	389 (60%)	135 (21%)	123 (19%)	

[1] B. P. below 140/90 mm. Hg.
[2] Usually means decrease in diastolic pressure of more than 20 mm. Hg or persistence of only systolic hypertension.
[3] Includes ten postoperative deaths.

647 patients, 60% were reported cured following corrective surgery (B.P. below 140/90 mm. Hg), 21% were considered improved (in general, this meant a decrease in diastolic pressure of more than 20 mm. Hg or persistence of only systolic hypertension), and 19% were failures (Table 8).

These studies confirm that there has been a great improvement in the selection of patients and in surgical techniques, and they establish beyond doubt that the presence of an obstructive renal vascular lesion is not *per se* the cause of hypertension in all cases. Similar lesions of equally severe degree can, in fact, be found in normotensive subjects. In a necropsy study (*29*), HOLLEY and co-workers have demonstrated a high frequency of obstructive lesions in the renal arteries of normotensive subjects (Table 9).

Table 9. *Arteriosclerotic narrowing of renal arteries*[1]

Renal artery	Normotensive	Hypertensive
Abnormal	127 (50%)	29 (76%)
Normal	129	9
	256	38

[1] Necropsy study [HOLLEY et al. (*29*)].

EYLER and co-workers (*30*) have obtained similar findings by angiography in quite a large proportion of normotensive subjects (Table 10). It is therefore our belief that, where failures have been

Table 10. *Incidence of renal artery abnormalities*[1]

Renal artery	Normotensive	Hypertensive
Abnormal[1]	98 (32%)	121 (62%)
Normal	206	75
	304	196

[1] Atherosclerotic plaques, post-stenotic dilatation, fibromuscular hyperplasia [EYLER et al. (*30*)].

reported, the cases in question have been patients in whom the hypertensive process preceded the appearance of the arterial occlusive lesion. In our view, the patients who have benefited from surgery consist either of those with a mixed type of hypertension, i.e. renovascular hypertension superimposed on a previously established essential type with a varying degree of nephrosclerosis, or, alternatively, of a group in whom a milder type of hypertension may persist owing to the presence of arteriolar lesions produced by severe hypertension exsisting over a period of many years – as seems to be the case in patient P.P. (Figs 3 and 4).

The studies we have reported from our laboratory illustrate the importance of determining blood renin activity. If renin activity is higher than normal in the exipheral venous blood, it can safely be assumed to be excessive in the renal venous blood as well and therefore to correspond with a high juxtaglomerular cell count and granularity. This measurement of renin activity makes it unnecessary to undertake a pre-operative open biopsy of the involved kidney as suggested by the earlier work of CROCKER et al. (*31*) and ITSKOVITZ et al. (*21*), who were the first to demonstrate the significance of a high juxtaglomerular cell count and granularity as regards the prognosis of renovascular surgery.

In cases where renin activity in the peripheral blood is within the normal range – as illustrated in patient R.M. (Fig. 6), in whom five determinations done on five different days were all within the normal range prior to operation – it becomes necessary to determine renin activity in renal venous blood obtained by catheterisation, as suggested by the studies of HELMER (*32*) and more recently by KIRKENDALL et al. (28). If renin activity is within the normal range both in the peripheral venous blood and in the renal venous blood of the involved kidney, the decision as to whether to resort to arterioplasty (endarteriectomy, by-pass, patch) will depend on the individual circumstances of the case and will have to be based primarily on haemodynamic considerations. It must be remembered that GUPTA and WIGGERS demonstrated in 1951 (*33*) that a reduction in the aortic lumen of more than 45–55% is required to produce distally any changes in arterial pressure (Fig. 9). In 1956, HAIMOVICI and ESCHER confirmed that a reduction of up to 60% in the diameter of the aorta induced insignificant blood-pressure changes distally and that a reduction in the diameter of the lumen of between 60% and 70% was necessary to produce significant manometric changes (*34*). Therefore, a decrease in systolic pressure beyond the stenosis of more than 30 mm. Hg would indicate, according to GUPTA and WIGGERS, a reduction of 55–65% in the arterial lumen (Fig. 9). This can be quite significant, and surgery should accordingly be considered in such cases, not only in order to afford possible relief from the hypertensive condition, but also to improve renal function and thus save the kidney from further atrophy and disuse.

Many studies have demonstrated a) an improvement in renal function, as measured by various parameters (glomerular filtration

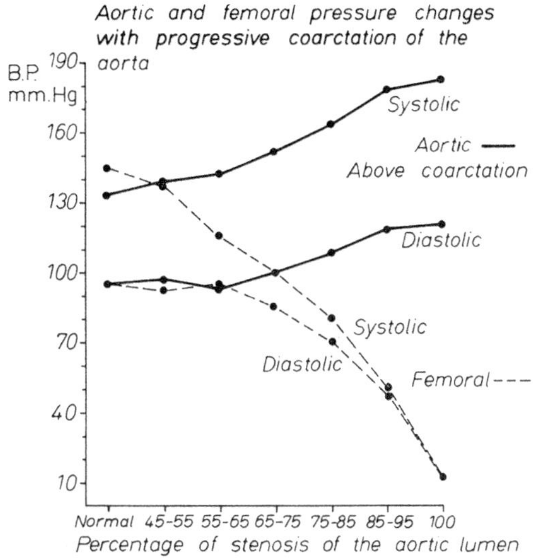

Fig. 9. The studies illustrated here show a progressive fall of 30 mm. Hg in femoral systolic pressure with increasing stenosis of the aortic lumen up to about 60%, although the diastolic pressure does not change. The major question is whether a systolic gradient of 30 mm. Hg or less, with the concomitant decrease in pulse pressure, is sufficient to initiate the release of renin from the involved kidneys [reproduced by courtesy of the American Heart Association, Inc., from GUPTA and WIGGERS, (*33*)].

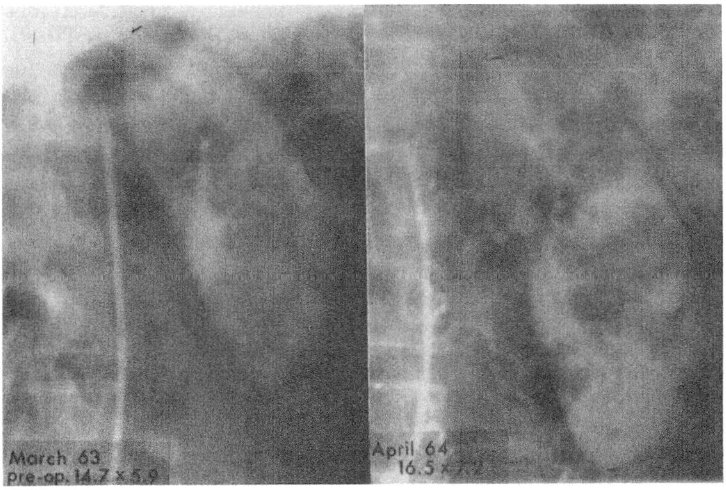

Fig. 10. Patient A. R. (see Figs 1 and 2). The venous phase of the angiogram shown on the right, after one year of normotension and adequate renal blood supply, illustrates the significant increase in renal mass (1.8 × 1.3 cm.) as compared with the size of kidney before corrective surgery.

rate, renal blood flow), following arterioplasty in patients with renal artery obstruction, and b) an increase in kidney mass, as in the case of patient A. R. (Fig. 10). In addition, it should be noted that the lesions of ischaemic tubular atrophy are reversible, as recently exemplified by one of our patients with a Leriche syndrome and an almost complete thrombosis of the left renal artery. When endarteriectomy was performed on this patient in 1959, there was a slight improvement in his hypertensive condition, and the diffused and very marked ischaemic tubular atrophy revealed by the biopsy done at that time completely disappeared following surgery, as confirmed by detailed histological examination of the same kidney obtained at autopsy in 1965 following death from acute myocardial infarction (*35*).

We have refrained from doing pre-operative open biopsy of the involved kidney in a search for possible renal arteriolar changes, because of the added suffering and risks to the patient, and because the indications for surgery are sufficient if the obstruction is severe enough to produce a systolic gradient greater than 30 mm. Hg. It must be pointed out that two patients from Group 2 were cured following surgery, despite the presence of significant arteriolar changes in the kidneys in question.

The importance of determining renin activity in patients with renal artery obstruction and with biochemical and clinical features of primary aldosteronism has been established by KIRKENDALL et al. (*36*), CONN et al. (*37*), our own group (*38*), and BROWN et al. (*39*), following demonstration of undetectable or minimal arterial angiotensin levels in cases of primary aldosteronism secondary to adrenocortical adenoma (*40*, *41*) and following the suggestion made by ourselves (*42*), KIRKENDALL et al. (*36*), LARAGH et al. (*43*), and CONN (*44*) that, thanks to its simplicity and rapidity, measurement of renin activity might well prove of value in the differential diagnosis of this condition *versus* that due to renal artery stenosis.

Summary

We have presented the results of our studies in 37 patients suffering from hypertension associated with renal artery obstruction. In the group of 14 patients with a significant systolic pressure gradient, a high blood renin activity and/or high juxtaglomerular cell count and granularity, and absence of arteriolar lesions in the involved kidney, 12 were cured and two were significantly improved. In the second group, two out of eight patients presenting similar features, but also with arteriolar changes in the involved kidney, were cured; and in the third group, only one out of ten patients with a significant pressure gradient, but with normal blood renin activity and/or juxtaglomerular cell count and granularity, was cured. In the light of these findings, a review of the literature and a physiopathological discussion are presented.

Zusammenfassung

Die Resultate unserer Untersuchungen bei 37 Patienten, die an Hochdruck litten und gleichzeitig eine Nierenarterienstenose hatten, werden vorgelegt. In einer Gruppe von 14 Patienten mit signifikantem, systolischem Druckgradienten, einer hohen Reninaktivität im Blut und/oder hoher juxtaglomerulärer Zellzahl und Granulation, aber ohne Schädigungen der Arteriolen in der betroffenen Niere, wurden 12 geheilt und zwei erheblich gebessert. In der zweiten Gruppe wurden zwei von acht Patienten geheilt, die ähnliche Erscheinungen, jedoch außerdem arterioläre Veränderungen in der befallenen Niere hatten. In einer dritten Gruppe wurde einer von zehn Patienten mit signifikantem Druckgradienten aber mit normaler Reninaktivität im Plasma und/oder juxtaglomerulärer Zellzahl und Granulation geheilt. Im Hinblick auf diese Befunde wird eine Übersicht über die Literatur gegeben und die Pathophysiologie besprochen.

Résumé

Nous avons présenté le résultat de nos études chez 37 malades porteurs d'une hypertension associée à une obstruction de l'artère rénale. Dans le groupe de 14 malades présentant un gradient élevé de pression systolique au niveau de la sténose, une haute activité de rénine dans le sang ou un pourcentage élevé de cellules juxta-glomérulaires granuleuses, ainsi qu'une absence de lésions artériolaires dans le rein intéressé, 12 ont été guéris et deux notablement améliorés. Dans le deuxième groupe, deux des huit malades présentant des caractéristiques semblables, mais également des altérations artériolaires dans le rein intéressé, ont été guéris. Dans le troisième groupe, un seul des dix malades présentant un gradient élevé de pression, mais une activité de rénine dans le sang normale et une numération normale des cellules juxta-glomérulaires granuleuses a été guéri. A la lumière de ces observations on présente une revue de la littérature et une discussion physiopathologique.

Acknowledgements

This work was generously supported by grants from the Ministries of Health of Ottawa and Quebec (Federal-Provincial Plan), the Medical Research Council of Canada, the National Institutes of Health, U.S.A. [Grant HE-06420-64 (Endo)], the Life Insurance Medical Research Fund, Rosemont, Pa., and the CIBA Company Limited, Montreal.

It is a pleasure to acknowledge the painstaking and devoted help of the following: Mrs. A. Brossard and Mrs. D. Lopez, dietitians; Miss F. Salvail, Miss L. Dagenais, and Miss L. Gauthier, R. N.; Mr. C. Grisé, Miss M. Tremblay, Mrs. L. Carbonneau, Mrs. S. Olivieri, and Mrs. P. Desrosiers, R. T.; and Miss I. Morin for the illustrations.

References

1. Blackman, S. F., Jr.: Bull. Johns Hopkins Hosp. **65**, 353 (1939). — 2. Kaplan, N. M., and J. G. Silah: J. Clin. Invest. **43**, 659 (1964). — 3. Veyrat, R.: Personal communication. — 4. Connor, T. B., M. Berthrong, W. C. T. Thomas, Jr., and J. E. Howard: Bull. Johns Hopkins Hosp. **100**, 241 (1957). — 5. Rapoport, A.: N. England J. Med. **263**, 1159 (1960). — 6. Stamey, T. A., I. J. Nudelman, P. H. Good, F. N. Schwentker, and

F. HENDRICKS: Medicine **40**, 347 (1961). — 7. TREMBLAY, G. Y., R. VEYRAT, J. DE CHAMPLAIN, R. BOUCHER, R. LEFEBVRE, P. ROY, P. CARTIER, and J. GENEST: Transact. Ass. Amer. Physicians **77**, 201 (1964). — 8. BOUCHER, R., R. VEYRAT, J. DE CHAMPLAIN, and J. GENEST: Canad. Med. Ass. J. **90**, 194 (1964). — 9. BOUCHER, R.: To be published. — 10. TURGEON, C., and S. C. SOMMERS: Amer. J. Path. **38**, 227 (1961). — 11. CASTLEMAN, B., and R. H. SMITHWICK: J. Amer. Med. Ass. **121**, 1256 (1943). — 12. NOWACZYNSKI, W., E. KOIW, and J. GENEST: Canad. J. Biochem. Physiol. **35**, 425 (1957). — 13. SMITH, H. W., W. GOLDRING, and H. CHASIS: Bull. N. Y. Acad. Med. **19**, 449 (1943). — 14. SMITH, H. W.: Amer. J. Med. **4**, 724 (1948). — 15. SMITH, H. W.: J. Urol. **76**, 685 (1956). — 16. KINCAID-SMITH, P.: Austral. Ann. Med. **10**, 166 (1961). — 17. SPENCER, F. C., T. A. STAMEY, H. T. BAHNSON, and A. COHEN: Ann. Surg. **154**, 674 (1961). — 18. WYLIE, E. J., D. PERLOFF, and J. S. WELLINGTON: Ann. Surg. **156**, 592 (1962). — 19. HUNT, J. C., E. G. HARRISON, O. W. KINCAID, T. E. BERNATZ, and C. D. DAVIS: Proc. Staff Meet. Mayo Clin. **37**, 181 (1962). — 20. STEWART, B. H., M. S. DEWEESE, J. CONWAY, and R. J. CORREA: Arch. Surg. **85**, 617 (1962). — 21. ITSKOVITZ, H. D., E. A. HILDRETH, A. M. SELLERS, and W. S. BLAKEMORE: Ann. Int. Med. **59**, 8 (1963). — 22. GLENN, J. F.: J. Urol. **90**, 22 (1963). — 23. DUSTAN, H. P., I. H. PAGE, E. F. POUTASSE, and L. WILSON: Circulation **27**, 1018 (1963). — 24. THOMPSON, J. E., D. J. AUSTIN, and C. G. WHEELER: Surgery **55**, 42 (1964). — 25. DEBAKEY, M. E., G. C. MORRIS, R. O. MORGEN, E. S. CRAWFORD, and D. A. COOLEY: Amer. J. Surg. **107**, 84 (1964). — 26. POUTASSE, E. F.: Amer. J. Surg. **107**, 97 (1964). — 27. SMITHWICK, R. H., R. C. NEWTON, D. H. CROCKER, and J. H. HARRISON: Amer. J. Surg. **107**, 104 (1964). — 28. KIRKENDALL, W. M., A. E. FITZ, M. S. LAWRENCE, and D. A. CULP: Abstract, Amer. Heart Ass. Meeting, Miami Beach, October 1965; and Personal Communication. — 29. HOLLEY, K. E., J. C. HUNT, A. L. BROWN, Jr., O. W. KINCAID, and S. C. SHEPPS: Circulation **26**, 731 (1962). — 30. EYLER, W. R., M. D. CLARK, J. E. GARMAN, R. L. RIAN, and D. E. MEININGER: Radiology **78**, 879 (1962). — 31. CROCKER, D. W., R. A. NEWTON, E. M. MAHONEY, and J. H. HARRISON: N. England J. Med. **267**, 794 (1962). — 32. HELMER, O. M.: Circulation **25**, 169 (1962). — 33. GUPTA, T. C., and C. J. WIGGERS: Circulation **3**, 17 (1951). — 34. HAIMOVICI, H., and D. J. W. ESCHER: Arch. Surg. **72**, 107 (1956). — 35. GENEST, J.: to be published. — 36. KIRKENDALL, W. M., A. E. FITZ, and M. L. ARMSTRONG: Dis. Chest. **45**, 337 (1964). — 37. CONN, J. W., E. L. COHEN, and D. R. ROVNER: J. Amer. Med. Ass. **190**, 125 (1964). — 38. DE CHAMPLAIN, J., J. GENEST, and R. VEYRAT: Transact. Ass. Amer. Physicians. To be published 1965. — 39. BROWN, J. J., O. L. DAVIES, A. F. LEVER, W. S. PEART, and J. I. S. ROBERTSON: Brit. Med. J. 1964/II, 1636. — 40. GENEST, J., W. NOWACZYNSKI, E. KOIW, R. BOUCHER, P. BIRON, and M. CHRÉTIEN: Memorias del IV Congresio Mundial de Cardiologia, Tome IV-A, Galve, Mexico, October 1962. — 41. GENEST, J., P. BIRON, M. CHRÉTIEN, R. BOUCHER, and E. KOIW: J. Clin. Invest. **41**, 1360 (1962). — 42. GENEST, J.: Canad. Med. Ass. J. **90**, 430 (1964). — 43. LARAGH, J. H., T. J. CANON, and R. P. AMES: Ann. Int. Med. **59**, 117 (1963). — 44. CONN, J. W.: J. Amer. Med. Ass. **190**, 134 (1964).

Discussion

TAQUINI: I should like to call your attention to some haemodynamic facts. In dealing with pressure gradients, it is necessary to know the flow. There is a difference between a gradient with a flow of, let's say, 500 ml. and the same gradient with a flow of 250 ml. To compare gradients in different situations, it is necessary to know the renal flow in each of them.

Similarly, with regard to Dr. PAGE's comment on the changes in the renin content following haemorrhage, before and after blocking renal innervation, it would be necessary to know the flow in both cases. It is known that bleeding, both in animals and in man, produces vasoconstriction in the renal territory, which cannot be present after the renal nervous system has been blocked. Differences in the degree of renal ischaemia could explain, in part at least, some of the differences found before and after blockade.

TCHERDAKOFF: In our patients we measured pressure gradients before surgery by catheterisation and during surgery in the usual way, and we found a tremendous disparity between the pressure gradients before and during surgery. I should like to know whether Dr. GENEST found the same kind of thing.

PETERS: I should like to put forward a working hypothesis as to the primary stimulus to increased renin secretion and an eventual increase in renin activity of kidney tissue. I shall be glad if anyone can spot any inconsistencies.

A sudden decrease in renal perfusion pressure, due, for instance, to bleeding, appears to trigger off a reflex which results in an increase in renal resistance[1]. Constricting the renal artery may be supposed to elicit a similar reflex vasoconstriction. Increased renin secretion, shown to occur after haemorrhage[2] as well as after clamping one renal artery[3], may be a consequence of this reflex renal vasoconstriction. Reflex vasoconstriction in the kidney would, on the other hand, diminish or abolish the initial pressure gradient above and below a clamp on the renal artery; the initial decrease in perfusion pressure caused by constricting the renal artery may thus escape detection. Dr. PAGE has just told us that ganglionic blocking agents and local anaesthetics applied to the kidney suppress the increase in renin secretion caused by constricting one renal artery; the suppression could be due to an inhibition of the vasoconstrictor reflex. Similarly, the protection of the dog's kidney against the late consequences of temporary total ischaemia by denervation or by dibenamine[4] may be due to an inhibition of reflex vasoconstriction. If my hypothesis is correct, denervation and dibenamine should

---

[1] KRAMER, K.: In: Shock, Pathogenesis and Therapy. An International Symposium. Ed. by K. D. BOCK. Springer, Berlin, 1962, p. 134.

[2] ZIEGLER, M., and F. GROSS: Proc. Soc. Exper. Biol. Med. **116**, 774 (1964).

[3] GROSS, F., G. SCHAECHTELIN, H. BRUNNER, and G. PETERS: Canad. Med. Ass. J. **90**, 258 (1964).

[4] BALINT, P.: In: Acute Renal Failure. A Symposium. Ed. by S. SHALDON and G. C. COOK. Blackwell Scientific Publications, Oxford, 1964, p. 12.

also inhibit the increase in renin secretion after clamping or after haemorrhage.

Clamping one renal artery in the rat is followed by an increase in renin secretion, if the opposite kidney is left untouched. If the opposite kidney is removed, renin secretion in the clamped kidney remains unchanged. If the opposite kidney is present, constriction of the renal artery is probably followed by renal vasoconstriction. G.F.R. falls markedly after clamping. The fall in G.F.R. and, presumably, renal vasoconstriction are much less pronounced after clamping the renal artery in the unilaterally nephrectomised rat[1].

If reflex renal vasoconstriction is responsible for increased renin secretion, drugs or procedures which abolish renal vasoconstriction after haemorrhage (or after clamping) should also prevent a rise in renin secretion. Thus, infusions of mannitol and of other hypertonic solutions have been shown to prevent reflex renal "shut-down"[2] and should be expected to suppress increases in renin secretion.

KINCAID-SMITH: I have been looking for examples of disappearance of the histological changes of ischaemic atrophy following vascular surgery, but I haven't been able to find any, and I was very interested in Dr. GENEST's example. However, I do not quite understand how the kidney could have increased in size on the measurements which he gave us. The kidney which he showed us initially measured 12 cm. in length on a radiograph, in spite of quite severe histological changes of ischaemic tubular atrophy. In my experience, if ischaemic tubular atrophy of that degree was wide-spread, the kidneys have been very small, and one would expect a measurement of 8 or 9 cm. in length on an x-ray. The kidney at autopsy measured 10 cm., which corresponds roughly to 12 cm. radiographically, because there is a difference between the radiograph and the autopsy measurement; in other words, it was still about the same size. I would suggest therefore that the histological changes in the biopsy were not representative of changes throughout the kidney, but represented a small area of ischaemic atrophy, such as can occur in stenosis of the main renal artery.

DOLLERY: I should like to ask Dr. GENEST whether he has taken into account the over-all changes in renal blood flow. Dr. PAGE has pointed out the dangers of inferring too much from concentrations. In one example that Dr. GENEST illustrated, there was almost complete infarction of the body of the kidney. In this instance, the total renal blood flow must have been very greatly reduced, and a high concentration of renin in the renal vein on that side might still have meant that the ischaemic kidney was producing less renin than the other, normal kidney. I think it is very important to bear this in mind, particularly as there are now methods of measuring renal blood flow directly by means of a double-lumen catheter in the renal vein.

DUSTAN: I should like to ask Dr. GENEST about the circumstances under which he sampled the renal venous blood. The reason for my question is that we have found great disparity in renin activity in renal venous blood when sampling is performed by renal vein catheterisation as opposed to that done during operation. The anaesthesia itself seems to evoke renin release, as also does the small amount of exploration that is necessary before the renal venous blood can be sampled.

---

[1] PETERS, G., H. BRUNNER, and F. GROSS: Nephron **1**, 295 (1964).

[2] PETERS, G., and H. BRUNNER: Amer. J. Physiol. **204**, 555 (1960).

GENEST: In response to Dr. TCHERDAKOFF's question, we have not measured systolic gradient before and during surgery. It would be interesting to do so, although I should have a reservation as to whether the gradient would remain the same at different levels of blood pressure, since the patient's blood pressure during anaesthesia is usually a good deal lower than before operation.

Regarding Dr. KINCAID-SMITH's question, the differences in kidney measurements are due to the fact that one measurement was done on the angiographic film, which, because of the technique used with the x-ray source at 36—40 inches from the film, is always greater by 20% to 25% than the actual size of the kidney, and the other was done at autopsy. It is difficult to compare one with the other. Even if the left kidney, measured on the angiogram done in 1959, was 12 cm. in length, this in itself does not preclude the presence of ischaemic tubular atrophy. All we can say is that, in the biopsy taken, there was diffuse ischaemic tubular atrophy throughout the specimen obtained. We cannot say anything about the rest of the kidney. It is for this reason that we were so careful in studying the histology of this kidney at the time of autopsy, especially in the region of the biopsy. No ischaemic tubular atrophy lesion could be found anywhere in the whole kidney six years after endarterectomy of the occluded renal artery.

In answer to Dr. DOLLERY: we have not made simultaneous measurements of renal blood flow and renin activity. We are quite convinced that the very high levels of renin activity in renal venous blood are well above the changes that could be due to decreased renal blood flow. You will also have noticed from the figures I showed that the renal venous renin activity levels correlate very well with the renin content of the involved kidney.

As to Dr. DUSTAN's question, the renin activity measurements are, we believe, most valuable. Two factors other than the renovascular one may influence these levels: one is the sodium balance of the patient. None of our patients was oedematous nor were they receiving natriuretic agents. The second factor is anaesthesia itself, which, as Dr. STRONG and Dr. TREMBLAY in our department have shown in dogs as well as humans, does produce a significant, although slight to moderate, increase in renin activity in the majority of patients. Dr. STRONG also studied the effect of physical manipulation of the kidney in the dog. This did not result, after five minutes of massaging the kidney, in any significant increase in renin activity in renal venous blood.

Some variations in renin activity levels do occur on unrestricted diets, but they are much less marked if the patient's sodium intake is constant from day to day.

Conservative treatment of renovascular hypertension

By

HARRIET P. DUSTAN, T. F. MEANEY, and I. H. PAGE

Enthusiasm for surgical treatment of hypertension followed the demonstration that nephrectomy or arterial reconstructive procedures can cure hypertension associated with occlusive renal arterial disease. Experience has tempered this enthusiasm for several reasons. Surgical treatment carries a high risk of myocardial infarction and strokes in patients with renal atherosclerosis and associated coronary and cerebral vascular disease. Also, the non-atherosclerotic renal arterial diseases can affect such long segments of the main artery and primary branches that reconstructive operations are not feasible; when the stenosis is unilateral, nephrectomy can be performed, but these lesions often occur bilaterally, requiring some type of revascularization operation. Further, there are some patients in whom either the hypertension or the occlusive disease is so mild that operative treatment does not seem warranted until one or the other worsens. Finally, there is as yet no sure way of determining whether the stenosis plays an important role in a patient's hypertension, and, until a method is available, recommendation for surgical treatment must be based on clinical judgement alone.

Patients with this type of renal hypertension deserve adequate blood-pressure control, because they can suffer from the complications of elevated arterial pressure just as frequently as patients with essential hypertension. In the opinion of some, renovascular hypertension does not respond to antihypertensive drugs. Our experience (*1*) is in sharp contrast, for we have shown that drug treatment is usually as effective as in essential hypertension. In addition to the uncertainty about the effectiveness of drugs, there has been the concern that, even though blood pressure might be controlled, renal arterial disease would progress to the point of producing irreparable renal atrophy.

This report describes the effects of antihypertensive drug treatment and the course of renal arterial disease in 23 hypertensive patients with occlusive lesions who were treated for periods of one to eight years.

Clinical material and methods of study

Of the 23 patients, ten were males who, at the time of this study, ranged in age from 41 to 71 years; the thirteen women were between 32 and 75 years of age. All had been originally referred for the evaluation and treatment of hypertension. Six had been under treatment for essential hypertension for three to eight years prior to performance of the first renal arteriogram. In the rest, this procedure had been included in the initial investigation. Renal excretory function was estimated at yearly intervals from levels of blood urea, serum creatinine, and from clearances of creatinine, urea, or mannitol. Urinary protein excretion was measured quantitatively at yearly intervals. Intravenous urograms were performed at yearly intervals, and in the past three years renal laminograms have also been obtained. Renal arteriograms were done either by translumbar aortic injection or by selective renal arterial injection of sodium diatrizoate (*2, 3*). Arteriography was repeated at least once after one or more years of treatment, and in one patient as many as six times.

Diagnoses of the types of renal arterial disease were made from arteriographic features (*4, 5*). Although this is not so certain a method of diagnosis as is microscopic examination of a resected renal artery, our continuing experience has shown it to be very valuable. In a study such as this, there is no way of knowing whether these lesions developed during the course of essential hypertension or were the initiating factor in the patients' hypertension.

Of the 23 patients studied (Table 1), 18 were considered to have atherosclerotic renal arterial disease. Five were thought to have non-atherosclerotic lesions: one, either intimal fibroplasia or fibromuscular hyperplasia; two, medial fibroplasia; and two, subadventitial fibroplasia. The only lesions having similar arteriographic

Table 1. *Arteriographic diagnoses in hypertensive patients treated medically*

Lesion	No.	Age
Atherosclerosis	18	42—75
Intimal fibroplasia, fibromuscular hyperplasia	1	41
Medial fibroplasia	2	46—48
Subadventitial fibroplasia	2	32—39

features are intimal fibroplasia and fibromuscular hyperplasia. The other three types — atherosclerosis, medial fibroplasia, and subadventitial fibroplasia — are distinct from each other. The last two lesions have previously been classified as fibromuscular hyperplasia (*6, 7*). Only one of this group was operated upon; because hypertension has disappeared, one assumes that it had a renal origin.

Analysis of the sequential urograms and arteriograms was used in assessing the natural history of renal arterial lesions. Renal lengths were obtained from each urogram. Increasing disparity in size of the two kidneys, if such had been present at the original examination, or appearance of disparity were considered to reflect progressive arterial narrowing. In the analysis of arteriograms, renal arterial stenosis was graded 0 to 4, depending on the degree of narrowing: 0 – no disease, 1 – less than 25% narrowing, 2 – 25 to 50% narrowing, 3 – greater than 50% narrowing, but excluding complete occlusion, 4 – complete occlusion. An increase in the grading of stenosis or development of post-stenotic dilatation was taken as a sign of advancing arterial disease.

Pretreatment levels of arterial pressure were obtained from averages of measurements, by sphygmomanometer, made four times daily during the initial hospitalization. The effects of treatment were judged in 21 patients from averages of arterial-pressure measurements obtained at home twice daily. Two patients did not measure their blood-pressure levels at home, and in these, readings obtained during re-evaluation hospital visits were used. Since most patients receiving antihypertensive drugs have reasonably stable weekly averages of home readings, the level of arterial pressure used in this analysis of the effectiveness of drug treatment was an average of the readings obtained at home during the month prior to the final study.

A variety of drugs was used. Hydrochlorothiazide was most frequently given (14 patients), and guanethidine was used often (9 patients). Other drugs used were reserpine, α-methyldopa, hydralazine, chlorisondamine, bretylium, pargyline, mecamylamine, and triamterene. The goal of treatment was to reduce supine diastolic arterial pressure to as near normal levels as possible; presence of orthostatic hypotension, without reduction in supine diastolic pressure, was not considered adequate treatment.

Results

Control of hypertension. The effectiveness of antihypertensive drug treatment was graded according to the level of diastolic arterial pressure present during the month prior to the final evaluation (Table 2). Fifteen patients were considered to have good blood-pressure control with an average of 174/93 mm. Hg, as opposed to a pretreatment average of 202/115 mm. Hg. In five, arterial pressure was not so well controlled, and the treatment average for the group was 167/103 mm.Hg, while the pretreatment level had been 203/123 mm. Hg.

Table 2. *Effect of antihypertensive drug treatment in 23 patients with renal arterial stenosis*

	Supine diastolic pressure averages		
	100 mm. Hg or less	101—105 mm. Hg	105 mm. Hg or more
No.	15	5	3
Control: B. P.. . .	202/115	203/123	185/109
Treatment: B. P. . .	174/93	167/103	200/119

In three patients, arterial pressure was higher at the time of final study than before treatment and averaged 200/119 mm. Hg in contrast to 185/109 mm. Hg before drug therapy was begun. These patients deserve special comment, because their treatment was inadequate. One was a 39-year-old woman who had subadventitial fibroplasia of the right renal artery. Her initial therapy with 100 mg. guanethidine daily reduced supine arterial pressure from 195/114 to 173/98 mm. Hg, but caused troublesome diarrhea and disabling exercise hypotension. Decrease in the amount of guanethidine to 50 mg./day relieved the symptoms, but did not maintain good blood-pressure control. At the end of the year of treatment, arterial pressure averaged 212/115 mm. Hg. At that time, surgical repair of the right renal artery was performed, followed by relief of hypertension; for example, in the month prior to the third anniversary of the operation, home blood pressures averaged 126/76 mm. Hg. The other two patients have been unable to take adequate amounts of effective drugs; in one, a man of 71 years, this was because of recurrent, disabling exercise hypotension, and in the other, a woman of 48 years, because of a variety of side effects which she considered intolerable.

Natural history of renal arterial lesions. Some indications of the natural history of these occlusive lesions could be gleaned from the arteriograms, intravenous urograms, and renal function studies performed during the treatment period. In this group of patients, evidence of progression of renal atherosclerosis was found more frequently than that of the non-atherosclerotic lesions. Eighteen patients were judged, on arteriographic features, to have atherosclerotic renal arterial disease, and signs suggesting increasing stenosis were found in 11 (Table 3). In two, this suggestion came only from a progressive decrease in length of one kidney, although arteriographically the stenosis did not seem more severe. In four, only on arteriography did the lesions appear more stenotic; however, these patients had bilateral lesions and both seemed more

Table 3. *Progression of renal atherosclerosis in 18 patients treated medically*

Patients with progressive lesions		11
Signs of progression:		
Urographic	2	
Arteriographic	4	
Both urographic and arteriographic	5	
Time of progression		14 to 72 months
Patients with non-progressive lesions		7
Duration of study		18 to 56 months

severe. Five patients had both arteriographic evidence of progressive stenosis and decrease in renal size. Renal excretory function has decreased in three patients, with increases in serum creatinine from 1.0 to 2.4 mg./100 ml. (Tables 4 and 5). Two of the others have shown a slight reduction in excretory function.

Table 4. *Serum creatinine as index of renal excretory function in 23 medically treated patients with renal arterial stenosis*

Lesion	No.		Creatinine — mg./100 ml. mean	range
Atherosclerotic	18	before treatment	1.3	0.8—2.3
		after treatment	1.8	0.9—3.8
Fibrosing	5	before treatment	0.9	0.5—1.2
		after treatment	1.1	0.7—1.3

Table 5. *Changes in serum creatinine in 18 patients with renal atherosclerosis*

Increases — mg./100 ml.			
0	0—0.49	0.49—0.99	>0.99
2	11	2	3

The time of progression of these atherosclerotic lesions was variable; in one patient progression was evident on the first reevaluation examination, 14 months after the original study. In another it was seen only after six years. This patient had had a left nephrectomy in 1956, because an orificial atherosclerotic plaque with superimposed thrombosis had produced a non-functioning kidney; arteriography preoperatively had also shown roughening of the first portion of the right renal artery. Repeat arteriograms in 1958, 1959, and 1960 failed to show any change in this lesion. In 1962, however, development of moderate azotemia suggested the possibility of progressive arterial disease, and this suggestion was borne out by the arteriographic finding of severe occlusive disease. Although this lesion had progressed rapidly over a period of 19 months (from August, 1960, to March, 1962), it has not become more severe since then, for arteriography in March, 1964, showed no change, and results of renal function tests in May, 1965, were no different from those obtained in 1962.

Regardless of evidence of increasing stenosis in 11 patients, there were seven whose lesions appeared stable. Neither arteriograms nor intravenous urograms gave any sign that the plaques had increased in size, and results of renal function tests have remained unchanged. Failure to observe worsening was not necessarily a reflection of a short period of observation. Although four patients have been followed for less than two years, three have been studied repeatedly during 46 to 56 months of treatment.

The five patients with non-atherosclerotic renal arterial diseases have been followed up for periods ranging from one to eight years, and only one showed any evidence of progression (Table 6). This

Table 6. *Progression of fibrosing renal arterial lesions in five patients treated medically*

Patients with progressive lesions		1
Signs of progression:		
Urographic	0	
Arteriographic	1	
Both urographic and arteriographic	0	
Time of progression		28 months
Patients with non-progressive lesions		4
Duration of study		12 to 84 months

was a woman, aged 48 years, thought to have bilateral medial fibroplasia. The first arteriograms, done in November, 1962, had shown aneurysmal dilatations characteristic of this lesion (*1*). Another arteriogram in December, 1963, gave a suggestion that these had become larger, and, finally, the examination of March, 1965, clearly showed progression of the lesion. One other patient in this group is of particular interest. In 1957, at the age of 24, she was found to have bilateral renal arterial disease, much more severe on the right than on the left. The lesion on the right was excised, and an end-to-end anastamosis of the proximal and distal arterial segments performed. Examination of the excised renal artery showed subadventitial fibroplasia. In the seven years since the operation, the disease on the left has shown no change; six arteriograms have been performed during this time, and the appearance of the lesion in February, 1965, was the same as on the preoperative arteriogram of February, 1957. None of these patients with fibrosing renal arterial lesions has shown any decrease in renal excretory functions (Table 4), and in none has proteinuria developed.

Discussion

Any study of hypertension associated with renal arterial stenosis has the disadvantage that there is no way of knowing whether the occlusive lesions are responsible for the elevated arterial pressure. This is just as true of a study of the effects of surgical treatment as it is of one, such as this, concerned with drug therapy. Patients who are cured of hypertension by surgical relief of stenosis are classified as having had renal hypertension, but those who are not cured cannot yet be so classified, even though the stenosis may have initiated the arterial-pressure elevation which was later maintained by another mechanism.

This report of the effectiveness of antihypertensive drugs in patients with occlusive renal arterial disease confirms and extends our earlier observations (*1*). Although there was no way for us to determine whether the lesions were "significant", this study does show that stenoses are not rapidly progressive.

The responsiveness of renal hypertension to antihypertensive drugs that have different mechanisms of action indicates that there are several factors, in addition to the renal pressor system, that operate to keep arterial pressure elevated in patients with occlusive lesions. In our experience, this type of hypertension can sometimes be controlled with a chlorothiazide diuretic alone, suggesting that volume and electrolyte factors play a role just as they do in renoprival hypertension (*8*, *9*, *10*). Further, the ability of guanethidine and ganglioplegic drugs to reduce arterial pressure in these patients points to a neurogenic mechanism which helps maintain the hypertension. Such a mechanism functions in chronic renal hypertension in the dog, for McCUBBIN et al. (*11*) have shown resetting of the carotid sinus baroceptors, so that they operate to sustain the hypertension rather than reduce it. More recent work (*12*) has presented evidence of the effect of angiotensin on sympathetic nervous activity in the dog. Such an effect may explain the responsiveness to guanethidine of one of our patients who later became normotensive following excision of the stenotic renal arterial segment. Finally, the demonstrations of relationships between adrenal and renal functions suggest that a steroid hormonal factor may, in some way, participate in renal hypertension.

The information available from this study concerning progress of renal arterial lesions deals with atherosclerosis primarily, for there were few patients with the non-atherosclerotic, fibrosing lesions. In the latter group, more patients and much longer periods of follow-up are necessary to establish the natural history of these diseases. Certainly, it had been our clinical impression that they are but slowly, if at all, progressive, and this impression has obtained support from the present demonstration that only one out of five non-atherosclerotic lesions showed any change; even in the longest follow-up period of eight years, no apparent worsening has occurred.

Eleven of the 18 patients with atherosclerotic stenosis showed evidence of progressive disease. However, in only three were there significant decreases in renal excretory function, and in one of these, the disease advanced only after four years of close observation. Further, there were seven patients in whom atherosclerotic plaques seemed unchanged over periods of study as long as five years. Thus, these results show that the presence of atherosclerotic stenosis is not, in itself, an indication for immediate operation. Renal conserving operations have been strongly urged, in the past, in order to protect against progressive renal atrophy. However, from this study it can be seen that renal atrophy is not rapidly progressive, thus allowing time for the preparation of a carefully considered plan of therapy based on response to antihypertensive drug treatment and knowledge of the natural course of each patient's stenosis.

Occasionally, the first arteriogram done for investigation of hypertension in a patient with extrarenal evidence of atherosclerosis shows a completely obstructed renal artery. We have recently found that complete occlusion by atherosclerotic lesions represents a thrombosis or arterial dissection (*5*). Because the arteriogram cannot give any indication of the time when occlusion occurred, there has been a tendency to believe that this is the ultimate fate of any atherosclerotic stenosis. It is probably this lack of knowledge about the natural history of renal atherosclerotic lesions that has been responsible for the zeal with which renal conserving operations have been recommended. Complete occlusion has not occurred in any of the 18 patients reported in this study. An additional patient, not under treatment and therefore not included here, was found to have complete obstruction six months after the first arteriogram had shown an atherosclerotic stenosis. Actually, we have had more experience with complete occlusion following endarterectomy than with the naturally occurring form.

Summary

The effectiveness of antihypertensive drug treatment and the natural history of occlusive lesions were studied in 23 hypertensive patients with renal arterial stenosis treated for periods ranging from one to eight years. Diagnoses of stenotic lesions were based on arteriographic features. Eighteen patients were considered to have atherosclerotic lesions, five patients, non-atherosclerotic or fibrosing.

For the most part, drug treatment maintained good arterial-pressure control. In 15 patients, supine diastolic pressure averaged 100 mm. Hg or less, and in five it was maintained between 101 and 105 mm. Hg. In three patients, hypertension was not well controlled over long periods, because they either could not or would not take adequate amounts of drugs.

Progress of renal arterial lesions was judged from sequential intravenous urograms, renal arteriograms, and estimates of renal excretory function. Eleven of the 18 patients with atherosclerotic renal arterial occlusive disease had signs of progressive stenosis over periods ranging from one to six years. In seven, no evidence of progression was found, even after almost five years of follow-up. Decreases in renal excretory function paralleled the radiographic findings.

The five patients with non-atherosclerotic renal arterial stenoses were followed for between one and eight years, and only one showed arteriographic signs of progressive disease after two years of study. Renal excretory function has not decreased.

This study indicates that conservative treatment of renal hypertension is effective and practical and has not been accompanied by rapidly advancing renal atrophy.

Zusammenfassung

Bei 23 während ein bis acht Jahren behandelten hypertonischen Patienten mit Nierenarterienstenose wurden die Wirksamkeit einer antihypertensiven Therapie und der Verlauf der auf den Verschluß zurückzuführenden Schädigungen untersucht. Die Diagnosen der stenosierenden Prozesse gründeten sich auf arteriographische Merkmale. Bei 18 Patienten wurden atherosklerotisch bedingte Läsionen angenommen, bei fünf nicht atherosklerotische oder fibrotische.

Bei den meisten Patienten ließ sich durch eine medikamentöse Behandlung eine gute Kontrolle des Blutdruckes erreichen. Bei 15 Patienten betrug der diastolische Blutdruck im Liegen durchschnittlich 100 mm Hg oder weniger, bei fünf konnte er zwischen 101 und 105 mm Hg gehalten werden. Bei drei Patienten gelang es nicht, den Blutdruck während längerer Zeit zu senken, weil sie die verschriebenen Präparate nicht in genügenden Dosen nehmen konnten oder wollten.

Das Fortschreiten der Nierenarterienläsionen wurde auf Grund von intravenösen Urogrammen, renalen Arteriogrammen und Bestimmungen der exkretorischen Nierenfunktion verfolgt. Elf der 18 Patienten mit atherosklerotischen Verschlüssen der Nierenarterie wiesen während Perioden von ein bis sechs Jahren Zeichen einer fortschreitenden Stenose auf. Bei sieben fand sich kein Anhalt für ein Fortschreiten des Prozesses, selbst bei einer

Verfolgung bis zu nahezu fünf Jahren. Die Abnahme der exkretorischen Funktion ging im allgemeinen den radiographischen Befunden parallel.

Die fünf Patienten mit nicht atherosklerotisch bedingten Nierenarterienstenosen wurden während ein bis acht Jahren beobachtet; nur einer von ihnen ließ nach zwei Jahren arteriographische Zeichen einer fortschreitenden Erkrankung erkennen. Die exkretorische Nierenfunktion hatte dabei nicht abgenommen.

Diese Studie zeigt, daß die konservative Behandlung des renalen Hochdruckes wirksam und zweckmäßig ist, und daß sie nicht von einer rasch fortschreitenden Nierenatrophie begleitet ist.

Résumé

On a étudié chez 23 hypertendus présentant une sténose de l'artère rénale et traités pendant des périodes allant de un à huit ans, l'efficacité des traitements médicamenteux antihypertenseurs et l'évolution des lésions obstructives. Le diagnostic de la lésion sténosante a été fait sur les caractéristiques de l'artériographie. Dix-huit malades ont été considérés porteurs de lésions athérosclèreuses, cinq de lésions non athérosclèreuses ou fibrosantes.

Dans la plupart des cas le traitement médicamenteux a maintenu les chiffres de la pression artérielle à un niveau satisfaisant. Chez 15 malades, la pression diastolique en position couchée était de 100 mm Hg ou moins, et chez cinq, elle se trouvait entre 101 et 105 mm Hg. Chez trois malades, l'hypertension n'a pas été contrôlée de façon satisfaisante pendant de longues périodes, parce qu'ils ne voulaient ou ne pouvaient prendre des doses convenables de médicaments.

Les progrès des lésions artérielles rénales ont été appréciés par des urographies intra-veineuses répétées, des artériographies rénales et des évaluations de la fonction excrétoire rénale. Onze des 18 malades avec obstruction artérielle rénale athérosclèreuse ont présenté des signes de sténose progressive sur des périodes allant de un à six ans. Chez sept malades, aucun signe évolutif n'a été constaté, même après une surveillance de près de cinq ans. Les diminutions de la fonction excrétoire rénale ont évolué de façon parallèle aux données radiographiques.

Les cinq malades présentant des sténoses artérielles rénales non athérosclèreuses ont été suivis de un à huit ans, et seulement dans un cas l'artériographie a montré des signes d'évolutivité de la maladie après deux ans d'observation. La fonction excrétoire rénale n'avait pas diminué.

Cette étude indique que le traitement conservateur de l'hypertension rénale s'est montré efficace et pratique et ne s'est pas accompagné d'une évolution rapide vers l'atrophie rénale.

Acknowledgements

This study was supported, in part, by a grant, H-6835, from the National Heart Institute, Bethesda, Md.

We wish to express our appreciation for the generous supplies of drugs made available for this study. Dr. W. E. WAGNER of CIBA Pharmaceutical Company, Summit, N. J., made available guanethidine, reserpine, chlorisondamine, hydrochlorothiazide, and hydralazine; Dr. E. FOLTZ of Merck, Sharp and Dohme, α-methyldopa and mecamylamine; Dr. D. SEARLE of Burroughs Wellcome and Co., bretylium; and Mr. D. CHEETHAM of Smith, Kline and French Laboratories, triamterene.

We wish to thank Miss E. DAVY, Miss I. PATTERSON, and Miss R. HORVATH for their help in the long-term study of these patients and Miss C. MONROE for skilful secretarial work.

References

1. DUSTAN, H. P., I. H. PAGE, and E. F. POUTASSE: Circulation **27**, 1018 (1963). — 2. POUTASSE, E. F.: J. Amer. Med. Ass. **178**, 1078 (1961). — 3. MEANEY, T. F., and H. P. DUSTAN: Circulation **28**, 1035 (1963). — 4. McCORMACK, L. J., T. J. NOTO, E. F. POUTASSE, and H. P. DUSTAN: Clin. Res. **12**, 363 (1964). — 5. McCORMACK, L. J., E. F. POUTASSE, T. F. MEANEY, T. J. NOTO, and H. P. DUSTAN: Submitted for publication. — 6. WYLIE, E. J., and J. S. WELLINGTON: Amer. J. Surg. **100**, 183 (1960). — 7. WELLINGTON, J. S.: Amer. J. Path. **43**, 955 (1963). — 8. MERRILL, J. P., C. GIORDANO, and D. R. HEETDERKS: Amer. J. Med. **31**, 931 (1961). — 9. MERRILL, J. P., and E. SHUPAK: Canad. Med. Ass. J. **90**, 328 (1964). — 10. DUSTAN, H. P., and I. H. PAGE: J. Laborat. Clin. Med. **64**, 948 (1964). — 11. McCUBBIN, J. W., J. H. GREEN, and I. H. PAGE: Circulation Res. **4**, 205 (1956). — 12. McCUBBIN, J. W., and I. H. PAGE: Circulation Res. **12**, 553 (1963).

Some observations on the filtration fraction, on the transport of sodium and water in the ischemic kidney, and on the prognostic importance of R.P.F. to the contralateral kidney in renovascular hypertension

By

T. A. Stamey

Many investigative units have had five to ten years' experience in the diagnosis and treatment of hypertension due to occlusive disease of the renal arteries. The basic technique for advancing our knowledge has been reliable and reproducible differential renal function studies. Without meaningful renal function data it is virtually impossible to assess the significance of occlusive disease, and it is clearly impossible to gain any insight into the basic problems of renal hemodynamics and nephron transport in the ischemic kidney.

I need not remind this group of distinguished physicians firstly, that the basic functional characteristic of unilateral occlusive disease associated with curable, renovascular hypertension is excessive reabsorption of sodium and water in the ischemic kidney, secondly, that this increased reabsorption occurs primarily in the proximal tubule — an observation which explains why there are greater differences between the two kidneys in the concentration of para-aminohippuric acid ($U_{P.A.H.}$), inulin ($U_{In.}$), and creatinine ($U_{Cr.}$) than in the concentration of sodium (U_{Na}) — and, finally, that not only does an infusion of urea, saline, and antidiuretic hormone (A.D.H.) stabilize urine flow for accurate assessment of renal function, but the urea increases the diagnostic disparity between the two kidneys in excessive water reabsorption (*1*).

Functionally significant, *unilateral* occlusive disease of the main renal artery is always associated with large differences in the rate of urine flow (V.) and in total water reabsorption (as measured by differences in $U_{P.A.H.}$, $U_{In.}$, or $U_{Cr.}$). Under the conditions of the urea, saline, and A.D.H. infusion, there is at least a 3 : 1 decrease in V. and a 100% increase in $U_{P.A.H.}$ in the ischemic kidney (*1*). It is important that these large differences are characteristic, because some reports which have indicated smaller differences in V. and

$U_{P.A.H.}$ (or $U_{Cr.}$ or $U_{In.}$) have failed to recognize that essential hypertension, in patients with normal arteriograms and equal kidney sizes, is frequently associated with differences of as much as 50% in V. and a 10–40% increase in $U_{P.A.H.}$ (*1*). Thus, these reports of unilateral occlusive disease of the main artery associated with small excretory differences in renal function probably represent functionally insignificant main renal artery stenosis superimposed on essential hypertension.

The clinical (*2–4*), as well as the experimental (*5–8*), evidence indicates that a large artery must be narrowed by at least 50% before a pressure gradient is produced across the stenosis. The slope of the systolic curve, distal to the stenosis, may be decreased, but the maximal pressure at the height of the systolic curve is the same. Since blood flow is proportional to pressure and indirectly proportional to resistance ($F. \propto P./R.$), one can only conclude that short constrictions in large arteries constitute a negligible resistance in terms of the total vascular bed, changing neither flow nor pressure, as long as the constriction is not too great (less than 50% of the cross-sectional area).

When the obstruction of the main renal artery finally reduces the cross-sectional area enough to constitute a significant resistance in relation to the distal arteriolar bed, the pulse pressure falls distal to the stenosis; at first, only the systolic pressure decreases, but with further constriction, a diastolic gradient develops as well. Blood flow, however, may not fall in the presence of a decreased mean pulse pressure if the resistance of the arteriolar bed distal to the stenosis decreases. This ability to decrease the distal arteriolar resistance (the degree of arteriolar constriction) in the face of an increasing proximal resistance may be a property common to all vascular beds, but it is clearly true of the renal vascular bed, where these changes are readily measured. Selkurt showed more than ten years ago that glomerular filtration rate (G.F.R.) and renal plasma flow (R.P.F.) in the dog's kidney did not fall until the pressure distal to the stenosis was reduced by at least 40 mm. Hg; water and electrolyte excretion did not change until R.P.F. and G.F.R. decreased (*9*, *10*). For obvious reasons no comparable studies have been made in the human kidney, but there are many patients with aortographic evidence of partial renal artery occlusion who do not have hypertension. For example, in a review of 409 patients in whom angiography had been done for a variety of vascular problems, Eyler et al. were able to match varying degrees of renal vascular abnormalities in hypertensive patients with similar changes in normotensive patients (*11*). Holley et al., in a necropsy study,

Table 1. *B. R., 55-year-old, white female with functionally insignificant fibromuscular hyperplasia of the right renal artery*, March 5, 1964

Time	Column 1 Urine flow			Column 2 Concentration of inulin ($U_{In.}$)			Column 3 Clearance of inulin ($C_{In.}$)			Column 4 Concentration of P.A.H. ($U_{P.A.H.}$)			Column 5 Clearance of P.A.H. ($C_{P.A.H.}$)			Column 6 Filtration fraction ($C_{In.}/C_{P.A.H.}$)		
	R.	L.	R./L.	R.	L.	R./L.	R.	L.	R./L.	R.	L.	R./L.	R.	L.	R./L.	R.	L.	R./L.
min.	ml./min.			mg./100 ml.			ml./min.			mg./100 ml.			ml./min.					
—37	1 ml. of 0.25 % heavy Nupercaine injected into fourth lumbar space for saddle anesthesia.																	
—25	Plasma No. 1 drawn.																	
—24	Infusion of 8 % urea in normal saline started at 9.6 ml./min. to deliver 1.5 mg./ml. of inulin, 1.0 mg./ml. of P.A.H., and 5 mU./kg./hr of A.D.H.																	
—22	19.9. ml. of 10 % inulin and 2.2 ml. of 20 % P.A.H. injected i.v.																	
—13	Blood pressure 138/96 mm. Hg.																	
—12	5 mU./kg. of A.D.H. injected i.v.																	
0	No. 7 Fr. polyethylene catheter passed easily to left midureter; right kidney urine collected from open stopcock of cystoscope.																	
8	Blood pressure 138/100 mm. Hg.																	
25	Plasma No. 2 drawn.																	
33	Blood pressure 144/100 mm. Hg. Left kidney urine slightly blood-tinged; right kidney urine collected across the bladder crystal clear.																	
18—28	4.82	4.22	1.14	208.5	234.5	0.89	47.17	46.47	1.01	95.5	108.7	0.88	200.07	199.50	1.00	0.24	0.23	1.04
28—38	5.63	4.67	1.21	164.7	177.8	0.93	43.53	38.98	1.12	79.4	82.7	0.96	194.28	167.94	1.16	0.22	0.23	0.96
38—48	7.67	6.56	1.17	121.6	142.9	0.85	43.80	44.02	0.99	59.2	71.6	0.83	197.52	204.13	0.97	0.22	0.22	1.00
Av.18-48	6.04	5.15	1.17	164.9	185.1	0.89	44.84	43.16	1.04	78.0	87.7	0.89	197.29	190.52	1.04	0.23	0.23	1.00
51	Plasma No. 3 drawn.																	
53	800 ml. of 8 % urea in normal saline absorbed.																	

Time	Column 7 Concentration of creatinine ($U_{Cr.}$)			Column 8 Excretion rate of creatinine ($U_{Cr.}V.$)			Column 9 Concentration of sodium (U_{Na})			Column 10 Excretion rate of sodium ($U_{Na}V.$)			Column 11 Clearance of sodium ($U_{Na}V./P_{Na}$)			Column 12 % of filt. sod. excr. ($C_{Na}/C_{In.} \times 100$)		
	R.	L.	R./L.	R.	L.	R./L.	R.	L.	R./L.	R.	L.	R./L.	R.	L.	R./L.	R.	L.	R./L.
min.	mg. %			mg./min.			μEq./ml.			μEq./min.			ml./min.					
—25							Plasma No. 1 = 134.3											
25							Plasma No. 2 = 133.8											
18—28	7.2	8.1	0.89	34.8	34.4	1.01	89.99	87.67	1.03	433.8	370.0	1.17	3.23	2.75	1.17	6.84	5.92	1.15
28—38	5.9	6.2	0.95	33.4	29.0	1.15	88.00	87.62	1.00	495.4	409.2	1.21	3.69	3.05	1.21	8.47	7.81	1.08
38—48	4.5	5.5	0.81	34.5	36.3	0.95	91.39	86.76	1.05	701.0	569.1	1.23	5.22	4.24	1.23	11.91	9.62	1.24
Av.18-48	5.9	6.6	0.89	34.2	33.2	1.03	89.79	87.35	1.03	543.4	449.4	1.21	4.04	3.34	1.21	9.07	7.78	1.17
51							Plasma No. 3 = 135.0											

found that 49% of 256 unselected normotensive patients had some degree of main renal artery occlusion (*12*).

The following patient is representative of our experience of functionally insignificant lesions:

B. R., a 55-year-old, widowed, white female, was hospitalized in March, 1964, for urologic investigation of some upper calyceal changes in the left kidney (Fig. 1). In June, 1963, she had left flank pain, radiating to the left groin and lasting three to four hours. Similar episodes occurred in July and August, and microscopic hematuria was noted. An intravenous pyelogram (I.V.P.) in August showed acute obstruction of the upper calyx, but no visible stone. Although she became asymptomatic, repeat pyelograms in October, 1963, and January, 1964, showed persistent calyceal distortion in the upper calyx of the left kidney (Fig. 1); the previous obstruction of the calyx had disappeared. Her past history revealed the passage of a single ureteral calculus in 1954. A small basal cell carcinoma was removed from her chin in December, 1960; her blood pressure at that time was recorded as 115/75 mm. Hg.

Before her admission to the hospital in March, 1964, she was seen in consultation on an outpatient basis; her blood pressure then was 120/80 mm. Hg. Upon admission to the hospital, it was recorded 19 times in four days. The highest systolic pressure, except during the period of the differential function study, was 120 mm. Hg; the highest diastolic pressure was 80 mm. Hg. Urinalysis and all blood findings, including serum creatinine and blood urea nitrogen (B.U.N.), were normal. The urine culture was sterile. Because the left upper calyceal changes were compatible with a small cyst or tumor, a left selective renal arteriogram was performed (Fig. 2); this study did not reveal either a cyst or a tumor. A selective arteriogram of the right renal artery, however, showed fibromuscular hyperplasia with typical sausage-like constrictions (Fig. 3). These changes in the right renal artery were confirmed by different injections in three oblique positions.

Differential function studies, using an infusion of urea, saline, and A.D.H. were performed on March 5, 1964. These studies, which are summarized in Table 1, showed that the right kidney had a

---

Fig. 1. A 10-minute film from the intravenous pyelogram in patient B.R. The left upper calyces show evidence of distortion.

Fig. 2. A transfemoral, selective arteriogram of the left kidney in patient B.R. The left renal artery is normal; the arterial pattern in the renal cortex does not suggest a cyst or tumor.

Fig. 3. A transfemoral, selective arteriogram of the right kidney in patient B.R. There is marked fibromuscular hyperplasia of the right renal artery.

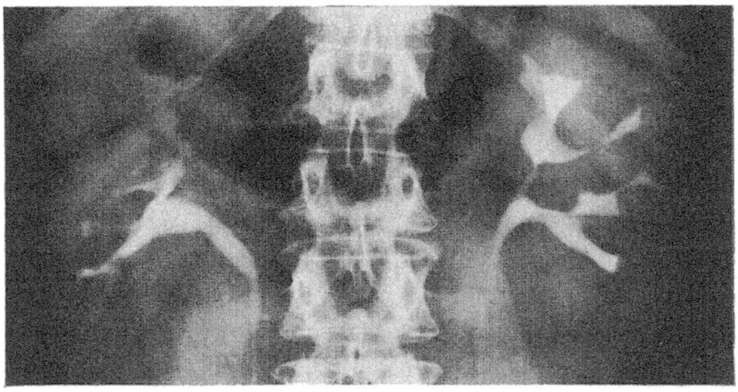

Fig. 1

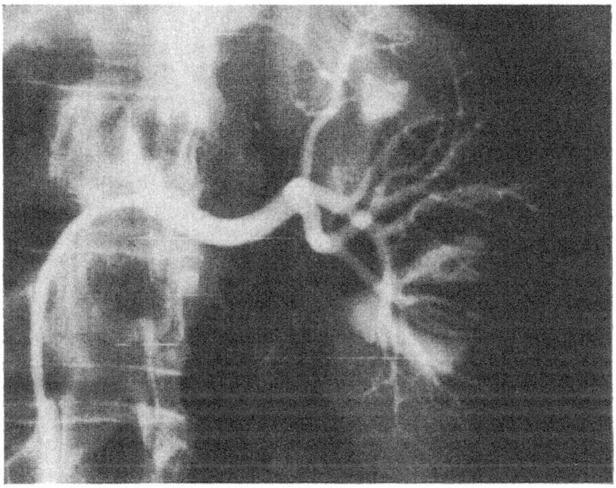

Fig. 2

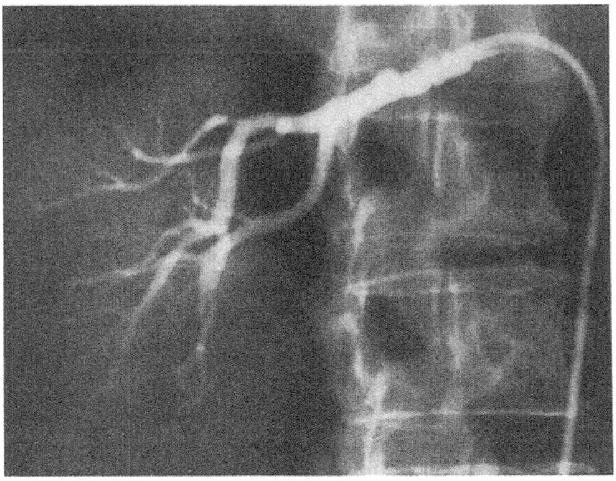

Fig. 3

greater R.P.F. and G.F.R. than the left. The right kidney excreted more water and more sodium than the left kidney, and the concentrations of inulin, P.A.H., and creatinine were slightly less in the urine from the right kidney. There was not a single characteristic in these studies to suggest a functionally ischemic kidney. The patient had functionally insignificant occlusive disease of the right renal artery which was not affecting the kidney and not producing hypertension.

I realize that these introductory comments are now a matter of history, especially for those physicians who have used careful differential function studies in the investigation of the hypertensive patient. In this paper, however, I should like to consider three observations, derived from differential renal function studies, which are not so widely appreciated.

1. The filtration fraction (F.F.) in the ischemic kidney is always less than the F.F. in the contralateral kidney.
2. The greatest increase in reabsorption of water in the ischemic kidney occurs in those kidneys which have the smallest reduction in R.P.F. and G.F.R. (*1*).
3. In *unilateral* occlusive disease of the renal arteries, cure of the patient's hypertension depends not only upon the presence of a functionally significant lesion (marked differences in sodium and water reabsorption), but also upon the degree of small-vessel disease in the contralateral kidney as measured by the clearance of P.A.H.

1. The filtration fraction of the ischemic kidney

It is well recognized that the filtration fraction (G.F.R./R.P.F.) in the hypertensive patient is increased, and, in general, the more severe the hypertension, the higher the F.F. (*13*). The factors responsible for these changes in afferent and efferent arteriolar constriction at the glomerulus are completely unknown. In 1963, in an attempt to explain our clinical observation that juxtaglomerular cell hyperplasia was not present in those ischemic kidneys which had ceased to form glomerular filtrate, we considered the possibility that the primary stimulus for the renin-angiotensin system was not a change in some baroceptor stretch mechanism at the afferent arteriole, as suggested by TOBIAN (*14*), but rather a change in Na concentration at the site of the macula densa (*1*). This hypothesis had three advantages: it assigned a physiologic role to the striking anatomic position of the macula densa; it related the renin-angiotensin system to an endocrine stimulus (Na concentration) rather than to a system based upon mechanoreceptor or baroceptor control; and it explained not only all the experimental perfusion evidence relating to juxtaglomerular cell hyperplasia (a fall in G.F.R. markedly affects the concentration of Na in the tubule), but also the influence of diet (high and low salt) and of adrenalectomy on juxtaglomerular cell hyperplasia in terms either of a direct change in Na concentration within the glomerular filtrate or of a change in G.F.R.

We pointed out that if a decrease in Na concentration in the tubular fluid at the macula densa is the primary stimulus for an increase in circulating renin and angiotensin, then a plausible explanation for the increase in F.F. in hypertensive patients would be that this constitutes a homeostatic response (*1*). If, for example, in the hypertensive patient with partial occlusion of one renal artery, the fall in Na concentration at the macula densa stimulates the renin-angiotensin system, the increased angiotensin would produce still more vasoconstriction leading to a further fall in R.P.F. and G.F.R., which would, in turn, act as further stimulus to the secretion of renin. Since angiotensin must vasoconstrict the efferent arteriole more than the afferent arteriole (in order to increase the F.F.), the resulting disparity in vasoconstriction could serve to help maintain the G.F.R. at any given reduction in R.P.F. caused by angiotensin vasoconstriction. To the extent that further falls in G.F.R. are dampened, further stimuli to renin production through changes in G.F.R. and Na concentration are prevented. In this sense, the elevated F.F. in the hypertensive patient may be a homeostatic mechanism for "softening" the effects of further changes in the Na-renin system by stabilizing G.F.R.

In an attempt to examine the effect of angiotensin in the afferent-efferent balance at the glomerulus, two observations have been made:

a) When angiotensin is infused in hypertensive patients with an elevated F.F., the F.F. increases still further. Although the angiotensin infusion decreases both G.F.R. and R.P.F., the fall in R.P.F. always exceeds the fall in G.F.R.; in some instances, the decrease in G.F.R. is hardly detectable, while the fall in R.P.F. may be 20–30% or more.

b) A study of hypertensive patients with functionally significant, unilateral, occlusive disease of the main renal artery presented an opportunity to compare the afferent-efferent balance of the glomeruli in the Goldblatt kidney with the glomeruli in the contralateral kidney. Since the Goldblatt kidney releases its renin into the venous circulation (through both the renal vein and lymph), the arterial circulation should present a uniform concentration of angiotensin to the glomerular beds of both kidneys. The Goldblatt kidney, however, always has a reduced blood flow, and therefore *less* angiotensin will reach the glomerular bed than in the contralateral kidney. The data in Table 2 are representative F.F. values from 11 patients with unilateral occlusive disease of the main renal artery. Although the F.F. is usually elevated in both kidneys, these figures show that the F.F. in the Goldblatt kidney is always less elevated than that of the contralateral kidney. It is a reasonable assumption that this difference is due to less angiotensin reaching the glomerular bed of the Goldblatt kidney.

Table 2. *The filtration fraction of the Goldblatt kidney compared to the contralateral kidney*

Patient	Goldblatt kidney			Contralateral kidney			F.F. Goldblatt kidney / F.F. contralateral kidney
	G.F.R. ml./min.	R.P.F. ml./min.	F.F.	G.F.R. ml./min.	R.P.F. ml./min.	F.F.	
1. R.Y.	93	384	0.24	106	372	0.28	0.86
2. B.G.	67	269	0.25	81	306	0.26	0.96
3. L.S.	51	181	0.28	71	236	0.30	0.93
4. A.H.	72	196	0.37	110	278	0.40	0.93
5. A.C.	40	274	0.15	65	367	0.18	0.83
6. E.R.	29	138	0.21	61	243	0.25	0.84
7. V.T.	40	189	0.21	78	343	0.23	0.91
8. E.P.	28	94	0.30	60	183	0.33	0.91
9. H.P.	31	138	0.22	67	276	0.24	0.92
10. J.B.	31	190	0.16	82	434	0.19	0.84
11. E.L.	8	53	0.15	31	154	0.20	0.75
						Average	0.88

The observation that the F.F. of the ischemic kidney is less elevated than that of the contralateral kidney means that the cause of an elevated F.F. cannot be explained in terms of some direct mechanical response or reflex to occlusive vascular disease; if a simple reduction in R.P.F. were somehow the cause of the increase in F.F., the Goldblatt kidney with its greater decrease in R.P.F. should have had the higher F.F.

Finally, the smaller increase in the F.F. of the ischemic kidney explains why we have always observed that the diagnostic differences between the two kidneys in $U_{P.A.H.}$ are greater than the differences in $U_{In.}$ or $U_{Cr.}$. P.A.H. is secreted in the ischemic kidney into a smaller volume of glomerular filtrate (in relation to the R.P.F.) than occurs in the contralateral kidney. Thus, before water reabsorption begins, the concentration of P.A.H. in the proximal tubule of the ischemic kidney is greater than the concentration of P.A.H. in the contralateral kidney; on the other hand, the concentration of inulin and creatinine, before water reabsorption, will be the same in the proximal tubules of the two kidneys.

2. The relationship of reduced G.F.R. to excessive water reabsorption

The greatest amount of excessive water reabsorption, per unit of reduction in glomerular filtrate, occurs in those vascular lesions with the *smallest* reduction in R.P.F. and G.F.R. (*1*). The functional differences between the Goldblatt kidney and the contralateral kidney in 13 patients with unilateral main renal artery disease are schematically presented in Fig. 4. In none of these patients was the

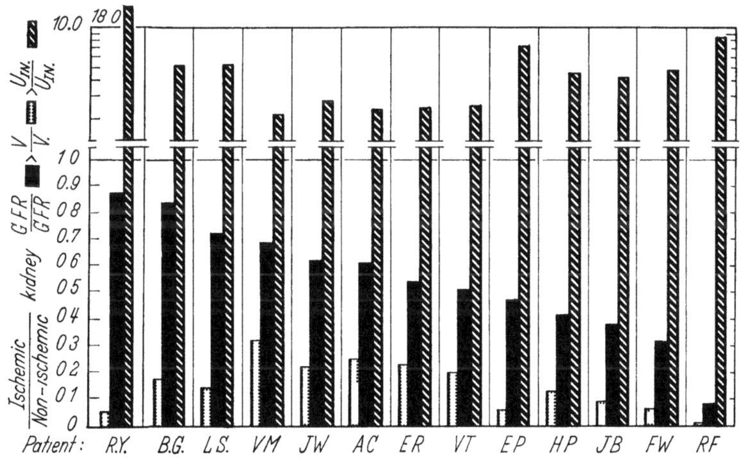

Fig. 4. The relationship of reduced G.F.R. to excessive water reabsorption. These 13 patients are arranged from left to right according to the increasing differences in G.F.R. between the ischemic Goldblatt kidney and the contralateral, non-ischemic kidney. All patients had unilateral main renal artery occlusions. The differences between the two kidneys in urine flow rate, V./V., and the concentration of inulin, $U_{In.}/U_{In.}$, are indicated by the appropriate columns. The ischemic kidney in patient E.P. received all of its R.P.F. from collateral circulation emptying directly into the main renal artery (*1*).

difference in size between the two kidneys more than 1–2 cm., except in R.F. and L.S., whose Goldblatt kidneys were 2.5 cm. smaller than the contralateral kidneys. In patients R.Y. and B.G. there was no difference in renal mass between the left and right kidney. The differences between the two kidneys in G.F.R., V., and $U_{In.}$ are expressed as a ratio of the ischemic kidney to the contralateral, "non-ischemic" kidney (a ratio of 1.0 would indicate no difference between the two kidneys). The patients are arranged from left to right according to the increasing differences in G.F.R. between the ischemic Goldblatt kidney and the contralateral, "non-ischemic" kidney. The average patient with functionally significant, unilateral renal artery obstruction shows about 50% reduction in G.F.R. (and R.P.F.) when the Goldblatt kidney is compared to the contralateral kidney, and a 4 or 5 : 1 difference in V. On the right side of Fig. 4, it is not surprising that the differences in V. become increasingly larger, because greater differences in G.F.R. are present[1]. What is surprising, however, is the patients with small differences in G.F.R. on the left side of the figure (R.Y., B.G., and L.S.). In a report on our first seven patients with renovascular hypertension (*15*), the smallest difference in R.P.F. and G.F.R. was a 37% decrease in the Goldblatt kidney as compared to the contralateral kidney; we expressed some concern as to whether small reductions in R.P.F. would show the same characteristics of excessive water reabsorption. To our surprise, hypertensive patients with smaller reductions in R.P.F. and G.F.R. have consistently shown the largest differences in excessive water reabsorption (Fig. 4).

This observation should be carefully considered for two reasons. For one thing, it explains why differential renal function studies are a sensitive method for the detection of unilateral main renal artery disease. When peripheral resistance can no longer decrease and thereby maintain renal blood flow in the presence of a falling mean arterial pressure, the first detectable change in R.P.F. and G.F.R. to the glomerular bed will produce a marked increase in the reabsorption of filtered sodium and water. This observation explains why small differences in V. (50% or less) and $U_{P.A.H.}$ (10–40%) are virtually impossible in Goldblatt kidneys with unilateral obstruction of the main renal artery. If the occlusive disease is advanced enough to produce the first reduction in R.P.F. and G.F.R., then large differences in V. and $U_{P.A.H.}$ will be present (Fig. 4). The more advanced the occlusion and the larger the reductions in R.P.F. and G.F.R., the greater the part played by the reduced G.F.R. *per se* in restricting the output of water from the ischemic kidney.

[1] Although the differences in V. and U_{In} for patient E.P. seem somewhat out of line, this is the only patient among the 13 who had total occlusion of the main renal artery; all of the R.P.F. was derived from collateral circulation which emptied into the main renal artery (1).

The second and more important reason for considering the left side of Fig. 4 is that these small reductions in R.P.F. and G.F.R. produce marked changes in Na and water transport within the kidney. To the extent that Na and water are related to the general problem of hypertension, these small reductions (probably even a reduction of 1%, if it could be measured) in R.P.F. and G.F.R. must be regarded as a physiologic event of some consequence. This is especially true in the controversy over the genesis of renal hypertension. Is it caused by a change in pulse pressure or by decreased R.P.F. and G.F.R.? SELKURT's data demonstrated that graded, mean arterial pressure decrements did not change R.P.F., G.F.R., or Na and water excretion, until a gradient of at least 40 mm. Hg in mean renal arterial pressure was produced (*9*). In a later publication (*10*), he showed that large changes in pulse pressure had no influence on Na and water excretion; when mean renal arterial pressure was severely reduced from control values of 149 to 88 mm. Hg, there were marked changes in Na and water excretion. Although SELKURT tended to discount a change in R.P.F. and G.F.R. during this 61 mm. Hg fall in mean pressure, his data actually show a fall in G.F.R. of 6–8% when the experimental and the control periods are compared. It is true that R.P.F. did not appear to change in SELKURT's studies; if, however, as in our patients with Goldblatt kidneys, the F.F. is less elevated in the experimental kidney than in the control (as, indeed, his data show), it is quite possible not to detect the earliest fall in R.P.F. in the experimental kidney when a decrease in G.F.R. is readily apparent. If one were unaware of this difference in F.F., it would be possible to assign more importance to the apparent lack of change in P.A.H. data and to discount the small fall of 6–8% in G.F.R.

Failure to appreciate these large changes in Na and water transport produced by the smallest change in R.P.F. and G.F.R. (Fig. 4) partly accounts for the usual objections raised in this symposium to the use of the word ischemia. Our group has emphasized repeatedly that there is no acceptable evidence to support the baroceptor-pulse pressure theory of renin secretion (*1*). Recent experiments in the anesthetized dog served to underline the fact that a change in pulse pressure *per se* produces no change in the rate of renin release into the renal vein (*16–18*). Although SKINNER et al. maintain from these experiments that it is not a change in pulse pressure that is responsible for the release of renin, but instead a fall in *mean* pulse pressure, it is quite apparent from their published data that when mean pulse pressure finally fell in their experiments, they were dangerously close to the first change in R.P.F. (and G.F.R., which was not measured). In fact, the data reported in their first article (*16*), entitled "Renal baroceptor control of renin secretion", clearly show that large changes in pulse pressure with a small fall in mean pulse pressure produced no change in renin secretion, while the first detectable increase in renin occurred when R.P.F. was just starting to fall. When one considers the recent Cleveland data (*16*–*18*), recalls the fact that SELKURT could show no change in Na and water transport by decreasing pulse pressure, or even mean pulse pressure, by up to 40 mm. Hg (*9*), and remembers that the earliest fall in R.P.F. and G.F.R. in the human kidney is associated with remarkable changes in the renal handling of Na and water (*1*), it is hard to accept that a pulse pressure-baroceptor mechanism is at the basis of Goldblatt hypertension. Since changes in pulse pressure and moderate changes in mean pulse pressure (up to 40 mm. Hg) have no effect on Na and water transport in the kidney, it is far easier to believe that the primary stimulus is a reduction in R.P.F. and G.F.R. and that the word ischemia is, indeed, the correct term.

3. The prognostic importance of R.P.F. to the contralateral kidney

In the past eight years, 23 patients have been operated upon for unilateral, functionally significant occlusive disease of the renal arteries. All patients showed unequivocally positive results in differential function studies, and renal arteriography revealed unilateral lesions. The arteriograms were of excellent quality and the contralateral vasculature was thought to be normal. Excluded from this study are all patients who had bilateral main renal artery disease, all patients in whom the contralateral kidney was grossly abnormal on a congenital basis (pelvic kidney, etc.), and all patients in whom the success of vascular repair of the kidney was questionable (all patients who had undergone reparative surgery had postoperative arteriograms as well as differential renal function studies).

With these exclusions, our total operative experience in the past eight years of patients with unilateral lesions is summarized in Table 3. The average preoperative and postoperative outpatient blood pressures for each patient are given together with the data on preoperative R.P.F. to the contralateral kidney; the duration of follow-up appears immediately beside the postoperative blood pressure. All 23 patients should have been cured of their hypertension. In fact, only 13 became normotensive; five others (Nos *7*, *14*, *15*, *17*, and *22*) were unquestionably improved. Five patients (22% of the 23 patients) showed no change in their blood pressure except

Table 3. *The prognostic importance of R.P.F to the contralateral kidney in the cure of unilateral, renovascular hypertension*

Patient, age, race, and sex	Preoperative B. P. (Av.) mm. Hg	Postoperative B. P. (Av.) mm. Hg	R.P.F. to contralateral kidney ml /min./1.73 m.²
1. F. W. (50, W. M.)	240/140	100/60 (12 months)	518
2.* J. W. (20, W. M.)	170/120	110/70 (18 months)	460
3.* V. M. (24, C. F.)	210/120	120/80 (36 months)	456
4.* J.V.W. (24, W. F.)	160/110	122/76 (26 months)	435
5.* J. B.[1] (12, W. F.)	200/150	130/70 (12 months)	433
6.* W. G. (19, W. M.)	165/120	125/85 (24 months)	400
7. A. C. (50, W. M.)	210/115	146/96 (18 months)	367
8.* V. T. (18, W. F.)	170/110	112/70 (12 months)	343
9. G. K. (32, W. F.)	204/112	112/76[2] (3 months)	328
10. B. G. (44, W. M.)	170/120	138/80 (36 months)	306
11.* C. M.[1] (54, W. F.)	210/150	110/72 (24 months)	291
12. A. H. (55, W. M.)	240/120	135/85 (16 months)	278
13.* H. P. (43, W. F.)	220/120	124/80 (36 months)	276
14. J. K. (45, W. M.)	220/130	140/95[2] (14 months)	271
15. R. F.[1] (52, W. M.)	240/140	160/102 (6 months)	249
16. K. P. (47, W. M.)	210/115	130/85 (8 months)	247
17. L. S. (25, W. F.)	230/120	160/110 (12 months)	236
18. F. L.[3] (59, W. F.)	259/124	230/120 (7 months)	210
19. P. K.[3] (72, W. F.)	252/116	258/110 (3 months)	198
20. E. P. (37, W. F.)	260/140	200/140 (12 months)	183
21. E. L. (57, W. M.)	220/120	200/120 (18 months)	157
22. M. A.[1] (36, W. F.)	220/140	170/111 (24 months)	152
23. E. R. (65, W. F.)	245/120	250/120 (36 months)	89

Legend: W. F. = white female, W. M. = white male, and C. F. = negro female.

* = In all patients, except those marked with an asterisk, atherosclerosis was the cause of the functionally significant, unilateral main renal artery obstruction.

Patients Nos 2, 3, 5, 8, 11, and 13 had fibromuscular disease as the cause of their main renal artery obstruction.

The occlusive disease in the main renal artery of patients 4 and 6 was caused by an aneurysm.

[1] = Patients with malignant hypertension: funduscopic examination showed papilledema, hemorrhages, and exudates. F. W., patient No. 1, had hemorrhages and exudates, but no papilledema.

[2] = G. K., patient No. 9, had a B. P. of 170/102, seven months following her nephrectomy, in spite of being normotensive for three months. Her husband had lost his job, however, and she was extremely upset.

J. K., patient No. 14, had a B. P. of 150/105, 48 months following nephrectomy.

[3] = Patients Nos 18 and 19 had such marked obstructions of their main renal artery that the Goldblatt kidney did not excrete urine on function study or contrast medium on intravenous pyelography.

Patients Nos 1, 5, and 21 had surgical correction of their arterial obstruction as shown by postoperative arteriograms and repeat function studies. The remaining 20 patients had either a primary nephrectomy at the original operation or a secondary nephrectomy if vascular repair was unsuccessful.

for a transient fall in the first few days following surgery. From Table 3 it is clear that the 22% of patients (Nos 18, 19, 20, 21, and 23) who did not respond to surgery had a markedly reduced R.P.F. to the contralateral kidney (less than 210 ml./min./1.73 m.^{2}). The only patient who showed some response to surgery and had a low contralateral R.P.F. was patient M.A. (No. 22), a seriously ill, 36-year-old, white female with weight loss, papilledema, hemorrhages, exudates, and marked proteinuria. At surgery, wedge biopsy of the contralateral kidney showed fresh arteriolar necrosis in the majority of the glomeruli; thus, some of the reduction in R.P.F. (152 ml./min.) was acute, rather than chronic, and possibly reversible to some extent. In fact, in the months following surgery, R.P.F. to the contralateral kidney increased from 152 ml./min. to 190 ml./min. This patient remains hypertensive, but her fundi are now Grade I only, and she is in reasonably good health. Three of the four other patients who were unquestionably improved (Nos 14, 15, and 17), but definitely not cured, had R.P.F.'s of 271, 249, and 236 to the contralateral kidney.

All of the patients with unilateral non-atheromatous vascular disease had excellent contralateral R.P.F.'s and all were cured of their hypertension. These eight patients constitute the majority of the 13 who became normotensive. Thus, of the 23 patients with unilateral disease, 15 had arteriosclerotic vascular disease as the cause of their main renal artery occlusion; only five of these 15 patients were actually cured, while another five were certainly improved. These figures may serve as a reminder that the solution to the problem of renovascular hypertension ultimately depends upon solving the basic problem of arteriosclerosis. In the meantime, however, if surgery for renovascular hypertension is limited to those patients who have not only functionally significant lesions (marked excessive water reabsorption), but also an excellent R.P.F. to the contralateral kidney (greater than 250 ml./min.), the cure rate should approach 80–90%. It is equally apparent that surgery is contraindicated in those patients with unilateral lesions who have an R.P.F. of less than 250 ml./min./1.73 m.^{2} in the contralateral kidney. The presence of malignant hypertension may be an exception to this observation.

Patients Nos 18 and 19 had such marked obstructions in their main renal artery that the Goldblatt kidney failed to excrete either urine during ureteral catheterization or contrast medium during intravenous pyelography. The contralateral R.P.F. was low in each instance; simple nephrectomy in these two patients failed to influence the blood pressure.

The plasma clearance of P.A.H. should be measured in all patients in whom differential renal function studies are carried out. Not only is $C_{P.A.H.}$ the sole valid measure of vascular disease in the contralateral kidney, but, in addition, the difference in $U_{P.A.H.}$ between the two kidneys will, as already pointed out, invariably be greater than the differences in $U_{Cr.}$ or $U_{In.}$. Furthermore, since the elevated F.F. in hypertensive patients tends to maintain the $C_{Cr.}$ or $C_{In.}$ at levels out of proportion to the fall in $C_{P.A.H.}$, $C_{Cr.}$ in the contralateral kidney will often be within the normal range when $C_{P.A.H.}$ will be unquestionably reduced. As a final argument for measuring the clearance of P.A.H., it should be borne in mind that the biochemical reaction for determining P.A.H. is a more accurate method than the alkaline picrate technique for determining creatinine, especially serum creatinine.

Patient E.L. (No. 21, Table 3) is discussed in detail below, because the studies on this patient illustrate three aspects of occlusive disease of the renal artery in relation to renal function which need to be emphasized:

1. Renal angiography, no matter how excellent the technique adopted may be, does not yield a reliable estimate of small-vessel disease. Lobular vessels may appear anatomically normal in the presence of severe arteriosclerosis.

2. Excessive Na and water reabsorption is dependent upon a reduction in R.P.F. and G.F.R. to the total nephron population of one kidney as compared with the contralateral kidney. Patient E.L.'s case demonstrates that the reduced R.P.F. and G.F.R. caused by a unilateral main renal artery obstruction may be superimposed upon bilateral small-vessel disease and still result in large differences in Na and water transport.

3. Correction of the disparity in reduced G.F.R. to the functioning nephrons in one kidney results in disappearance of the preoperative, disparate pattern of excessive Na and water reabsorption, even though bilateral small-vessel disease is present and the blood pressure remains elevated.

E. L., a 57-year-old, white male, was first seen by us in January, 1964. In 1958, he had a transient episode of dizziness with numbness and weakness in his right arm and leg; his blood pressure was normal. He was digitalized for episodic, atrial fibrillation in 1962, and again his blood pressure was found to be normal. Daily frontal headaches began in August, 1963, and at that time it was noted that his blood pressure varied between 180/110 and 220/120 mm. Hg. His hypertension did not respond to hydralazine therapy. In November, 1963, after an extremely severe frontal headache, he

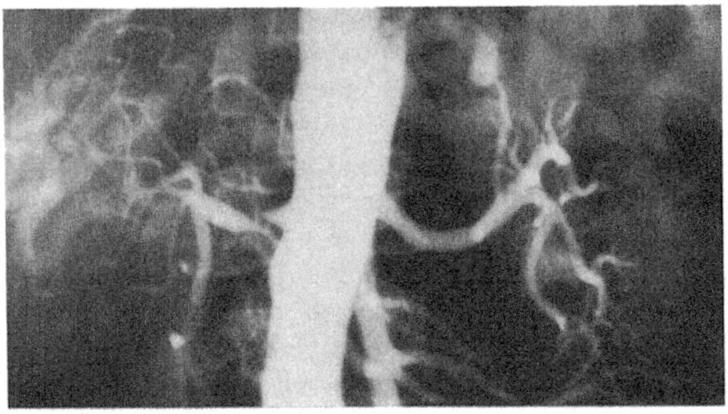

Fig. 5

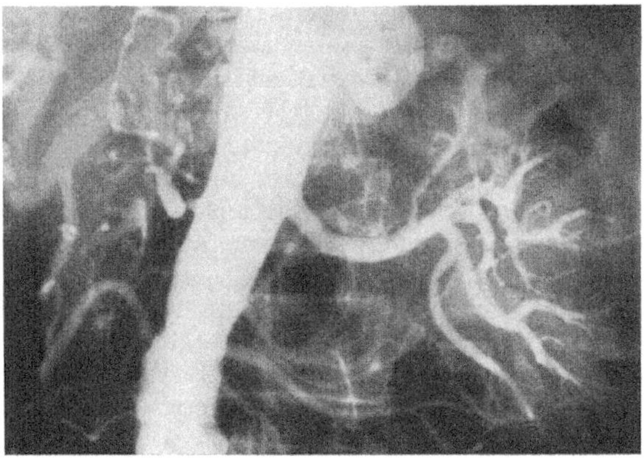

Fig. 6

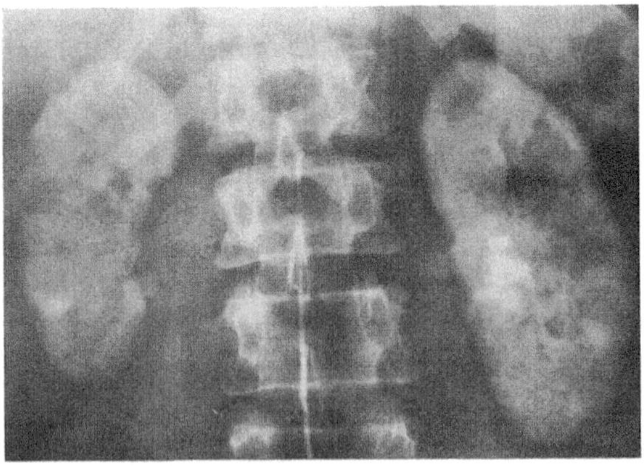

Fig. 7

became dizzy and incoherent for 48 hours. An E.E.G. and bilateral carotid arteriograms were recorded and thought to be normal. In December, 1963, he had several days of painless, gross hematuria. An I.V.P. showed delayed excretion of contrast medium in the right kidney; the 10-minute film showed a normal collecting system, but no excretion was apparent on the 5-minute film. The right kidney was 2 cm. smaller than the left (see Fig. 7).

Upon admission to the hospital in January, 1964, the patient was found to be slender and slightly underweight; his blood pressure was 200/110 mm. Hg. Examination of the fundi showed marked arteriolar narrowing with one or two old exudates in each eye; there were no hemorrhages or papilledema. The chest x-ray showed a slightly enlarged heart, and a right bundle branch block was evident on the E.K.G. Urine cultures were sterile, the urinalysis was normal except for 5 mg.% of protein, and first-morning urine specimens had specific gravities which were never greater than 1.016. The 15-minute excretion of phenolsulfonphthalein was 25%. Serum chemistries were normal except for a serum creatinine of 2.6 mg.% and a uric acid of 7.7 mg.%. His hematocrit was 45%.

Percutaneous, transfemoral aortography showed a marked stenosis at the ostium of the right renal artery (Figs 5, 6 and 7); the contralateral vasculature to the left kidney appeared normal. On February 3, 1964, an 8 mm. knitted Dacron graft was placed from the lower aorta into the distal end of the right renal artery. A large pressure gradient (greater than 100 mm. Hg) was present before placing the graft, and no gradient was detectable at the end of surgery. The left kidney appeared normal grossly, but a wedge biopsy was taken for microscopic study.

Differential renal function studies were performed before and nine days after surgery; they were repeated 16 weeks and 11 months after surgery (Table 4). All four differential function studies shown in Table 4 were carried out under the same conditions: a saddle block anesthesia and a standard infusion, at a rate of 10 ml./min., of 8%

Fig. 5. A transfemoral arteriogram in patient E.L. The right renal artery has a severe occlusion at the aortic ostium. The left renal artery and its branches appear normal. The aorta is markedly atherosclerotic.

Fig. 6. An oblique, transfemoral arteriogram in patient E.L. The left renal artery and its branches are magnified because the left kidney-to-film distance is increased. The left renal vasculature appears reasonably normal.

Fig. 7. The nephrogram phase from the transfemoral arteriogram series in Fig. 5. The right kidney is smaller than the left.

Table 4. *E. L., 57-year-old hypertensive white male with right renal artery stenosis*

Time	Urine flow ml./min.			R.P.F. ml./min.			G.F.R. ml./min.			$U_{P.A.H.}$ mg. %			UNa mEq./l.		
	R.	L.	R./L.	R.	L.	R./L.	R.	L.	R./L.	R.	L.	R./L.	R.	L.	R./L.
Preoperative	0.4	7.8	0.05	53	154	0.34	8	31	0.26	402	58	6.97	22	91	0.24
9 days postop.	2.1	4.0	0.52	66	151	0.44	11	28	0.39	84	101	0.83	107	93	1.15
16 weeks postop.	1.7	4.8	0.34	48	120	0.40	9	25	0.36	86	74	1.16	92	92	1.00
11 months postop.		(Total) 5.5			(Total) 207			(Total) 45		161	159	1.01	105	101	1.04

urea in saline, containing P.A.H., inulin, and A.D.H. (*1*). The data shown in Table 4 (uncorrected for 1.73 m.²) represent the average of three consecutive, 10-minute collection periods, which showed less than a 6% variation in urine flow rate differences between the two kidneys in consecutive periods. There was no bladder leakage in the first three studies, but in the last study (11 months after surgery), marked bladder leakage occurred; because of this, the last study appears as a measurement of total renal function (R.P.F. and G.F.R.), except for the differences in $U_{P.A.H.}$ and U_{Na}.

Renal arteriography was repeated 16 weeks and 11 months after surgery. Fig. 8 is representative of both studies. Repeat intravenous pyelograms made postoperatively showed equal calyceal appearance times in both kidneys.

Following surgery, the patient's blood pressure never changed from the preoperative levels. He received no therapy for his hypertension in the first year after surgery. The patient has continued to work as a crane operator, and except for occasional periods of increased forgetfulness and mild obtundation, he has remained in good general health. His serum creatinine 11 months after surgery was 2.3 mg.%, his serum cholesterol was 285 mg.%, and his urinalysis was unchanged.

Representative sections from the wedge biopsy of the contralateral left kidney are shown in Figs 9 and 10. Severe arteriosclerosis was present in all the large arteries of this biopsy. The appearance of these arteries on biopsy, especially of those in Fig. 10, should be compared carefully with the arteriogram of the left kidney (Figs 5 and 6). These studies should make us all proceed with caution when we attempt to assess the presence or absence of small-vessel disease by renal angiography.

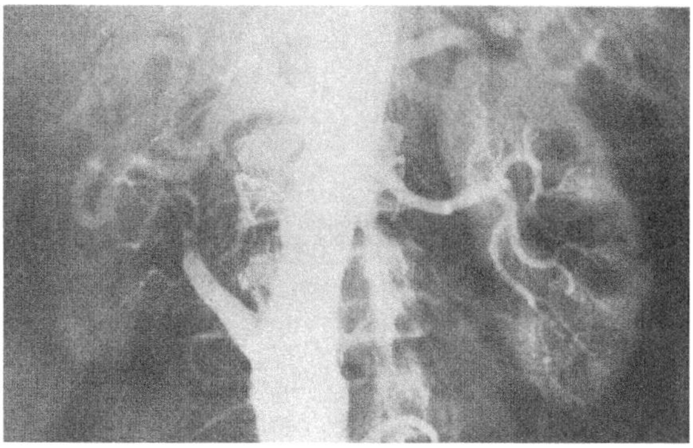

Fig. 8. A postoperative, transfemoral arteriogram in patient E.L. made 11 months after surgery. A similar picture was obtained 16 weeks after surgery. The Dacron graft, placed end-to-end in the renal artery, is functioning well.

The renal function data contained in Table 4 show the classic preoperative pattern of functionally significant, unilateral main renal artery disease. There is a 20 : 1 difference in V., but only a 4 : 1 difference in G.F.R. $U_{P.A.H.}$ is increased by seven times in the right kidney, while U_{Na} is reduced to one quarter of that in the contralateral kidney. What is important, however, is that this pattern is superimposed on marked bilateral disease (indeed, the preoperative serum creatinine was 2.6 mg. %). Since the obstruction in the right renal artery could have produced any degree of reduction in R.P.F. and G.F.R., the presence of small-vessel disease can be assessed only from the data on R.P.F. and G.F.R. in the contralateral kidney. In this patient it is clear that the R.P.F. of 154 ml./min. (corrected to 157 ml./min./1.73 m.^{2} in Table 3) to the contralateral left kidney represents a severe reduction in renal function produced by small-vessel disease. Since, from the standpoint of hypertension, it should make no difference to a kidney whether arterial obstruction is in the main renal artery or in the lobular arteries, it is not surprising that a low R.P.F. in the contralateral left kidney precluded a change in blood pressure following surgery on the right kidney.

The function studies (Table 4) made nine days after surgery show the pattern usually found immediately following vascular

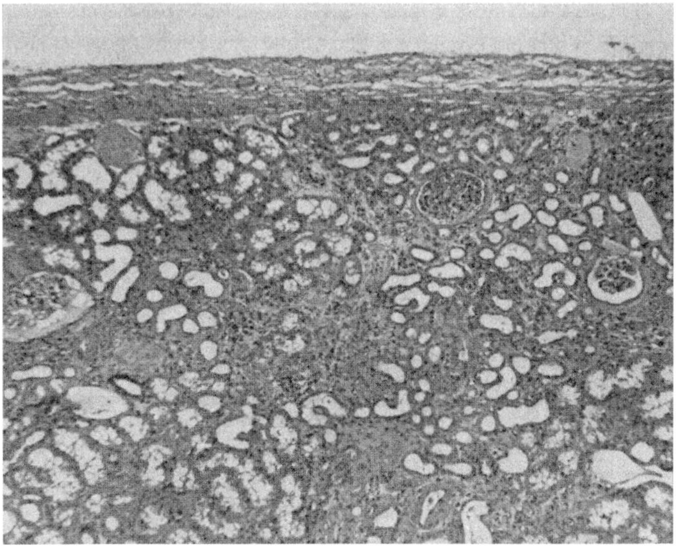

Fig. 9. A representative section from the wedge biopsy of the contralateral left kidney in patient E.L. Note the interstitial fibrosis, some hyalinized glomeruli, and the leucocytic infiltrates.

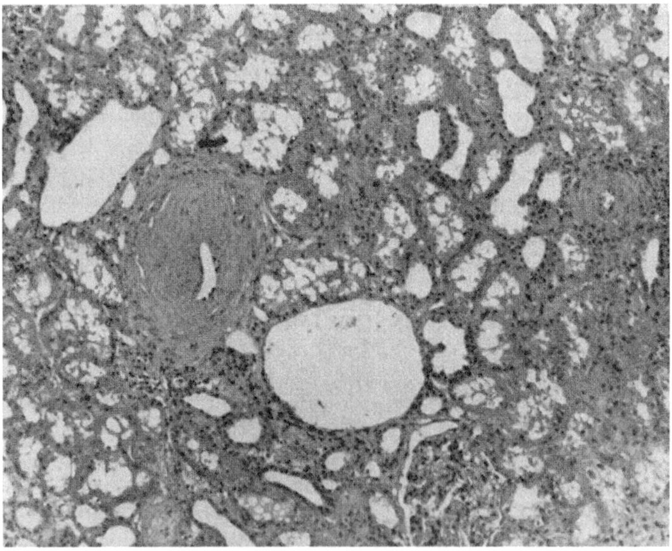

Fig. 10. A typical arteriosclerotic artery from the wedge biopsy of the left kidney in patient E.L. Note that the size of the artery is larger than the glomerulus in the lower part of the field. There is a smaller artery, also markedly narrowed by arteriosclerosis, at the upper, right margin of the figure.

repair (*1*), i.e. the comparative increase in Na and water reabsorption present preoperatively in the right kidney is converted temporarily to a relative failure to reabsorb Na and water compared with the left kidney. $U_{P.A.H.}$ changed from a 6.97% increase to a 17% decrease (0.83) and U_{Na} from a preoperative ratio of 0.24 to a postoperative ratio of 1.15. It should be noted that, although the change in R.P.F. and G.F.R. after nine days is definitely significant, it is a very small change indeed (12.4% increase in R.P.F. and 13.7% increase in G.F.R.). However, although small, this increase in R.P.F. and G.F.R. was enough to re-establish equivalent volumes of glomerular filtrate to the remaining functioning nephrons in the right kidney as compared with the left kidney; all evidence of disparate excessive Na and water reabsorption disappeared. The fact that a small additional reduction in G.F.R. to all the nephrons in the right kidney (13.7 %, comparing the postoperative increase to the preoperative G.F.R.) produced large differences in Na and water reabsorption in this patient is similar to the observations in the patients on the left side of Fig. 4, except that in this instance (E.L.) the main renal artery obstruction was superimposed on bilateral, symmetrical small-vessel disease. From these studies it is reasonable to believe that the marked increase in reabsorption of filtered Na and water, characteristic of occlusive disease of the renal arteries, is caused by a disparity in G.F.R. between the two kidneys, and that small differences in G.F.R. produce large changes in Na and water transport.

Summary

Differential renal function studies performed in patients with unilateral occlusive disease of the renal arteries have produced several additional observations which relate to R.P.F., G.F.R., and Na and water transport in the ischemic kidney. These observations are as follows:

(1) The filtration fraction (F.F.) in the ischemic kidney is always less than the F.F. in the contralateral kidney. This smaller increase in the F.F. of the Goldblatt kidney is probably due to less angiotensin reaching the glomerular bed of the ischemic kidney. Some evidence is presented to support the hypothesis that the elevated F.F. in hypertensive patients may be caused by angiotensin; if this is true, the increase in F.F. could serve as one mechanism for stabilizing G.F.R. in order to prevent further stimulation of the Na-renin system. This difference in the F.F. between the Goldblatt kidney and the contralateral kidney also explains why $U_{P.A.H.}$ differences, as a measure of excessive water reabsorption, are always greater than $U_{Cr.}$ or $U_{In.}$ differences.

(2) The greatest increase in reabsorption of water in the ischemic kidney occurs in those kidneys which have the smallest reduction in R.P.F. and G.F.R. This observation not only explains why differential function studies are a sensitive index of reduced R.P.F. and G.F.R. to functioning nephrons, but also emphasizes why the smallest reduction in R.P.F. and G.F.R. must

be considered a physiologic event of some consequence in relation to Na and water transport. Since a decrease in pulse pressure or even a decrease in mean pulse pressure of up to 40 mm. Hg does not change Na and water transport within the kidney, it is unlikely that a pulse pressure-baroceptor mechanism controls the renin-angiotensin system; a reduction in R.P.F. and G.F.R., by decreasing Na concentration in the tubule and thereby stimulating renin secretion, is the more likely stimulus.

(3) In unilateral occlusive disease of the renal arteries, cure of the patient's hypertension depends not only upon the presence of a functionally significant lesion (marked differences in Na and water reabsorption) but also upon the absence of small-vessel disease in the contralateral kidney as measured by the clearance of P.A.H. If surgery for unilateral renovascular hypertension is limited to those patients who have functionally significant lesions in one kidney and an R.P.F. greater than 250 ml./min./m.^{2} in the opposite, contralateral kidney, the cure rate should approach 80—90%. The higher the contralateral R.P.F., the better the prognosis.

(4) Renal angiography, however excellent the technique, does not yield a reliable estimate of small-vessel disease. Interlobar vessels may appear anatomically normal in the presence of severe arteriosclerosis.

(5) Studies are presented which demonstrate that the reduction in R.P.F. and G.F.R. caused by a unilateral main renal artery obstruction may be superimposed upon bilateral small-vessel disease and still produce large, unilateral differences in Na and water transport. Correction of the disparity in reduced G.F.R. to the functioning nephrons in one kidney results in the disappearance of the preoperative, disparate pattern of excessive Na and water reabsorption, even though bilateral small-vessel disease is present and the patient remains hypertensive.

Zusammenfassung

Differenzierende Nierenfunktionsuntersuchungen bei Patienten mit einseitiger Verschlußerkrankung der Nierenarterien haben verschiedene zusätzliche Veränderungen ergeben, welche in Beziehung zur Nierendurchblutung, zum Glomerulumfiltrat sowie zum Natrium- und Wassertransport in der ischämischen Niere stehen. Es handelt sich um folgende Beobachtungen:

1. Die Filtrationsfraktion (F.F.) in der ischamischen Niere ist immer niedriger als diejenige in der kontralateralen Niere. Dieser geringere Anstieg der F.F. in der Goldblattniere beruht wahrscheinlich darauf, daß in der ischämischen Niere weniger Angiotensin das Glomerularbett erreicht. Es werden einige Hinweise gegeben, um die Hypothese zu stützen, daß die erhöhte F.F. bei Hochdruckpatienten durch Angiotensin hervorgerufen sein kann. Falls dies zutrifft, könnte der Anstieg der F.F. als ein Mechanismus zur Stabilisierung des Glomerulumfiltrates dienen, um einer weiteren Anregung des Natrium-Renin-Systems vorzubeugen. Der Unterschied in der F.F. zwischen der Goldblattniere und der kontralateralen Niere erklärt auch, warum die Unterschiede in der $U_{P.A.H.}$ (als ein Maß für die exzessive Wasserrückresorption) immer größer sind als die Unterschiede von U_{Cr} oder U_{In}.

2. Der größte Anstieg der Rückresorption von Wasser in der ischämischen Niere findet sich in den Nieren, in denen die Durchblutung und das Glomerulumfiltrat am wenigsten abnehmen. Diese Beobachtung erklärt nicht nur, warum die differenzierenden Funktionsuntersuchungen ein empfindlicher Index für die im Verhältnis zu den tätigen Nephren herabgesetzte Nierendurchblutung und das Glomerulumfiltrat sind, sondern unterstreicht auch,

warum die geringste Verminderung der Nierendurchblutung und des Glomerulumfiltrates als ein physiologischer Vorgang anzusehen ist, der Auswirkungen auf den Natrium- und Wassertransport hat. Da eine Abnahme des Pulsdruckes oder sogar des mittleren Pulsdruckes um bis zu 40 mm Hg den Natrium- und Wassertransport innerhalb der Niere nicht verändert, ist es unwahrscheinlich, daß ein Pulsdruck-Barorezeptor Mechanismus das Renin-Angiotensin System kontrolliert; eine Verminderung der Nierendurchblutung und des Glomerulumfiltrates, die eine Abnahme der Natriumkonzentration in den Tubuli hervorruft und dadurch die Reninsekretion anregt, ist der wahrscheinlichere Reiz.

3. Bei einseitiger Verschlußerkrankung der Nierenarterien hängt die Heilung des Hochdruckes nicht nur von der Anwesenheit einer funktionell bedeutsamen Schädigung ab (deutliche Unterschiede in der Natrium- und Wasserrückresorption), sondern auch vom Fehlen einer Erkrankung der kleinen Gefäße in der kontralateralen Niere, die mit Hilfe der P.A.H.-Clearance festzustellen ist. Wenn die Operation bei der einseitigen renovaskulären Hypertension auf diejenigen Patienten beschränkt wird, die funktionell bedeutsame Schädigungen in einer Niere haben und eine Durchblutung von mehr als 250 ml/min/m² in der kontralateralen Niere, dann sollte die Heilungsquote 80—90% erreichen. Je besser die Durchblutung der kontralateralen Niere ist, desto besser ist die Prognose.

4. Auch bei noch so guter Technik ist die Angiographie der Niere keine zuverlässige Methode für die Feststellung einer Erkrankung der kleinen Gefäße. Die interlobären Gefäße können auch bei Anwesenheit einer schweren Arteriosklerose anatomisch normal erscheinen.

5. Es werden Untersuchungen mitgeteilt, aus denen hervorgeht, daß die Verminderung der Nierendurchblutung und des Glomerulumfiltrates infolge einseitiger Verlegung der Hauptnierenarterie eine bilaterale Erkrankung der kleinen Gefäße überlagern, aber trotzdem noch erhebliche einseitige Unterschiede im Natrium- und Wassertransport verursachen kann. Eine Korrektur des Mißverhältnisses von vermindertem Glomerulumfiltrat zu funktionierenden Nephren in der stenosierten Niere führt zum Verschwinden der präoperativ exzessiven Rückresorption von Natrium und Wasser auf der stenosierten Seite, und zwar auch dann, wenn eine bilaterale Erkrankung der kleinen Gefäße vorliegt und der Patient hypertonisch bleibt.

Résumé

L'étude différentielle des fonctions rénales de malades présentant une affection obstructive unilatérale de l'artère rénale, a conduit à plusieurs constatations nouvelles au sujet du R.P.F., du G.F.R. et du transport de l'eau et du Na dans le rein ischémique. Ces constatations sont les suivantes:

1. La fraction de filtration (F.F.) dans le rein ischémique est toujours inférieure à la F.F. dans le rein contro-latéral. Cette augmentation plus modérée de la F.F. dans le rein de Goldblatt est probablement due à ce qu'une quantité moindre d'angiotensine atteint le réseau glomérulaire du rein ischémique. Des arguments sont présentés en faveur de l'hypothèse selon laquelle les taux élevés de la F.F. chez les hypertendus pourraient être dus à l'angiotensine; si cette hypothèse est exacte, l'accroissement de la F.F. pourrait être l'un des mécanismes tendant à stabiliser le G.F.R. en vue d'empêcher une stimulation supplémentaire du système sodium-rénine. Cette différence dans la F.F. entre le rein de Goldblatt et le rein contro-latéral explique également pourquoi les différences dans la $U_{P.A.H.}$, prise comme

mesure de la réabsorption excessive d'eau, sont toujours plus grandes que les différences dans la $U_{Cr.}$ ou la $U_{In.}$.

2. La plus grande augmentation de la réabsorption d'eau dans le rein ischémique se produit dans les reins qui présentent la plus petite réduction du R.P.F. et du G.F.R. Cette observation non seulement explique pourquoi les études fonctionnelles différentielles sont un indice sensible de la diminution du R.P.F. et du G.F.R. dans les néphrons en fonction, mais aussi souligne pourquoi la plus petite diminution du R.P.F. et du G.F.R. doit être considérée comme un fait physiologique d'importance dans le transport de l'eau et du sodium. Puisqu'une diminution de la pression différentielle ou même de la pression moyenne, allant jusqu'à 40 mm Hg, ne modifie pas le transport d'eau et de sodium dans le rein, il est peu vraisemblable qu'un barorécepteur sensible à la pression différentielle contrôle le système rénine-angiotensine; une réduction du R.P.F. et du G.F.R., entraînant une diminution de la concentration en Na dans le tubule, d'où stimulation de la sécrétion de rénine, est le stimulus le plus vraisemblable.

3. Dans les obstructions unilatérales de l'artère rénale, la guérison de l'hypertension ne dépend pas seulement des lésions à traduction fonctionnelle manifeste (différence importante dans la réabsorption de l'eau et du Na), mais aussi de l'absence d'affection des petits vaisseaux du rein contro-latéral, appréciée par la clearance du P.A.H. Si la chirurgie de l'hypertension d'origine vasculaire rénale unilatérale reste limitée aux malades qui présentent des lésions à traduction fonctionnelle significative dans un rein et un R.P.F. supérieur à 250 ml/min/m² dans l'autre rein, le taux de guérison devrait atteindre 80 à 90%. Plus le R.P.F. contro-latéral est élevé, plus le pronostic est bon.

4. L'angiographie rénale, même avec une excellente technique, n'est pas un bon moyen d'exploration des affections des petits vaisseaux. Les artères interlobaires peuvent apparaître morphologiquement normales en dépit de l'existence d'une artériosclérose sévère.

5. On présente des études démontrant que la réduction du R.P.F. et du G.F.R. provoquée par une obstruction unilatérale du tronc de l'artère rénale peut se surajouter à une affection bilatérale des petits vaisseaux et entraîner, là encore, des modifications importantes unilatérales dans le transport de l'eau et du sodium. La correction de cette disparité entre les deux reins, créée par la diminution du G.F.R. par rapport aux néphrons fonctionnels du rein ischémié, a pour conséquence la disparition du tableau dyssymétrique préopératoire de réabsorption excessive de sodium et d'eau, alors même que subsiste l'affection bilatérale des petits vaisseaux et que le malade reste un hypertendu.

References

1. Stamey, T. A.: Renovascular Hypertension. Williams and Wilkins, Baltimore, 1963. — 2. Hancock, E. W., W. M. Madison, Jr., M. H. Proctor, W. H. Abelmann, and G. W. B. Starkey: N. England J. Med. **258**, 305 (1958). — 3. Haimovici, H., and D. J. W. Escher: Arch. Surg. **72**, 107 (1956). — 4. Patel, D. J., R. L. Lange, and H. H. Hecht: Amer. J. Med. **26**, 761 (1959). — 5. Mann, F. C., and by invitation J. F. Herrick, H. E. Essex, and E. J. Baldes: Surgery **4**, 249 (1938). — 6. Gupta, T. C., and C. J. Wiggers: Circulation **3**, 17 (1951). — 7. Cannon, J. A., E. L. Lobpreis, G. Herrold, and H. L. Frankenberg: Ann. Surg. **152**, 635 (1960). — 8. Haimovici, H.: Surgery **36**, 1075 (1954). — 9. Selkurt, E. E., P. Hall, and M. P. Spencer: Amer. J. Physiol. **159**, 369 (1949). — 10. Selkurt, E. E.: Circu-

lation **4**, 541 (1951). — 11. Eyler, W. R., M. D. Clark, J. E. Garman, R. L. Rian, and D. E. Meininger: Radiology **78**, 879 (1962). — 12. Holley, K. E., J. C. Hunt, A. L. Brown, Jr., O. W. Kincaid, and S. G. Sheps: Amer. J. Med. **37**, 14 (1964). — 13. Friedman, M., A. Selzer, and H. Rosenblum: J. Amer. Med. Ass. **117**, 92 (1941). — 14. Tobian, L.: Physiol. Rev. **40**, 280 (1960). — 15. Stamey, T. A., I. J. Nudelman, P. H. Good, F. N. Schwentker, and F. Hendricks: Medicine **40**, 347 (1961). — 16. Skinner, S. L., J. W. McCubbin, and I. H. Page: Science **141**, 814 (1963). — 17. Skinner, S. L., J. W. McCubbin, and I. H. Page: Circulation Res. **15**, 64 (1964). — 18. Skinner, S. L., J. W. McCubbin, and I. H. Page: Circulation Res. **15**, 522 (1964).

Discussion

Hood: I should like to make one comment on and ask two questions about Dr. Dustan's paper. Among a little more than 300 arteriographic lesions, about 200 cases were interpreted as having haemodynamic significance, either on the strength of complete occlusion or of elaborate separate kidney function studies. We were rather conservative from the outset, and of these 200 patients only about 60 have been operated upon. Of these 60, about 40 had some form of drug treatment afterwards. All the others have naturally been treated during these years. Our experience is the same as yours; there is very little to suggest that they present any special problem as regards treatment. But there remains the question of potential progression and/or sudden occlusion. We found that two cases, while on the waiting-list for the surgeon, developed a thrombosis of the kidney. We had two other cases who promptly went into oliguria, and the pre-arteriographic probability diagnosis was a small kidney with a total or nearly total obstruction and fresh thrombosis in the bigger and better kidney, which up till then had caused no trouble. In both cases this pre-arteriographic probability diagnosis was proven true. One patient was too bad to do anything about, so we did not perform arteriography; she died within 12—16 hours. The other one was operated upon directly after the arteriography; the bigger kidney was opened up, and a long thrombus removed. The patient promptly produced urine, achieving 2,000 ml. in 24 hours. Thus, there is this question of acute occlusion and complete loss of kidneys.

Now I should like to turn to my two questions. In proximal renal artery stenosis we have a statistically significant increase in plasma triglyceride levels. We have 24% who show definitely abnormal levels. Now we should like to normalise these levels, and in the majority of cases we are able to do so, either by diet or by the combination of diet and Atromid. We are going to study the rate of progression in these cases, much along the lines that you suggested. As the Cleveland Clinic has been interested in triglyceride and atherogenesis, I should like to ask whether you have done anything similar.

My second question: we have been using serum creatinine levels over a number of years in trying to estimate the progress of a lesion. The snag we have encountered here is that, using the Bonsness and Tausky method five years ago manually and using the machine now, all our kidney cases — with the exception of the very worst ones — actually appear to have improved. On this basis we could publish "improvement" in a variety of kidney disorders. Did you measure your serum creatinine in the 1959/60 patients manually? I presume you are using the machine now.

Dustan: As far as triglyceride levels, cholesterol, and lipids are concerned, Dr. Hood, I cannot give you any information in this group of patients, since I did not include such considerations in my analysis. I would, however, comment on the patient in this group who had no evidence of progression of renal arteriosclerosis. This man's serum cholesterol level had been kept, by diet, at approximately 200 mg./100 ml. over a period of about four years. Although he had not shown any evidence of change in his renal arterial lesion, coronary arterial disease had progressed considerably during that period. As far as serum creatinine levels are concerned, we have been using the Technicon for approximately five years. We were originally, however, rather concerned by the observation which you have cited, that there were some differences in the values obtained by the manual method as opposed to the Technicon method.

SMIRK: Dr. DUSTAN, you investigated patients in various age groups. Now, when you studied the renal function of the affected kidney, did you find that defects of function are more advanced in the older patients?

DUSTAN: I think they probably are. I have the impression that such patients tend to have more peripheral disease in the form of segmental atrophy than younger persons. This is not necessarily the case, because subadventitial fibroplasia is a severely stenosing lesion and can produce very large decreases in function on the affected side. I suppose, therefore that one cannot make a generalisation, but I have been impressed by the fact that some patients with atherosclerotic stenoses have more evident peripheral disease.

SMIRK: A second question is: when, with the passage of time, there is an increase in the degree of renal arterial stenosis, is there at the same time a greater difficulty in maintaining control of the blood pressure by drugs?

DUSTAN: It has not been our experience that an increase in stenosis has been reflected by an increased difficulty in controlling hypertension.

BROD: I should like to take up the statement made by Dr. DUSTAN about the possibility of controlling patients with renal artery stenosis very efficiently by conservative management. Actually we have operated upon 28 patients, to my knowledge, and only in 23% of the patients have we seen any real benefit from the operation. All the rest remained unaffected. This, in conjunction with the risk involved in the operation, leads us today to propose conservative management in the great majority of our patients with renal artery stenosis. I should like to ask Dr. DUSTAN whether she has seen any worsening of renal function in the stenosed kidney after bringing down the blood pressure by hypotensive agents.

I should also like to ask both Dr. DUSTAN and Dr. STAMEY, or anybody else in the audience, whether they have seen actually anybody dying in uraemia as a result of progression of the stenosis to a complete obstruction. And finally I should like to ask Dr. STAMEY how he would evaluate cases in which there is no stenosis of a single renal artery, but where the kidney is supplied by two or three vessels, each of which is relatively narrow in comparison with one single normal renal artery.

STAMEY: We have not had the opportunity to perform differential function studies on a hypertensive patient who has a seemingly normal, single renal artery on one side and multiple, small arteries feeding the contralateral kidney. I know of two patients, both children, in whom there is little doubt that removal of the kidney with multiple, small-appearing arteries alleviated a very serious hypertension. Function studies, however, were not done on these two patients. I assume that renal function studies, in this type of problem, would show at least a pattern of segmental stenosis; if all the arteries are sufficiently narrowed, the pattern should be identical to main renal artery occlusion. Dr. BROD has raised a good question here, because differential function studies represent the critical examination, since blood flow cannot be judged on the basis of aortography.

Dustan: Dr. Brod, we have not seen decreases in the renal function following control of hypertension. This is really very clear, even in people with single kidneys supplied by severely stenotic renal arteries or in people with severe bilateral stenoses. It is an interesting possibility, but we have not observed it.

Lee: I think that the juxtaposition of these two papers on the programme and especially Dr. Stamey's closing comments more than justify an attitude that has been developing recently in the New York area. We are backing off, very decidedly, in recommending surgery for many of these cases. The younger group with primarily fibrosing lesions do remarkably well postoperatively in the great majority of instances. But in almost an equal number of the older age group, where the lesion is primarily arteriosclerotic, we have one cure out of 16 patients and a few deaths. We are therefore reluctant to recommend a surgical procedure in which the cure rate is less than triumphant and where appropriate medical management may now be possible.

Genest: Dr. Dustan, I should like to express one reservation concerning the way one reports the average result of drug treatment, using only the blood-pressure readings during the last month of treatment in a patient followed for one to eight years under a given drug regimen. I wonder if you have any data comparing the mean results of blood-pressure response during the last month of drug treatment with those obtained during the entire period of drug administration?

Dustan: Yes, I have, Dr. Genest. For this analysis I averaged the blood pressures recorded during the last month of the first year and compared them with those obtained in the last month of the total period of evaluation. The pressures recorded during the last month of the first year tended to be a little higher than those at the end of the period of observation. I think this has been the usual experience in treating hypertension — either the drugs become more effective or, alternatively, the doctors know better how to treat elevated arterial pressure.

Stamey: I should like to comment on Dr. Lee's statement. I think we have learned too much in the past ten years to adopt a nihilistic attitude towards surgery for this disease. I suspect, Dr. Lee, that most of the 16 patients operated for atherosclerotic occlusions, in which there was only one cure, did not have positive differential function studies.

Lee: They did. These were done in all patients but one.

Stamey: These results, then, are a little discouraging, because there certainly are some patients, usually in the younger age group of 30—45 years, who have functionally significant atherosclerotic occlusions with good renal plasma flow to the contralateral kidney; these patients should show excellent results after surgery. Likewise, some of the older patients who develop malignant hypertension, superimposed on chronic hypertension, have had an excellent remission of their malignant phase following surgery for occlusive disease. I certainly agree with you that the best results have been obtained in patients who had unilateral, fibromuscular disease, but these patients, as I have tried to show today, have higher renal plasma flows to the contralateral kidney than any patients in our series. Thus, for the highly selected patient I believe surgery is the best therapy. The biggest mistake, however, has been to operate on stenoses that were of no functional significance to the kidney; our own mistake was to not recognise earlier the importance of small-vessel arteriosclerosis in the contralateral kidney and of its detection by pre-operative assessment of the renal plasma flow to that kidney.

LEE: The "split function" tests were carried out on about 100% of the subjects. And I should like to emphasise again that the arteriosclerotic patients were not the so-called "malignant" type and were decidedly in the older age group.

Hypertension and nephritis

By

C. Wilson

In the various types and stages of nephritis, hypertension occurs in a wide variety of circumstances, and it would be surprising if a single factor were responsible for the elevation of blood pressure in all these situations. In renal disease, variations in blood volume, electrolyte status, anaemia, acid-base balance, and myocardial efficiency vary widely and independently, and any of these may influence cardiac output or peripheral resistance, the two factors which determine the blood-pressure level.

It is perhaps not unreasonable to assume that in nephritis the disorder of physiological control of the blood pressure bears some relationship to that which leads to hypertension after renal artery constriction in the experimental animal. At any rate, an analysis of the humoral and haemodynamic factors in experimental hypertension provides an opportunity to examine these same factors in the more complex situation of nephritis in man.

On this basis, a useful starting point is the feed-back mechanism which appears to regulate volume control when renal artery perfusion pressure is reduced by reduction in blood volume on the one hand or by renal artery constriction on the other (Fig. 1).

While this seems to be an acceptable hypothesis for volume control, it is obvious that the pathological situation of renal artery constriction, by reducing perfusion pressure, provides a false signal for sodium and water retention. The crucial question is whether this signal produces an inappropriate response in volume control which may cause or contribute to the rise in blood pressure.

One method of approach is to examine the various hypertensive syndromes which are encountered in different stages of nephritis, in an attempt to discover whether associations can be found between changes in blood volume and blood pressure.

The most obvious of such situations is acute glomerulonephritis, where there is good evidence that plasma volume is acutely elevated, presumably owing to impaired ability of the kidney to eliminate sodium or water, or both. Hypervolaemia in acute nephritis has been demonstrated by direct measurement of plasma volume, and its variation with urine output is most clearly shown by following the change in haematocrit and plasma protein during removal of oedema when diuresis occurs. Hypertension in acute nephritis is usually only moderate in degree and in most cases is rapidly reversible, return to normal levels running closely parallel with the elimination of oedema.

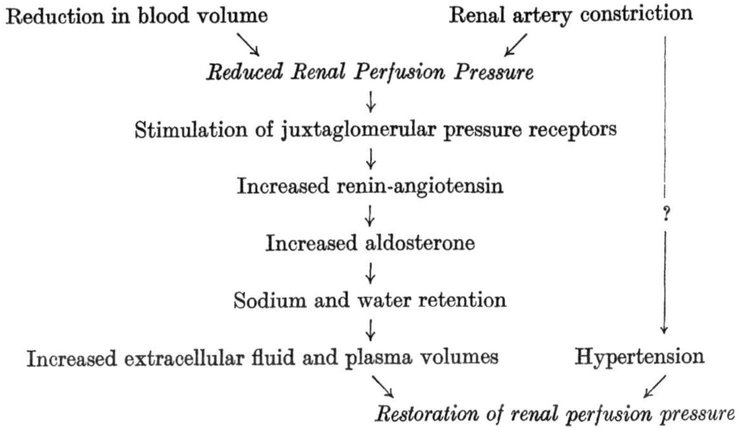

Fig. 1. Homoeostatic response to renal artery constriction.

The relationship of the hypervolaemia to hypertension is by no means uniform, but, in general, patients with a marked increase in venous pressure and pulmonary congestion have a severe degree of hypertension (Table 1). In such cases, DE FAZIO and his colleagues (1959) measured the cardiac output and found it significantly increased; the calculated peripheral resistance was, however, at or near normal levels. It appears therefore that in this common form of nephritic hypertension, elevation of blood pressure is, at any rate in some cases, associated with a high-output state due to hypervolaemia rather than to a primary increase in peripheral resistance, and that reversal of hypertension occurs when diuresis, spontaneous or induced, restores the blood volume to normal.

The most extreme situation of impaired sodium and water excretion in acute nephritis occurs with the development of anuria. The situation here, as regards plasma volume and hypertension, is often complicated by fluid depletion due to vomiting and reduced fluid intake and by the possible effects of uraemia on cardiac output. MERRILL and SCHUPAK (1964) have shown that correction of uraemia by dialysis may improve cardiac output, and this is often associated with a rise in blood pressure. Furthermore, in the anuric patient, a small increase in blood volume may cause a disproportionately large rise in blood pressure. In acute nephritis, and

Table 1. *Systemic and pulmonary congestion in acute nephritis*

Age	Raised jugular venous pressure	Dyspnoea	Pulmonary congestion	Blood urea mg. %	Blood pressure mm. Hg	Hypertensive encephalopathy
7	+	++	+	87	195/130	+
32	+	++	+	24	190/110	
28	+	++	+	51	170/110	
6	+	++	+	37	130/105	
4	+	+	+	40	?	
43	?	+	+	51	180/110	
43	+	++		21	190/120	
23	?	+	+	102	150/100	
42	?	++	?	54	210/105	+
25	+	+	+	111	150/90	
9	+	+	+	25	175/125	
13	+	+	+	57	160/80	
49	+	+	+	40	165/80	
15	+		+	172	165/90	
29	+	+	+	376	180/110	

certainly in those cases with anuria, oedema is usually slight in degree, and it is somewhat surprising that in the presence of increased venous pressure, and of some reduction of osmotic pressure of the plasma proteins, fluid is not more effectively transferred from the vascular to the extravascular compartment. These observations suggest that, whatever the origin, there is a failure of volume control which may be causing or contributing to the rise in blood pressure.

A further manifestation in acute nephritis is the occurrence of attacks of hypertensive encephalopathy, in which loss of vision, convulsions, and coma may be preceded by frontal headache and rising blood pressure. This complication has been studied by Byrom (1954) in rats with experimental renal hypertension, and there is unequivocal evidence that the attacks are accompanied by intense cerebral vasoconstriction. In the anuric patient, such attacks may be precipitated by overhydration and even by blood transfusion; moreover, the response of hypertensive encephalopathy to venesection may be very dramatic. These clinical and experimental observations suggest that the aggravation of hypertension and the regional cerebral vasoconstriction which accompany attacks of encephalopathy may result from expansion of blood volume.

Turning now to hypertension in chronic nephritis, long-term observation in these patients reveals a form of hypertension – sometimes continuing for many years – which in its clinical features resembles benign essential hypertension. At first, the high blood pressure may be only moderate and even intermittent (Fig. 2), and in this phase the hypertension may be very responsive to treatment with mild hypotensive drugs, such as reserpine. After a variable interval, however, a progressive rise in blood pressure occurs, often over a few months, and the hypertension becomes fixed at a high level. If effective hypotensive therapy is not promptly given, malignant hypertension may supervene. This hypertensive transformation is invariably associated with deterioration in renal function, and not infrequently with oedema and signs of systemic and pulmonary congestion, as in acute nephritis. Whilst heart failure is undoubtedly present in the late stages, some of the early congestive symptoms may well be attributable, again as in acute nephritis, to fluid retention and hypervolaemia, and correction of these may result in a reduction in blood pressure.

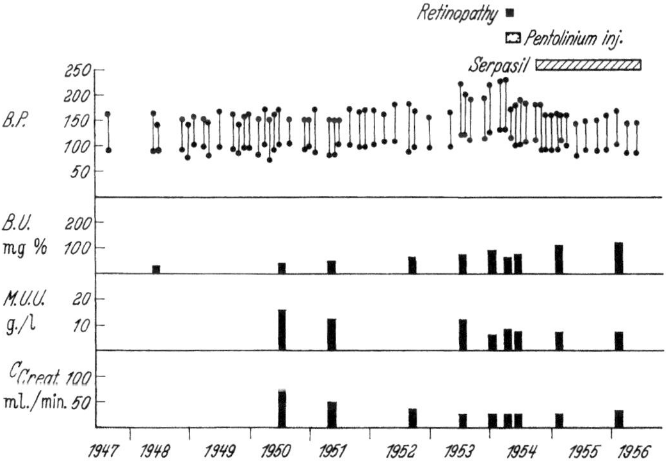

Fig. 2. Course of hypertension in a case of chronic nephritis. B.P.: Blood pressure; B.U.: Blood urea; M.U.U.: Maximum urine urea concentration; CCreat.: Creatinine clearance.

The reasons for the development of malignant hypertension are still obscure. Nevertheless, it seems probable that impairment of renal function is an important factor, since the incidence of malignant hypertension in patients with chronic nephritis is much higher than in those with essential hypertension (Table 2). Uraemia as such is obviously not necessary, since unilateral renal artery stenosis can lead to malignant hypertension, both in man and in the experimental animal, in the absence of nitrogen retention. Recent experience in the treatment of patients with renal failure and malignant hypertension by intermittent dialysis has shown that blood pressure can be restored to normal by fluid depletion, and it

Table 2. *Malignant hypertension in chronic glomerulonephritis and in essential hypertension*

	Total cases	Malignant hypertension	%
Chronic type I nephritis	78	36	48.7
Chronic type II nephritis ("membranous")	41	26	63.4
Essential hypertension (Kimmelstiel and Wilson, 1936)	250	10	4.0

appears probable (as Merrill has suggested) that reduction of the excess volume of water in the body compartments, rather than sodium depletion alone, is the important factor. Shaldon (1965), in treating malignant hypertension by intermittent dialysis, has recently produced evidence that, although both sodium and water must be depleted in order to lower the blood pressure, total exchangeable sodium may return to normal levels without return of hypertension.

The most problematic form of hypertension in chronic nephritis is the prolonged benign phase, during which renal function is apparently normal and there is no evidence of oedema or hypervolaemia. In this phase the high blood pressure clinically resembles benign essential hypertension. There is some evidence that in this form of hypertension, volume control is not normal. Hejl and his colleagues (1962) have shown that in hypertensive subjects, plasma expansion with dextran or saline causes a greater increase both in venous pressure and in cardiac output than in normotensive subjects, and this provides a possible explanation for the accelerated water and electrolyte diuresis in hypertensive subjects after plasma expansion. This abnormal response to plasma expansion implies either a failure of relaxation of venous tone in these circumstances or else a delayed transfer of fluid from the vascular to the extravascular compartment. In either case it is apparent that the equilibrium between plasma and interstitial fluid is disturbed.

This survey of volume-pressure relationships in acute and chronic nephritis suggests that disturbance of volume control may play a significant role in the production of hypertension, but the correlation is in many ways imperfect, and more definitive evidence is required. At the London Hospital, my colleagues LEDINGHAM and FLOYER have attempted to obtain such evidence, using the experimental model provided by renal artery constriction in the rat, and I should like to refer briefly to some of their observations. This model, in which one kidney is removed and the renal artery of the remaining kidney is clipped, provides a much less complicated situation than human renal artery stenosis, for in these patients, metabolic and haemodynamic changes may arise from the presence of the opposite kidney and the variable degrees of structural damage in the ischaemic kidney. These factors, I am sure, account for some of the discordant results obtained in different patients and by different observers.

In studying haemodynamic relationships in experimental hypertension one of the most important considerations is to separate clearly the developing phase of hypertension from the established phase, which is the usual clinical situation. The reason for this is that feed-back mechanisms, which are the essential basis of homoeostasis, by their nature lead to a restoration of, or at any rate an approximation to, the status quo. In the specific case of renal artery constriction in experimental animals, it is known that the resulting hypertension restores renal artery perfusion pressure to normal or near normal levels, and this will also apply to the other intermediate variables which may have played a significant role in the development of hypertension. For example, if increased plasma volume, or cardiac output, or renin production were involved in the elevation of the blood pressure after renal artery constriction, these factors would be expected to return to normal once the hypertension was established. Their participation in the establishment of the new level of equilibrium might then only be demonstrable while the hypertension was developing, or if the situation were suddenly changed, e.g. by removal of the renal artery constriction, or during a phase of sudden plasma expansion. In these situations, the sequence of events involved in the homoeostatic readjustment might be discovered.

LEDINGHAM and COHEN (1964) in our department have made a study of plasma volume and cardiac output following renal artery constriction in the rat. In order to study developing hypertension, cardiac output was measured in unanaesthetised rats by an electromagnetic flow-meter implanted round the ascending aorta. Extracellular fluid volume and plasma volume, which were measured over the same period, were found to increase following renal artery constriction. Cardiac-output studies showed a corresponding rise in cardiac output during the first five to ten days after renal artery constriction. From these observations it was concluded that when hypertension develops there is a greater and more prolonged rise in extracellular fluid and plasma volumes than in normotensive controls, and that this is associated with increased cardiac output. Other observations (LEDINGHAM, 1953) showed, however, that the extracellular fluid volume gradually returned to normal after about 40 days, although hypertension persisted at its previous level. This is consistent with the concept of an altered level of homoeostasis, in which renal artery perfusion pressure is restored, extracellular fluid volume and cardiac output return to normal, but arterial pressure and peripheral resistance are established at a new level. Any tendency of the blood pressure to fall will set in train the same sequence of events as that which led to the development of hypertension. An essential assumption in this hypothesis is that increase in cardiac output leads to peripheral myogenic arteriolar constriction due to autoregulation of peripheral blood flow. There is considerable evidence that myogenic constriction of arterioles occurs in response to increased arterial pressure, and indeed the observations of DE FAZIO and his colleagues (1959) in acute nephritis support the view that such a mechanism may be responsible for the hypertension in this condition. The above experimental model in the rat provides a parallel to the human situation in which acute nephritis fails to resolve and passes into the chronic phase with residual hypertension due to persistent structural renal damage.

Turning now to this chronic phase of renal hypertension, I have already referred to the abnormal response of venous pressure, cardiac output, and diuresis to plasma expansion in established hypertension in man. This phenomenon has been studied by FLOYER (1962) in the experimental model in the phase of chronic hypertension produced by renal artery constriction in the rat. Using the haematocrit as a measure of plasma volume, FLOYER (1962) observed that in hypertensive rats, following intravenous saline infusion, hypervolaemia persisted longer than in normotensive animals. This observation is consistent with the finding by HEJL and his colleagues (1962) of a more marked rise in venous pressure and cardiac output after plasma expansion in human hypertension than in normal human subjects. It also supports the concept of a disturbance of volume control in the hypertensive state, which prevents appropriate transfer of fluid from the plasma to the interstitial tissue. This impairment of fluid exchange between vascular and extravascular compartments could be due to altered properties of the capillary membrane or to changes in the extracellular fluid which offered a resistance to transfer of water from the plasma. Such an alteration in the properties of the extracellular fluid might well persist when the measurable extracellular fluid volume had returned to normal. Recently, FLOYER (1965), using the

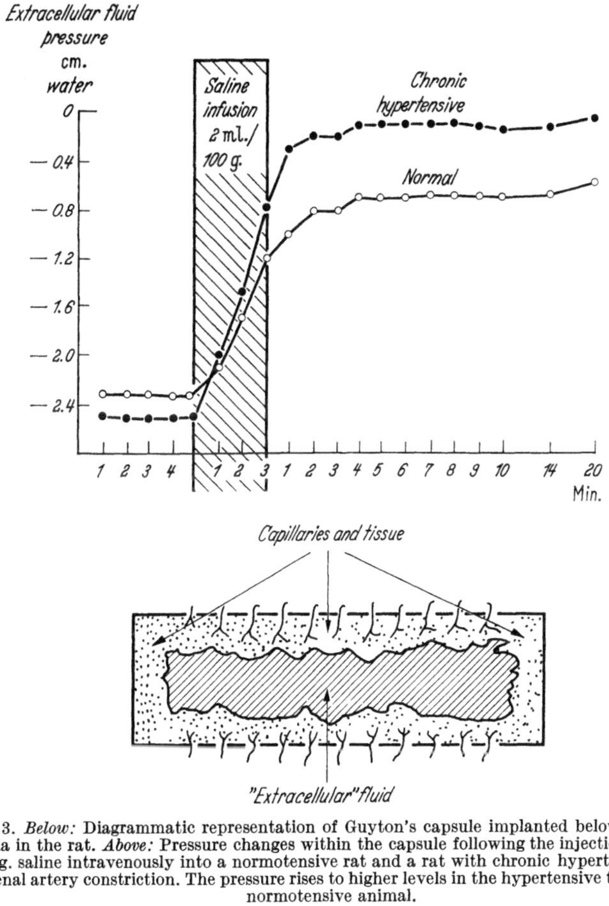

Fig. 3. *Below:* Diagrammatic representation of Guyton's capsule implanted below the deep fascia in the rat. *Above:* Pressure changes within the capsule following the injection of 2 ml./ 100 g. saline intravenously into a normotensive rat and a rat with chronic hypertension due to renal artery constriction. The pressure rises to higher levels in the hypertensive than in the normotensive animal.

implanted subcutaneous capsule introduced by GUYTON, attempted to measure extracellular fluid pressure changes following plasma expansion in the hypertensive rat (Fig. 3). Assuming that changes within the implanted capsule reflect changes in the extracellular fluid, his observations indicate that in the hypertensive animal a given expansion of extracellular fluid volume produces a greater increment in pressure than in the normotensive, and this might well provide an explanation for the slower correction of hypervolaemia in these circumstances. This reduced ability of the circulation to adapt to changes in the volume of its contents provides a possible explanation for many of the phenomena of hypertension in nephritis to which I have already referred. The occurrence of a similar abnormal response to plasma expansion in patients with essential hypertension may indicate the presence of a renal component leading to persistent diastolic hypertension in this condition.

In conclusion, I would suggest that in the altered homoeostatic situation of renal hypertension, restriction of fluid exchange between the vascular and extravascular compartments may lead to a disturbance of volume control which could contribute to the maintenance of hypertension by way of increase in cardiac output and increased arteriolar resistance imposed by autoregulation of the peripheral blood flow.

These are preliminary observations, based on somewhat sparse data. The analysis of homoeostatic readjustments in arterial hypertension is highly complex, and we are groping for new techniques, in the hope that these may enable us to understand what we are treating.

Summary

Stimulation of renin and aldosterone secretion results from reduced renal perfusion pressure and provides an effective feed-back mechanism for volume control. The crucial question is the relationship of this homoeostatic response to the hypertension which follows renal artery constriction. Plasma volume and extracellular fluid volume increase promptly after renal artery constriction, and this might initiate hypertension through augmented cardiac output. In this communication the author discusses the relationship between hypertension and changes in blood volume in glomerulonephritis, with special reference to acute nephritis and malignant hypertension. Evidence is presented which suggests that in renal hypertension the exchange of fluid between the vascular and extravascular compartments may be disturbed, so that adaptation of the circulation to plasma-volume expansion is impaired. This may lead to a disturbance of volume control and to persistent elevation of blood pressure by way of increased cardiac output and autoregulation of the peripheral resistance.

Zusammenfassung

Anregung der Renin- und Aldosteronsekretion als Folge eines verminderten Nierenperfusionsdruckes stellt einen wirksamen Rückkoppelungsmechanismus für die Volumenkontrolle dar. Die entscheidende Frage ist, welche Beziehung zwischen dieser homöostatischen Reaktion und dem Hochdruck besteht, der auf eine Konstriktion der Nierenarterie folgt. Das Plasmavolumen und das extrazelluläre Flüssigkeitsvolumen nehmen nach Nierenarteriendrosselung rasch zu, und auf diese Weise könnte der Hochdruck durch ein erhöhtes Herzminutenvolumen ausgelöst werden. In der vorliegenden Mitteilung wird die Beziehung zwischen Hochdruck und Änderungen im Blutvolumen bei Glomerulonephritis besprochen, unter besonderer Berücksichtigung der akuten Nephritis und des malignen Hochdruckes. Es werden Befunde vorgelegt, die vermuten lassen, daß beim renalen Hochdruck der Austausch von Flüssigkeit zwischen den intra- und extravasalen Räumen gestört sein kann, so daß die Anpassung des Kreislaufes an eine Plasmavolumenzunahme verschlechtert ist. Auf dem Wege über ein erhöhtes Herzminutenvolumen und eine Autoregulation des peripheren Widerstandes kann dadurch eine Störung der Volumenkontrolle und ein anhaltender Anstieg des Blutdruckes auftreten.

Résumé

La réduction de la pression de perfusion du parenchyme rénal provoque une stimulation de la sécrétion de rénine et d'aldostérone qui représente un efficace mécanisme de "feed-back" pour la régulation du volume. La question clé est la relation entre cette réponse homéostasique et l'hypertension consécutive à une constriction de l'artère rénale. Le volume du liquide extracellulaire et du plasma augmente rapidement après constriction d'une artère rénale, et ceci pourrait déclencher une hypertension par augmentation du débit cardiaque. Dans cette communication, l'auteur discute les relations existant entre l'hypertension et les modifications du volume sanguin dans la glomérulonéphrite, en particulier en ce qui concerne la néphrite aiguë et l'hypertension maligne. Des arguments sont présentés suggérant que dans l'hypertension rénale les échanges de liquide entre les compartiments vasculaire et extravasculaire peuvent être troublés, de sorte que l'adaptation de la circulation à l'expansion du volume plasmatique est perturbée. Ceci peut conduire à des troubles de la régulation du volume et à une élévation persistante de la pression artérielle par augmentation du débit cardiaque et autorégulation de la résistance périphérique.

References

Byrom, F. B.: Lancet 1954/II, 201. — De Fazio, V., R. C. Christensen, T. J. Regan, L. J. Baer, Y. Morita, and H. K. Hellems: Circulation **20**, 190 (1959). — Floyer, M. A.: Communication to Med. Res. Soc. London, November 1962. — Floyer, M. A.: International Club on Arterial Hypertension, First Meeting, Paris, July 1965. — Hejl, Z., J. Hofman, and M. Ulrych: Lancet 1962/I, 515. — Kimmelstiel, P., and C. Wilson: Amer. J. Path. **12**, 45 (1936). — Ledingham, J. M.: Clin. Sc. **12**, 337 (1953). — Ledingham, J. M., and R. D. Cohen: Canad. Med. Ass. J. **90**, 292 (1964). — Merrill, J. P., and E. Schupak: Canad. Med. Ass. J. **90**, 328 (1964). — Shaldon, S.: Reported at meeting of Association of Physicians. London, May 1965.

Introduction to the General Discussion

By

F. C. Reubi

This morning's session was devoted to renovascular and other forms of renal hypertension. In introducing the general discussion, I should like to comment briefly on two very important topics: renal artery stenosis and nephritic hypertension.

Renal artery stenosis raises two interesting problems. The first is related to the pathogenesis of hypertension and concerns the possible role of the renin-angiotensin system. Undoubtedly, the hypothesis presented by Dr. Genest is extremely attractive. It seems, however, that many of us are not entirely convinced that in this condition the blood pressure rises as a consequence of increased blood levels of renin. Whereas Dr. Genest's data seem to support his hypothesis, some other facts are rather difficult to explain on this basis. I should like to quote only one example. In 1962, Bartter and his associates (*1*) described two cases of severe hypokalaemia due to hyperkaliuria. In both cases a marked hyperplasia of the juxtaglomerular apparatus was found, but the granularity of the J.G. cells was not significantly increased. These patients had elevated blood levels of renin, angiotensin, and aldosterone, but their blood pressure was normal. We have recently observed a similar case with some hyperplasia of the J.G. apparatus, very few granules in the J.G. cells, increased renin and aldosterone levels in the blood, marked hypokalaemia, and a perfectly normal blood pressure. It seems difficult to accept Bartter's view that hypertension is absent just because the vessels of these patients do not respond to angiotensin. Perhaps the aldosterone-stimulating factor is not angiotensin. This would mean that the J.G. apparatus forms substances other than renin and that the exact meaning of the J.G. granules is still unknown.

The second problem is a clinical one. Is it possible to prove in a given case that renal artery stenosis, as demonstrated by angiography, is responsible for the observed hypertension? Is it possible to predict when surgery will bring down the blood pressure? Which test is entirely reliable?

A large number of tests has been developed in an attempt to answer our first question. On the whole, the results have been rather disappointing. The best evidence would be the demonstration of a pressor substance in the renal venous blood draining from the affected kidney. In the case of a unilateral stenosis, the production of any pressor substance may be actually reduced on the other side, owing to a feed-back mechanism. This means that the pressor activity of the mixed peripheral blood may remain uncharacteristic. We feel, therefore, that any attempt to demonstrate increased pressor activity in the blood should involve bilateral catheterisation of the renal veins. The comparison of the relative activity of the two renal venous samples might disclose a marked disparity. Such a finding would strongly suggest that a renal pressor mechanism is operating on the side of the highest activity. Instead of estimating renin and/or angiotensin, it might be easier to measure the pressor response of the anaesthetised, nephrectomised rat to the injection of the unpurified plasma samples. This technique has recently been recommended by GROLLMAN and his associates (*2*).

Dr. STAMEY's paper makes it clear that surgery will not bring down the blood pressure if the functions of the contralateral kidney are markedly reduced. The P.A.H. clearance of the separate kidneys seems to be an extremely suitable method of predicting whether the operation will be successful or not. From our personal experience, we can only confirm Dr. STAMEY's statement.

Concerning the other forms of renal hypertension, I should like to limit my comment to the volume-control hypothesis presented by Dr. WILSON.

That, in acute glomerulonephritis, hypertension is merely due to water and salt retention is an attractive hypothesis. Renal ischaemia seldom occurs in these cases, and increased plasma renin or angiotensin levels have never been demonstrated. In a majority of patients salt restriction alone brings down the blood pressure within a few days, while oedema disappears. Not all the observed facts, however, can be explained on this basis. The slow heart rate of acute nephritis makes it very different from hypervolaemic cardiac failure. In spite of an increased plasma volume, cardiac output is often normal in acute hypertensive nephritis; this points to a peripheral vasoconstriction. On the other hand, patients with the nephrotic syndrome may have at the same time a perfectly normal blood pressure and a heavy salt and water retention. Admittedly, they have, as a rule, a decreased plasma volume, owing to the shift of fluid into the extravascular space, and this might account for this difference. — But there is still another condition with fluid and salt retention and without diastolic hypertension: in most cases of acute renal failure of any origin, with or without manifest over-hydration, there is a marked increase in stroke volume, heart rate, and cardiac output. The systolic blood pressure may be somewhat elevated, while the diastolic values are low, the mean blood pressure being within the normal range only to diminish in the terminal stage.

In chronic nephritis the blood-pressure elevation, when it exists, is largely due to peripheral vasoconstriction, as long as the glomerular filtration rate is not too severely impaired. There is little to indicate that in these cases salt and water retention plays any part in this phenomenon. The question arises whether the peripheral vasoconstriction is not simply due to the release of renin or of another pressor substance by the kidney. This release might be elicited by renal ischaemia or tissue damage.

There is little doubt that, in the terminal stage of chronic renal disease, salt and fluid restriction or long-term treatment with the artificial kidney may reduce the blood pressure. It is not clear, however, whether the reduction is due merely to sodium or to water loss. An over-all group correlation with the exchangeable sodium and with the body weight exists, but does not hold true for every individual case. It has also been suggested that an unknown pressor substance might be removed from the blood by repeated haemodialyses. Anyway, it should be stressed that the lowering of the blood pressure upon salt deprivation does not mean that hypertension is due to salt retention. It would be equally unjustified to claim that essential hypertension is largely due to sympathetic over-activity just because most cases respond well to α-methyldopa or guanethidine. As in almost every type of high blood pressure, we feel that, in nephritic hypertension, salt and water are only one factor, and that, depending on the conditions studied, this factor may be more or less important.

I hope there will be some more comments on this subject.

References

1. BARTTER, F. C., P. PRONOVE, J. R. GILL, and R. C. MCCARDLE: Amer. J. Med. **33**, 811 (1962). — 2. MCPHAUL, J. J., D. A. MCINTOSH, L. F. WILLIAMS, E. J. GRITTI, W. G. MALETTE, and A. GROLLMAN: Arch. Int. Med. **115**, 644 (1965).

General Discussion

WILSON: The heart rate is not always slow in acute nephritis; it may be rapid. I do not think there is any consistent change in the heart rate in acute nephritis.

REUBI: If there is cardiac failure, it is fast, if there is no cardiac failure . . .

WILSON: I think the occurrence of heart failure in acute nephritis is a very controversial issue. There is congestion — systemic and pulmonary — which may be attributable to hypervolaemia. I agree that renal hypertension is not necessarily due to sodium and water retention. After all, one can anastomose the ureter with the inferior vena cava in the rat (after removing the opposite kidney), and renal artery constriction still causes hypertension. What I was suggesting was that there may be some abnormality in fluid exchange between the vascular and the extravascular compartments, in the hypertensive state.

BROD: Following the Prague Symposium on Hypertension and some comments made by Dr. HOOD, my colleagues HEJL, PRÁT, and DEJDAR[1], and HORNYCH and I have become interested in the problem of renal artery stenosis. At that time we didn't want to believe that the frequency of renal artery stenosis might be high. We have subsequently studied 354 unselected patients with hypertension (today we have over 500) who had been aortographed and have found that renal artery stenosis can be encountered even in patients with normal blood pressure; it is somewhat more frequent in patients who have a labile hypertension (Stage I), and much more frequent in patients with fixed hypertension (Stages II and III). However, if we break down these groups according to age, we find that in the normotensive group severe renal artery stenosis is encountered only after the age of 60, i.e. in the seventh decade of life. The same is more or less true of labile hypertensives. On the other hand, in patients with fixed hypertension, renal artery stenosis can be encountered in any decade. We therefore believe that it is in Stages II and III of hypertension that one should really think of renal artery stenosis. This, of course, brings us back to the problem whether renal artery stenosis is the cause or the consequence of hypertension. If it is true that Stages II and III develop from Stage I, then one would really expect — if renal artery stenosis is the cause of hypertension — to find it already in Stage I; but one doesn't.

In screening for patients with renal artery stenosis, it is obviously necessary to consider every patient with Stage II and Stage III hypertension; but as we cannot aortograph every patient in this large group, we should have some means of deciding where we really should aortograph. The radioisotope renogram can be useful in this connection[2]. Where it is normal, renal

---

[1] HEJL, Z., V. PRÁT, and R. DEJDAR: Proc. 2nd Internat. Congress of Nephrology, Prague, August 1963. Excerpta Medica Foundation, Amsterdam, 1964. International Congress Series No. 78.

[2] HORNYCH, A., B. VAVREJN, A. OPPELT, V. PRÁT, Z. HEJL, R. DEJDAR, E. KOTKOVÁ, and P. CHARVÁT: in press.

artery stenosis is unlikely to be present. In the whole group of normal renograms we have found only two patients with a renal artery stenosis. On the other hand, where there is some abnormality in the radio-isotope renogram, renal artery stenosis is encountered relatively frequently. Of course, there are false positives, but this doesn't matter. Thus, Stage II and III hypertensives with abnormal isotope renograms are an indication for aortography.

Finally, I should like to ask Dr. WILSON what he thinks about hypertension in patients who have had acute glomerulonephritis or pyelonephritis, in whom hypertension persists for years after the disease has burnt out and is the main pathological feature, the renal functions now being practically normal and the family history negative. How would he classify this hypertension and how would he explain it?

WILSON: I did refer to this similarity between the benign type of renal hypertension and benign essential hypertension. I suggested that both forms might be related to a disturbance in the exchange of fluid between vascular and extravascular compartments. The accelerated diuresis following plasma loading indicates that there is in fact an abnormality there that we have to explain.

HOOD: I have a question to put to Dr. WILSON. To get an idea of the very earliest steps in the relationship between fluid gain and hypertension in acute nephritis, and prompted by some findings in a new experimental model of acute nephritis, I should like to ask you whether you yourself have ever observed a case from, let's say, the onset of a streptococcal angina to the development of the clinical features and made observations on blood pressure and weight — in other words, before the onset of the clinical features of acute nephritis?

Secondly, I should like to make a comment on Dr. REUBI's remarks. It would be nice to have a test that could be picked up in the renal vein. We have adopted the Helmer method, but we have used another bio-assay with simultaneous duplicate tests in two separate chambers with the rat uterus. We have so selected the volume of plasma introduced simultaneously into these two chambers that it will not cause a twitch in either of the two uteri in any single normal human or in any single patient with kidney disease unaccompanied by hypertension. The test is considered to be positive if the two uteri twitch at the same time. The test sample is sandwiched between standard doses of angiotensin and samples of normal plasma. This is repeated on three frozen plasma samples, on at least three to eight occasions. With this type of technique we would get a 40% positive response in renovascular hypertension and no positive response in chronic pyelonephritis. When we performed the test in 23 patients and attempted to do a bilateral renal venous catheterisation, the very small flows in some of these renal artery stenoses naturally caused us some difficulty. Thus, we could only obtain bilateral samples in eight cases, and there was no side difference between any of those; there was no difference between the renal veins or the femoral arteries. We tried to strengthen our test by giving an acute infusion of hexamethonium, bringing the blood pressure down and repeating the sampling after 90 minutes, but even then we could find no difference in the response.

WILSON: I have seen one case in which oedema and hypertension developed after streptococcal infection without albuminuria. Renal biopsy was carried out, but unfortunately failed. However, other workers have reported the development of hypertension and oedema without albuminuria in cases in which renal biopsy showed no, or very slight, changes. I think this supports the hypothesis of hypervolaemic hypertension.

HARTMANN: I should like to ask Dr. WILSON whether he has any information about mild glomerulonephritis and labile hypertension. The reason for my question is that we compared a group of 162 young people suffering from labile hypertension with another group of 105 young people; the average age in both groups was 24 years. In the hypertensive group, we found that 57% had an antistreptolysin titre above 400 units. This figure is very similar to those found in chronic glomerulonephritis and chronic rheumatic fever. If there is any connection between a mild glomerulonephritis, possibly indicated by this high titre of antistreptolysin, and the labile hypertension, the question arises whether one should in the future give penicillin prophylaxis to this group of juvenile patients with so-called essential hypertension.

WILSON: You must find some evidence to make the diagnosis of acute nephritis, e.g. the presence of hypervolaemia or abnormalities in the urine deposit or on renal biopsy.

TCHERDAKOFF: Most of the ways of selecting patients, as far as diagnosis and prognosis of renal artery disease are concerned, have been mentioned this morning, but I do not believe that anyone has yet mentioned the results of the angiotensin infusion test as described by KAPLAN and SILAH[1]. We have performed such a test in a few patients, and I must say we have been rather disappointed; first, because we found no parallel between the results of the test and the plasma renin content, and, secondly, because there were discrepancies between the results of the test and the results of surgery. I should be very much interested to know whether other groups have had similar experience.

SMIRK: I should like to comment on a statement by Dr. REUBI, namely that the decrease in blood pressure brought about by drugs such as hexamethonium is not to be regarded as proof that a nervous mechanism is responsible for the hypertension. I agree, because it is also possible that there is an increase in the reactivity of the blood vessels to a normal amount of nervous stimulation. We are not committing ourselves to either view, but have had experience of the very great difficulty in distinguishing between these two. For this reason we have used the expression "neurogenically maintained"[2], which does not commit the person who uses the expression either to the opinion that nervous stimulation of blood vessels is increased or to the view that the effect is due solely to enhanced vascular reactivity to nervous stimulation. But sensing Dr. REUBI's interest in this, may I ask whether he agrees or has some other explanation?

With regard to what was said by Dr. BROD, I should like to mention briefly that we found the basal blood pressure formed a higher proportion of the casual blood pressure in people with frank renal hypertension as contrasted with essential hypertension.

GENEST: Has anyone any comments concerning the question raised by Dr. TCHERDAKOFF about the angiotensin infusion test?

DOLLERY: Dr. BRECKENRIDGE[3] in our group has carried out the angiotensin infusion test in 50 hypertensives. He found that it was repeatable and

[1] KAPLAN, N. M., and J. G. SILAH: N. England J. Med. **271**, 536 (1964).
[2] DOYLE, A. E., and F. H. SMIRK: Circulation **12**, 543 (1955).
[3] BRECKENRIDGE, A.: Lancet **1965/II**, 209.

little affected by treatment with sympathetic blocking drugs. However, using KAPLAN's criteria he obtained both false positive and false negative results. The sensitivity to angiotensin appeared to be randomly distributed amongst hypertensions of various aetiologies. The test doesn't seem to be helpful.

GENEST: I think it should be pointed out that the state of sodium balance is most important in assessing the response to the angiotensin infusion, as was shown by our former collaborator, Dr. VEYRAT[1]. In carrying out this test, one should take care to determine the sodium intake in order to assess correctly the blood-pressure response to angiotensin.

STAMEY: There is a practical application for the KAPLAN infusion test. Dr. WAX, in Dr. D. McDONALD's unit at Rochester[2], has shown that if angiotensin is infused during the course of a radio-active hippuran-I^{131} renogram, the diagnostic characteristic of the ischaemic kidney — the prolonged $T^1/_2$ of the excretory phase — is enhanced. The excretory or third phase of the renogram curve is dependent primarily on urine flow rate (at least at reasonable levels of R.P.F.); angiotensin is the only agent I know that can increase the differences between the two kidneys in urine flow rate in the absence of an osmotic diuresis. Urea also increases the flow-rate differences, but the osmotic increase in urine flow rate from the ischaemic kidney washes out the accumulated radio-activity in the pelvis and calyces of the ischaemic kidney, thereby blunting the differences in the excretory phase of the renogram. For this reason, the observation made by WAX and McDONALD that angiotensin increases the difference in the renogram between the ischaemic kidney and the contralateral kidney is an important contribution to the use of the renogram as a screening procedure for hypertensive patients. Those who like to use the KAPLAN test may find it practical to combine this test with the I^{131} renogram.

KIRKENDALL: We have had experience with the angiotensin infusion test and have been disappointed as to its usefulness. We studied normal subjects, patients with essential hypertension, and ones with renal artery stenosis, using the procedure suggested by KAPLAN and his group. One difference has been that we have recorded intra-arterial pressures during the studies. We found that, although the normal subjects required slightly more angiotensin than hypertensives to raise diastolic blood pressure by 20 mm. Hg, almost exactly the same amount, on the average, was used to achieve the same elevation in the patients with essential hypertension and those with renal artery stenosis. We were also unable to find a correlation between the amount of angiotensin needed to elevate the blood pressure and renin levels in nine persons. We did find that one patient with primary aldosteronism required small amounts of angiotensin to raise diastolic blood pressure by the standard amount. We have concluded that the angiotensin infusion test is of no value to us in predicting renin levels — except possibly in patients with primary aldosteronism — or the presence of significant renal artery stenosis.

PEART: As to the question of sensitivity which has been raised by this discussion around the KAPLAN and SILAH paper, I should just like to say that there is one very good study, and I think only one, in which a proper assessment of what was meant pharmacologically by sensitivity has been

---

[1] VEYRAT, R.: Canad. Med. Ass. J. **90**, 215 (1964).

[2] WAX, S., and D. McDONALD: Surg. Forum **15**, 498 (1964).

reported. This paper was published in Australia by JOHNSTON and JOSE[1]. Dose-response curves have been drawn up and, confirming what Dr. GENEST said, the patients whose curves show very distinct alterations are those in whom the sodium balance is altered, particularly, for example, the cirrhotics with ascites that LARAGH et al.[2] first asserted to be less sensitive to angiotensin. Now, in many other cases, this alleged lack of sensitivity has been "demonstrated" by giving either an infusion or a dose at one time and then finding that the rise in pressure obtained at another time is different. This method is in fact invalid; it cannot be applied in the rat, the cat, or the rabbit, nor can it be used in man, because the principle of a pharmacological assay obtains in man, just as much as in any other animal. I think you could predict that this test was going to be misleading, just from reading the paper, and I have not been surprised to find that many who have used it have found a similar lack of correlation in anything that has been measured.

ZAIMIS: The term "increased or decreased sensitivity" covers many different mechanisms, such as the rate of excitation of the smooth muscle, the rate of contraction of the contractile elements, the rate of recovery of the cell membrane potentials, or the rate of the relaxation of the contractile elements. Therefore, only through a better understanding of the kinetics of smooth muscle contraction—of which we know very little at present— shall we be able to see in the proper perspective the changes which are today referred to under the general label of "sensitivity".

Mammalian smooth muscle, when stimulated electrically or by drugs, contracts and remains contracted as long as the stimulus lasts. However, BORN[3] produced evidence suggesting that the development of tension by smooth muscle involves two mechanisms. One is responsible for the immediate rise in tension which occurs when the muscle is stimulated, and this mechanism continues to function in anoxia and in the presence of 2,4-dinitrophenol. The second mechanism is responsible for the sustained tension which the muscle shows both spontaneously and following stimulation, and this mechanism is abolished when metabolism is interfered with. For example, in the absence of glucose or of oxygen the smooth muscle contracts, but its ability to sustain the increased tension is reduced or completely abolished. In our department, we have been able to demonstrate that certain hypotensive drugs are also able to interfere with the ability of the smooth muscle to sustain contraction. These observations are, to my mind, significant, because they may lead us not only to a better understanding of the mode of action of certain hypotensive drugs, but also to some understanding of the changes occurring in the arterial smooth muscle in hypertensive patients.

---

[1] JOHNSTON, C. I., and A. D. JOSE: J. Clin. Invest. **42**, 1411 (1963).

[2] LARAGH, J. H., P. J. CANNON, and R. P. AMES: In: Aldosterone. A Symposium. Ed. by E. E. BAULIEU and P. ROBEL. Blackwell Scientific Publications, Oxford, 1964, p. 427.

[3] BORN, G. V.: J. Physiol. **131**, 704 (1956).

Drug treatment of hypertension

Public lecture

By

I. H. PAGE

It is hard to believe that when several of us who are here began work on hypertension, there was no treatment for it worthy of the name. True, we had many suggested remedies, such as extract of watermelon and cucumber seeds, mistletoe and garlic; and one enterprising business man sold "whiffless garlic". Red meat and too much sex were forbidden! No one really believed in the low-salt diet. About 1928, potassium thiocyanate began to be used by a few, but it caused many toxic manifestations and was more effective against headaches than as a means of lowering arterial pressure.

I wonder if you recall some of the regimens that were recommended confidently in the early thirties? Treatment was, of course, supposed to be based on etiology, and the causes were "worry, fear, lead, rheumatic and other infections". Treatment consisted of psychotherapy, careful regulation of the mode of life, well-balanced diet, baths not below 34 degrees, ovarian gland preparations, iodides, and "the bowels to be kept free". Clearly no one at the time was in favor of sin.

You have probably forgotten that at that time a majority of physicians believed that lowering blood pressure would result in reduced renal blood flow and eventual uremia. It was the old Cohnheim theory that hypertension was a compensatory phenomenon, and hence elevated blood pressure was necessary to force blood through the narrowed blood vessels.

When I started to work on hypertension with Dr. D. D. VAN SLYKE at the Rockefeller Institute in 1931, one of the first problems I explored was the relationship between urea clearance and the height of the blood pressure. VAN SLYKE had shown a rough relationship between clearance and renal blood flow. Indeed, it was the only clinically applicable method at the time for gaining some notion of renal blood flow. I shudder to think of the method I used to lower the patient's blood pressure: it was intramuscular colloidal sulfur! That was the day when all manner of substances were being put into colloidal solution and used in treatment. Colloidal silver or Argyrol was the most successful by far, and this found its place usually among college men and soldiers following indiscretions. But colloidal sulfur did lower blood pressure temporarily and, to my surprise, did not lower urea clearance or, presumably, renal blood flow. This at least gave me heart that research into the field of anti-hypertensive agents had some merit.

The past 35 years have, in a sense, been the golden age of research in hypertension. You are all fully conversant with the great advances in the experimental parts, because you have contributed so much to them. But, as you also know, it has been the great period of search for adequate methods of reducing elevated blood pressure to normal or near normal levels.

We still have some way to go in persuading some physicians and the public that adequate treatment is time-consuming and exacting. We need a little more perfectionism, even when the perfectionist is defined as one who takes infinite pains and often gives them to others. Unfortunately also, there are still many highly questionable remedies being sold to the public. Remember that the great Sir CLIFFORD ALLBUTT firmly believed in d'Arsonvalization as a valuable remedy. The modern version is washing the blood with electrons.

Serious attempts to lower blood pressure with drugs began just a little after sympathectomy was introduced. The story of that stormy period when the surgeons made their first foray into our then placid field is a most interesting one, but that must be reserved for another day.

One of the first drugs to receive widespread attention was rutin. It was recommended to cure increased capillary fragility, and consequently it was soon being combined with vitamin C for treatment of diabetic retinitis, the fragility said to occur with potassium thiocyanate, and for the prevention of cerebral hemorrhage. It was "the drug of the year". Fortunately for most of us, we used it before it lost its remedial powers!

Largely due to the efforts of FREDERICK ALLEN, low-salt diets had some limited vogue. ALLEN did not present sufficiently convincing evidence to persuade most people of the merits of so tasteless a diet. GEORGE PICKERING has a lovely quotation apropos of low-salt diets. The King in *Alice Through the Looking Glass* says, "There is nothing like eating hay when you're faint. . . . I didn't say there was nothing better. I just said there is nothing like it."

But this was not the end of it. A strong trend developed for strict low-salt diets which erupted into the Kempner rice-diet. The rice-diet had a certain aura and allure to it. It was recommended with almost religious fervor. You had to start by believing! Then the quaint idea of a "rice house" sounded just sufficiently wicked to be attractive. Lastly, there were certain social rewards. We had a patient in Washington who created quite a stir by arriving at a diplomatic dinner party with her bag of rice. Unsalted rice and fruit juice was a form of medical mayhem. There is no doubt that as a low-salt, low-cholesterol, low-caloric diet it had merit, but not enough to have it adopted as a way of life in the society of abundance that we now live in. More and more it has come to be the feeling that the Chinese can have it!

I think you can see that with the passage of time and much research, some of the fundamental groundwork was, perhaps unconsciously, being laid for more successful treatment. Certainly, the early attempts to be rid of excessive sympathetic activity by surgical means foreshadowed later developments with guanethidine and the like. And low-salt diets focused attention on the need for control of sodium in treatment of hypertension.

As I look back, I think the most important contribution made by surgical sympathectomy was the reversal of malignant hypertension. In 1931 I made a clinical study of this syndrome. It did not take me long to realize how quickly fatal it was. Consequently, when Dr. G. HEUER began doing anterior nerve root sections for me, I referred patients with malignant hypertension to him on the theory that we had much to gain, perhaps, but certainly nothing to lose. To my astonishment, within days after operation I saw the eyegrounds clear, reversal of the inverted T waves, and shrinkage in the size of the heart. I believe this was the first time reversal had been seen. From 1932 on I was converted to the idea that lowering blood pressure was a desirable thing. Several years later we were able, with kidney extracts, to reverse malignant hypertension, but the repeated intramuscular injections were very painful. We did not find the mechanism by which the extracts worked, but that there was a degree of success cannot be doubted by those who had experience at the time.

The ganglion blocking agents, beginning with tetraethylammonium chloride, were the next step, and, as you recall, the blockade was for both sympathetic and parasympathetic impulses. The clinical result was usually a severe fall in pressure, especially an orthostatic one. But the side effects, chiefly a result of parasympathetic blockade, were often fearful to behold and even worse to experience. These, I am sure, I need not detail for you, because they are too recent in most of our minds and too vivid as well; they will not be forgotten. Again emphasis was placed on the importance of the neural component of hypertension.

I have spoken of hypertension almost as though all of it had the same mechanism. We have known for a long time this is not true, but still we had very few methods for differentiating one from the other. The hypertension of pheochromocytoma and that associated with adrenal cortical disease called attention to an endocrine hypertension, and SELYE found an experimental counterpart by giving desoxycorticosterone acetate to salt-treated rats. The neural component was highlighted in the hypertension resulting from cutting the buffer nerves, and, finally, the renal facet took on its true importance with GOLDBLATT's demonstration of hypertension produced by a clamp on the renal artery. It had been known since the time of RICHARD BRIGHT that hypertension is often associated with disease of the kidneys. So it has become increasingly clear that clinical hypertension is a great mix of diseases with differing mechanisms. But this need not necessarily worry us. Since most, if not all, of the mechanisms involved in the production of the varied types of hypertension are normally functional, it means that there are many ways to approach the problem of bringing the pressure to normal. For example, even though there is good evidence that there is a renal component in hypertension produced either by a clamp on the renal artery or by enclosing the parenchyma in cellophane, still elevated arterial pressure can be greatly lowered by drugs blocking sympathetic nerve transmission.

This brings me to a point that, I suppose, still needs discussion, because everyone is not agreed that blood pressure should be lowered to normal. After it had been made clear that tissue perfusion was not reduced when arterial pressure declined to normal, there seemed to be no contraindication to hypotensive agents. It had also been shown that reduction in pressure was associated with reversal of the signs of malignant hypertension, and that in some cases of heart failure, reduction in pressure quickly abolished the decompensation. Then there was long-term evidence that in some patients the progressive downward course of renal excretory efficiency was slowed or halted. And, finally, for the first time the insurance statistics in the United States show a fall in deaths from hypertension. I agree that none of this evidence is conclusive in proving the value of antihypertensive agents but, combined with what we know of hemodynamic effects on the heart and blood vessels, I find it hard to believe that we are not on the right track. It is, like smoking and lung cancer, unproved, but certainly there is enough smoke to suggest fire.

Does blood pressure in the prone position need to be reduced to fully normal levels? A few years ago I should have said no, if only because the drugs then available made this achievement virtually impossible. But now this argument is usually no longer valid; hence I believe that every effort should be made to come as close to a normal prone arterial pressure level as possible. I say this chiefly because I suspect the next great movement in our field will be attempts to prevent the acceleration of atherogenesis that occurs as a result of hypertension. Often, we have been able to reduce blood-pressure levels, but the patient dies of atherosclerosis, albeit much later. Dr. H. DUSTAN and I have already seen this. Many of our patients have had coronary artery catheterization, performed by Dr. M. SONES, and the results offer convincing evidence of the common involvement of these vessels with atherosclerosis. I am sure that the cerebral vessels must be injured as well, leading to the high incidence of stroke in these patients. The widespread distribution of atherosclerosis in patients with hypertension is regularly impressed upon us when we see the inside of vessels during operations for the purpose of removing obstructions to blood flow in the renal arteries.

The next step in the drug treatment of hypertension was the introduction of hydralazine or Apresoline. This interesting drug came from the CIBA laboratories and marked an important advance in treatment. Curiously, we still are not sure of this drug's full mechanism of action. In some patients it was very effective and in others not. Perhaps its most dramatic effect was the production of what came to be known as "Apresoline or hydralazine disease". This occurred in a few people and usually when the dose was high. As you recall, there was a rheumatoid-arthritis-like phase and another lupus-like stage. Both were serious and both ordinarily reversed when the drug was stopped. It seemed the perfect model of a collagen disease resulting from a synthetic chemical. Unfortunately, it has not been possible to reproduce it in animals, so that study of this truly fascinating condition has not received the attention that is surely its due.

At that stage of our knowledge, in order to achieve reasonable reduction in blood pressure, it was necessary to use very large doses of the antihypertensive drugs then available. This all too often led to many undesirable side effects. Treatment was both expensive and uncomfortable.

Meanwhile, work had gone on, slowly but surely, on the structure and synthesis of angiotensin. When it became available for everyone to study, there was suddenly the hope that an anti-angiotensin or anti-renin would be the answer to renal hypertension. The same hope was held out for an anti-serotonin. But none of these, except anti-renin, has so far been found. I believe, however, that somebody, some time, somewhere, will stumble on one. Certainly the search among the analogs of angiotensin has yielded nothing. What an enormous help it would be if an effective agent were found to block the action of angiotensin!

I think some recent results from our laboratory will be very helpful in this search, because they add the facets of synthesis and release of angiotensin to that of the direct antagonism. Drs ROBERTSON, SMEBY, BUMPUS, and I were able, with a new organ-culture technique of ROBERTSON, to grow the juxtaglomerular cells *in vitro*. These cells were shown to contain renin and release it to the supernatant culture medium. Thus, a controllable system is provided for study.

I speak of blocking *the* action of angiotensin too lightly. It is not certain whether its stimulating action on the adrenal cortex or its direct pressor action should be nullified. Which would be most helpful? But there is still another action which might interest you, since it is far less well known.

My colleagues, DE MOURA, OLMSTED, MCCUBBIN, and I have studied the continuous infusion of sub-pressor amounts of angiotensin into unanesthetized dogs for several weeks. After a few days, the blood pressure and peripheral resistance of these dogs begin to rise, and within some ten days the pressure may reach average levels of 200/120 mm. Hg with peak diastolic levels of 200 mm. Hg. But the curious thing about these animals is that when they are placed in a completely quiet room or when they sleep, arterial pressure falls to normal. In short, angiotensin infusion seems to sensitize normal dogs to external stimuli with the result that hypertension develops. Control infusions without angiotensin do not induce hypertension. In contrast to these experiments where sub-pressor doses of angiotensin were given, OLMSTED and I have given continuously large doses for five weeks. Pressure is maintained at high levels, but only by slowly and steadily increasing the amount of angiotensin infused. Clearly these large doses are not necessary to elicit hypertension in dogs in an environment that is filled with the stimuli that are usual for dogs.

We suppose that the increased cardiovascular reactivity induced by angiotensin is the same as that which MCCUBBIN and I found with tyramine. Tyramine acts indirectly by liberating norepinephrine. You may recall we suggested that angiotensin increased the effectiveness of endogenous norepinephrine as a transmitter and that this provided a bridge between the humoral renal facet and the neural aspect of the hypertension.

The next drug to appear on the horizon, *Rauwolfia serpentina*, originated in India and did not become widely used in the west until early 1950. I think most of you will remember the very large doses we all used, which resulted ultimately in a variety of severe side effects, such as depression and even Parkinsonism. But the hypotensive and sedative effects of reserpine were definite and soon convinced us that this was an important drug. The search for analogs became intense, and the air was full of claims about one having less side effects than another. But after the dust settled, reserpine remained the most useful of this group of drugs.

Perhaps the most interesting part of the story of reserpine was the demonstration that it causes release of most of the bound serotonin and norepinephrine in the brain. Around this phenomenon has grown up a large pharmacological literature concerned not only with binding of biogenic amines but also with the mental effects of their storage and release. It was at about this time that the notion of tranquilizers began to take root. You know what an enormous business this has become. Tranquilizers are said to be like money – it doesn't make you happy, but it quiets the nerves. There was a time not long ago when the public press was full of suggestions for reducing the stress on human beings, so that we should all become happy and tranquil. But, as someone has said, all this would amount to would be "Miltown under the spreading atrophy". Never forget that stress is man's challenge to greatness.

By now we had low-salt diets, hydralazine, ganglion blocking agents, and reserpine to treat our hypertensives. Surgery on the sympathetic system was largely disappearing.

With the continued development of the science of drug therapy of hypertension in the early fifties, we became interested in treating the syndrome usually called "hypertensive encephalopathy". As you know, this was the term FISHBERG preferred and one that PICKERING used to denote cerebral thrombotic episodes. Our interest was rather to find a drug that would quickly, and surely, control the preternaturally high blood pressure. This turned up in the form of sodium nitroprusside. It has the enormous disadvantage of being so cheap that drug houses cannot afford to sell it; hence it has not been widely used despite its great usefulness. I know of no drug that more effectively lowers blood pressure, but it must be given intravenously, and therefore the patient needs constant supervision. But during hypertensive episodes of the severity of which I speak, this is necessary anyway.

The headache, restlessness, and final coma with severe rise in diastolic blood pressure are overcome within a matter of hours when blood pressure is reduced and kept at a normal level by nitroprusside. There are, of course, other ways of treating this syndrome, but I have yet to be convinced that any other is quite so certainly effective. It is a commentary on something that supposedly authoritative publications, such as *The Medical Letter* in the United States, fail even to mention this form of treatment while presenting in some detail several much less effective ones. Such is the power of convenience and dependence on second-hand information.

One of the more remarkable developments in the treatment of hypertension occurred in 1934 when it was recognized that the dye prontosil was antibacterial. The active substance was the metabolite sulfanilamide. During the course of attempts to decrease the renal clearance of penicillin it was unexpectedly found that some of the sulfa derivatives interfered with reabsorption of uric acid. From this came probenecid for gout. A side effect of sulfanilamide was interference with tubular reabsorption of sodium, with mild inhibition of carbonic anhydrase. From this observation came the important diuretic chlorothiazide, synthesized by NOVELLO and SPRAGUE in 1957. Hypoglycemia was another side effect, and from it came the first clinically useful oral hypoglycemic agent. Sulfanyl guanidine induced thyroid hyperplasia, calling attention to the structural similarity of the sulfonamide group to thiourea. Among the latter's derivatives thiouracil proved a valuable inhibitor of thyroid-hormone synthesis.

It seems to me this is the most remarkable example of the value of molecular modification of drugs of which I know. It gave our field a powerful new diuretic which allowed us to reduce the dosage of other antihypertensive drugs by as much as a half and still get a good result. The disastrous side effects of the large doses needed for effective lowering of blood pressure disappeared overnight!

Diuretics have since ancient times been thought useful for circulatory diseases. You will recall that Dr. SYLVIUS at the University of Leyden knew of the diuretic properties of oil of juniper. He believed he could improve the extracts by putting the berries in pure alcohol and distilling the mixture. The result was success beyond his dreams. Within a few years, all Holland found itself suffering from ills that could be cured only by Dr. SYLVIUS' medicine.

Chlorothiazide and dihydrochlorothiazide have now become commonplace in the treatment of hypertension. Countless attempts to produce more useful analogs have been made but, so far, with little success. Aldosterone antagonists have been used to a very limited degree, especially in those patients where chlorothiazide produces severe hypokalemia. The pteridine derivative triamterene often corrects the potassium deficit. Spironolactones have been used, but their relative ineffectiveness and expense do not suggest an important future.

Two years after the appearance of the thiazide diuretics, Mull, Maxwell, and Plummer synthesized guanethidine. This drug has the great advantage of both depleting the transmitter norepinephrine and preventing its release at the myoneural junction. It does not produce concurrent parasympathetic paralysis.

So much has been written about the mode of action of both guanethidine and diuretics that there is no need to take up your time describing them. I think most clinicians would choose guanethidine if they were forced to work with only one drug; it is that valuable! After six years of widespread use, almost no significant side effects have appeared. Some patients require addition of other antihypertensive drugs, such as reserpine or hydralazine, and dihydrochlorothiazide to achieve adequate control of blood pressure.

Let me digress a moment to emphasize again the need for adequate control of blood pressure. To be adequately controlled, it is our belief that blood pressure should be at, or near, normal in the prone position. Many drugs produce orthostatic hypotension, and it is too easy to accept blood pressures measured in the standing or even sitting position as evidence of good control. While many do not agree with me, I believe patients do best when kept in bed in the hospital during their introduction to antihypertensive drugs. Severe orthostatic hypotension may then be elicited without unusual danger, and at the same time lying pressure can be brought to approximately normal levels. After several weeks, the dosage of the drugs can be slowly reduced while the patient is trying to adjust to the severe postural fall in blood pressure. An attempt is made to find the delicate balance between disabling postural hypotension and normal prone arterial pressure. In this way, I believe, drugs are used to their maximum effectiveness. I think this method of administration is especially effective in the treatment of malignant hypertension, when a period of two months or more of hospitalization is usually necessary to insure that the eyeground changes have cleared and blood pressure stays at normal levels.

We also teach our patients to take their own blood pressure twice a day. We are often asked whether all this attention of the patient to his own blood pressure doesn't make him neurotic. The answer is no, although some people today feel if you are not neurotic, you must be illiterate.

We ask them to send us a written monthly report of these measurements. In addition, we ask them to enter the hospital for more extensive study at least once a year, or more often if indicated. In short, we are advocating very careful control of blood-pressure levels along with assurance that the drugs we are giving are producing the effects we expect. My experience has been that far too many physicians give an antihypertensive drug without first being sure that the drug is effective in the particular patient and then being sure that the effectiveness is maintained.

Nineteen-sixty saw the introduction of still another antihypertensive agent by SJOERDSMA. In this case it was the outcome of extensive studies of the metabolism of norepinephrine in Sweden, Canada, Germany, and the United States, but we are still not clear on the mechanisms of action of the drug itself, α-methyldopa. Initially there was much confident discussion claiming it to be a decarboxylase inhibitor. Clearly, this is not the mechanism of its prime antihypertensive action.

α-Methyldopa is certainly a useful drug and, as with the others, its effectiveness is increased by combining it with a diuretic. In our experience, however, there have been a number of patients in whom even doses as high as 4 g./day are ineffective. This uncertainty does not recommend the drug for the treatment of malignant hypertension where prompt lowering of blood pressure is vital.

The latest drug to appear is one of the monamine-oxidase inhibitors. This group of substances had been widely used in the treatment of depression. As a side effect, hypotension had frequently been noted. Indeed, years ago we used iproniazid as a treatment for hypertension but gave it up when evidence of toxicity appeared. While there is no doubt that in some patients a drug such as pargyline will lower blood pressure, it also greatly augments the pressor response to substances such as tyramine. The eating of tyramine-containing foods, such as aged Cheddar and Stilton cheese, is followed by a dangerous rise in arterial pressure.

Oddly enough, Chianti wine and some beers also contain a fair amount of tyramine. There is also potential danger when using monamine-oxidase inhibitors with certain tranquilizers and hypotensive drugs. Norepinephrine or serotonin may be released in the nervous system by some of these drugs. Ordinarily, the stimulating effect of these amines is controlled by destruction of the enzyme, but if the oxidase is already inhibited, there is trouble ahead. The combination may produce extreme excitement, hypertensive crisis, and some very weird behavior. It is a strange turn of the wheel of fate that a man can come home "potted" after an evening of tranquilizers and Stilton cheese.

It seems to us that the side effects and potential hazards of this group of drugs outweigh the limited advantages they might have. Today a proposed antihypertensive drug must be better than those we already have, and this cannot be said of pargyline.

There is still another possible approach to the problem of blocking the action of the transmitter, norepinephrine. This is the result of the investigations of UDENFRIEND, showing that tyrosine hydroxylase converts tyrosine to dopa, and dopamine-β-oxidase converts dopamine to norepinephrine. There is evidence that the first step is rate-limiting, since tissues contain much less tyrosine hydroxylase than dopamine-β-oxidase and decarboxylase. Several competitors for the receptor site on the enzyme have been studied, but all have had serious toxic side effects making them useless for treatment.

There are other drugs now available which in our opinion have not been proved to have enough merit over those I have described. These include such agents as benathedine, guanoxan, and bretylium. An interesting drug belonging to the benzothiadiazine group that actually causes retention of sodium and water is diazoxide. Given intravenously, it causes a quick fall in arterial pressure lasting three to four hours. Unfortunately, it also produces hyperglycemia. Another drug that lowers pressure quickly and effectively when given intravenously is trimethaphan (Arfonad). It is expensive and I fail to see any advantage over sodium nitroprusside.

Lastly, I want to speak briefly about the possible reversibility of hypertension. If there is a secreting tumor or an obstructive renal lesion causing the elevation in blood pressure, it would not be expected that a lasting reduction of blood pressure would continue after the antihypertensive drugs were withdrawn. The reversal of the malignant syndrome that I first saw following the reduction in blood pressure resulting from anterior nerve root section gave hope that if drug treatment effectively maintained normal pressure for long periods, possibly the reduced pressure levels would be maintained without further use of antihypertensive drugs. This has proved to be true in some of our patients. In some of those treated for the past fifteen years with long-maintained normal blood-pressure levels all drugs were discontinued and often a placebo substituted. The pressure has promptly risen in some, but in others, either no rise or a very slight one occurred, and this has been maintained for more than three years. In short, hypertension in some people seems to be reversible if antihypertensive drugs are used persistently and effectively for long periods.

What about the future? At the moment it seems that we have almost come to the end of the effort to improve diuretics and perhaps even drugs that block sympathetic transmission. We badly need those that will nullify the actions of angiotensin. Whether anti-renin will be useful is entirely unknown. The anti-aldosterone drugs have not proved very effective. Whether this means that the aldosterone mechanism is not important in most patients or that the blockade is not very effective is difficult to say.

Drugs which act to slow the heart and reduce cardiac output have not been adequately studied and may be found to be useful. I do not think we have studied sufficiently the effects of drugs that blunt the harshness of our environment. We are convinced that angiotensin in very small amounts sensitizes the body to external stimuli that elevate blood pressure. Then there also must be substances that will aid in the resetting of the vascular barostats downward, just as there seem to be naturally occurring ones that participate in the resetting upwards during the course of hypertension.

There are times when we think antihypertensive therapy has been simply a Pyrrhic victory, because the residual atherosclerotic damage remains. Healing has been seen in the vessels of patients with malignant hypertension, and I am not wholly pessimistic about the possibility that it may be induced in atherosclerotic ones. I think it would be wise to look at the problem of atherosclerosis as though it were a solvable one. I suggest that the next great chapter will be the combining of the treatment of arterial hypertension with measures to prevent atheropoiesis.

Let me conclude on a happy note. Surely we deserve to preen ourselves on the accomplishments of the past three decades. Contrary to some, I think we now know a lot about hypertension. In my view, both hypertension and atherosclerosis represent a class of diseases only recently recognized for what I think them to be, namely "diseases of regulation". In a system so complex as is needed to regulate accurately the supply of blood to the tissues, it is not surprising that we have yet to uncover many of the regulating mechanisms.

It is hard to understand why hypertension has so long been neglected despite the fact that, among civilized men, it is now the second greatest killer. Knowledge of its mechanisms and treatment is only beginning to be properly taught in medical schools. It is little wonder that treatment has been neglected in the practice of medicine.

All this is in the process of change. People are at last becoming interested and deeply concerned about it. Only recently the President of the United States appointed a Commission for the Study of Heart Disease, Cancer, and Stroke. Much as I deplore the idea that research and medical care might be initiated and directed by committee, still it shows interest, which is something we had very little of before.

May I be permitted a word in behalf of our long-suffering patients? We demand much of them and I firmly believe that those who follow directions minutely do better than the careless. But there are important areas of living in which we physicians know no more than others. Often when we don't know what to do we proscribe instead of prescribe – we forbid this or that of the things people often most enjoy. I suppose this characteristic is a hangover from the days when anything that was pleasurable was sinful. Whether we forbid smoking, alcohol, and such, may make a good deal of difference as to whether people will think life worth living. I should therefore remind you that smoke and alcohol were the oldest known preservatives and that Winston Churchill was 100 proof of this observation!

The past three decades have indeed been a golden age in the understanding and treatment of hypertension. The period has been singularly free from exploitation either of the patient's pocketbook or the scientist's reputation. The work will, I believe, stand as a model of clear thinking, prudent financing, and lack of exaggerated claims. We must all admit that there have been those within our family who have often unwittingly disturbed our equable working relationships. Fortunately, the disturbances have been short-lived and quickly forgotten. If during the next thirty years as much is accomplished, the disastrous effects of hypertension on civilized man may well be at an end. May I be forgiven if, in speaking for our field, I say that we have done well.

Closing remarks

By

C. Bartorelli

We have arrived at the end of this symposium and the time has now come to summarise the conclusions of our joint work. I think it would be presumptuous for someone who has been actively concerned in the organisation of this meeting to stress how productive the work has been. We shall leave it to the readers of the published proceedings to judge that for themselves. From the point of view of the participants, there is no doubt that meetings of this type, at which persons representing, as we do, different backgrounds and disciplines have the opportunity of comparing and discussing their opinions and experience, are extremely useful. The presence at these sessions of physiologists, pharmacologists, and clinicians is a clear sign that in medical disciplines every step forward is nowadays a product of teamwork, and I am sure that each of us, on returning home, will have something to take back to his colleagues in the form of more accurate views, widened experience, or new ideas.

As to the scientific conclusions of this symposium, I shall speak for myself and try to describe the present status of my opinions on antihypertensive therapy, after listening to so many authoritative reports and lively discussions.

First of all, I should like to touch on the problem of surgical treatment, as we have heard a few divergent views on this subject. Nobody will deny, however, that the perspectives of the surgical management of hypertension have shifted strikingly in recent years. Even in the early fifties, radical removal of sympathetic ganglia, sometimes associated with adrenalectomy, was still thought to be – and probably was – the most effective way of dealing with essential arterial hypertension. Failures and side effects of this approach are only too well known; but the medical treatment of fifteen years ago was no more successful and no less troublesome. The efficacy of the new hypotensive drugs that have come on the scene since 1950 has made this type of surgery obsolete, except in rare cases involving contra-indications or resistance to drug therapy, which, I must confess, I myself have never encountered. This does not mean, of course, that surgery no longer has a place in antihypertensive treatment. On the contrary, its scope has recently extended into an entirely new field, that is to say to types of hypertension that were unknown until a few years ago. Indeed, the shift in the indication for surgical treatment of hypertension from essential, or primary, to secondary hypertension is also due to the recent clinical definition of syndromes such as primary aldosteronism and, particularly, renovascular hypertension.

The dilemma with which we were faced when we were obliged to choose between medical and surgical therapy has thus been resolved as far as essential hypertension is concerned; unfortunately, it presents itself anew in connection with renal artery stenosis. A considerable proportion of patients maintain high blood pressure after reconstructive surgery, revascularisation of the affected kidney, and even nephrectomy. Of course, we should like to be able to forecast the outcome of surgery, and it is therefore very encouraging to have heard at this symposium that separate renal function tests, besides being so useful in diagnosis, also seem to be indicative of the probable results of surgical treatment. An attempt to remove or by-pass the obstruction in renal circulation should therefore be made in most cases of renovascular hypertension, whenever the hypertension is of early onset and the functional conditions of the contralateral kidney are still well preserved. At any rate, there is some consolation in the knowledge that patients who have not benefited by surgery, or are poor operative risks, are generally responsive to the usual antihypertensive drugs.

As far as essential hypertension is concerned, the treatment of choice is always medical. When arterial pressure is high enough to threaten vascular disease, a hypotensive drug regimen should always be started. The physician now has at his disposal various drugs which are capable of effectively lowering arterial pressure, whether it has risen suddenly and transiently in an acute outburst or is chronically elevated. Failure to control even the highest blood pressures and the severest cases of hypertension can rarely be ascribed to a lack of effect on the part of the drugs employed or to intolerable side effects – especially since the method of associating several drugs with different mechanisms of action, and of potentiating their effects by diuretics, permits relatively low doses of each drug to be given. Unsuccessful treatments, which are unfortunately all too numerous, commonly result from failure to persuade either the family doctor or the patient (and often both) that hypotensive therapy must be pursued with the greatest perseverance and care for an indefinite period of time. The reward for so much patience and trust is great indeed, both for the patient and the physician. We have recently seen a change in the prognosis of hypertension so striking as to render rapidly obsolete the attribute that used to designate the severest stage of this disease. Malignant hypertension is no longer malignant in prognosis when appropriate hypotensive therapy brings blood pressure back to lower values before too much irreversible damage is inflicted upon the kidney. In addition, the survival of less severely ill patients is remarkably prolonged by effective antihypertensive treatment. The exhaustive long-term studies that have been described by several authors during this symposium may usefully be consulted to substantiate these conclusions, so important are they for the practitioner.

What further improvements in the medical management of hypertension may be expected in the near future? A better understanding of the biochemical changes induced by hypotensive drugs, both in short-term and long-term administration, and a fuller knowledge of their side effects – especially of those appearing only after prolonged administration – will indisputably contribute towards an improvement in our way of dealing with existing drugs and the development of better compounds. The sophisticated methods of evaluating the clinical effectiveness of hypotensive drugs, which have been discussed repeatedly during our meeting, as well as improved tests for assessing body functions in patients, will help in screening new drugs and in judging the benefit they give the patient.

However, what would really constitute an important step forward in the treatment of hypertension would be the discovery of some means of dealing with the vascular disease that is so often associated with high blood pressure. The features of these vascular lesions and their relationship to hypertension have been clearly illustrated at this symposium. No doubt, lowering the blood pressure slows down the progress of vascular disease, but unfortunately arteriosclerosis continues to develop, though at a slower rate. Stopping its progress should be one of the aims of future research.

Finally, a few words on pathogenesis. I cannot help thinking that the acquisition of more information on the causes and mechanisms of arterial hypertension would necessarily be reflected in a terrific improvement in its treatment. Although pathogenesis was not the subject of this meeting – and in my opening remarks I explained why – a few promising leads deriving from current research into this problem have been apparent during our sessions.

The long-standing interest in renal hypertension has yielded more and more precise information on the structural, functional, and biochemical aspects of renal participation in blood-pressure control and in the regulation of water and electrolyte metabolism. On the other hand, the nervous system, which has long been the Cinderella of experimental hypertension, is becoming more and more of a pole of attraction for hypertension research as experimental methods permitting more careful exploration of its importance in the regulation of circulation are being developed. Histochemical, physiological, and pharmacological approaches to this kind of study have been stressed during our discussions. Furthermore, studies in the intact conscious animal in entirely physiological conditions have contributed to the filling of the gap between research on neural and renal mechanisms of hypertension.

It remains to be seen whether some of these current trends will yield further and more decisive results between now and our next meeting to discuss hypertension. All of us here, I know, hope and trust that they will. – And on this note of optimism I declare the meeting closed.

List of authors

Subject index

ANTIHYPERTENSIVE THERAPY

PRINCIPLES AND PRACTICE

AN INTERNATIONAL SYMPOSIUM

PROCEEDINGS

EDITED BY

F. GROSS

WITH THE ASSISTANCE OF

S. R. NAEGELI AND A. H. KIRKWOOD

BASLE

WITH 225 FIGURES

SPRINGER-VERLAG NEW YORK INC., 1966

The Symposium took place at Siena, Italy
28th June - 3rd July, 1965
under the chairmanship of
C. Bartorelli, Siena
and was sponsored by
CIBA

 Library of Congress Catalog Card Number 66-17 551
Softcover reprint of the hardcover 1st edition 1966

ISBN 978-3-642-49456-7 ISBN 978-3-642-49737-7 (eBook)
DOI 10.1007/ 978-3-642-49737-7

Title No. 1329

GPSR Compliance

The European Union's (EU) General Product Safety Regulation (GPSR) is a set of rules that requires consumer products to be safe and our obligations to ensure this.

If you have any concerns about our products, you can contact us on ProductSafety@springernature.com

In case Publisher is established outside the EU, the EU authorized representative is:

Springer Nature Customer Service Center GmbH
Europaplatz 3
69115 Heidelberg, Germany

Batch number: 10723245

Printed by Printforce, the Netherlands